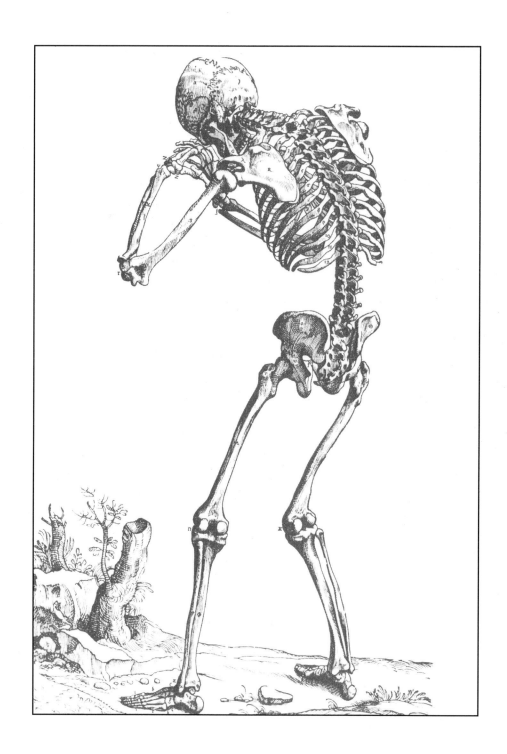

FOURTH EDITION

SPEECH AND HEARING SCIENCE
Anatomy and Physiology

Willard R. Zemlin

*Professor Emeritus of Speech and Hearing Science
and the School of Basic Medical Sciences, University of Illinois*

Allyn and Bacon
Boston London Toronto Sydney Tokyo Singapore

Executive Editor: Stephen D. Dragin
Editorial Assistant: Christine Svitila
Marketing Manager: Kathy Hunter
Editorial Production Service: MARBERN HOUSE
Manufacturing Buyer: Megan Cochran
Cover Administrator: Linda Knowles
Compositor: Omegatype Typography, Inc.

Library of Congress Cataloging-in-Publication Data

Zemlin, Willard R.
    Speech and hearing science : anatomy and physiology / Willard R.
  Zemlin.—4th ed.
        p.   cm.
    ISBN 0-13-827437-1
    1. Speech.   2. Hearing.   I. Title.
    [DNLM: 1. Speech.   2. Hearing.   WV 501Z53s 1997]
  QP306.Z4   1997
  612.7′8—dc21
  DNLM/DLC   96-53899
                                              CIP

Printed in the United States of America

17 2020

6 HEARING 414

7 EMBRYOLOGY OF THE SPEECH AND HEARING MECHANISM 512

8 CIRCULATION 549

Thirty-five years ago a new professor at the University of Illinois began his first class in anatomy and physiology. He gave that class a purple, mimeographed outline of the topics he would cover. That was the beginning of the book you are about to read, learn, study, and use as a reference for the rest of your professional life. In the first hardcover edition of that text, Dr. Zemlin stated in the preface that, if the text were successful, it would serve as a starting point to stimulate students' interest. That first text was printed and the goal is still relevant today. This volume has grown with the knowledge base in the field; what was speculation has become theory and practice supported by data today.

More than one generation of speech-language pathology and audiology students have learned the anatomic and physiologic bases of speech using earlier editions of this text. Some have used the text as a starting point for their own research, and all have developed their own conceptualization of how the speech and hearing mechanism works after studying these chapters. Most students find this volume daunting at first. For many who use this text, anatomy is a foreign language that first must be learned before understanding its full meaning. Like any foreign language, once the basic language is mastered, there is an ease of use that allows more complete comprehension. Students will be surprised at how, by the end of a semester's study of anatomy and physiology, both their specific comprehension as well as their "feel for the subject" will increase.

To those of you who have just begun this field of study, it is well to understand that the profession believes that knowledge of the normal processes of speech and hearing should precede the study of the abnormal processes. Understanding that normal function should precede recognition of abnormal function is only one paradigm in scientific thought, but our profession is firmly founded in this belief. Speech science focuses on the way the speech and hearing mechanism works in the "normal" state. As clinicians, you will want to know what movements and coordinated efforts are necessary to produce speech accurately, so that, if a patient/client

sounds different than you would expect, you can figure out how that individual has created that deviant sound. The knowledge of the movement and coordination differences found in a person's speech is the basis for correcting the deviance. The study of how the speech musculature works, then, is vital to your becoming successful speech pathologists.

This text will provide you with the basis for understanding disorder. It is as comprehensive a source as there is available on these topics. You must be patient and learn the material well. In all likelihood, you will use this text in your beginning undergraduate courses and again in your advanced graduate courses in specific speech disorders. When you finally become professional speech-language pathologists or audiologists, you will use this book as a reference over and over again. As a professional speech-language pathologist, I used my edition until the covers were broken and its pages, dog-eared. All three previous editions have served me well in my professional career.

The scope of practice within the profession has grown to such an extent that speech-language pathologists and audiologists are now found in intensive care units, radiology laboratories, respiratory care departments, and in neurology and otolaryngology offices. We, as a profession, are working with sicker and sicker patients who depend on our knowledge of speech physiology. It is essential, then, that our understanding of the anatomy and physiology of speech is detailed and comprehensive. Our patients' lives do depend on it. When you complete your study and become professionals in the field, you will become "speech physiology experts" on which other professionals depend. Your construct of how we produce speech will be formed while studying these pages. You could not have a better, more comprehensive learning experience. Learn the "language of anatomy," and learn all you can.

Patricia K. Monoson
Associate Dean and Professor of Speech Pathology
College of Health Related Professions
University of Arkansas

One problem associated with writing a textbook such as this one pertains to the breadth and depth of the substance within it. What to include and how much to include must be weighed, for one thing, against a typical college semester, or an academic year, in addition to the question of just how much a student can be expected to absorb within the confines of a semester.

Communication is an incredibly complex process, by no means fully understood. We, as humans, are complex and a description of the structure and function of the speech and hearing mechanism must of necessity also be complex, if it is to be at all complete.

Students today typically enroll for one semester of anatomy and physiology of speech and hearing, and a second semester of acoustics and neurology, or some combination of these subjects. The point is this: the introductory course is almost always the one and only exposure to speech and hearing science the student will ever receive.

Each of us who is concerned with the rehabilitation of speech, language, and hearing should be able to visualize the anatomical structures involved, to understand their usual functions, and to hypothesize how they might function under adverse circumstances. In this text, I have attempted to provide comprehensive and relatively detailed information upon which to base these constructs, but, once they have been established in your mind, you needn't be concerned about retaining the details that helped you develop them. At the same time, I have attempted to provide a reference book for use later in your academic and professional life. This explains the many references cited, the depth of coverage, and the chapters on embryology and circulation.

I have also included, where appropriate, short clinical notes and supplemental notes that may be useful. One may legitimately question the wisdom of putting a section on embryology at the end of the text. Why put at the end, what takes place at the beginning? When a student has been exposed to the material of the text, the structures and terminology will be familiar and the topic of embryonic development perhaps a little easier to grasp.

For the preparation of specimen materials I am indebted to my laboratory partners, students who lent not only helping hands, but also their enthusiasm. Their presence brightened an otherwise drab and lonely laboratory. I am especially indebted to my laboratory partners who collaborated in preparation of specimen materials for this, the fourth edition. Becky Taylor and Fang Ling Lu worked alongside me while I was a guest of Memphis State University as part of their Center for Excellence program. My thanks to Dr. Dan Beasley, Dr. Leonard Murrell of the Department of Anatomy, University of Tennessee Center for the Health Sciences opened the anatomy laboratory facilities to us and made us feel welcome. Timothy Jones of the Department of Anatomy was very helpful.

Dr. Elaine Paden, University of Illinois, once again gave me her valuable support by reviewing manuscript, old and new, as I was preparing this edition. Book production has changed dramatically since the production of the third edition. Stephen Dragin of Allyn and Bacon enlisted the competent services of Marjorie Payne, Marbern House. Yoram Mizrahi of Omegatype Typography, Champaign, Illinois, was responsible for producing the manuscript. All in all a pleasant experience.

Once again I am especially grateful to my wife, Eileen, for her role in the preparation of the manuscript, for her professional opinions and advice, for her encouragement, and much more. Her name does indeed belong on the cover along with mine, but she hesitates to be seen with me in public.

W. R. Z.

Study Guide/Workbook	Available from
to Accompany	Stipes Publishing Co.
Speech and Hearing Science:	10–12 Chester Street
Anatomy and Physiology,	Champaign, IL 61820
4th ed.	(217) 356-8391
ISBN: 0-87563-730-2	Fax: (217) 356-5753
	E-mail: stipes@soltec.net

Introduction and Orientation

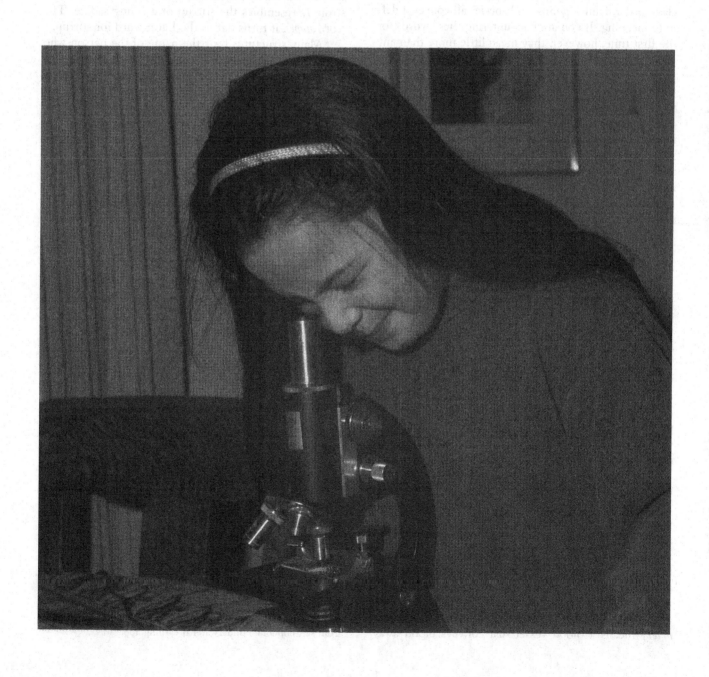

INTRODUCTION

At the present time, human beings occupy the space at the top of the phylogenetic ladder. We are of the

PHYLUM------------------------------------Chordata
SUBPHYLUM -----------------------Vertebrata
CLASS ----------------------------Mammalia
ORDER --------------------------Primate
SUBORDER --------------Anthropoid
FAMILY------------------Hominidae
SPECIES -----------------Sapiens

To a biologist or a zoologist, the words phylum, class, order, family, genus, and species all convey a definite meaning. If you are encountering these words for the first time, however, they mean little more than any other aggregate of esoteric jargon. But the words are of paramount importance. In large part, learning a new topic or academic discipline consists of learning a new working vocabulary.

The classification scheme used to describe human beings or *Homo sapiens* tells us that we are animals and not vegetables. We have hollow nervous systems and a vertebral column. In addition, we have hair and suckle our young. We are the most highly developed of the mammals, to the extent we are human in form, and we are *very, very* wise.

A dictionary definition of man (referring to all humankind) is: "An individual of the highest type of animal existing or known to have existed, different from other high types of animals, especially in his extraordinary mental development." To paraphrase this definition: We alone are the only animals so highly developed we are able to tell ourselves that we are superior to all other animals.

The pages to follow will present the speech and hearing mechanisms unique to humans in an attempt to account for normal speech and hearing processes on anatomical, physiological, and neurological bases. The purpose of this chapter is to define anatomy and physiology and to familiarize the reader with some terminology appropriate to anatomical and physiological descriptions.

Anatomy and physiology are very old sciences, and their language often stems from Latin or Greek roots. An example of a root is *port*, from which we get transport, export, import, etc. A word root plus a vowel constitutes a **combining form** such as *thermo*, *micro*, and *speedo*. As we progress I will try to provide the derivations of various words we encounter. You are probably already familiar with many frequently used anatomical terms and with word roots common to both scientific and nonscientific vocabularies. For example, the word *artery* means a blood vessel that conveys blood away from the heart to any part of the body. The anatomical term for the "windpipe" is *trachea*, and it means "rough artery." Why?

Anyone interested in anatomy and physiology will find a medical dictionary a comforting and valuable ally; the student also will be greatly aided by turning to the glossary at the back of this textbook, or to a dictionary, for the meaning of each new word.

Anatomy is a descriptive science, and many of the names given to structures are descriptive. Examples are the names for the auditory ossicles. *Ossicle* is a term denoting a small bone, but it is usually reserved for the small bones of the middle ear, namely, the malleus, incus, and stapes. The *malleus* is so named because of its resemblance to a sculptor's mallet, while the *incus* is that which is struck by the mallet, or the anvil, and the *stapes* strongly resembles the stirrup of a riding saddle. The word *stapes*, it turns out, is the Latin word for stirrup.

Many structures bear the name of the person who presumably discovered or extensively studied them. The Eustachian tube was described by the sixteenth-century physician Bartolomeo Eustachio, the Fallopian tubes by the sixteenth-century physician Fallopius of Modena, and the laryngeal ventricle of Morgagni by the seventeenth-century anatomist Giovanni Batista Morgagni. Anatomists and other scientists are making serious efforts to abandon **eponyms** wherever meaningful terms can be used instead. Today, the Eustachian tube is called the auditory tube, a term that conveys much more information. And this explains the change in attitude. To an anatomist, the term Poupart's ligament is meaningless, but the term *inguinal* (L. *inguinalis*, groin) *ligament* is meaningful. Descriptive terms are helpful. If you are familiar with anatomy, you will immediately recognize that the sternocleidomastoid muscle arises from the sternum and clavicle and that it inserts into the mastoid process of the temporal bone. Muscles are often named after their points of attachment, but many are named after certain descriptive properties or, in other words, their morphological characteristics. Other muscles are named, at least in part, after their location in the body. We will elaborate some general principles pertaining to the naming of muscles later in this chapter.

Definition of Anatomy

Anatomy is the study of the structure of organisms and the relations of their parts. The etymology of the word tells us that anatomy means dissection, usually of human cadavers, and the word *cadaver* is an ancient Latin acrostic,[1] *caro data vermibus*, literally "meat given to worms."

---

[1] A series of lines or verses in which the first, last, or other particular letters form a word or phrase. Another **acronym** is SCUBA, from **s**elf-**c**ontained **u**nderwater **b**reathing **a**pparatus.

Dissection of a cadaver is but a means to an end—to furnish the student with firsthand knowledge of the structure of anatomy of living persons. But dissection is an extremely time-consuming process that requires patient guidance and expert tuition. We rely heavily upon our predecessors' experiences.[2]

Today anatomy demands much more than the gross descriptions that can be obtained by the classical dissection techniques. The scope of interest has widened considerably since the time of Galen, Vesalius, and da Vinci, and techniques have changed as well. Electromyography; bright-field, polarized-light, and electron microscopy; tissue culture; the use of radioisotopes; and computer analysis of data are among the tools of the trade for anatomists and physiologists today. In recent years, neurodiagnostic techniques such as computed tomography (CT scans or CAT scans), positron emission tomography (PET scans), single photon emission tomography (SPECT scans), and magnetic resonance imaging (MRI) are capable of supplementing tradition anatomical studies. (Kuehn, et al., 1989; Love and Webb, 1992; Perrier, et al., 1992; and Moore, 1992.) A number of specialized fields have emerged within the discipline of anatomy. Some of the specializations are

1. **Descriptive** or **systemic** anatomy, in which the body is considered as being composed of a number of systems, each consisting of rather homogeneous tissues which exhibit some peculiar functional unity.

2. **Regional** or **topographical** anatomy, which deals primarily with the structural relationships of the various parts of the body. Thus, we have head and neck anatomy, anatomy of the extremities, and so forth.

3. **Applied** or **practical** anatomy, which is concerned with the application of anatomy to a specialized field, such as surgery.

4. **Microscopic anatomy,** which is concerned with the details of structure as revealed through the microscope. It includes *cytology*, which is the study of cells, and *histology*, which is the study of the microscopic structures of tissues.

5. **Developmental anatomy,** which specializes in the growth of the organism from the single cell to birth.

6. **Geriatric anatomy,** a relatively modern field that investigates the morphophysiology of the aged (long-lived) individual.

7. **Anthropological anatomy,** which deals with the anatomic features of peoples and with the natural history of various races and ethnic groups.

8. **Artistic anatomy,** which is the study of external morphology of the living body for purposes of artistic representation.

9. **Comparative anatomy,** which, as the name suggests, is the study of the structure and the comparative structures of all living organisms.

Anatomic Variability

Virtually all the specifiable parameters of human structure, function, sensitivities, and capacities can be placed on a continuum of one sort or another, with the extremes representing statistical polarities that require interpretation.

We readily acknowledge that genetic traits are transmitted from generation to generation, and we are content to accept the fact that morphological uniqueness is a product of inherited characteristics, at least to a large extent. Evidence of this is seen in eye color, skin color, morphotypes, and, perhaps, dispositions. However, we tend to overlook the fact that uniqueness is also transmitted to our deep structures. We are all different, but we differ in ways we are not, and will never be, aware of.

The closer one looks, the more variation between specimens one finds, and so a great deal of variability in morphology is not surprising. And, where we have variability in structure, we can expect to find variability in function. Where we have variability in structure and function, the question of criteria for deviance and deviant behavior becomes an exceedingly difficult one.

Woodburne (1973) alerts his readers to the question of variability and he states,

Regularity is commonly equated with normality, but the latter word tends to carry a connotation of correctness which the facts themselves do not support. Even worse, the term "abnormal" carries overtones of "deformity" and does not correctly describe the simple fact of differences in form and arrangement. These terms and their common implications are to be avoided in considering anatomical variation.

Definition of Physiology

Biology (Gk. *bios*, life) is the science that deals with the phenomenon of life and living organisms in general. Within the broad field of biology, a number of specialized disciplines can be identified. One of them is known as **physiology** (Gk. *physis*, nature), and it can be defined as a science dealing with the functions of living organisms or their parts, as distinguished from **morphology** (Gk. *morphe*, form), which is concerned with their form

---

[2]There are some shortcomings in the study of the dead, or **necrology,** as it is sometimes called. DiDio (1970) states, "Death has inherent in it the condition of change; in addition, the fixative and embalming fluid, to a greater or lesser extent, modify the normal appearance of the organs. Moreover, the diseases the organism had during its lifetime caused other alterations that should be identified and properly evaluated before establishing the so-called normal pattern."

and structure. As in anatomy, a number of areas of specialization can be found. just a few subdivisions of physiology are

1. **Animal physiology,** which deals with the functions of living animals as a whole. Specialized branches exist within animal physiology, such as *mammalian, hominal* (human), etc.

2. **Applied physiology,** in which physiological knowledge is applied to problems in medicine and industry. *Auditory physiology* as it relates to noise pollution is an example.

3. **Cellular physiology,** in which the physiology of life processes of individual cells or small groups of cells is studied. Cellular reproduction and nerve impulse conduction are examples of areas of interest.

4. **Experimental physiology,** in which experiments are carried out in a laboratory environment with animals or human subjects.

5. **Pathologic** (Gk. *pathos,* disease) or **morbid** (L. *moridus,* sick) **physiology,** which is the study of functions that have been modified by disease processes.

6. **General physiology,** which is the science of general laws of life and functional activity.

7. **Special physiology,** which is the physiology of particular organs: *cardiology* (Gk. *kardia,* heart) and *endocrinology* (Gk. *endo,* within, + *krinein,* to separate) the study of organs that secrete internally.

8. **Vegetable physiology,** which is the physiology of plants.

ANATOMICAL NOMENCLATURE

Anatomy and physiology, like so many other sciences, have their own language, but one that is not at all exclusive. The word **nomenclature** comes from the Latin words *nomen* (name), the plural form of which is *nomina,* and *calare* (to call). Nomenclature means terminology, or an organization and classified system of terms.

The founder of a formalized system of anatomical nomenclature is said to be Sylvius, a sixteenth-century anatomist. He was the teacher of Andreas Vesalius (1514–1564) who is regarded by many as the founder of anatomy as we know the science today. Illustrations from his monumental *De Humani Corpus Fabrica,* which was published in 1543, are shown in the inside front and back covers.

Since the time of Vesalius, anatomical terms for various structures proliferated until by the end of the nineteenth century about 50,000 terms applied to about 5000 structures. Clearly something had to be done, and in 1895 a series of international meetings of anatomists was begun in Basel, Switzerland, for the purpose of adopting a uniform anatomical nomenclature. It was known as the **Basel Nomina Anatomica,** or BNA. The BNA gave all the terms in Latin, which at that time was almost a universal language. The system failed to gain worldwide recognition, however, and a number of modified systems appeared. In 1935 the Germans revised the BNA to form the JNA (Jena Nomina Anatomica). The British also revised the BNA, and their revision was known as the BR (British Revision).

A new International Anatomical Nomenclature Committee (IANC) was formed in 1950. One of its principles states

The terms should be in Latin for international meetings and scientific publications with international circulation; the terms may be translated into their vernacular equivalents for national and local meetings, journals and teaching purposes.

We can take advantage of this principle—a liberalized Anglicization of the Basel Nomina Anatomica will be used in this book, but wherever possible, descriptive terms will be defined either in the text or the glossary.

Many of the terms used in this text refer to the human body in a standardized reference position called the anatomical position.

The Anatomical Position

The anatomical position is used as a reference for descriptive purposes. This is the position shown in Figure 1-1 of the living body standing erect, facing the observer, eyes front, arms at the side with palms of the hand and tips of the feet directed forward. Anyone who attempts to assume this position will find it somewhat unnatural, but nevertheless it is used as a reference, even if the subject is lying face down (*prone*), face up (*supine*), or in any other position. In reference to the anatomical position, sometimes the head is described as being in the **Frankfort plane** in which the lower border of the **orbit** (eye socket) is on the same horizontal plane as the upper border of the **external auditory meatus** (the small opening into the ear).

Confusion may arise over the use of certain terms for the upright human and also for lower animals that walk on all fours, or live in water and don't walk at all. Since humans are erect, the ventral and anterior surfaces as shown in Figure 1-2 are the same, whereas ventral and anterior have quite different meanings with respect to a horse. A similar problem arises in the description of a developing embryo (Gk. *embryon,* a swelling within). Because the growing embryo must

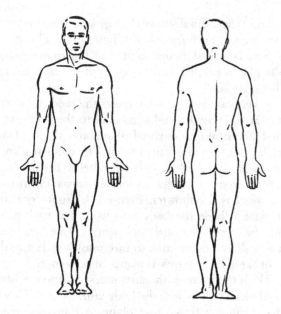

FIGURE 1-1

The anatomical position. The living body, standing erect, facing the observer, eyes front, arms at the side with the palms of the hand and tips of the feet directed forward.

conform to the limitations imposed by the uterine space, it becomes curved over on itself very early in its development, by a process called **flexion**. The terms **anterior** and **posterior, superior,** and **inferior** become cumbersome, so the terms **ventral** and **dorsal, rostral** (L. *rostrum,* beak) and **caudal** (L. *cauda,* tail) are generally used, as shown in Figure 1-3.

General Anatomical Terms

Some general terms for locations and for anatomical surfaces or **facies** (any presenting aspect or surface) are listed next. All the terms can be listed as contrasting pairs, and some of the terms can be used interchangeably.

1. **Ventral** (L. *venter,* belly), away from the backbone, or toward the front of the body.
2. **Dorsal**[3] (L. *dorsum,* back), toward the backbone, or away from the front of the body.
3. **Anterior** (L. *anterior,* before), toward the front, or away from the back. This term is usually used with reference to the free extremities or the head, but it is sometimes used interchangeably with ventral.
4. **Posterior** (L. *posterus,* behind), toward the back, or away from the front. This term is also used with reference to the free extremities or the head, but may be used interchangeably with dorsal.
5. **Superficial,** toward the surface as distinct from superior.
6. **Deep,** away from the surface, as distinct from inferior.
7. **Superior,** upper, as distinct from superficial.

[3]In the hands and forearms, **palmar** or **volar** (L., a concave surface) are substituted for **ventral** and **anterior,** while the term **dorsal** is retained for the back of the hand. The sole of the foot is called **plantar,** while **dorsal** is retained for the top or opposite surface of the foot.

FIGURE 1-2

Terms of direction. For an upright human, the terms rostral and cranial, posterior and dorsal, and anterior and ventral can be used interchangeably. For an animal on all fours, these terms have specific meanings.

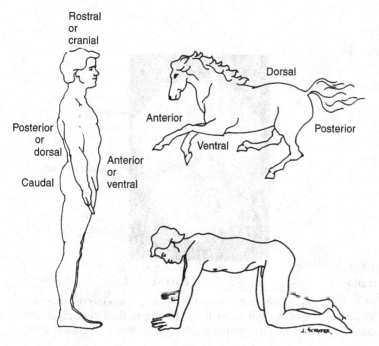

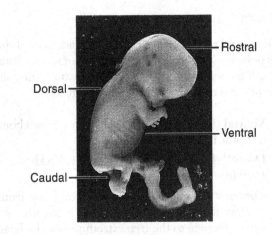

FIGURE 1-3

A human embryo. The terms rostral-caudal and ventral-dorsal are generally used as terms for direction.

8. **Inferior,** lower, as distinct from deep.

9. **Cranial** (L. *cranium*, skull), toward the head. The term rostral is sometimes used.

10. **Caudal,** toward the tail, away from the head. Its use is usually restricted to the trunk.

11. **External** (L. *externus*, outside), toward the outer surface. This term is most often used to describe body cavities or the body wall, but is sometimes used interchangeably with superficial.

12. **Internal** (L. *internus*, inside), toward the inner surface. This term is also used to describe body cavities or the body wall, but is sometimes used interchangeably with deep.

13. **Medial** (L. *medialis*), toward the axis or midline.

14. **Lateral** (L. *latus*, side), away from the axis or midline.

15. **Proximal** (L. *proximus*, next), toward the body or toward the root of a free extremity.

16. **Distal** (L., *distant*), away from the body or the root of a free extremity.

17. **Central,** pertaining to or situated at the center.

18. **Peripheral** (Gr. *peri*, around), toward the outward surface or part.

Planes of Reference

Three planes of reference are commonly used in anatomy. They are the **sagittal,** the **frontal,** and the **transverse** planes. A vertical plane or cut that divides the body into right and left halves (mirrored images in the embryo) is called the **sagittal plane** because it corre-

sponds to the sagittal suture (L. *sagitta,* arrow) that is so easily seen in an infant skull (Figure 1-4). This plane may also be called medial sagittal or midsagittal plane, while planes parallel to it, away from the midline, are called sagittal.

A vertical plane that intersects the median sagittal plane at right angles and is parallel to the forehead is called a **frontal** or a **coronal plane,** and all the planes parallel to it are also called frontal or coronal planes. This is because they are either parallel to the forehead (L. *frons,* front) or to the coronal (L. *corona,* crown) suture, which is also shown in Figure 1-4. Frontal or coronal planes divide the body into front and back parts. Both the frontal (coronal) and sagittal planes are vertical as well as longitudinal, so care must be taken in the use of these latter terms as planes of reference.

With the body in the anatomical position, a horizontal plane that divides the body into upper and lower parts is called a **transverse plane.** A transverse plane that divides the body into upper and lower halves is called the midtransverse plane.

These planes of reference, which are shown in Figure 1-5, may also be employed in descriptions of individual organs or parts of the body; their use is not restricted to the body as a whole.

The anatomical position, planes of reference, and some general terms are all summarized pictorially in Figure 1-6.

The fundamental unit of structure and function is the **cell,** and no description of the human body would be complete without at least referring to these basic building blocks in the formation of almost all animal tissue.

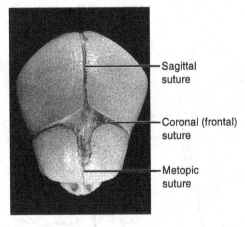

FIGURE 1-4

An infant skull as seen from above, showing the sagittal, coronal, and metopic (pertaining to the forehead) suture. The metopic suture is often obliterated in the adult skull.

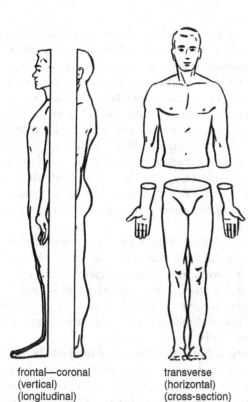
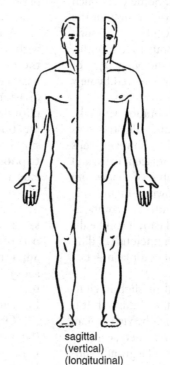

FIGURE 1-5

Planes of reference. The frontal-coronal and sagittal planes are also vertical or longitudinal planes, while the transverse plane is horizontal, cross-sectional, or perpendicular to the longitudinal planes.

frontal—coronal
(vertical)
(longitudinal)

transverse
(horizontal)
(cross-section)

sagittal
(vertical)
(longitudinal)

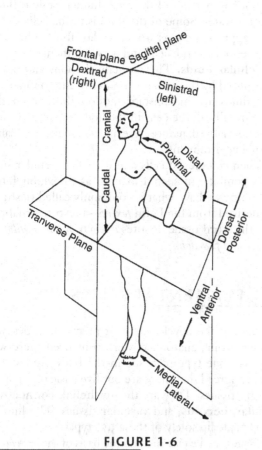

FIGURE 1-6

Pictorial summary of planes and general terms.

CELLS

Cells (L. *cella*, a small cavity) are highly organized masses of **protoplasm** (Gk. *protos*, first + *plasma*, a thing formed or molded) which possess the peculiar property we have come to call life. The following criteria determine the category of the living:

1. **Irritability** (L. *irritare*, to tease), the ability to be stimulated or affected by (to react to) a change in the environment.

2. **Growth.**

3. **Spontaneous movement,** or the movement that originates from within the organism.

4. **Metabolism,** which is the use of food and oxygen to build or repair tissue, to produce heat and energy.

5. **Reproduction,** or the ability to produce new protoplasm.

Cells are unusually small and are measured in microns. One micron is one-thousandth of a millimeter or 10^{-3} mm. A single cell would need to be about 100 microns in diameter in order to be just visible to the naked eye. Red blood cells are about 7 to 8 microns in diameter.

There are about 100 trillion cells in the human body, and since they are individual units of living matter, they are subject to a limited life span. Some cells, such as those in the nervous system, may live throughout the life of the organism that hosts them, while others, such as blood cells, have a life span of about four months. Other cells, such as those comprising the outer layer of skin, are continuously dying and being replaced by new cells.

An isolated cell placed in a fluid solution will take on a spherical shape, and so cells are often illustrated as if they were spherical. In living tissues, however, cells are subjected to the forces exerted by adjacent cells, and they may appear in any one of a number of shapes and configurations. A schematic cell is shown in Figure 1-7.

The basic substance that enters into the composition of all living cells is called **protoplasm;** it can be divided into two principal constituents, a **nucleus** (L. dim. of *nux*, nut) and its enveloping mass of **cytoplasm**—i.e., cell-plasma.

The nucleus is usually spheroidal or slightly elongated and conforms to the general shape of the cell. It is surrounded by a nuclear envelope which by virtue of an **endoplasmic reticulum** (L., dim. of *rete*, net) seems to be continuous with the cell membrane. The ground substance of the nucleus contains **chromatin** (Gk. *chroma*, color) deposits which consist largely of **deoxyribonucleic acid,** or **DNA.** It contributes to the formation of **chromosomes** (Gk. *chroma* + *soma*, body) during cell division and is, therefore, responsible for transmission of genetic traits. The nucleus also contains a **nucleolus** (L., dim. of *nucleus*) which contains **ribosomes.** They are necessary for protein biosynthesis by the cell.

The **cytoplasm** of a living cell appears rather homogeneous when viewed under the conventional bright-field microscope. It consists of about 70 to 85 percent water and about 20 percent protein substance. It is surrounded by a semipermeable membrane called the outer plasma membrane. It controls the exchange of certain molecules and ions between the cell and its environment.

A number of identifiable structures can be found within the substance of the cytoplasm. One of them is the **centrosome,** usually found near the nucleus. It has been clearly associated with mitotic (asexual) cell division. Another cytoplasmic organelle is the **mitochondrion** (Gk. *mitos*, thread + *chondrion*, granule). The function of these complex structures can be stated quite simply—to provide energy in the form of **adenosine triphosphate,** or **ATP,** a substance we will encounter later in a brief examination of the contractile process of muscle tissue.

The endoplasmic reticulum mentioned earlier seems to form the structural matrix of the cytoplasm, part of which constitutes a separate organelle, the **Golgi apparatus;** its function is believed to be *temporary storage of secretary substances.* It is very prominent in secretory cells. The endoplasmic reticulum also seems to form an intracellular transport network.

Other organelles within the cytoplasm include lipid (fat) droplets, vacuoles (L. *vacuus*, empty + *ole*, dim. ending), glycogen particles, crystalline inclusion bodies, lysosomes (which are digestive organs of the cell), and certain inert substances.

About 56 percent of the adult human body is fluid, most of it water. Some of the fluid is inside cells and is known appropriately as **intracellular fluid.** Fluids in the spaces outside the cells and between them are called **extracellular fluids.** They contain the ions and nutrients required by the cells to sustain life and to function. These fluids are in constant motion throughout the body. Virtually all the cells in the body, in spite of their highly specialized nature, live in essentially the same "internal environment."

When colonies of cells and their intercellular substances combine in such a manner as to exhibit functional unity, we have what is commonly called **tissue,** a word derived from the Latin *texere*—a texture or fabric. Today the word tissue denotes *a colony of cells similar in structure and function.*

ELEMENTARY TISSUES

Long before the development of precision optics and the microscope, anatomists were convinced there was more than one type of tissue in the body. Today it is generally agreed that there are but five basic types of elementary tissues. They are the **epithelial, connective, muscular, nervous,** and **vascular** tissues. The human body is made up solely of these five types.

Tissues can be classified on the basis of the *presence or absence of intercellular substances,* as well as their *characteristics,* and they can also be classified according to the *form of the cell.* Here is one scheme, used by DiDio (1970).

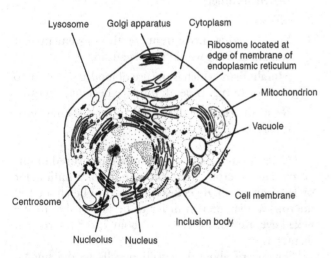

Lysosome   Golgi apparatus   Cytoplasm

Ribosome located at edge of membrane of endoplasmic reticulum

Mitochondrion

Vacuole

Cell membrane

Inclusion body

Centrosome

Nucleolus   Nucleus

FIGURE 1-7

Schematic representation of a cell showing the nucleus and cytoplasm and the principal constituents of each.

A. Tissue without intercellular
   substance—epithelium
B. Tissue with intercellular substance
   1. Semifluid—connective
   2. Solid
      a. Cartilage
      b. Bone
   3. Fluid
      a. Blood
      b. Lymph
C. Tissue with elongated cells
   1. Partially elongated—nervous tissue
   2. Totally elongated—muscular tissue

Epithelial Tissue

Epithelial (Gk. *epi*, upon + *thele*, nipple) tissues are characteristically arranged in mosaics, forming sheets of tissue that cover the external surface of the body, line the tubes or passages leading to the exterior, and almost without exception, line the internal cavities in the body. These tissues, which are formed by closely approximated cells, have very little intercellular substance. Epithelial tissue has a free surface and rests upon a **basement tissue;** that is, it rests upon a stratum of connective tissue. Epithelial tissue is subjected to various functional demands, depending upon its location. On the surface of the body it is subjected to drying and abrasion. In the body cavities,

however, where it is subjected to little abrasion, it is covered with a fluid film and forms smooth gliding surfaces. As might be expected, there is a relationship between functional requirements and the shape of epithelial cells. Indeed, the shapes of the cells provide clues as to their function, whether it be *protective, secretory, sensory, glandular,* or *absorptive.* Epithelial tissues may be classified into three groups, the criterion being primarily location. They are **epithelial tissue proper, endothelial tissue,** and **mesothelial tissue.**

Epithelial Tissue Proper

This tissue forms the **epidermis** (outer layer of the skin) and the **internal membranes** that are *continuous with the skin,* such as mucous membranes lining the digestive, respiratory, urinary, and generative (pertaining to reproduction) tracts or tubes. The shape of epithelial cells is varied, ranging from flat, pavement-like (**squamous**) to rodlike (**columnar**) cells. Intermediate forms are **cuboidal.** When columnar cells line a curved surface with a small radius, they may appear **pyramidal.**

In addition, epithelial tissue may be composed of a single layer of cells (**simple**) or of several layers of cells (**stratified**). Some epithelial cells are specialized to serve as sensory cells for exteroceptors, in the eye and ear especially. These cells are usually columnar, often characterized by numerous small hairlike **cilia** on their free surface. Some examples of epithelial tissues are shown in Figure 1-8.

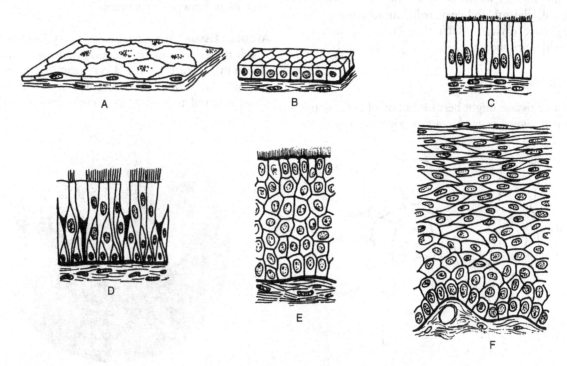

FIGURE 1-8

Examples of epithelial tissues. The shape of epithelial cells varies from flat, scalelike to rod-like columnar cells. (A) Simple squamous, (B) cubodial, (C) simple ciliated columnar, (D) pseudostratified ciliated, (E) ciliated stratified columnar, (F) stratified squamous.

An important variation of simple columnar epithelium may be seen in the form of **goblet cells.** These cells, found in the intestinal and respiratory tracts, are actually single-cell mucous glands that secrete mucin.

Endothelial Tissue

This tissue is confined almost exclusively to the inner lining of the walls of the blood and lymph vessels, and unlike internal epithelial tissue, it has no continuity anywhere with the epidermis. Endothelial tissues are composed of but a single layer of rather flat cells (**simple squamous**), so they present an extremely smooth surface that reduces the possibility of fragmenting blood cells that might cause blood clots.

Mesothelial Tissue

This is a specialized form of epithelial tissue which lines the primary body cavities. There are four such cavities in the human: the **peritoneal cavity** (L., Gk., *peritonaion,* from *per,* around + *teinein,* to stretch), which is located in the abdomen; the two **pleural cavities,** which house the lungs; and the **pericardial cavity,** which houses the heart. Mesothelium is often referred to as **serous membrane,** which indeed it is. Serous membranes consist of a sheet of areolar (loose, connective) tissue whose free surface is covered by a single layer of flat cells not unlike those of endothelium. The free surface of serous membrane is extremely smooth and slippery. The three serous membranes in the body cavities are called the **peritoneal, pleural,** and **pericardial membranes,** after the respective cavities which they line. The primary body cavities are shown schematically in Figure 1-9.

Connective Tissue

Connective tissues might best be described as those tissues which *connect or bind structures together, support the body,* and *aid in bodily maintenance.* The various types of connective tissue, in contrast to epithelium, have relatively few cells and a proportionately large amount of intercellular substance, which consists of various types of fibers, ground substance, and tissue fluid. The noncellular components of connective tissue are collectively called the **matrix.** Interestingly enough, connective tissue is subdivided, not on the basis of the characteristics of the living cells in the tissue, but rather on the basis of the nonliving intercellular substances. For example, areolar (meshlike) tissue is characterized by soft intercellular substance, while the intercellular substance in cartilage is firm, yet somewhat flexible. In bone, the intercellular substance consists of deposits of inorganic salts and is hard and rigid. Generally speaking, connective tissues can be divided into **loose, dense,** and **special** types. Loose connective tissue includes **areolar** and **adipose** tissues, which are characterized by scattered fibers, whereas dense connective tissues are characterized by numerous tightly packed fibers. Examples include **tendons, ligaments, fasciae,** and **reticular** (netlike) tissues. Specialized connective tissue with solid or rigid intercellular substances include the various types of **cartilage** and **bone.**

Loose Connective Tissue

Loose connective tissue is extensively distributed throughout the body. Its primary function is to bind parts together, at the same time allowing considerable movement between structures.

Areolar Tissue Areolar tissue is a very loose tissue, in which the cells lie in an irregular network of fibers, as shown in Figure 1-10. It is a very primitive form of tissue and, due to its rather irregular structure, is sometimes referred to simply as "loose connective tissue."

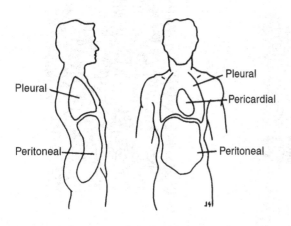

FIGURE 1-9

The three primary body cavities are the peritoneal, pleural, and pericardial.

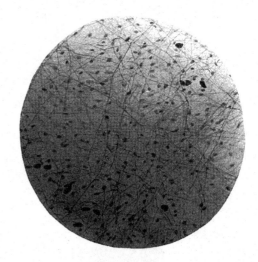

FIGURE 1-10

A microphotograph of areolar tissue.

Areolar tissue is commonly found just beneath the skin. Indeed, it forms the "bed" for skin and mucous membrane and is found almost everywhere in the body. Because it is invariably associated with other types of tissue, it is difficult to illustrate, or to demonstrate in isolation. The word *areolar* stems from a Latin word which denotes a space.

Adipose Tissue Adipose tissue is very similar to areolar tissue, but it has a *high concentration of fat cells*. It is frequently found just beneath the skin, in a layer of tissue called **subcutaneous fascia**. The fat cells are large and have an ovoid or spherical shape. The cytoplasm is displaced to the periphery of the cell, and the nucleus, usually flattened, is pressed against the cell wall. When seen in fixed preparations, as in Figure 1-11, fat cells assume the shape of a signet ring.

Dense Connective Tissue

Dense connective tissue is characterized by an abundance of closely packed fibers. In many dense connective tissues, **collagenous (Gk. *koila*, glue + *gen*, to beget) fibers** predominate. When boiled in water, they yield gelatin. Other dense connective tissues are characterized by **elastic fibers** which return to their normal length after having been stretched. **Reticular fibers** are also found in dense connective tissues.

It is on the basis of the intercellular substance that dense connective tissue can be designated as white and unyielding (**white fibrous tissue**), or yellow and elastic (**yellow elastic tissue**). Dense connective tissues (fibrous) make up **tendons, aponeuroses, ligaments,** and **fasciae.**

Tendons Tendons are tough, nonelastic cords, largely composed of closely packed **parallel fibers.** *A tendon can always be associated with a muscle.* It is by means of tendons that most muscles attach to bone, cartilage, or in a few instances, to one another, as in the case of the digastric and omohyoid muscles in the neck. In certain regions, such as on the anterior and lateral abdominal wall, muscles attach by means of very broad tendinous sheets called **aponeuroses,** which by definition are white flattened tendinous expansions serving mainly as an investment (covering) for muscle, or connecting muscles with the parts that they move upon contraction. There are a number of instances, then, when broad tendons are referred to as aponeuroses.

Ligaments Ligaments (L. *ligare*, to bind) are also characterized by tightly packed parallel fibers, but with an abundance of elastic fibers. This gives them the special property that makes them particularly suitable for joining bone to bone, bone to cartilage, and cartilage to cartilage.

The term ligament, as it is used in gross anatomy, has *two meanings*, which is something we ought to recognize. The term ligament means *a band of tissue that connects bones or supports viscera*. When applied to structures related to a joint, a ligament is *a strong fibrous cord or sheet*. When applied to a serous membrane (as in the case of the ligaments of the peritoneum in the abdominal cavity), a ligament is merely *a sheet of epithelial membrane with little or no tensile strength*. In addition, the term **membrane** is used where ligament seems to be far more appropriate. For example, the shafts of the radius and ulna of the forearm are bound together by an extremely tough expanded ligament called the *interosseous membrane*. And to further complicate matters, the *inguinal ligament* located in the groin is actually a tendinous structure associated with the external layer of the anterolateral abdominal musculature, but more about that later.

Fascia Fascia (L., a band or bundle; pl. *fasciae*) as used in anatomy applies to all of the dense fibrous connective tissues not otherwise designated as tendons, aponeuroses, or ligaments, even though the irregularly arranged fibers in fascia distinguish it from the other dense fibrous tissues on a histological basis.

Fascia varies considerably in thickness and density throughout the body, and it is usually found in the form of membranous sheets. Fasciae are commonly associated with muscles. They are *responsible for the organization of muscle fibers into functional mechanical mediators of movement*. The **subcutaneous fascia** is a continuous sheet of fascia found over the body, located between the skin and deeper structures. It is actually a two-layered structure. The outer one commonly contains accumulations of fat, and so its thickness varies considerably among individuals; **deep fasciae** and **subserous fasciae** are also identified. The term fascia is also used in a more

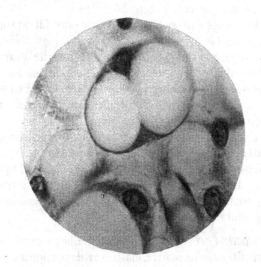

FIGURE 1-11

A microphotograph of adipose tissue.

restrictive sense to identify local regions of connective tissue that are not tendons, aponeuroses, or ligaments. It is very pervasive tissue that we nevertheless tend to ignore in anatomical descriptions. In many areas it appears to be no more than a gossamer feltlike network, but it does keep us from coming apart.

Reticular Tissue Reticular tissue, shown in Figure 1-12, is a very delicate matrix of cells which have processes that extend in all directions to join the processes of neighboring cells. In spite of its feltlike nature, it is nevertheless classified as a dense connective tissue. A primitive type of tissue, it often forms a supporting framework for the **parenchyma** of such organs as the lymph nodes and liver. Parenchyma pertains to the essential or functional elements of an organ.

Special Connective Tissue

Connective tissues play several roles in the body, defensive at the cellular level and structural due to extracellular properties. The principal role of special connective tissue, namely, bone and cartilage, is structural.

Cartilage Cartilage, like the other connective tissues, is composed of cells, ground substance, and intercellular fibers. The cells of cartilage, called **chondroblasts** (Gk. *chondros*, cartilage), are found in irregular spaces called **lacunae** (L. dim. of *lacus*, small lake or cavity) within the ground substance. The properties of the fibers and ground substance impart special characteristics to cartilage. For example, the cartilage which covers the articular surfaces of bone is capable of withstanding compression forces of over 20,000 kilograms per square centimeter. Surprisingly, this same cartilage tears easily.

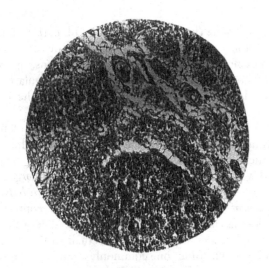

FIGURE 1-12

A microphotograph of reticular tissue.

In the early stages of development, cartilage forms the entire skeleton of the body, and in the adult it forms the skeletal framework for such structures as the larynx, trachea, bronchi, and ears.

Cartilage is capable of growth, and indeed forms the "growing skeleton" of youngsters. Because cartilage is flexible, it may grow by proliferation of chondroblasts, and the growth may be *interstitial* (expansive growth due to cell multiplication), or it may be *appositional* (growth due to deposition or formation at the periphery).

Depending upon the nature and relative concentrations of fibrous substances, cartilage may be subdivided into three types: **hyaline, elastic,** and **fibrous.**

Hyaline Cartilage. Hyaline (Gk. *hyalos*, glass) cartilage, shown in Figure 1-13, appears as a bluish-white translucent substance in the fresh state, strongly resembling milk glass. It covers the articular surfaces of joints and forms the framework for the lower respiratory tract. The apparently homogeneous intercellular substance actually contains a great amount of collagenous fibers. The arrangement of the collagen fibers is often described as a series of arches extending radially toward the surface, where they turn horizontally before returning vertically. Experiments dating back to 1848 have shown that, if the articular surface of a cartilage is pierced by a round pin and then withdrawn, a longitudinal split line remains and the pattern of the split lines is constant and distinctive. The splits have been shown to follow the predominant direction of the collagen fibers in the horizontal layer or zone. Early researchers proposed that the split line orientation reflected the direction of the most habitual movement. Other investigators deny any preferred orientation of collagen in articular cartilage (McCall, 1968; Freeman, 1973). The ground substance seems to be concentrated in the areas immediately surrounding the lacunae and is almost absent in the matrix between the cell areas.

Hyaline cartilage has a relatively poor blood supply so nutrition is provided in large part through diffusion. Poor nutrition may be responsible for the dramatic changes that occur with age. Hyaline cartilage loses its transparency and appears yellowish and cloudy. In addition, a certain amount of **calcification** or **ossification** (turning to bone) may occur.

Except for the articular surfaces of cartilages, all cartilage is invested by a tough fibrous membrane called **perichondrium.** When muscles or tendons impinge upon cartilage, the union is made possible by virtue of the perichondrium. A similar fibrous membrane invests bone, and it is called **periosteum.**

Elastic Cartilage. Because of the large numbers of elastic fibers in its matrix, elastic cartilage appears somewhat yellow and opaque. It is flexible and elastic and seems almost rubbery in consistency. As in hyaline car-

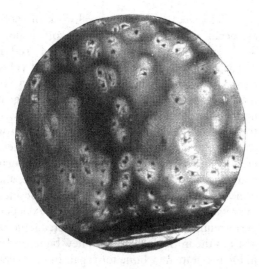
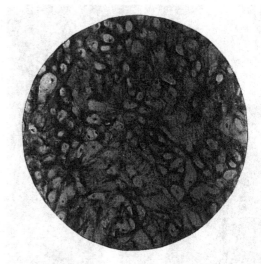

FIGURE 1-13

Hyaline and elastic cartilage.

tilage, the ground substance contains collagenous fibers. Elastic cartilage can be found in the ear, external auditory meatus, epiglottis, and auditory (Eustachian) tube and in some small cartilages of the larynx. All of the structures in which elastic cartilage is found have something to do with the production or reception of sounds. Calcification of the elastic cartilages rarely, if ever, occurs. Elastic cartilage is shown in Figure 1-13.

Fibrocartilage (Fibrous Cartilage). Fibrous cartilage is characterized by a dense network of collagenous fibers and cartilage cells. Variable amounts of hyaline matrix may be found in fibrous cartilage, particularly in the cell territories. Fibrous cartilage may be found in some joints in the body, especially in the form of intervertebral discs of the vertebral column.

Bone Bone (L. *os*, Gk. *osteon*), the other specialized dense connective tissue, is characterized by a rigid matrix, or intercellular substance. Bone or **osseous tissue** is composed of cells (**osteoblasts** and **osteocytes**), collagenous fibers, and ground substance. The rigidity of bone is due to the rather large amounts of inorganic salts that are deposited in its matrix. These salts, which are about 85 percent calcium phosphate and 10 percent calcium carbonate, with traces of calcium fluoride and magnesium fluoride, constitute about two-thirds of fresh bone weight.

In bone, as in cartilage, the intercellular substance predominates over the cells, and it is the intercellular substance, of course, that is responsible for the physical properties of bone. All through life, bone is subjected to tremendous compression and disrupting forces (tension), especially when we walk, run, jump, and lift heavy objects. In terms of its tensile strength (resistance to

stretch), bone can be compared to fresh white oak, and it resists compression about as well as concrete.

Classification of Bones. Grossly, two kinds of bone may be identified—**dense** or **compact** bone, and **spongy** or **cancellous** bone. The histological character of the cells and intercellular substance, however, is the same in both compact and spongy bone. They differ only in the degree of porosity and in architecture.

Compact bone, if inspected with the eye, appears white, homogeneous, and without any particular structure. Spongy bone, on the other hand, appears porous. It consists of delicate spicules of bone or **trabeculae** (L., dim. of *trabs*, a beam, or supporting structure) that intersect to form a very complicated meshwork. The trabecular arrangement is largely influenced by mechanical demands placed on the individual bone. Compact bone forms the outer shell, or **cortex** (L. bark, shell) of most bones, while the remaining interior is composed of spongy bone. Usually the demarcation between compact and spongy bone is somewhat ill-defined; rather, a gradual transition between the two takes place. A longitudinal section of a long bone (femur) reveals both the compact and spongy bone, as illustrated in Figure 1-14. The interdigitating trabeculae are shown in Figure 1-15.

The primary characteristic of bone is its lamellar structure; that is, the fibers and ground substance are laid down in thin layers, or **lamellae** (L., dim. of *lamina*, a plate). When a cross section of compact bone is examined microscopically, as in Figure 1-16, it is seen to be pierced by longitudinal canals called the **Haversian canals.** They anastomose with each other to form an elaborate canal system that accommodates blood vessels and nerves. The Haversian canals are surrounded by concentric **lamellae,** not unlike the growth rings of a

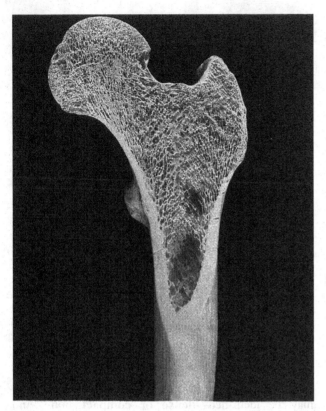

FIGURE 1-14

A longitudinal section through a femur showing spongy and compact bone.

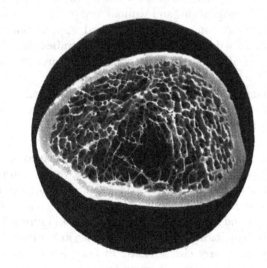

FIGURE 1-15

Trabeculae as seen in a cross-section through a femur.

tree. The bone cells or osteocytes are located within oval **lacunae,** which are between the lamellae. Small canals (**canaliculi**) extend from the lacunae to communicate with the canaliculi of adjacent lacunae.

The spaces within the meshwork of spongy bone are occupied by bone marrow, the soft tissues of bone. Two types of marrow are recognized: **red marrow,** which manufactures red blood cells, and **yellow marrow,** which is pure adipose tissue. In the very young, red marrow predominates, but with increasing age more red marrow is transformed into yellow marrow, which in the aged gradually turns into gelatinous marrow.

Except at their articular surfaces, all bones are covered by a tough, fibrous membrane called **periosteum,** and although it is closely adherent to bone, and invests every irregularity, it can be stripped off. Besides providing attachments for muscle tendons, the deeper layer of periosteum contains **osteoblasts** (osteogenic cells) that assist in the initial formation of new bone, and that later in life generate new bone for repair in the event of fractures or disease. The superficial layer of periosteum is richly supplied with the capillaries that are responsible for the food supply to the bone tissue. This is why bones in the fresh state have a characteristic pink hue.

Depending upon their shape, bones are classified as **long, short, flat, irregular,** or **accessory.** The length of a long bone is simply greater than its width, so some of them, as in the fingers and toes, are really quite short. Short bones, on the other hand, are usually cuboidal in shape and have several articular surfaces. They are found in the wrist and ankle. Flat bones (as in the skull) have a plate of compact bone on their outer and inner surfaces, and these plates are separated by a thin marrow space. In the skull, the marrow space is known as **diploe** (Gk. fold). As the name implies, irregular bones are not amenable to classification. Examples include the hip bones and the vertebrae that make up the spinal column.

Accessory and **sesamoid** bones can also be identified. The most common of the accessory bones are called **Wormian** bones. They are found in the skull, between the suture lines. Sesamoid bones are small bony structures found within tendons. They protect tendons from abuse and also have certain mechanical properties that contribute to movement about a joint.[4]

In addition, certain bones, particularly those adjacent to the nasal cavities of the head, are hollow and are known as **air-containing** bones. If nothing else, the air spaces (sinuses) reduce the weight of the bones slightly.

The 206 or so bones in the adult human skeleton are divided into an **axial** and **appendicular** skeleton. The spine is the axis of the body, and the axial skeleton includes those bones associated with the spinal column, its extensions and processes, or in other words, the vertebrae, skull, hyoid bone, and rib cage, as shown in Figure 1-17.

---

[4]The patella or kneecap is a sesamoid bone formed in the tendon of the quadriceps femoris muscle.

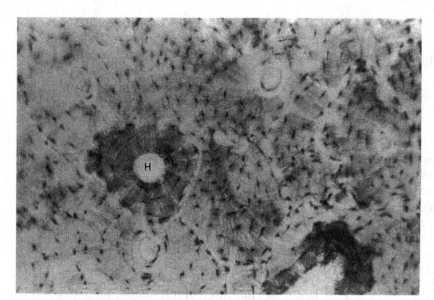

FIGURE 1-16

Microscopic view of bone. A Haversian canal (H) is surrounded by concentric lamellae. Osteocytes are found within the lacunae.

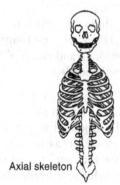

Axial skeleton

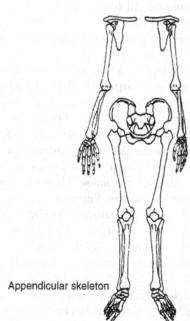

Appendicular skeleton

FIGURE 1-17

The axial and appendicular skeletons.

The appendicular skeleton, as the name implies, pertains to those bones of the appendages, or the bones of the **pectoral** (upper limb) girdle and the **pelvic** (lower limb) girdle.

Descriptive Terminology. Points or regions where tendons attach to the periosteum and where ligaments attach to bone are often characterized by identifiable landmarks that can serve as points of reference. Bones may be pierced by arteries, veins, and nerves, and the perforations also may form useful landmarks.

Frequently used anatomical terms for descriptions of skeletal structure often refer either to elevations or to depressions of bones.[5]

Elevations

Condyle—a rounded or knucklelike process.

Crest—a prominent ridge.

Head—an enlargement at one end of the bone, beyond its neck.

Process—a bony prominence.

Spine—a sharp projection.

Trochanter—a very large bony projection.

Tubercle—a small rounded projection.

Tuberosity—a large rounded projection.

Depressions

Fissure—a cleft or deep groove.

Foramen—an opening or perforation in a bone (or cartilage).

Fossa—a pit or hollow.

Fovea—a small pitlike depression.

---

[5]These terms do not apply exclusively to osseous structures.

Groove—a furrow.

Meatus—a tube or passageway.

Neck—a constriction near one end (the head) of a bone.

Sinus—a cavity within a bone.

Sulcus—a groove or a furrow.

A long bone is shown in Figure 1-18. The long, smooth, and slender portion of the bone is known as the **shaft** or **diaphysis** (Gk. point of separation between the stalk and branch). The articular ends of the bone are called the **epiphyses** (Gk. an on-growth), and they are covered by a cap of hyaline cartilage. An epiphysis may be the **head** of a bone, an **articular facet** (Fr. *facette*), or a **condyle,** depending upon its shape and its relationship with other bones. Other useful landmarks are also shown in the figure.

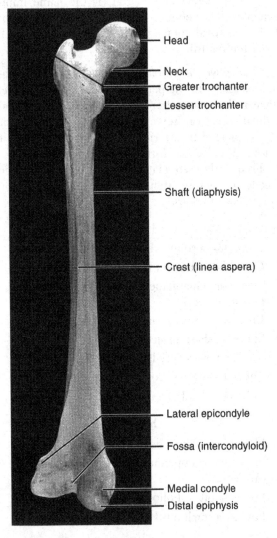

— Head
— Neck
— Greater trochanter
— Lesser trochanter

— Shaft (diaphysis)

— Crest (linea aspera)

— Lateral epicondyle

— Fossa (intercondyloid)

— Medial condyle
— Distal epiphysis

FIGURE 1-18

Illustration of a long bone (femur).

Classification of Joints. The functional connections that exist between the various bones of the skeleton are called **articulations** or **joints** (L. *junctio,* a joining). Although we may tend to associate movement with the word joint, some articulations are virtually immovable, and the bones themselves will fracture before the joint yields. Other joints permit a very slight movement, at the expense of some strength, while others are freely movable (in certain directions), with completely separated articular surfaces. The articular surfaces may contact one another, but there is no anatomical continuity between them.

Joints can be categorized either on a functional basis or on an anatomical basis, and either way there are three major categories.

On a *functional basis* there are **synarthrodial** (Gk. *syn,* with, together + *arthrosis,* joint) or immovable joints, **amphiarthrodial** (Gk. *amphy,* on both sides) or slightly movable or yielding joints, and **diarthrodial** (Gk. *dis,* twice, double + *arthron,* a joint) or freely movable joints.

On an *anatomical basis* there are **fibrous** joints which are immovable (synarthrodial), **cartilaginous** joints which yield (amphiarthrodial), and **synovial** joints which are freely movable (diarthrodial).

Synarthrodial (Fibrous, Immovable) Joints. Synarthrodial joints include all those in which the bones are almost in direct contact and are joined together by a thin intervening connective tissue, so as to restrict or prevent movements. There are four varieties of synarthrodial joints: **suture, schindylesis, gomphosis,** and **syndesmosis.** All four varieties are represented by articulations of the bones of the skull, and some are exclusive to the skull, and so are important to us.

The **suture** (L. a seam) is only found in the skull, and an example of a true suture is shown in Figure 1-19. It is a **serrated suture** in which the edges of the bones are serrated (L. a saw) like the teeth of a saw. The bones are separated only by a thin fibrous tissue which is continuous with the periosteum externally and with the dura mater internally. Other sutures appear more in the form of interdigitating toothlike projections on the opposing edges of the bones. They are called **dentate sutures.** In the **suture limbosa,** the bones interlock on beveled surfaces. A suture allows little or no movement. Sometimes two originally separate bones become united by an osseous union, and the joint becomes obliterated. Such a condition is called a **synostosis.**

Another type of synarthrodial joint is called the **schindylesis.** It is found where a single plate of bone is inserted into a cleft that has been formed by the separation of two laminae in another bone. This is a rather uncommon joint, best exemplified by the articulation of the sphenoid and the perpendicular plate of the ethmoid with the vomer bone.

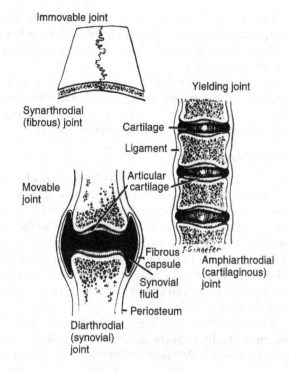

FIGURE 1-19

Three major types of joints. The immovable is a synarthrodial or fibrous joint, the yielding is an amphiarthrodial or cartilaginous joint, and the movable is a diarthrodial or synovial joint.

The **gomphosis** is a type of joint found mainly in the head. The word originally was derived from the idea of a peg driven into wood. The gomphosis is well represented in the skull, because it is by means of a gomphosis that the root of a tooth is held in place.

The **syndesmosis** is a form of joint where two bones are united by interosseous ligaments. The word is derived from a Greek term denoting a band. It is found between the tibia and fibula of the lower leg, and in the middle ear.

Amphiarthrodial (Cartilaginous, Yielding) Joints. This type of articulation is quite commonly found in the skeleton. The amphiarthrodial joint permits a certain amount of movement, or give. In this joint, the contiguous bone edges are united by interposing cartilage. Two types of amphiarthrodial joints can be found in the skeleton: **synchondrosis** and **symphysis.**

The **synchondrosis** is broadly represented in the skeleton. It is a rather rigid cartilaginous joint that ossifies with increasing age. As such it is often regarded as a temporary joint. Synchondroses are commonly found in the skull at birth, and for some years after. Precocious synchondroses at the base of the skull can be a very serious matter, resulting in mental retardation. Synchondroses can also be found between the epiphyses and diaphyses of long bones during the early years of life.

The **symphysis** is another type of amphiarthrosis that is broadly represented in the skeleton, because it is found between the individual vertebrae and between the two pubic bones. In this joint the contiguous edges of bone are connected by discs of fibrocartilage. The articular facets are covered by hyaline cartilage, with the fibrocartilage between them. An amphiarthrodial joint is shown schematically in Figure 1-19.

Diarthrodial (Synovial, Movable) Joints. These joints are broadly represented in the body, and they have widely variable degrees and directions of free movement. The bones are joined by a band of fibrous tissue called the **articular capsule,** within which is a joint cavity. An articular capsule is shown schematically in Figure 1-19. The internal layer of the articular capsule secretes a small amount of **synovial fluid,** which lubricates the joint cavity. The opposed ends of bones in a diarthrodial joint or, in other words, the articular facets are covered by a layer of hyaline cartilage. In some diarthrodial joints, the joint is divided by an **articular disc** or **meniscus,** the periphery of which is continuous with the fibrous capsule, while its free surfaces are invested by a synovial membrane. These joints permit more than one type of movement at the same time, such as gliding and rotation.[6]

Diarthrodial joints, which are illustrated in Figure 1-20, are classified according to their types of movement.

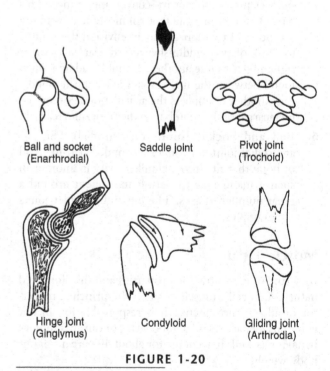

FIGURE 1-20

Six classes of diarthrodial joints.

[6]The low level of friction in synovial joints has been described as equivalent to "ice on ice."

Classification systems vary, but there are at least six types of diarthrodial joints.

1. **Gliding Joint.** (Arthrodia) Gliding joints are those in which the articulating surfaces are alternately slightly convex and concave, or the surfaces may be flat. They permit only gliding or sliding movements. They are found between the articular processes of the vertebrae and in the joints of the hand and foot.

2. **Hinge Joint.** (Ginglymus) Hinge joints permit movement in one plane, usually forward and backward, with a considerable range of movement. The interphalangeal joints (in the fingers) are good examples of these hinge joints.

3. **Pivot Joint.** (Trochoid) The trochoid (Gk. *trochos*, wheel) is so named because of its resemblance to a pulley or pivot. Movement between the first two cervical vertebrae is an example of rotation at a pivot joint.

4. **Condyloid.** (Ellipsoid) The word condyle is from the Greek word for knuckle. Here an oval-shaped articular facet fits into an elliptical-shaped cavity. Such a joint permits all types of movement except rotation. The wrist joint is an example.

5. **Saddle Joint.** In this unique joint both articulating surfaces present a concave-convex appearance. This type of joint permits all types of movement, with the exception of rotation. A way to envision this joint is to think of two saddle-shaped articular surfaces, at right angles to one another. A double saddle joint is found between the malleus and incus in the middle ear. Another example is the articulation between the metacarpal of the thumb with the trapezium (carpal).

6. **Ball and Socket Joint.** (Enarthrodial) The enarthrodial joint consists of a rounded ball-like end of bone that fits into a cuplike cavity in another in such a manner as to permit movement around a great number of axes. The hip and shoulder joints are examples.

Muscle Tissue

By virtue of its contractile properties and the elongated nature of its cells, muscle tissue is the principal mediator of all our movements. It is responsible for all our voluntary behavior and a good share of our involuntary behavior as well. It accounts for about 40 percent of our body weight.

The word muscle has an interesting history, and it stems originally from the Greek word for the common little mouse (*mus musculus*) that seems to prefer to live in people's houses. Apparently, at one time in the early history of anatomy, someone thought that a muscle preparation, along with its tendon, resembled a mouse with its tail, and so we have it. *Mylo-* is a combining form from the Greek *mys*, denoting a muscle, while the combining form meaning flesh is *sarco-*.

Muscle tissue may be classified on either a histological or an anatomical basis; in both classifications, three types of muscle tissue may be identified: **striated** (skeletal), **smooth** (visceral), and **cardiac** (heart).

Striated Muscle

Striated muscle, shown in Figure 1-21, consists of long fibers which, when viewed under a microscope, are seen to be crossed by evenly spaced transverse bands, hence the term **striated**. Striated muscle is supplied by the somatic division of the peripheral nervous system, and since we have voluntary control over it, striated muscle is **voluntary muscle.** Because striated muscle attaches primarily to the skeletal system, this tissue may also be called **skeletal muscle.**

Throughout the remainder of this text we shall be concerned chiefly with the actions of striated muscles. There are about 329 of them in the human body, and *all but two are paired muscles.* They are the **procerus** muscle, which wrinkles the area between the eyebrows when we frown, and the **diaphragm.** Muscles vary greatly in their size. The tiny stapedius muscle in the middle ear, for example, is only 2 or 3 mm in length, while the sartorius, which crosses over the front of the thigh, is over 60 cm in length.

The smallest functional unit of muscle tissue is the **muscle cell** or **muscle fiber** (terms that are synonymous). They range from 0.01 to 0.1 mm in diameter and from 1 to 120 mm in length. As shown in Figure 1-22, muscle fibers are cylindrical in shape with somewhat blunt ends. An individual muscle fiber is multinucle-

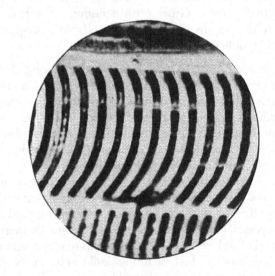

FIGURE 1-21

Photomicrograph of striated muscle.

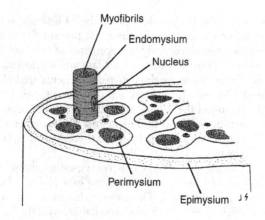

FIGURE 1-22

Schematic of a muscle fiber and connective tissue associated with it.

ated[7] and composed of hundreds, or even thousands, of long filamentlike **myofibrils** which are imbedded in a form of specialized protoplasm called **sarcoplasm.** The myofibrillae and sarcoplasm are enclosed by a delicate, elastic, transparent, and homogenous membrane called **sarcolemma** (Gk. *sarco + lemma,* husk). Numerous irregularly spaced nuclei lie imbedded within the substance of the sarcolemma. The sarcoplasm of a muscle fiber is impregnated with numerous fat droplets which may be more or less abundant, depending upon the extent to which the individual is nourished. Muscle fibers contain a protein called **myoglobin,** which is similar to the hemoglobin in blood. Myoglobin binds oxygen and increases the rate of oxygen diffusion into the muscle fiber. Muscles containing large amounts of myoglobin are dark red in color; otherwise, they are pale.

Each muscle fiber is terminated rather bluntly and is covered by a fibrous tissue called **endomysium,** which serves to bind the muscle fibers and to separate them from adjacent muscle fibers. Where an individual fiber terminates within a muscle, the endomysium becomes continuous with the endomysium of the neighboring muscle fibers. It is in this manner, then, that individual muscle fibers are bundled together to form a functional muscle.

Groups of muscle fibers (more properly called **fasciculi**) are similarly ensheathed and separated from other groups by a fibrous tissue more coarse and more pronounced than endomysium. It is called **perimysium.** Whereas fasciculi are ensheathed by perimysium, an entire muscle is encased by a still coarser fibrous envelope called **epimysium.** A fibrous intermuscular septum (fascia) separates and compartmentalizes muscle groups.

---

[7]Presumably embryonic muscle cells are formed by successive fusion of many cells.

At the ends of a muscle, the fibers are attached by a tendon to either the periosteum of bone or the perichondrium of cartilage. Connective tissue fibrils (collagen) insert into folds in the sarcolemma. *Muscle fibrillae are not continuous with the fibrillae of the connective tissue.* For comparative purposes, striated, smooth, and cardiac muscle tissue is shown schematically in Figure 1-23.

Smooth Muscle

Smooth muscle, a more primitive type of tissue than striated (skeletal) muscle, is found wherever movement is relatively independent of voluntary control. Smooth muscle is innervated by the autonomic nervous system; because of the independent role it seems to play, it is sometimes called **involuntary** muscle. It can be found in such organs as the stomach and intestines, blood vessels, and bronchial tubes. Because of the location of smooth muscle, some anatomists call it **visceral** muscle. As can be seen in Figure 1-23, there are no transverse striations or bands on the muscle cells, which accounts for its being referred to as smooth or unstriated.

Smooth muscle consists of **fusiform** (spindle-shaped) **cells,** which contain a single nucleus within the central portion of the sarcoplasm. The cells bear faint longitudinal striations. Depending on their location, the cells may appear long and slender, short and blunt, or irregular and twisted. The cells are small, ranging from 3 to 8 microns in diameter and from 15 to 200 microns in length. The external surface of the cytoplasm functions as a very definite cell wall, but it does not serve as a well-defined sarcolemma. Contraction of smooth muscle is slow and sustained, testimony to its primitive nature. Whenever a smooth muscle fiber is stimulated to contract, the contractile impulse is transmitted to adjacent fibers, without the benefit of nerve tissue, so the contraction passes wavelike over the entire muscular organ. This is called **ephaptic conduction.**

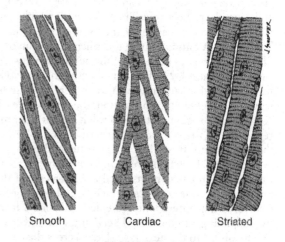

Smooth   Cardiac   Striated

FIGURE 1-23

Striated, smooth, and cardiac muscle shown schematically.

Cardiac Muscle (Myocardium)

Cardiac muscle, which is found only in the heart, seems to have some of the properties of both smooth and striated. It is involuntary, but striated. The cells contain myofibrils that are essentially the same as those of striated muscle, but the muscle fibers do not possess a definite sarcolemma. Fibrous connective tissue is articularly abundant in cardiac tissue. Cardiac tissue is also intrinsically self-excitable.

The physiology and anatomy of muscle tissue is an extremely complex and challenging area of science—so much so that it commands the attention of an entire discipline called **kinesiology,** which is by definition the science of movement.

Muscle Contraction

Scientists have known since before the mid-nineteenth century that skeletal muscle is striated. More recently, with better and better microscopes, we have learned that individual muscle fibers are composed of from several hundred to several thousand delicate filaments called **myofibrils.** In spite of their extremely small diameter (about 1 micron), each myofibril has in turn, lying side by side, about 200 long protein molecules called **myosin** and about twice as many protein molecules called **actin.** As shown by laboratory synthesis of contractile tissue, when nourished by ATP (adenosine triphosphate), the myosin and actin filaments comprise the **basic contractile unit.** Adenosine triphosphate, you may recall, is the product of the mitochondria within the substance of the cytoplasm (or sarcoplasm) of cells.

The distribution of myosin and actin filaments is very orderly, and when viewed microscopically, the myofibrils show the same pattern of cross-striation as the muscle fibers of which they are a part. As shown schematically in Figure 1-24, there are alternately fairly wide light and dark bands, which are known as I and A bands, respectively. The light bands which contain only the thin actin filaments are called the **I bands.** The **A bands** contain the much thicker myosin filaments as well as the ends of the actin filaments. As shown in Figure 1-24, the interval between any two **Z lines** is called a **sarcomere.** A sarcomere is an individual contractile unit. In addition, the middle of each A band has a region that is somewhat lighter than the remainder of the A band, but nevertheless it is darker than the I band. It is called the **H zone,** and as shown in Figure 1-24, contains only myosin filaments. The thin actin filaments are attached at either end of the sarcomere to the Z lines, which are short fibrous structures that interconnect the actin filaments from two adjoining sarcomeres. The Z lines extend from one myofibril to the next, completely across the entire muscle fiber, thereby causing the sarcomeres to lie side by side. And finally, a thin dark band can be seen in the center of the H zone. It is called the **M line** and is the result of the linkages of the thick myosin filaments, which retain the orderly arrangements of the thick filaments. Thus, the thin actin filaments are linked to the Z lines while the thick myosin filaments are linked to the M lines. A cross section through a myofibril in the region of the A band shows the thick filaments to be surrounded by six thin filaments, and any given thin filament is surrounded by three thick filaments. The architecture is very crystalline.

A single thick filament is composed of about 200 myosin molecules, each consisting of a globular head and a cylindrical tail. These molecules are arranged so the thick filament is divided into halves, with the heads of the molecules in each half oriented toward the Z line. These heads form cross-bridges which when activated move in an arclike manner, like the oar of a rowboat, and engage or bind to a complementary binding site on an actin filament. The numerous cross-bridge links cause the thin filaments to slide toward the center of the A band, thus shortening the length of the sarcomere. A single stroke of a cross-bridge produces only a small amount of thin filament movement, but the numerous cross-bridges within a single sarcomere undergo many cycles of movement during a single contraction.

As shown in Figure 1-24, molecules of actin are arranged in two chains that form a double helix. Two additional proteins can be found on the thin filaments. They are **troponin** and **tropomyosin,** and both are bound to the thin actin filament. Tropomyosin is a rodlike molecule that is arranged end to end along the chains of actin in such a way that they partially cover the myosin binding sites and prevent actin from binding to the myosin cross-bridges. The tropomyosin molecule is held in this position by a molecule of troponin, which itself is bound to both the tropomyosin and actin. Troponin also binds to calcium, when present.

Within the fluid of the sarcoplasm is an extensive **endoplasmic (sarcoplasmic) reticulum.** The reticulum forms a segmented tubular sleeve around each myofibril (see Figure 1-25). One segment of the reticulum surrounds an A band, while the adjacent segment surrounds an I band. At the ends of these sarcoplasmic segments are enlargements (the **lateral sacs**) which contain calcium. At the A–I band junction of the sarcoplasmic reticulum can be found a transverse (T) tubule. This "T" system provides a means of transportation from the extracellular medium into the interior of a muscle fiber. When an **action potential** spreads over muscle fibers, the potential is transmitted to the interior of the cell by way of the T system. As the muscle action potential passes the lateral sacs of the sarcoplasmic reticulum, calcium is released, and it diffuses into the cell where it quickly binds to the troponin molecules. This causes a change in the shape of the tropomyosin so that the actin binding sites are uncovered. As a result, binding between the myosin cross-bridges and actin binding sites is now possible. As the swinging myosin cross-bridges engage the binding sites, the actin filaments are drawn toward the center

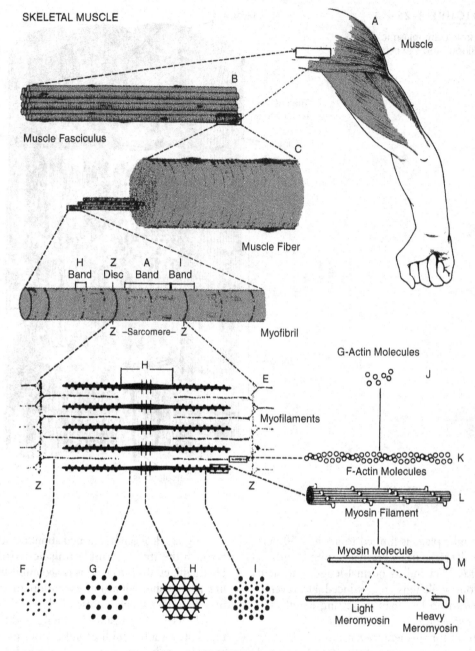

SKELETAL MUSCLE

Muscle

A

Muscle Fasciculus

B

Muscle Fiber

C

H Band   Z Disc   A Band   I Band

Z —Sarcomere— Z   Myofibril

G-Actin Molecules

J

E

Myofilaments

Z   Z

F-Actin Molecules

K

Myosin Filament

L

Myosin Molecule

M

N

Light Meromyosin   Heavy Meromyosin

F   G   H   I

FIGURE 1-24

Illustration of the levels of organization of human skeletal muscle. (From Bloom, W., and Fawcett, D., *A Textbook of Histology,* 9th ed., Philadelphia: Saunders, 1968.)

of the sarcomere. In a contracted muscle, the I bands are shortened in length, which causes the Z lines and the entire sarcomere to shorten (see Figure 1-26).

The release of calcium from the sarcoplasmic reticulum is very rapid, but the pumping out of the released calcium requires some time. This means that contraction continues for some time after the action potential. As calcium is pumped back into the lateral sacs of the reticulum, the binding sites are once again covered by the tropomyosin and muscle relaxation occurs. Energy for the calcium pump is provided by ATP, which also

provides the energy for the cross-bridge movement of the myosin molecules.

Length-Tension Relationship The length at which a muscle develops its greatest tension is termed l_0. This length is very nearly the same as the normal resting length. In a laboratory preparation as shown in Figure 1-27, a muscle may shorten by as much as 50 to 60 percent of its normal resting length. In the body, where muscles are attached to bones, the total range of length

FIGURE 1-25

The endoplasmic (sarcoplasmic) reticulum. (From Bloom and Fawcett, 1968.)

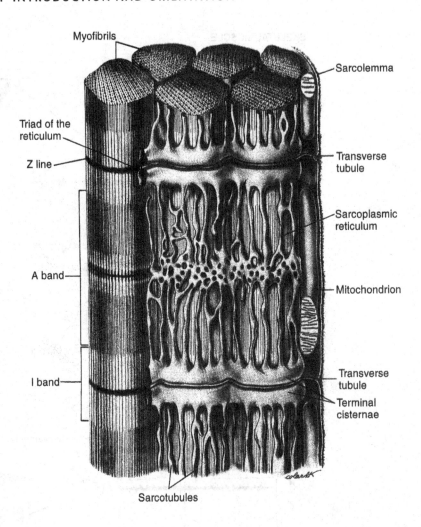

Myofibrils

Sarcolemma

Triad of the reticulum

Z line

Transverse tubule

Sarcoplasmic reticulum

A band

Mitochondrion

I band

Transverse tubule

Terminal cisternae

Sarcotubules

change that can take place is limited to about a 30 percent increase or decrease of its normal resting length. If a muscle is *stretched* beyond its normal length and then stimulated, its contractile tension is reduced. However, if a muscle is *shortened* to less than its resting length, the *maximum tension of contraction is also reduced.*

An explanation for this length-tension relationship can be found in the arrangement of the cross-bridges of the thick myosin filaments and binding sites of the thin actin filaments. When the muscle has been stretched excessively, the cross-bridges are unable to engage the actin binding sites. At normal resting length, however, the maximum number of bridges can engage the actin for maximum contractile strength, and when the actin filaments begin to overlap, the efficiency is again decreased and the strength of the contraction is reduced.

Muscle contraction does not necessarily result in a shortening of a muscle. Anyone who has attempted to lift something that simply won't budge has experienced an **isometric** contraction, in which the muscle does not shorten during contraction. An **isotonic** contraction occurs when a muscle shortens, but the tension of the muscle remains constant.

A great deal can be learned about muscle contraction through the study of **single muscle twitches** (Alipour-Haghighi, et al., 1987). This is accomplished by delivering a very short-duration excitation to the nerve of a muscle or by passing a pulse of electrical stimulus to the muscle itself. The result is a single, sudden contraction that lasts for a few milliseconds. An isometric method of recording twitch responses is shown in Figure 1-27B and a schematic of a single muscle twitch is shown in Figure 1-27C. Skeletal muscles come in a wide variety of sizes, from the miniscule stapedius muscle in the middle ear to the quadriceps femoris, which runs the full length of the thigh. Generally, the smaller muscles have short durations of contraction as compared with large muscles. An ocular muscle, for example, has a duration of contraction of less than 10 milliseconds; the gastrocnemius in the calf has a duration of contraction of about 30 milliseconds; while the soleus muscle, also in the calf, has a duration of contraction of about 100 milliseconds. Clearly the duration of contraction is related to the function of a muscle.

Strength The strength of muscle contraction is considerable. According to Guyton (1981), the maximum

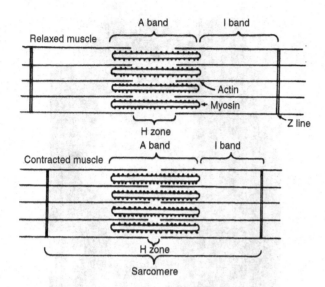

Z line (Ger. Zwiechenschiebe)
H zone (Ger. Heller)
Old term for A band is Q band (Ger. Querschiebe)

FIGURE 1-26

The contractile process shown schematically, in which the actin filaments are drawn toward the myosin filaments and slide in between them so the length of the sarcomere is reduced. The width of the A band remains unchanged but appears darker in the contracted state.

strength of contraction of a muscle operating at normal muscle length is about 3.5 kilograms per square centimeter of muscle belly area. If we apply that value to the large extensor muscle of the leg (the quadriceps femoris muscle) which has an area of about 100 square centimeters, the maximum contractile tension can exceed 350 kilograms at the patellar (kneecap) tendon. Small wonder that athletes sometimes "pull tendons."

Even when a muscle is "at rest" a certain amount of contractile tension often remains. This very slight amount of contraction, called **muscle tone,** is usually present in the postural muscles.

CLINICAL NOTE: "Floppy Infant" is a diagnostic term for infants who have **hypotonia** (diminished muscle tone) and muscle weakness.

Fatigue Prolonged and vigorous contraction of a muscle may lead to fatigue, a condition due in part to the inability of the metabolic processes to continue to provide the muscle cells with necessary energy. Nerve impulses may pass into the muscle tissue, and in fact, they may even spread out over the muscle in a perfectly normal fashion, but the contractions become weaker and weaker. However, if a muscle becomes excessively fatigued, it may remain contracted and rigid for minutes

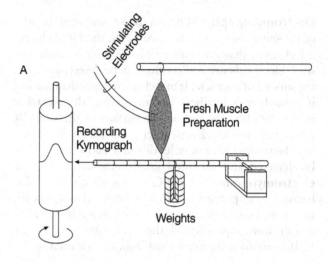

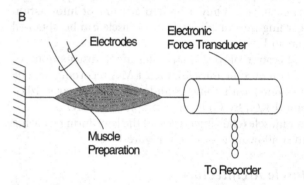

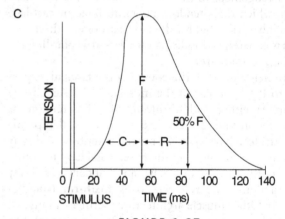

FIGURE 1-27

Methods of recording muscle contractions. Recording of an isotonic contraction is shown in **A;** recording of an isometric contraction is shown in **B;** and a schematic muscle twitch is shown in **C.**

at a time. This seems to be due to depletion of the ATP, and as a result there is a rigid union between the actin and myosin filaments.[8]

---

[8]Much the same process takes place several hours after death in a state called **rigor mortis.** Here, again, depletion of ATP causes muscle contraction to take place until bacterial action begins to destroy muscle protein. This usually takes about a day.

Electromyography When a nerve stimulus is adequate and causes a muscle to contract, the rapid chemical changes that take place (ion exchange) result in a small electrical current flow that can be detected all over the surface of a muscle. If muscle activity is adequate and if enough muscle fibers become active, the electrical energy can be detected on the surface of the skin. By placing electrodes directly over a muscle, or by inserting electrodes into a muscle, this bioelectric activity can be detected and recorded graphically to produce an **electromyogram.** The **EMG,** as it is usually called, has become an important research and clinical tool, but the data must be interpreted with some caution because, no matter how sophisticated the technique may be, an EMG can do little more than indicate the relative activity of a particular muscle or muscle group during a particular task. Only a limited amount of information regarding the contribution of a muscle can be obtained from an EMG.

Because of the unique location, distribution, or function of some muscles, their EMG recordings can be interpreted with some confidence. The electrocardiogram (EKG, ECG) is one example. An EMG of a masseter muscle (chewing muscle of the jaw) during chewing and swallowing is shown in Figure 1-28.

Muscle Architecture

The arrangement of the muscle fasciculi and the manner in which their tendons attach to bone or cartilage are highly varied, but for the most part one of three patterns is apparent. Muscles can be classed as **parallel, radiating,** or **pennate.**

In many muscles the course of the fasciculi is parallel to the long axis of the muscle. The fasciculi terminate at either end by means of a flat tendon, as illustrated in Figure 1-29. These muscles, called **parallel muscles,** have a great range of motion and may shorten by as much as one-half their total length. Sometimes these muscles may have an abundance of fleshy belly and may be referred to as **fusiform** (spindle-shaped). Other muscle architecture sacrifices a range of motion for an increase in power. Certain muscles, like the *pectoralis major* on the anterior chest wall, appear to be fan-shaped. The fasciculi diverge or converge as they approach their attachments. They are called **radiating** muscles, and an example is shown schematically in Figure 1-29. **Penniform** muscles, shown in Figure 1-29, are composed of fasciculi that converge onto a tendon, and depending upon their complexities, the muscles may be called **bipennate, multipennate,** or **circumpennate,** but they are, nevertheless, penniform. In these muscles the power is the combined power of all the contracting fibers, while the change in length is simply equal to the amount of contraction executed by any given obliquely directed fasciculus. In **parallel** muscles,

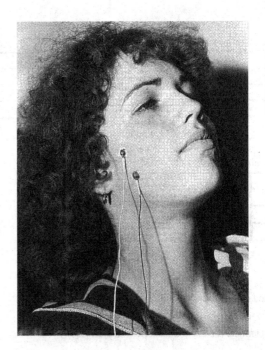

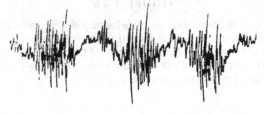

Chewing

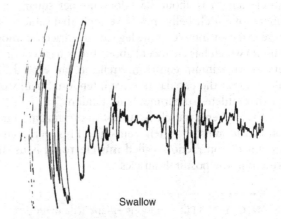

Swallow

FIGURE 1-28

Electromyographic recording of a masseter muscle during chewing and swallowing.

on the other hand, the power of the muscle is provided by the contraction of only the fibers contained in any transverse section, while the degree of shortening is equal to the sum total of the contraction of many fasciculi in series. Thus, to a large extent, architecture dictates the power of a muscle.

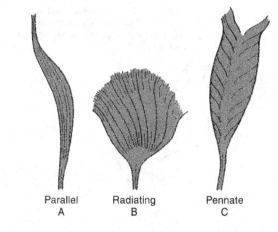

FIGURE 1-29

Various forms of muscle architecture.

In summary, the muscles composed of fasciculi running the length of the muscle have a great range of motion but relatively little power, while the radiating and penniform muscles have less range of motion, but a great deal more power. When a muscle contracts, it usually acts upon a movable joint to produce movement or to maintain posture. In most instances the characteristics of movement are determined by the mechanical arrangement of the structure to which a muscle is attached.

Muscle Attachments

Muscles usually have but two attachments, an **origin** and an **insertion.** The origin is conventionally the attachment that is fixed, or engages in the lesser movement, while the insertion can be thought of as the structure being acted upon. In the extremities, the *origin is the more proximal attachment*, while the *insertion is the more distal.* We ought to bear in mind that the criteria for the terms origin and insertion are somewhat relative, or at least dependent upon interpretation, and at times the definitions may fail completely. For example, the *thyrohyoid muscle*, which extends from the thyroid cartilage of the larynx to the hyoid bone, may upon contraction elevate the thyroid cartilage. Or in a different situation, the same muscle may depress the hyoid bone, and therefore would be called the *hyothyroid* muscle. And, as Woodburne (1973) points out, you can reach up and pull an object down, but in a different situation with virtually the same muscular activity, you can reach up and pull yourself up to the object.

Muscle Action

A common consequence of muscle contraction is the production of movements. This is particularly true of the extremities, and less true of the postural muscles, which in fact may contract to prevent movements. Skeletal muscles generally produce movement by acting

on a joint that lies between the origin and insertion of the muscle. That is, contraction of muscle tissue decreases the distance between the origin and insertion, with rotational or gliding action occurring about the joint. Thus, with some knowledge of the joint it bridges, we are in a position to predict the types of movement that will be produced by the muscle contraction. It is essential, however, that we guard against assuming that the action in a living body is exactly the same as the action inferred from observations of muscle attachments in a nonliving specimen. This is because muscles usually act in functional groups, and the laboratory is unable to demonstrate the effects of contraction of an opposing or complementary muscle in the muscle group. Knowledge of the nervous system is often helpful in the study of muscle actions; that is, there is often a correlation between the innervation of muscles and their actions.

A muscle-joint complex constitutes a **simple machine.** In other words, skeletal muscles are the source of a force applied to a lever system of some sort which produces bodily movements. In such a "biological lever" the bones act as **lever arms,** and the joint becomes the **fulcrum.** There are three classes of levers in mechanics, and they are all represented in the body.

Class I Levers A Class I lever is shown in Figure 1-30. There is an *applied force* at one end and a *resistance force* at the other, and the *fulcrum* about which the lever rotates is placed at some distance between the two ends of the

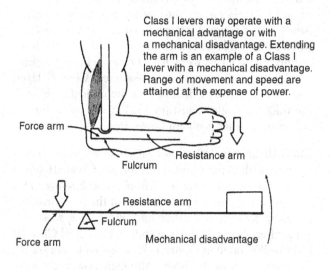

Class I levers may operate with a mechanical advantage or with a mechanical disadvantage. Extending the arm is an example of a Class I lever with a mechanical disadvantage. Range of movement and speed are attained at the expense of power.

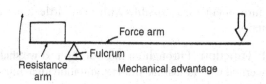

FIGURE 1-30

A Class I lever system.

lever. This lever system is exemplified by a child's teeter-totter. If the force arm is longer than the resistance arm, the lever will operate with a **mechanical advantage,** which simply means that a small applied force will move a large resistance force. If the force arm is shorter than the resistance arm, however, the system will operate at a **mechanical disadvantage,** so a large applied force will be required to overcome a small resistance force. It must be noted, however, that when the mechanical advantage is increased in a lever, the degree of movement is diminished by a proportional amount. The familiar crowbar and claw hammer for pulling nails are examples of Class I levers with mechanical advantage. It is even more important for us to appreciate the fact that when a Class I lever system operates with a mechanical disadvantage, the degree of movement in the resistance arm is increased.

In the case of a biological Class I lever, operating with a *mechanical disadvantage,* power of movement is lost, but *speed is gained,* and that is usually to our advantage. These levers are not well represented in the body, but some muscle-joint-bone systems that provide body stability employ them.

Class II Levers Class II levers are not at all well represented in the body. In fact, some anatomists argue that there are none! Class II levers consist of a *lever arm* with the *fulcrum* at one extreme end and an *applied force* at the other end. The *resistance force* is located somewhere between the fulcrum and the end of the lever arm. The ordinary wheelbarrow is an example. As illustrated in Figure 1-31, *these levers must operate with a mechanical advantage;* that is, the force required to displace a weight when a Class II lever is used is always less than the force required if no levers were used. Opening the jaw against resistance is an example of a biological Class II lever, and there is strong evidence that the ossicular chain in the middle ear also constitutes a Class II lever, but we will examine that problem more closely in Chapter 6.

Class III Levers Whereas Class II levers must always operate with a mechanical advantage, Class III levers must *always operate with a mechanical disadvantage.* This is because the *fulcrum* is at one end of the lever arm, the *resistance force* at the other end, with an *applied force* somewhere between the two ends. A biological Class III lever is illustrated in Figure 1-32. Class III levers are the most common in the body. Although power is lost in such a system, speed of movement is gained. As a result, rapid movements are possible with very little muscle contraction.

Muscle Function Throughout most of this text we shall be concerned with individual muscles and individual muscle actions. To some extent this is an unfortunate though conventional approach, for our brains do not mediate or monitor individual muscle actions; rather, they mediate and monitor skeletal and muscle group movement.

Class II levers always operate with a mechanical advantage. Opening the jaw against resistance is one example of a Class II lever.

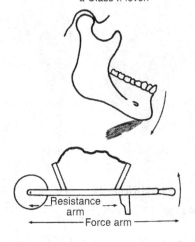

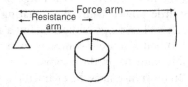

FIGURE 1-31

A Class II lever system.

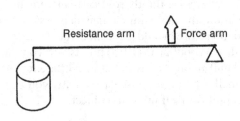

Class III levers always operate with a mechanical disadvantage. Although power is lost, speed of movement is gained.

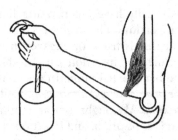

FIGURE 1-32

A Class III lever system.

A muscle can exert a force in just one direction, and it is incapable of exerting any force in the opposite direction. Thus, either muscle in a functional pair may be the **antagonist** of the other. Those muscles directly responsible for producing desired movements are called **prime movers;** those which act to maintain the body in an appropriate posture are called **fixation muscles.**

Descriptive Terminology Sometimes it is helpful to be able to describe the effects that a muscle contraction has on a specific joint, especially if the terms used are applicable to the entire body and can be related to the body in the anatomical position.

CLINICAL NOTE: Familiarity with the following terms will greatly enhance your ability to describe aberrant motor behavior.

Flexion is a term used to describe the bending of a part, or to describe the condition of being bent. A clenched fist is flexed.

Extension means a straightening. In the anatomical position, most of the structures, except the feet, are extended. For the feet, the terms dorsiflexion and plantar flexion are employed.

Dorsiflexion simply means bending in the direction of the dorsum of the foot.

Plantar flexion means bending in the direction of the sole of the foot.

Abduction means movement away from the body or, in the case of the digits, movement away from the axis of the extremity.

Adduction means movement towards the median plane or axis.

Medial rotation is a term that means to rotate a member toward the midplane of the body. Standing pigeon-toed is an example.

Lateral rotation means to rotate away from the midplane. Special terms are used to describe action of the feet and hands.

Pronation is a special term used with the hand and forearm. In the anatomical position the palm is forward. Pronation is rotation so the palm is downward or backward.

Supination is also a form of rotation, in such a way as to turn the palm upward or forward.

Eversion means rotation of the foot so the sole is turned outward.

Inversion means just the opposite of eversion, or rotation of the foot so the sole is turned inward.

Opposition is a term that applies mainly to the thumb, when it is rolled over onto the hand so the ends of the fingers can meet with the thumb in order to grasp something.

Circumduction is a circular movement, of course, and it requires flexion, extension, abduction, and adduction, in proper sequence. Rolling the eyes is a special case of circumduction.

Nomenclature of Muscles

A beginning anatomy student ought to pay particular attention to the names of muscles as they are encountered. Associations with the names of the muscles will often facilitate learning them, because the names of many muscles reflect some particular structural or functional characteristics.

Geometric names reflect the shape of a muscle, as in *trapezius* (trapezoid), *quadratus* (square), *lumborum*, *pyramidalis*, and *rhomboid*, while the **general form** of a muscle is reflected in such names as *gracilis* (slender or delicate), *serratus* (sawlike), *longus*, and *digastricus* (two-bellied). Muscles are also named for their **location in the body**, as in *temporalis* (temple), *intertransversarious* (between the transverse processes), *supraspinalis* (upon or above the spine or spinal process), *subclavius* (under the clavicle), and *intercostal* (between the ribs). **Descriptive terms** such as *major, minor, external, internal, rectus* (straight), and *oblique* are also very informative.

The names of some muscles reflect the **number of heads** at their origin, such as *biceps, triceps,* and *quadriceps*. The names of other muscles reflect their **attachments,** as in *sternocleidomastoid* (arising from the sternum and clavicle and inserting into the mastoid process of the temporal bone), *sternothyroid* (arising from the sternum and inserting into the thyroid cartilage), and *palatoglossus* (arising from the palate and inserting into the tongue). Other names may hint at their **function,** such as *levator scapulae* (lifts the scapula) and *tensor tympani* (increases tension of the eardrum).

Nerve impulses are the agents directly responsible for producing muscle contractions, and *muscle actions are determined in large part by the characteristics of the nerve supply to the muscles.*

Nervous Tissue

Nerve tissue is made up largely of a group of highly specialized cells which, in addition to being *elongated*, have the unique property of being extremely *irritable*. They respond to abrupt environmental changes by modifying their *electrochemical composition*. The contributions of the nervous system to speech production cannot be underestimated; consequently, the nervous system will be treated separately and at some length in Chapter 5.

Some muscles are well supplied with nerve tissue, others less so. We have seen how myofibrillae are capable of contraction in response to *chemical, electrical,* or *electrochemical stimuli*. Under normal circumstances, a muscle contracts in response to the electrochemical stimuli provided by the nervous system. The relation between nerve supply and muscle action is outlined in the following brief discussion of the motor unit.

The Motor Unit

The functional unit for producing muscle action is called a motor unit. As shown in Figure 1-33, it consists of a **nerve cell** (the body and its processes) and all the **muscle fibers** served by the nerve cell.

A nerve cell process, called an **axon** (Gk. *axle*, axis), divides into a number of **axon fibrils** just prior to terminating in the form of **muscle end plates,** which are in direct contact with muscle fibers. A single motor unit may include anywhere from a few to over a hundred muscle fibers.

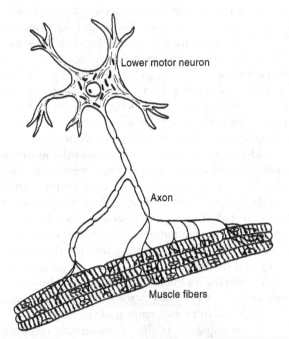

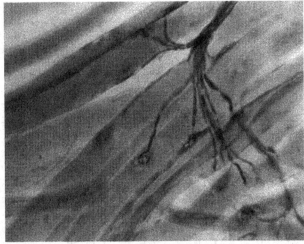

FIGURE 1-33

Schematic of a motor unit (top) and a photomicrograph of axon fibrils as they terminate on muscle fibers by means of motor end plates.

Muscle end plates may be likened to electrodes, for they transmit nerve impulses to the sarcoplasm of muscle fiber, which in turn responds by brief twitches, one twitch for each nerve impulse. A single muscle fiber is capable of "following" up to about fifty nerve impulses per second. It is interesting to note that all the muscle fibers in a single motor unit contract as a whole with one brief twitch for every impulse. Smooth, prolonged muscle contractions are accounted for by the mechanics of many motor units firing in *volleys*, repeatedly, so that their combined effects produce a seemingly constant contraction.

A critical inspection of a single motor unit muscle contraction reveals three distinct phases: the *latent period*, the *contraction period*, and the *relaxation period*. The interval between the onset of stimulus and onset of contraction is known as the **latent period.** The latent period is about 0.01 second in duration. Although no actual change in the length of muscle fibers occurs during the latent period, the chemical status of the fibers is changing rapidly. The latent period is followed by the **contraction period,** which lasts about 0.04 second. It is during the contraction period that work is being done by the muscle. The **relaxation period** is about 0.05 second in duration, during which there is a return to the previous relaxed state. It is important to realize that relaxation is purely passive, caused by the elasticity of the muscle fibers and by external forces exerted upon the ends of the muscle fibers. A fourth phase, known as the **refractory phase,** is sometimes recognized. During this phase, which lasts only about 0.005 second, chemical processes are occurring that restore the muscle to its normal resting state. Muscle fibers will not respond readily to a stimulus during the refractory period.

Voluntary muscle contractions may be graded from just a perceptible shortening to a maximum contraction. The *degree of muscle contraction* is dependent upon the number of active motor units within a muscle, as well as the rate of firing of the active motor units. There is strong evidence that single motor units behave in an **all-or-none** fashion; that is, once a stimulus has reached a certain critical level, all the muscle fibers of a motor unit contract. Within limits, the force exerted by the muscle fibers of a motor unit is directly related to the frequency of stimulus impulses, and the force exerted by an entire muscle is directly related to the number of active motor units. A weak stimulus activates fewer motor units; a strong stimulus activates more.

Innervation Ratio

There is also a relationship between the extent of nerve supply to a muscle (innervation) and the precision of muscle contraction. A muscle with a **high innervation ratio** (many muscle fibers to few nerve cells) will only be able to execute rather crude movements with large muscle contractions, while a muscle with a **low innervation ratio** (few muscle fibers to many nerve cells) will

be capable of smaller contractions with finer control. We can predict, simply by means of the innervation ratio of a muscle, whether it will execute small precise movements or large crude movements.

Vascular Tissue

Vascular tissue might be thought of as the "fluid tissues" of the body. It comprises almost 10 percent of body weight. Blood consists of **corpuscles** (cells) and **platelets** which are separated by a fluid intercellular substance called **blood plasma.** It is the intercellular matrix of vascular tissue.

The cells are erythrocytes (red cells) and leukocytes (white cells) (Gk. *erythros,* red; *kytos,* cell; *leukos,* white). **Erythrocytes** are nonnucleated, biconvex disclike elements, so there is some question as to whether or not they should be called cells; however, early in their development they do possess nuclei. **Leukocytes** are nucleated, while **blood platelets,** which are little protoplasmic dishes, contain neither nuclei nor hemoglobin, but they do produce an enzyme called **thromboplastin,** which is an important element in the clotting of blood.

Lymph (L. *lympha,* clear spring water), which is the immediate nutrient plasma of the tissue, appears to be a colorless watery-looking liquid, but it also may be yellowish and opalescent. The cells of lymph, called **lymphocytes,** resemble somewhat the leukocytes of blood.

The fluid tissues have many important functions. For example, they convey food and oxygen to all the living cells in the body and take on the waste materials generated by cellular activity. They distribute heat uniformly over the body and are instrumental in getting rid of the excess. In addition, the fluid tissues defend the body against disease-producing microorganisms.

The microenvironment of the cells of the body remains relatively constant due to the **circulatory system** (the blood-vascular system). In higher-order vertebrates this system consists of a gas pump and two fluid pumps. The **gas pump** is composed of the lungs–thorax complex, while the two **fluid pumps** are the right and left ventricles of the heart. These structures will be explored in chapters 2 and 8.

ORGANS

When two or more tissues combine in such a manner as to exhibit functional unity, they form an **organ.** By definition, an organ is a *somewhat independent part of the body that performs a special function.* The lungs, larynx, and tongue are some examples. Most organs are composed of various types of tissue, with one type predominating. The cells that compose the essential structure of an organ are known as the **parenchyma.** Other cells may be supportive, vascular, or nervous.

SYSTEMS

When two or more organs combine in such a manner as to exhibit functional unity, they are commonly called a **system.** There are at least nine recognized systems in the body, and very often eleven systems are listed. They are

1. The **skeletal system,** which is composed of the bones and their related cartilages. The study of the skeletal system is known as **osteology.**

2. The **articular system,** which is composed of the joints and ligaments. The study of the articular system is known as **arthrology.**

3. The **muscular system,** which forms the fleshy parts of the body. Acting on the skeletal and articular systems, the muscular system produces movement and locomotion. The study of muscles is called **myology.**

4. The **digestive system,** which is composed of the digestive tract and its associated digestive glands. The study of the internal organs of the thorax and abdomen (viscera) is known as **splanchnology** (Gk. *splanchnos,* viscus).

5. The **vascular system,** which is composed of the heart and blood vessels and the lymphatic system. The study of the vascular system is called **angiology.**

6. The **nervous system,** which is composed of the brain and spinal cord and all associated nerves, ganglia, nuclei, and sense organs. The study of the nervous system is known as **neurology.**

7. The **respiratory system,** which is composed of the air passageways and the lungs. The study of the lungs is called **pulmonology.**

8. The **urinary system,** which includes the kidneys and urinary passages. The study of the urinary system is **urology.**

9. The **generative** or **reproductive system,** which is closely associated with the urinary system and is sometimes included with it under the term **urogenital system. Gynecology** is the study of diseases of the genital tract of females, and pregnancy is sometimes regarded as a disease, or it may be managed by a specialty called **obstetrics.**

10. The **endocrine system,** which is composed of the ductless glands of the body. The study of this system is called **endocrinology.**

11. The **integumentary system,** which includes the skin, nails, and hair. The study of the integumentary system is called **dermatology.**

In addition, two or more of the above systems can be grouped together to form another system or apparatus. For example, the skeletal and muscular systems

constitute the **locomotor system.** The nervous and sensory systems form the **neurosensory system,** and the nervous and endocrine systems constitute the **neuroendocrine system.** There are also systems within systems. The **limbic system** as part of the nervous system is but one example. Since the early 1980's, the **immune** or **autoimmune system** has received a great deal of attention.

CLINICAL NOTE: The immune system functions like a well-orchestrated team, with each successive team member further weakening an incoming microbe. Initially, protein molecules called **antibodies** immobilize the invading microbe, which then enables a large **macrophage** to engulf the invader. The macrophage then "signals" white blood cells known as **T** cells that the immune system has been invaded. The **T** cells, so named because they mature in the thymus gland, finish off the infected cell either by killing the cell directly or by stimulating **B** cells (another type of white blood cell) to produce antibodies to kill the cell. The process is known as **antibody-related immunity.** The body contains as many as 100 million different kinds of antibodies and an equal variety of memory **T** cells and memory **B** cells. The memory cells provide long-term protection against a subsequent invasion by the same bacteria or virus.

Another type of immunity called **cell-mediated immunity** is particularly important in helping the body combat fungi, parasites, viruses, and tuberculosis. Cell-mediated immunity causes **T** cells to attack directly without the help of antibodies. A dramatic example of what can occur when the immune system fails is the autoimmune deficiency syndrome **(AIDS).** The **human immunodeficiency viruses HIV-1** and **HIV-2**—in particular **HIV-1**—are responsible for **AIDS.** Anyone who comes into physical contact with other humans should be aware that blood and body fluids containing visible blood are vehicles of the **HIV** virus. This also applies to semen and vaginal secretions. Blood and body fluids containing visible blood from all clients should always be handled as though they were infectious.[9]

With just a moment of thought it becomes apparent that no one of these systems is independent of the others. The speech mechanism draws heavily on some systems and less heavily on others, but either directly or indirectly it is dependent upon all the systems in the body. We shall be directing our attention to a good share of the *skeletal, muscular, nervous,* and *respiratory systems.* Sometimes our approach will be *regional* and sometimes it will be *systemic* and, at times, a little of

each. We shall be less concerned with the circulatory and endocrine systems, and probably will mention the reproductive and digestive systems only in passing.

SPEECH PRODUCTION

The Need for an Integrative Approach

Each of us, in our own minds, must generate a working construct of the speech and hearing mechanisms. Constructs are the personal property of the individuals responsible for generating them, and a valuable component in the battery of clinical and teaching tools we use in our professional lives. We must realize that constructs should never become stereotyped and inflexible. They should be constantly in a state of flux and subject to modification. *Stereotyped constructs lead to stereotyped and inflexible clinical management.*

In the pages that follow, we will become familiar with the structures comprising the speech and hearing mechanisms. We will also be faced with the responsibility of integrating these structures into a manageable working construct.

Speech production is sometimes described as consisting of four phases: **respiration, phonation, articulation,** and **resonance.** This compartmentalization of the speech act is very unfortunate. It is incomplete, for one thing, because it completely neglects the role of the hearing mechanism and other avenues of feedback.[10]

This compartmentalization also tends to convey the impression of an unrealistic, temporal sequence of events leading to the production of speech. That is, first we breathe, then we phonate, then we articulate, finally the process of resonance takes place, and lo and behold! Out comes speech! It's like putting beads on a string.

A model of speech production is shown in Figure 1-34. It illustrates the need for an integrative approach in generating a construct of speech production. Here, speech begins at the cortical level. The thought or response process leads to a sequence of neural impulses that are transmitted to the musculature of the breathing mechanism, to the larynx, and to the articulators. These neural impulses can be (but are not necessarily) delivered to all the musculature simultaneously, or to individual structures. This model recognizes both **temporal overlap** and the **mutual influence** the structures

---

[9]Hotline numbers: Center for Disease Control (CDC): 1-800-342-AIDS; Public Health Service Hotline: 1-800-447-AIDS.

[10]It is interesting to see how quickly speech deteriorates when a person cannot monitor the speech signal being produced. Small wonder that the speech of the deaf and severely hearing handicapped requires such long-term and patiently managed therapy.

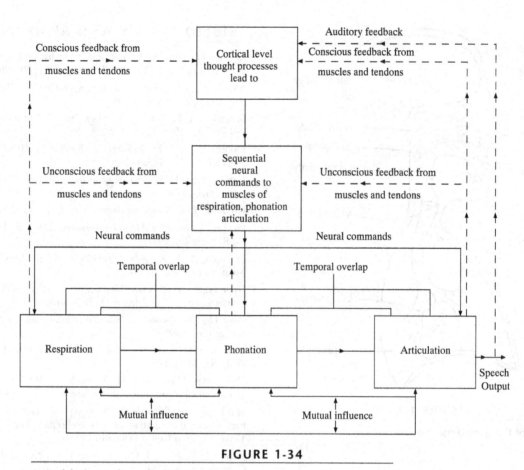

FIGURE 1-34

A model of speech production.

of the speech mechanism may have over one another. For example, we phonate and *at the same time* the articulators are actively producing a meaningful sequence of speech sounds. In addition, changes in air flow resistance that occur during phonation and articulation influence the respiratory system, and the articulatory process will, in many instances, influence the phonatory mechanism.

Specialized receptors in our joints, tendons, and muscles provide the brain with information about how well things are going. Some of this information never reaches the conscious level. Without **feedback, auditory** and **proprioceptive**, speech production would be as haphazard as throwing darts in the dark. We should also recognize that this highly integrated and incredibly complex chain of events can be interrupted (by disease, for example) at virtually any stage to interfere with the normal processes of speech production and reception.

Sound Production

Those parts of the body most closely associated with speech production include the **lungs**, the **trachea**, the **larynx**, the **nasal cavities**, and the **oral cavity** (mouth).

These structures, shown in Figure 1-35, form a versatile and intricate sound production system.

Two absolute requirements for the production of sounds of any kind are a **source of energy** and a **vibrating element.** The primary source of energy for speech production is air provided by the lower respiratory tract, in particular the lungs. They supply the sound vibrators (the vocal folds in the larynx) with power in the form of a fairly smooth unmodulated flow of air. We should note, however, that the conversion of a flow of air into sound may take place almost anywhere along the **vocal tract,** which is that portion of the speech mechanism lying above (and including) the vocal folds.

Usually we think of the vibrating folds as the primary source of sound for speech production, but there are others. By constricting the vocal tract somewhere along its length, the air stream may become turbulent to produce **fricative noise.** In addition, this turbulence may be generated with or without vibration of the vocal folds. Sounds may also be generated by momentarily blocking the flow of air through the vocal tract. A sudden release of the pressurized air may produce a mild explosion or a **plosive sound.** The vocal folds, the lips, the tongue, or the soft palate may act as valves to block the flow of air and to release it.

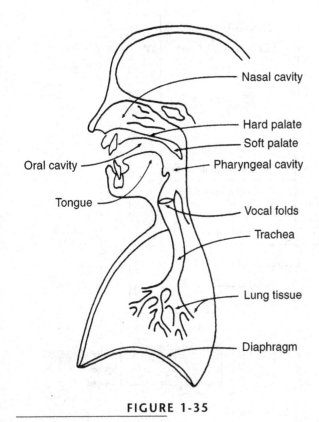

Nasal cavity

Hard palate

Soft palate

Oral cavity

Pharyngeal cavity

Tongue

Vocal folds

Trachea

Lung tissue

Diaphragm

FIGURE 1-35

Schematic of the speech mechanism.

The **quality** of many speech sounds may be greatly modified by changes in the configuration and thus the acoustical properties of the vocal tract. These changes are brought about mainly by modifications in the shape of the oral cavity.

A **physical analog** of the speech mechanism might consist of a *power supply, vibrating elements, a system of valves,* and a *filtering device.* No matter how the speech mechanism is represented, one of the first considerations is a power supply. Chapter 2 deals with the power supply, or the breathing mechanism.

It will be difficult initially to incorporate the breathing mechanism into our model. The *breathing mechanism* is an **air pump,** capable of supplying a variable air stream to the *larynx* and to the *articulatory mechanism,* each of which constitutes a **variable resistance** to the flow of air. Until we add these sources of resistance to our model, the breathing mechanism must stand alone.

BIBLIOGRAPHY AND READING LIST

Alopour-Haghighi, F., I. Titze, and P. Durham, "Twitch Response in the Canine Vocalis Muscle," *J. Sp. Hrng. Res.,* 30, 1987, 290–294.

ASHA. *AIDS/HIV. Implications for Speech-Language Pathologists and Audiologists,* December, 1990.

Basmajian, J. V., *Primary Anatomy,* 7th ed. Baltimore: Williams and Wilkins, 1976.

Bloom, W., and D. Fawcett, *A Textbook of Histology,* 9th ed. Philadelphia: W. B. Saunders, 1968.

Cunningham, D. J., *Textbook of Anatomy,* 9th ed. New York: Oxford University Press, 1951.

DiDio, L. J. A., *Synopsis of Anatomy.* St. Louis: C.V. Mosby, 1970.

Dorland's *Illustrated Medical Dictionary,* 25th ed. Philadelphia: W. B. Saunders, 1975.

Freeman, A. A. R., *Adult Articular Cartilage.* London: Pitman Medical, 1973.

Gray, H., *Gray's Anatomy,* 36th British ed. (P. L. Williams and R. Warwick, eds.). Philadelphia: W. B. Saunders, 1980.

Gray, H., *Gray's Anatomy,* 38th British ed. London: Churchill and Livingstone, 1995.

Guyton, A. C., *Textbook of Medical Physiology,* 6th ed. Philadelphia: W. B. Saunders, 1981.

Henderson, I. F., and J. H. Kenneth, *A Dictionary of Scientific Terms,* 7th ed. Princeton, N.J.: D. Van Nostrand, 1960.

Hultkranz, W., "Uber die Spaltrichtungen der Gelenkknorpel," Verhandlungen der Anatomischen Gesellschaft. Aus der Zwolfen Vesammlung in Kiel, 14 (Suppl.) 1898.

Judson, L. Y., and A. T. Weaver, *Voice Science.* New York: Appleton-Century-Crofts, 1965.

Kuehn, D., M. Lemme, and J. Baumgartner, *Neural Bases of Speech-Hearing and Language.* Boston: College Hill Press, 1989.

Love, R. J., and W. G. Webb, *Neurology for the Speech-Language Pathologist.* Boston: Butterworth–Heinemann, 1992.

McCall, J. G., "Scanning Electron Microscopy of Articular Surfaces." *Lancet,* 1968.

Moore, C., The Correspondence of Vocal Tract Resonance with Volumes Obtained from Magnetic Resonance Images," *J. Sp. Hrng. Res.* 35, 1992, 1009.

Moore, K. L., *Clinically Oriented Anatomy.* Baltimore: Williams and Wilkins, 1985.

Patten, B. M., *Human Embryology.* Philadelphia: Blakiston, 1946.

Perlman, A., I. Titze, and D. Cooper, "Elasticity of Canine Vocal Fold Tissue," *J. Sp. Hrng. Res.,* 27, 1984, 212–219.

Perrier, P., L. J. Boe, and R. Sock, "Vocal Tract Area Function Estimation from Midsagittal Dimensions with CT Scans and a Vocal Tract Cast: Modeling the Transition with Two Sets of Coefficients," *J. Sp. Hrng. Res.,* 35, 1992, 53–67.

Woodburne, R. T., *Essentials of Human Anatomy.* New York: Oxford University Press, 1973.

Breathing

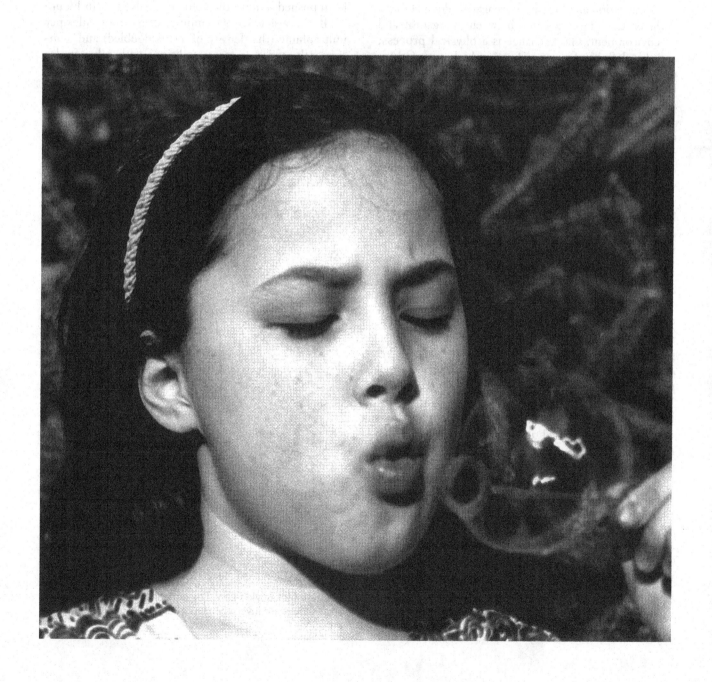

INTRODUCTION

Definition of Breathing

The very common words **breathing** and **respiration** may have many connotations. The word **breathe** stems from the Aryan root, *bhre*, to burn, and originally referred to steam, vapor, or exhaled air that was visible in the cold weather. It now means the air taken in and expelled by the expansion and contraction of the thorax. The Latin *spiritus halitus* pertains to air taken in and expelled during breathing, and from it we get such words as inhale and exhale and halitosis. Another Latin word, *spirare*, means to breathe, and from it come the common words such as inspire, expire, and respire.

Respiration and breathing are usually defined today as the process of gas exchange between an organism and its environment. Gas exchange is a **physical process,** and this definition may satisfy some biologists. Others may regard the respiratory process as the oxidation of food to produce water, carbon dioxide, and heat; so respiration becomes a **chemical process.**

For speech purposes, however, these definitions do not adequately define respiration. Speech production seems to require a primarily "nonrespiratory" function of the breathing apparatus, and it doesn't matter much whether the air is laden with carbon dioxide or not. The speech mechanism requires gas under pressure, and this brings us to the primary purpose of this chapter: to examine the **mechanical process** by which air is brought into the lungs and forced out again.

The Physics of Breathing

One of the best established laws in physics was given to us by Robert Boyle, a mid-seventeenth-century philosopher and chemist. **Boyle's law** states that *if a gas is kept at a constant temperature, pressure and volume are inversely proportional to one another and have a constant product.*

For an explanation of this law, we must turn to the **kinetic theory of gases.** The basis of kinetic theory is that gases are composed of large numbers of individual molecules that are engaged in unceasing motion. As shown in Figure 2-1A, when these molecules are confined in a vessel they move about randomly and at high speeds, colliding with one another and with the walls of the vessel. This bombardment exerts force on the walls of the vessel. *Provided volume and temperature are held constant, the force exerted on the walls of the containing vessel is a function of the number of gas molecules within the vessel.* In Figure 2-1B a greater number of gas molecules exerts a larger force on the walls than in A.

Figure 2-2A shows a volume of gas (V) in a cylinder which is under pressure (P). At the same time, a force

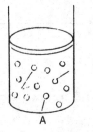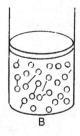

FIGURE 2-1

Illustration of pressure-gas-density relationship. In B, a greater number of gas molecules exerts a larger force on the walls than in A.

(F) is being exerted on a piston. When the piston has been pushed in until the volume is halved, as in Figure 2-2B, there is twice the number of gas molecules per unit volume (the density of gas is doubled) and, consequently, twice as many collisions with other molecules and with the walls of the vessel will occur per unit time. The force on the piston and on the walls is doubled, and the pressure is doubled, but *the product of pressure and volume remains the same*; that is, $(2P)V/2$ is a constant.

On the other hand, if the piston were raised so the volume is doubled, as in Figure 2-2C, the pressure exerted on the walls of the vessel must necessarily be reduced by one-half. Symbolically this means that $P/2(2V)$ is also a constant. Boyle's law may also be written as

$$P_1V_1 = P_2V_2$$

where

P = pressure
V = volume
$_1$ = initial state
$_2$ = final state

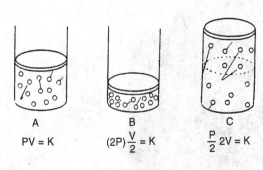

A
$PV = K$

B
$(2P)\dfrac{V}{2} = K$

C
$\dfrac{P}{2}2V = K$

FIGURE 2-2

Illustration of Boyle's Law. The equations show that pressure and volume are inversely proportional and have a constant product.

When air at atmospheric pressure is confined in an airtight container, equal amounts of pressure act on the outside and inside walls of the container, and the differential pressure is zero. A decrease in the volume of the container increases the pressure inside with respect to the outside, and an increase in the volume of the container causes the pressure to decrease with respect to the outside. *Pressures greater than atmospheric* are often called **positive** pressures, and *pressures less than atmospheric* are called **negative** pressures.

In mammals, the lungs lie inside an airtight thoracic cavity and communicate with the outside air by way of the *trachea, larynx, pharynx,* and the *oral* and *nasal cavities.* These structures constitute the **respiratory tract,** and it transmits air to the **organs of respiration,** the *lungs.* The *larynx,* shown schematically in Figure 2-3, forms the division between the **upper** and **lower respiratory tracts.**

The structure of the thorax is such that its volume can be increased or decreased, and we have already seen that an increase in volume will result in a negative pressure in the lungs with respect to the atmosphere. Consequently, air rushes into the lungs until the outside and inside pressures are equalized. This phase of breathing is known as **inspiration** or **inhalation.** Inhalation and exhalation as we have known it constitutes **pulmonary ventilation** as opposed to **external respiration,** which is gas exchange between the lungs and blood. **Internal respiration** is gas exchange between blood and the cells of the body.

The volume of air flow is proportional to the difference between atmospheric pressure and the pressure within the lungs, and can be described by the equation

$$F = k(P_1 - P_2) = k(P_{atm} - P_{alv})$$

where

F = air flow

k = proportionality constant

P_1 = initial pressure

P_2 = final pressure

P_{atm} = atmospheric pressure

P_{alv} = pressure within the lungs

A decrease in the volume of the thorax will result in positive pressure in the lungs, and provided the respiratory tract is open, air will rush out until once again the outside and inside pressures are the same. This phase of breathing is called **expiration** or **exhalation.** In the pages that follow we shall be concerned with the mechanisms by which the dimensions of the thoracic (or chest) cavity are increased and decreased during breathing, but only after we have accounted for the anatomy of the respiratory system and the properties of some of the structures that make up the breathing apparatus.

THE RESPIRATORY PASSAGE

The respiratory passage shown schematically in Figure 2-3 includes, in descending order, the **nasal** and **oral cavities,** the **pharynx, larynx, trachea,** and **bronchi.** These structures can form a continuous open passage leading from the exterior to the lungs, and it is in the lungs, of course, that the actual exchange of gas takes place. Here the red blood cells give up their carbon dioxide to the air and take on new oxygen. Although the *nasal, oral,* and *pharyngeal cavities* are definitely intrinsic parts of the breathing mechanism, they are also essential *organs of articulation* and *resonance.* Collectively, they form an exceptionally complex and highly variable system, which along with the larynx is called the **vocal tract,** but a great deal more will be said about that later. In the present context, then, suffice it to say that these cavities, *filter, moisten,* and *warm* the air prior to its entering the lower respiratory tract by way of the larynx.

The **larynx** is a modification of the uppermost tracheal cartilages. It forms a highly specialized valvular mechanism that may open or close the air passageway. An extremely important function of the larynx is to serve as a *protective device.* A sudden release of compressed air by the valvular mechanism will produce an

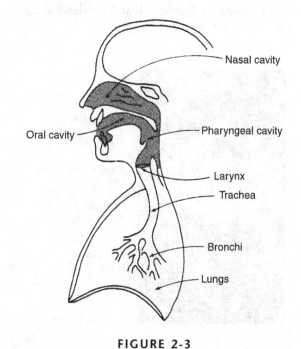

FIGURE 2-3

Schematic of the respiratory passage. Upper respiratory tract is shown as shaded area.

Labels in figure: Nasal cavity, Oral cavity, Pharyngeal cavity, Larynx, Trachea, Bronchi, Lungs

explosive exhalation that will clear the passageway of threatening mucus or a foreign object. The valvular action also permits *thoracic fixation* for circumstances that demand increased abdominal pressure in order to evacuate visceral contents. These include defecation (evacuation of fecal material from the rectum), emesis (Gk. *emein*, to vomit), micturation (urination), in addition to heavy lifting. For these reasons the larynx is extremely unique. It is a basic biological organ in addition to being highly specialized, capable of utilizing expired air for the production of voice.

Because the larynx is so complex anatomically and so important for speech production, it demands special attention. A detailed description of the larynx and some of its behavioral characteristics will be found in Chapter 3.

The Trachea

The trachea (Gk. *tracheia arteria*, rough artery)[1] varies so much from one individual to another that only a sort of generalized description can be given here. It extends from the larynx, at the level of the sixth cervical vertebra, to the bronchi below, which is at the level of the top of the fifth thoracic vertebra. The trachea shown in Figure 2-4 is about one-third natural size, which is about 11 to 12 cm in length and between 2 and 2.5 cm in diameter.[2]

The **trachea** is composed of from 16 to 20 horseshoe-shaped rings of hyaline cartilage, placed one above the other and separated by a small space that is occupied by a fibroelastic membrane. Each tracheal ring is incomplete in back where the trachea lies in direct contact with the esophagus. Two and sometimes three individual cartilages may be united either partially or completely. The intervening space between the ends of the tracheal rings is occupied by fibrous tissue and smooth muscle. This architecture accounts for the flexibility of the trachea and also permits the trachea to comply with, and yield to, the aerodynamic pressure changes that take place within the thorax.

The first tracheal cartilage is slightly larger than the rest, and it is connected with the inferior border of the cricoid cartilage of the larynx by means of the **cricotracheal ligaments.** The last cartilage of the trachea *bifurcates*, giving rise to the **main stem bronchi.** At the level

---

[1]At one time, early in the history of anatomy, it was thought that arteries contained air during life and that only the veins transported blood. This is because arterial blood drains into the venous system at death, and so at autopsy the arteries are usually devoid of blood. The windpipe was thought to be a rough artery, which was reasonable, because it contained air and not blood.

[2]In childhood, the diameter of the trachea in mm corresponds to age in years.

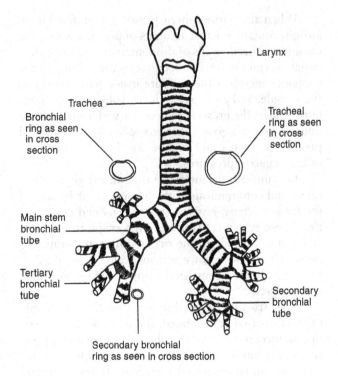

FIGURE 2-4

Schematic of the trachea and beginnings of the bronchial tree.

of bifurcation the trachea presents the **carina** (L. *carina*, keel of a boat), a ridgelike structure that is an important landmark for bronchoscopy. The gross structure of the trachea is shown in Figure 2-4, and the detailed structure is shown in Figure 2-5.

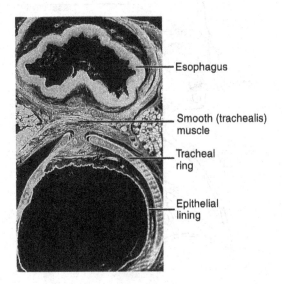

FIGURE 2-5

Photomacrograph of a transverse section through a trachea and esophagus.

The **fibrous membrane** of the trachea consists of two layers, one of which passes over the outer surface of the cartilaginous rings, while the other passes over the inner surface. In the spaces between the rings, however, the two layers blend to form a single **intratracheal membrane** which connects the tracheal rings one with another. The smooth muscle which is found in the space between the ends of the tracheal rings consists of an outer longitudinal layer and an inner transverse layer. The contractile state of these muscles varies and is dependent upon the oxygen requirements of an individual. The structure of the trachea is quite remarkable. Its cartilaginous framework provides rigidity to prevent collapse, while the ligaments and membranes provide the flexibility and mobility that permit it to be stretched (during inhalation, for example), twisted, or compressed.

The **mucous membrane** which lines the trachea is continuous above with that of the larynx and below with that of the bronchi. The surface layer of the membrane is composed of pseudostratified ciliated columnar epithelium. It rests upon a basement membrane beneath which is a submucous layer of connective tissue, blood vessels, and mucous glands. A microscopic view of the epithelial lining of the trachea reveals an occasional modified epithelial cell called a **goblet cell**. It is secretory and periodically releases mucus. This, along with mucus produced by mucous glands in the membrane, lines the trachea in the form of a continuous sheet. The **cilia,** which may be seen in the photomicrograph in Figure 2-6, perform an important function. They are continuously in motion, beating about ten times per second, at first quickly downward and then slowly upward. During their rapid downward movement the cilia "slip past" the mucus, and as they move slowly upward, the mucus is lifted as a continuous sheet upward toward the larynx. Every time we clear out a "frog in the throat," the cilia have performed their function of ridding the lower respiratory tract of accumulating mucus, smoke particles, and dust.

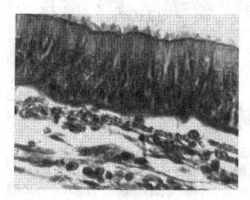

FIGURE 2-6

Photomicrograph of ciliated epithelial lining of the trachea.

> **CLINICAL NOTE:** One of the major causes of lung infection is related to a reduction of ciliary action. Normally, the mucus blanket is propelled toward the larynx at a rate of about 5 mm per minute. The smoke from a single cigarette can cause the cilia to be nonmotile for several hours. At the same time, cigarette smoke stimulates mucus secretion. The result may be a partial or even complete airway obstruction.
>
> The respiratory lining also contains protective **phagocytic cells** which ingest dust, bacteria, and other debris. These cells are also injured by tobacco smoke.

> **CLINICAL NOTE:** Because of such things as obstruction in the upper respiratory tract due to inflammatory disease, or to food lodged in the larynx, an emergency operation called a **tracheotomy** (*tracheo-* + Gk. *tome*, a cutting) is sometimes performed to provide an alternate pathway for air flow. An incision is made in the anterior neck, about 1 cm below the cricoid cartilage of the larynx, and the trachea is opened, usually between the second and third tracheal cartilages. The opening into the trachea is called a **tracheostoma** (*tracheo-* + Gk. *stoma*, mouth).

The Bronchi

The bronchi (Gk. *bronchos*, windpipe) are tubes that extend from the trachea to the lungs where they arborize to form what is often called the **bronchial tree.** The bronchi are divided to form three groups: the **main** or **main stem bronchi,** the **lobar** or **secondary bronchi** (supplying the lobes of the lung), and **segmental** or **tertiary** (L. *tertiarius,* third in order) **bronchi** (supplying segments of the lobes).

The **main stem bronchi** connect the trachea to the lung, and the point at which they enter is called the **hilum** (L. a small thing). Each main stem bronchus is slightly more than half the diameter of the trachea; however, the right bronchus is larger in diameter, shorter in length (about half), and more in direct line with the trachea than is the left. The right bronchus is larger because it supplies the larger lung. The significance of the less abrupt divergence of the right bronchus lies in the fact that *foreign bodies that may fall into the trachea are more liable to enter the right bronchus* than the left.

The construction of the **bronchi** is similar to that of the trachea. That is, they are composed of imperfect cartilaginous rings that are bound together by fibroelastic tissue. They are, however, more completely invested by smooth muscle fibers than is the trachea, and they are lined with pseudostratified ciliated columnar epithelium, and their walls also contain elastic and glandular tissue.

The **right bronchus** divides into three secondary bronchi, one for each lobe of the right lung. The secondary bronchi, in turn, subdivide into ten tertiary bronchi, each of which supplies a lung segment. The **left bronchus,** on the other hand, divides into two secondary bronchi, from which issue eight tertiary bronchi, each of which supplies an individual lung segment. The bronchi and partially dissected lungs are shown in Figure 2-7.

The Bronchioles

The **tertiary bronchi** divide repeatedly, becoming smaller until they verge on the microscopic. In an adult there are about 24 generations of divisions which comprise the bronchial tree, and it is interesting that although the bronchial tree may divide and subdivide, the combined cross-sectional area of any given subdivision is greater than the cross-sectional area of the parent division. The effect is to *minimize air friction* in the small diameters of the air passageway.

The final division of the bronchi gives rise to the **bronchioles,** tubes which are 1 mm or less in diameter. Repeated divisions of the bronchioles ultimately give rise to the **terminal bronchioles,** which communicate directly with the **alveolar ducts,** and they in turn open into the minute **air sacs** of the lung. As the bronchi and bronchioles divide, their cartilaginous framework becomes less and less prominent, while the amount of bronchial muscle tissue increases proportionately.

The Alveoli

The walls of the terminal bronchioles and air sacs are pitted with about 7,000,000 small depressions called alveoli. In anatomy, a small pit or depression is called an **alveolus,** and so the alveoli in the lungs are called **alveoli pulmonis** to distinguish them from the dental alveoli, for example.

The alveoli are lined by a single layer of epithelial cells resting on a thin basement membrane. The alveolar wall is invested by an elaborate capillary network (about 1000 miles of capillaries) separated from alveolar air by a barrier less than one-third the diameter of a red blood cell. The total area of the alveoli in contact with the capillary bed is in the order of 70–90 square meters (the size of a tennis court). This combination of immense area and thin barrier facilitates rapid exchanges of oxygen and carbon dioxide.

The epithelial cells lining the alveoli are called **Type I cells** to distinguish them from a much smaller number of **Type II cells** which produce a substance called **pulmonary surfactant** to be discussed later. The lining of the alveoli also contains the protective **phagocytic cells.** As shown in Figure 2-8, there are *pores* in the alveolar membrane that permit some collateral ventilation in the event of occlusion of an alveolar duct.

The Lungs (Pulmones)

The lungs get their name from an old English word, *lungen,* which means light in weight. They are located in the thoracic cavity and largely occupy it. The words **thorax** and **thoracic** stem from a Greek word that means "pertaining to the chest." In addition to the lungs, the thorax houses the heart, the great blood vessels, nerves, the esophagus, and lesser lymph and blood vessels. These latter structures are all accommodated in a space in the central region of the thorax known as the

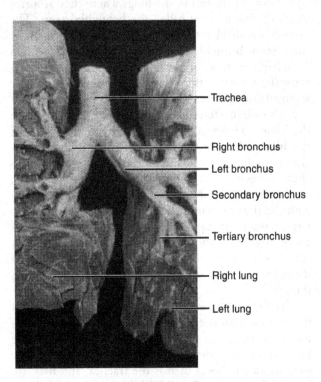

— Trachea

— Right bronchus

— Left bronchus

— Secondary bronchus

— Tertiary bronchus

— Right lung

— Left lung

FIGURE 2-7

Photograph of partially dissected lungs and bronchial tree.

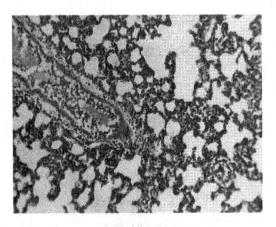

FIGURE 2-8

A segment of a terminal bronchiole and adjacent alveoli.

mediastinum, an interesting term which stems from the Latin expression *quod in medio stat*—"what is in the middle." As shown in Figure 2-9, the mediastinum is bounded on each side by a lung and by a pleural sac (to be described later). The mediastinum is divided by imaginary lines into an anterior, middle, posterior, and superior mediastinum.

The relatively unimportant anterior mediastinum contains a few mammary vessels and lymph nodes, while the middle mediastinum contains the heart, which is surrounded by a closed membranous sac known as the **pericardium.** The posterior mediastinum, behind the heart, contains part of the esophagus and trachea, some important nerve tracts, and the blood vessels that supply the head.

The lungs are probably best described as two irregular, cone-shaped structures. They are composed of spongy, porous, but highly elastic material that contains but a few smooth muscle fibers. This means that *lung tissue is passive* and cannot exert any force except that provided by the elastic properties of the lung, part of which can be accounted for by tissue elasticity—but that is only part of the story.

It has been estimated that only about one-fourth to one-third of the elasticity of the lung is due to the properties of the lung tissue itself. To account for the remainder of the elasticity, we shall have to look to the alveoli.

Properties of the Alveoli

The pulmonary alveolar epithelium which lines the alveoli is a uniquely thin tissue, to the extent the nuclei of the cells actually protrude into the air spaces. Because of the

secretory properties of epithelium, this tissue is moist. As a result, an **air-liquid interface** exists over the lining of the alveoli. In one sense the alveoli can be likened to tiny air-filled water bubbles. Due to the universal attraction of molecules for one another at this interface, a phenomenon called **surface tension** exists. The force produced by surface tension causes the liquid lining of the alveoli to behave much like stretched elastic, constantly trying to shorten and to resist further stretching.

Surface tension accounts for two seemingly opposing and paradoxical properties of lung tissue. First, it *accounts for the tendency of the alveoli to collapse*, and second, this *tendency to collapse is responsible for about two-thirds of the elasticity of lung tissue*. Indeed, the combined surface tension from some 7 million alveoli would require exhaustive muscular effort to overcome.

Fortunately, the Type II alveolar cells, mentioned earlier, produce a detergent-like substance called **pulmonary surfactant** which intersperses with the liquid molecules on the alveolar surfaces to *decrease surface tension* by 5–10 fold. A proper balance between alveolar fluid surface tension and surfactant is essential for normal respiratory function.

CLINICAL NOTE: An example of the consequences of insufficient surfactant production is a disease known as **respiratory distress syndrome** or **hyaline membrane disease,** which afflicts many premature infants. Because the surfactant-producing Type II cells are too immature to function properly, the infant's lungs are excessively resistant to expansion.[3] The infant is able to inspire only by exhaustive efforts, which may result in respiratory failure, lung collapse, and death.

Maturation of the Type II cells is facilitated by the hormone cortisol, which is produced by the mother late in pregnancy. Administration of cortisol to pregnant women is a means of combatting the disease. Postnatal administration of cortisol to infants is not effective.

Description of the Lungs

At birth the lungs are almost white in color, but pigmentation becomes more definite with age, and in the adult the lungs may appear grayish and mottled in black patches due to prolonged inhalation of dirt. Infant lungs are also large in proportion to the size of the thorax, and we shall see that this accounts for some rather interesting differences between the respiratory behavior of the infants and that of adults.

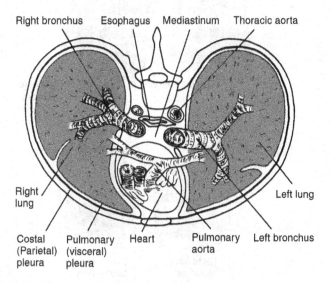

Right bronchus   Esophagus   Mediastinum   Thoracic aorta

Right lung

Left lung

Costal (Parietal) pleura   Pulmonary (visceral) pleura   Heart   Pulmonary aorta   Left bronchus

FIGURE 2-9

Schematic transverse section of thorax showing the lungs in relation to the heart and bronchi.

[3]The term **atelectasis** (Gk. *ateles*, imperfect + *tectasis*, expansion) refers to incomplete expansion of the lungs at birth or to collapse of the alveoli.

Normally the lungs lie freely within their pleural cavities and attach to the body only by their roots and the pulmonary ligaments (to be described later). The **roots,** of course, are formed by the bronchi, the pulmonary arteries and veins, the pulmonary plexus of nerves, and the lymphatic vessels. These structures are all encircled by connective tissue that contributes to the mediastinum.

The paired lungs are not exactly the same in size, shape, capacity, or weight. The right lung, larger than the left, is also somewhat shorter and broader. This is due to the **liver,** which occupies the upper right abdominal cavity, as seen in Figure 2-10. It forces the dome of the diaphragm higher on that side and this accounts for the shorter right lung. On the other hand, the **heart** occupies much of the left side of the thorax, and this accounts for the smaller left lung.

The lungs conform very closely to the outlines of the thoracic cage, and in specimens where the lungs have hardened *in situ*,[4] distinct impressions can be seen where the lungs made close contact with the ribs. Each lung has an apex and a base and costal and mediastinal surfaces, in addition to anterior, inferior, and posterior borders. The rounded **apex** shown in Figures 2-11 and

2-12 actually extends beyond the upper limits of the thorax, into the root of the neck to about 2.5 to 5 cm above the sternal end of the first rib. The **base** is broad and concave and conforms to the thoracic surface of the diaphragm. The **diaphragm** separates the base of the right lung from the bulk of the liver and separates the base of the left lung from the liver, stomach, and spleen. Some of these relationships can be seen in Figure 2-10.

The Lobes As may be seen in Figure 2-11, the **right lung** is partially divided into three lobes by two fissures. The oblique fissure separates the superior from the inferior lobe, while a horizontal fissure gives rise to a small middle lobe. The **left lung** is divided by an oblique fissure into a superior and an inferior lobe, but it has no horizontal fissure and, therefore, no middle lobe.

Weight Before respiration has occurred, the lungs have a *specific gravity* slightly greater than water, and they will sink. Once respiration has taken place, however, the lungs become partially filled with air, and even after removal from the body their specific gravity may

---

[4]*In situ* (L. in its original place).

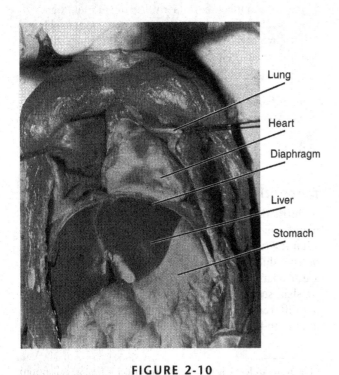

FIGURE 2-10

Abdominal and thoracic viscera, shown in relationship to the diaphragm.

Lung
Heart
Diaphragm
Liver
Stomach

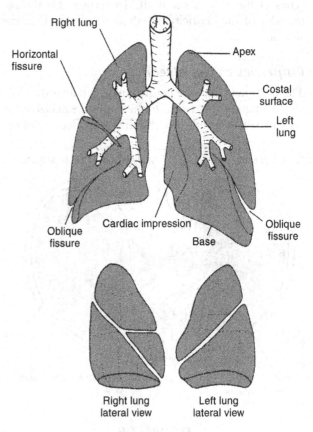

Right lung
Horizontal fissure
Apex
Costal surface
Left lung
Oblique fissure
Cardiac impression
Base
Oblique fissure

Right lung lateral view
Left lung lateral view

FIGURE 2-11

Illustration of the shape of the lungs and the lobes and segments of the lungs.

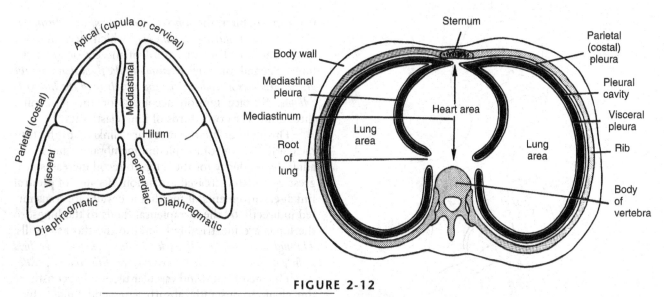

FIGURE 2-12

Schematic of parts of the pleurae and their reflections, as seen in a coronal section (A) and in a transverse section (B). (Transverse section from J. E. Crouch, *Functional Human Anatomy*, 3rd ed., 1978, Courtesy Lea & Febiger.)

be as low as 0.3, and so they will float.[5] These properties of lungs have value in forensic medicine.[6] For example, in the case of fetal death the lungs will sink, but in the case of neonatal death (within the first four weeks after birth) the lungs will float.

A pair of well-developed young adult male lungs has a *capacity* in excess of 5000 cubic centimeters (cc) of air; in a female about 4000 cc. Due to the imperfect elasticity of the lung tissue, collapsed (excised) lungs will not be entirely exhausted, but will contain about 500 cc of air. When fresh lungs are handled, they make a sound similar to the rustling of leaves (they crepitate). This is due to the presence of a small amount of air within the alveoli.

The Pleurae

The inner surface of the thoracic cavity, the thoracic surface of the diaphragm, and the mediastinum are lined with an airtight membrane called the **parietal** or **costal pleura** (Gk. rib, side). It is a thin, very delicate serous membrane that is almost identical to the peritoneum of the abdominal cavity. As shown in Figure 2-12, it is continuous with the **visceral pleura,** by means of reflections at the root of the lung (hilum), where a sleeve of pleura encloses the bronchi and pulmonary blood vessels. This sleeve forms a fold which is known as the **pulmonary ligament.**

Like other serous membranes, the pleurae are composed of a single layer of squamous mesothelial cells resting upon a delicate connective tissue membrane. The pleurae are also highly vascular, and they contain lymphatics and nerves. The visceral pleura is exceedingly delicate. It invests the lungs faithfully and closely follows their contours.

Functions of the Pleurae It is important to bear in mind that the right and left pleural sacs are completely separated, one from the other, and that the intervening space (the mediastinum) is occupied by the heart, blood vessels, and esophagus. One function of the pleurae is *to provide friction-free lung and thoracic surfaces.* The two moist surfaces glide on one another with every cycle of breathing. Rough or inflamed pleurae, as in **pleurisy,** and the accompanying friction, can account for the pain which occurs with each breath.

The pleurae also serve in a *protective capacity.* Since one lung is separated from the other by means of the airtight pleural sacs, a traumatic puncture of the thoracic wall results in the collapse of only one lung. If both lungs were to be enclosed within one airtight system (as they are in some lower animals), such a puncture would result in the collapse of both lungs, or the entire lung mass, followed quickly by death due to respiratory failure. Medically, a puncture that results in the collapse of a lung is called a **pneumothorax,** and it is shown schematically in Figure 2-13.

In the adult, the lung tissue does not quite fill the thoracic cavity, and so, in some areas, as shown in Figure 2-14, **pleural recesses** or **sinuses** can be found. In addition, the fluid-filled space between the visceral and

---

[5]The fact that lungs float is one reason they are used as food for alligators in zoos. Uneaten food floats on the surface where it can be removed, whereas other food might sink and contaminate the water.

[6]Legal medicine.

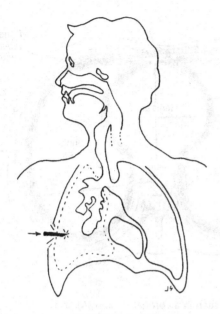

FIGURE 2-13

Schematic of a pneumothorax. The entrance of air into the pleural spaces results in a separation of the lung from the thoracic walls. Lung collapse shown greatly exaggerated.

parietal pleurae which we have identified as the **intrapleural space** is in actuality a nonexistent but potential space between the pleurae.

Mechanical Aspects of the Pleurae An appreciation of the mechanics of the pleural membranes is absolutely essential to understanding even the most basic rudiments of respiratory physiology. Earlier we learned that the lungs have a tendency to collapse and pull away from the thoracic walls. This can be accounted for by

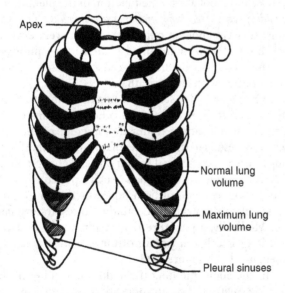

Apex

Normal lung volume

Maximum lung volume

Pleural sinuses

FIGURE 2-14

Schematic of pleural sinuses. In the adult the lung tissue does not quite fill the thoracic cavity.

two factors. First, the *inherent elasticity of lung tissue resists expansion during inhalation,* which accounts for about one-fourth to one-third of the elasticity of the lungs. Second, the *surface tension in the fluid that lines the alveoli produces a tendency for the alveoli (and the lungs) to collapse.* Surface tension accounts for the remaining three-fourths to two-thirds of lung elasticity.

Throughout life the lungs are "linked" to the thoracic walls by way of the pleural membranes, and in the adult the tendency for the lungs to recoil increases progressively with increased expansion. Because of **pleural linkage,** movements of the thoracic walls are transmitted indirectly by the intrapleural fluids to the lungs, so the lungs are inextricably bound to the thoracic walls. *Throughout every breath cycle the lung surfaces are held tightly in contact with the inner surface of the thoracic walls.*

The membranes and vascular tissues that constitute the pleurae constantly absorb gases and fluids which enter the **potential intrapleural spaces,** and this absorption in turn generates a subatmospheric pressure that binds the visceral and parietal pleural membranes together. The negative pressure of the intrapleural fluid has a value of about −10 to −12 mm Hg, and it is this negative **intrapleural fluid pressure** that acts as the linking force between the pleurae. This is the force that links the lungs to the thoracic walls.

The visceral pleura, then, is separated from the parietal pleura only by a thin layer of liquid. The lungs and thoracic walls are coupled by fluid that *assures friction-free surfaces* over which the lungs can glide during inhalation and exhalation. The liquid also provides immediate and complete transmission of the chest wall movements to the lungs.

During inhalation, when the chest cavity enlarges, this negative intrapleural pressure causes the lungs in turn to enlarge; during exhalation when the chest cavity is returning to its undilated state, the elasticity of the lungs is able to assert itself and the lungs become smaller. *The continuous absorption of intrapleural fluids and gases takes place mainly through the action of visceral pleurae.* This is because the **capillary pressure** of the pulmonary system is about 7 mm Hg less than that of the capillary pressure of the thoracic system.

The tendency of the lungs to pull away from the thoracic walls can be measured directly in the laboratory by means of a simple instrument called a **wet manometer.** As shown in Figure 2-15, a manometer consists of a calibrated U-shaped glass tube that contains mercury or some other liquid, usually water. One end of the tube is connected to a pressure source (either positive or negative). The difference in the height of the two mercury or water columns indicates the amount by which the pressure in either column differs from atmospheric. This difference is conventionally read directly in millimeters of mercury (mm Hg) or centimeters of water (cm H_2O or Aq).

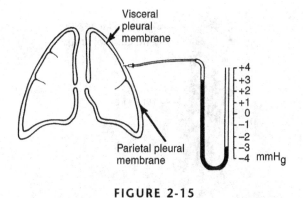

FIGURE 2-15

Schematic of a technique used to measure pleural-surface pressure by means of a manometer. The difference in the heights of the two columns registers the tendency for the lungs to pull away from the thoracic wall.

When a hypodermic needle is carefully inserted between the ribs, into the intrapleural space, the recoil of the lung is registered by the manometer. The negative pressure is called **pleural-surface (or intrapleural) pressure,** and at rest, with the airway open to the outside, a pressure of about –3 to –4 mm Hg is required to prevent the lungs from pulling away from the thoracic walls and collapsing by virtue of their own elasticity. We have seen that intrapleural fluid pressure amounts to –10 to –12 mm Hg, and so the lungs are maintained, tightly bound against the thoracic wall. As the lungs are stretched, however, the elasticity of the tissue, combined with the surface tension forces within the alveoli, generates an increased recoil, and an intrapleural pressure required to stretch the lungs can amount to values as large as –9 to –12 mm Hg, a value more than adequate to maintain the lungs in an expanded state.

In other words, the subatmospheric **intrapleural fluid pressure** is the *force that acts to bind the pleural membranes tightly to one another,* while the **pleural-surface (intrapleural) pressure,** which is the pressure we can measure, is important because it *registers the tendency for the stretched lungs to recoil and to pull away from the thoracic wall.*

We can summarize the mechanics of the pleurae by borrowing from Agostoni and Mead (1964):

It seems therefore that the essential mechanisms holding the lung against the chest wall are those keeping the pleural space gas free and nearly liquid free, while the mechanisms preventing a complete removal of liquid from the pleural space secures the lubrication of the coupling system.

Just why lung tissue should be subjected to stretching forces in the first place is something we might look into.

The Effects of Growth on Stretching Forces

At birth the lungs are proportionately quite large when compared to the size of the thorax. As a result, the lungs completely fill the thoracic cavity and are not placed under tension in the position of respiratory rest. This means that at the beginning of inspiration and at the end of expiration, the intrapleural or pleural surface pressure is the same as, or nearly the same as, atmospheric. Intrapleural fluid pressure is subatmospheric, however, so the lungs are linked to the thoracic wall, just as in the case of the adult.

Thus, at end-expiration the lungs are much the same as nonaerated lungs and they contain very little residual air, but as the thorax enlarges during inspiration, the lungs' surfaces follow the enlarging thoracic cavity and the lung tissue begins to be subjected to a **stretching force.** This force, however, is resisted by the inherent elastic properties of the lungs; they tend to pull away from the thoracic wall, just as in an adult, and the intrapleural pressure becomes negative with respect to atmospheric pressure. That is, *resistance to the stretching force accounts for negative intrapleural pressure,* and the *magnitude of this pressure is proportional to the degree of thoracic dilation.*

As an individual matures, the rate of the growth of the body in general, including the thorax, exceeds the growth rate of the lungs; nevertheless, the lung surfaces and the chest wall continue to remain in close contact, separated only by a thin film of serous intrapleural fluid.

With growth, the lungs, even at rest, are subjected to an ever-increasing stretching force. In the adult the lungs are subjected to such a stretching force that intrapleural pressure is always below atmospheric pressure at the position of respiratory rest; provided expiratory air flow encounters no substantial resistance (by a closed glottis, for instance). Intrapleural pressure is subatmospheric even at the end of a maximum expiratory effort. Because of the ever-present negative intrapleural pressure, the lungs cannot be completely evacuated voluntarily.

THE FRAMEWORK FOR THE BREATHING MECHANISM

The principal components of the skeletal framework for the breathing mechanism are the **vertebral** or **spinal column,** the **rib cage,** and the **pelvis,** and they are shown in Figure 2-16. These structures comprise the skeleton for the **torso** (L. *torsio,* to twist), which by definition is the trunk of the body without the head or free extremities. The framework for the respiratory system does include the skull, however, so our torso will be something of a compromise.

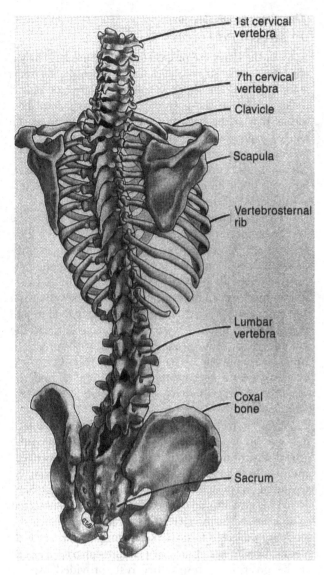

FIGURE 2-16

The skeletal framework for the breathing mechanism. (From Eileen and W. Zemlin, *Study Guide/Workbook to Accompany Speech and Hearing Science,* 3rd ed., 1988, Stipes Publishing Co.)

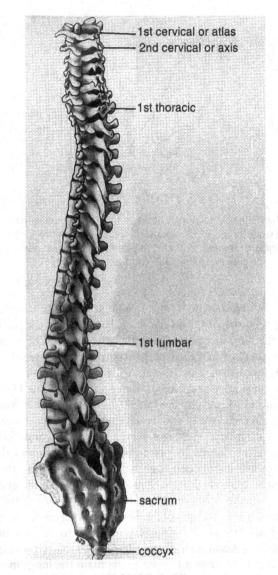

FIGURE 2-17

The vertebral column as seen in perspective from behind. (From Eileen and W. Zemlin, *Study Guide/Workbook to Accompany Speech and Hearing Science,* 3rd ed., 1988, Stipes Publishing Co.)

The Spinal Column

As shown in Figure 2-17, the spinal column consists of 32 or 33 individual **vertebrae** (L. *vertebra,* to turn) that are joined together by intervertebral cartilages and a very complex system of ligaments. There are seven **cervical** (L. *cervix,* neck), twelve **thoracic** (Gk. chest), five **lumbar** (L. *lumbus,* loin), five **sacral** (L. *sacrum,* sacred), and three or four **coccygeal** (Gk. *kokkyx,* cuckoo) vertebrae. The sacral vertebrae are fused solidly together and appear to be one bone, which is referred to as the **sacrum.** The coccygeal vertebrae are vestigial (not rudimentary) structures, which may vary in number from three to four and, occasionally, five. The individual coc-

cygeal vertebrae are usually thought of as a single structure called the **coccyx** (pronounced kok-siks).

Anatomy of the Vertebrae

The bulk of most vertebrae consists of a **corpus** or **body,** which is an unpaired anteriorly directed cylindrical projection. As shown in Figure 2-18, a pair of **legs** or **pedicles** arise from the body and are directed posteriorly. Two platelike structures project backward from these pedicles to fuse in the midline, thus completing an arch that encloses a space called the **vertebral foramen.** This arch, called the **neural arch,** offers protection to

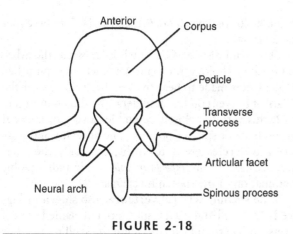

FIGURE 2-18

Schematic lumbar vertebra as seen from above.

the spinal cord, which in life occupies the space of the vertebral foramen.

A prominent projection, directed dorsally and more or less inferiorly from the neural arch, is called the **spinous process,** and collectively, these processes give us the **spinal column.** The spines of the vertebrae serve for the attachment of muscles and ligaments and, in addition, provide protection for the vertebral column. Paired **transverse processes** project laterally on either side of the vertebrae, and they, too, form points of attachments for muscles and ligaments, and in the case of the thoracic vertebrae, points of articulations for the ribs. There are, in addition, superior and inferior articular processes.

Articulations in the Vertebral Column

The two **superior** and two **inferior articular processes** articulate with adjacent vertebrae to form freely movable diarthrodial joints. The degree of movement at these joints is restricted by the nature of the ligamentous system and articulations between vertebral bodies.

There are two anatomically and functionally distinct types of articulations in the vertebral column. The bodies of the vertebrae are united by **intervertebral discs** and by the **anterior** and **posterior longitudinal ligaments.** The intervertebral discs are composed of fibrocartilage, and they are joined at their surfaces to thin layers of hyaline cartilage that cover the upper and lower surfaces of the bodies of the vertebrae. This joint, then, is an amphiarthrodial or yielding joint. The intervertebral discs vary considerably in their thickness, but collectively they constitute one-fourth of the column's length, which is normally between 72 and 75 cm.

The discs in the cervical and lumbar regions are thicker in front than behind, which explains the *concave curvature* of the column. In the thoracic region the discs are essentially uniform in thickness, but the bodies of the

vertebrae are somewhat wedge-shaped, being slightly thinner in front than behind. This accounts for the *convex curvature* of the thoracic region.

The **arches** of the vertebrae articulate by means of plane synovial joints which are enveloped by relatively thin and loose articular capsules; they are especially flexible in the cervical region. **Accessory ligaments** unite the laminae and the transverse and spinous processes of the vertebrae. The laminae of adjacent vertebrae are joined by the **ligamenta flava** (a term that describes their yellow color), while the tips of the spinous processes of the thoracic and lumbar vertebrae are connected by long, longitudinally directed **supraspinal ligaments.** The transverse processes are joined by **intertransverse ligaments,** which are well developed only in the lumbar region.

The **anterior** and **posterior longitudinal ligaments,** mentioned earlier, consist of an aggregate of both long and short fibers that extend throughout the length of the spinal column and bind the bodies of the vertebrae together. The short fibers attach to adjacent vertebrae while the longer fibers may pass over three or four vertebrae. The more conspicuous and prominent ligaments may be seen schematically in Figure 2-19.

Types of Vertebrae

The **cervical, thoracic,** and **lumbar** vertebrae are only grossly similar. Each presents certain distinguishable characteristics or landmarks. In spite of the complexity of the vertebral column, variations in the total number of vertebrae are less common than variations within different regions of the column. Vertebrae are often identified by letter to designate their type, followed by a number to indicate position. The seventh thoracic vertebra becomes T7 and the fifth lumbar becomes L5.

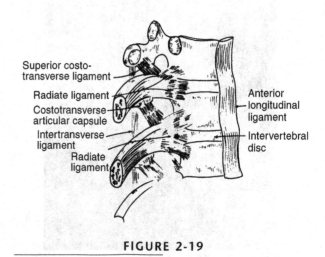

FIGURE 2-19

Schematic of costovertebral articulation as seen from the side.

Cervical Vertebrae The seven cervical vertebrae have a distinguishing feature, namely, **transverse foraminae.** In life they transmit vertebral veins and arteries, in addition to a bundle of nerves. A second distinguishing feature of cervical vertebrae (three through six) is a short bifurcated (cleft) spinous process. A fourth cervical vertebra is shown in Figure 2-20, and an x-ray of a cervical column is shown in Figure 2-21. Vertebrae C3

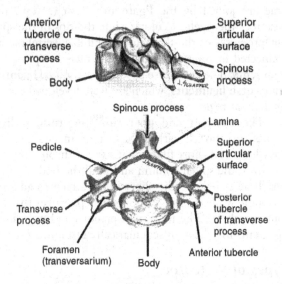

FIGURE 2-20

A fourth cervical vertebra as seen from the side (top) and from above (bottom).

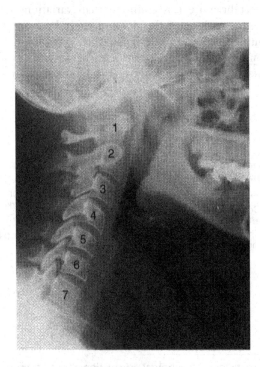

FIGURE 2-21

X-ray of the cervical column.

through C6 are typical, but C1, C2, and C7 deserve special attention.

The skull rests on **C1,** which is known as the **atlas.** In Greek mythology, the giant Atlas, who was punished by Zeus, was made to bear the weight of the sky (or the pillars of heaven) on his shoulders.[7] As shown in Figure 2-22, this vertebra closely resembles a ring of bone. It has no body or spinous process. The **anterior** and **posterior tubercles** are noteworthy, especially the anterior, because it is an *important landmark* in radiographic examination of the speech mechanism.

The **second cervical vertebra,** also shown in Figure 2-22, is called the **axis,** appropriately named since it forms a *pivot* around which C1 and the skull rotate. The axis presents an outstanding landmark, the **dens** (L. tooth) or **odontoid** (Gk. toothlike) process, which is an upward projection of the body. An anterior articular facet on the dens provides articulation with the anterior arch of the atlas, as shown in Figure 2-23.

The **seventh cervical vertebra,** shown in Figure 2-24, is distinctive because of the conspicuous *spinous process which can usually be palpated at the base of the neck.* Another feature of C7 is less conspicuous. The transverse foraminae are highly variable in their size and may even be absent.

[7]A classic Greek statue of Atlas depicts the sky or heaven as the Earth.

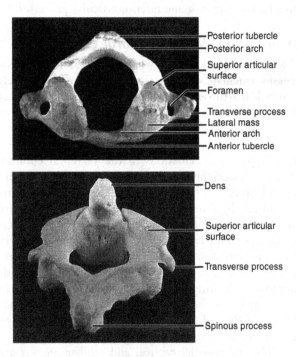

FIGURE 2-22

The first (atlas) and second (axis) cervical vertebrae. The first (top) is seen from above, and the second is seen in perspective from behind.

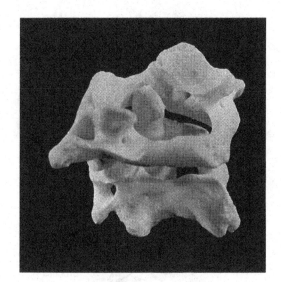

FIGURE 2-23

Articulated first and second cervical vertebrae.

Thoracic Vertebrae The thoracic vertebrae are twelve in number and are distinctive because of the **articular facets** on their transverse processes and vertebral bodies. These facets *provide points of attachment for the ribs.* The vertebrae increase in their overall size from T1 through T12. A typical thoracic vertebra as seen from above and from the side is shown in Figure 2-25. Another thoracic vertebra and its attachments with a rib are shown in Figure 2-26.

Lumbar Vertebrae The lumbar vertebrae, five in number, are very large. Their massive bodies make them particularly suitable for their *weightbearing functions.* These vertebrae are distinctive simply because they lack the features characteristic of the other vertebrae. They lack transverse foraminae, and they lack the articular facets on their transverse processes and vertebral bodies. In addition, their spinous processes are directed horizontally (see Figure 2-27).

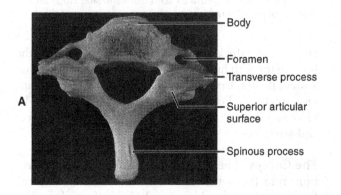

A
- Body
- Foramen
- Transverse process
- Superior articular surface
- Spinous process

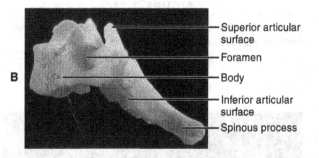

B
- Superior articular surface
- Foramen
- Body
- Inferior articular surface
- Spinous process

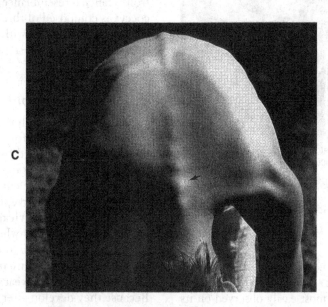

C

FIGURE 2-24

The seventh cervical vertebra (vertebra prominens) as seen from above (A) and from the side (B). In C the arrow points to the vertebra prominens.

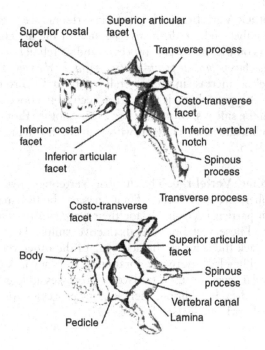

FIGURE 2-25

A typical thoracic vertebra as seen from the side (top) and from above (bottom).

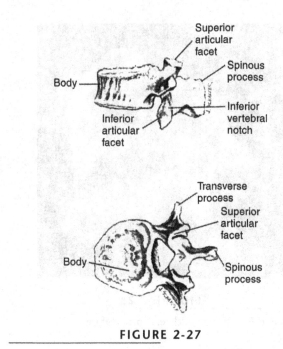

FIGURE 2-27

A typical lumbar vertebra as seen from the side (top) and from above (bottom).

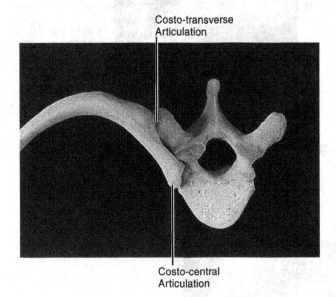

FIGURE 2-26

A thoracic vertebra and rib attachments as seen from above.

The Sacrum The sacrum is composed of five vertebral bodies that in the adult are united by four ossified intervertebral discs. This is most easily observed on its concave anterior or pelvic surface. The body of the first sacral vertebra has a prominent oval upper surface, and an especially thick intervertebral disc unites it with the body of the fifth lumbar vertebra. The dorsal surface has a **medial sacral crest** that constitutes vestiges of spinous processes. Four pairs of **sacral foramina** can be seen on a sacrum, and in life they transmit sacral nerves and arteries.

The Coccyx The coccyx, an inferiorly directed projection from the bottom of the sacrum, derives its name from a fancied resemblance to the beak of a cuckoo. The coccyx is composed of three or four fused vestigial vertebrae that articulate with the sacrum by means of a small intervertebral disc. A sacrum and a coccyx are shown in Figure 2-28.

Development of Spinal Curves

When viewed from behind, the vertebral column is almost straight, except for a slight lateral deflection to the right. When viewed from the side, the **infant vertebral column** has but one curve, which is the same as the thoracic and pelvic curves in the adult. This curve, called the **primary** curve, becomes modified as the infant matures. The **cervical** curve begins to develop at three or four months, when the child begins to hold its head up, and at nine months, when the child begins to sit upright. The **lumbar** curve begins to slowly develop when at about a year old the child begins to walk. Because they develop after birth, the cervical and lumbar curves, shown in Figure 2-29, are called **secondary** curves.

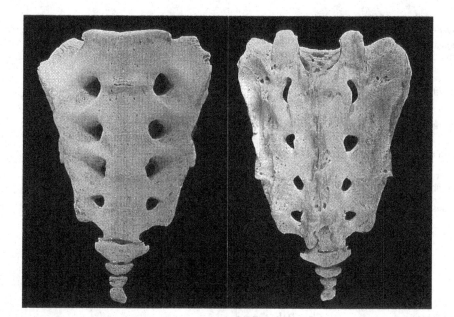

FIGURE 2-28

A sacrum and coccyx as seen from the front (left) and from behind (right).

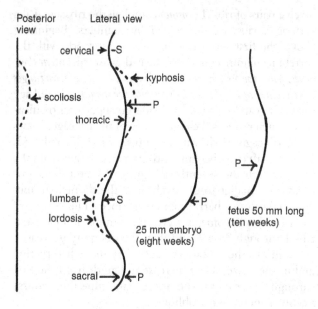

FIGURE 2-29

Primary, secondary, and abnormal vertebral curves, P = primary, S = secondary.

CLINICAL NOTE: Abnormal curvature of the vertebral column may be encountered in the clinical environment. An increase in the convex curvature of the thoracic region is called **kyphosis** (Gk. hunchback). It is sometimes caused by tuberculosis in one or more of the vertebral bodies. These bodies become eroded, weakened, and then distorted by the weight of the body. Muscular imbalance and poor posture may also be contributing factors. *Kyphosis can inhibit rib cage movement and reduce pulmonary compliance.*

Kyphosis can be contrasted with an exaggerated concave curvature in the lumbar region called **lordosis,** or *swayback.* Lordosis may also be due to tuberculosis and, in some cases, to poor posture and prolonged wearing of excessively high-heeled shoes.

Abnormal lateral curvature of the column, called **scoliosis** (Gk. curvation), may be caused by muscle imbalance, diet, paralysis, or poor posture. Early detection and treatment of scoliosis in children and adolescents can prevent permanent disability.

Sometimes, during the development of the embryonic vertebral column, *failure of fusion of the two sides of the neural arch* results in a defect known as **spina bifida** (L. *bifidus,* cleft into two parts).

The Sternum

The **sternum** or **breastbone,** shown in Figures 2-30 and 2-31, is a prominent midline structure located on the anterior, superior thoracic wall. An oblong structure, it consists of three parts: the **manubrium,** the **body,** and the **xiphoid** (or **ensiform) process.**

The uppermost segment of the sternum is known as the **manubrium** (L. *manubrium,* handle). It is a quadrilateral plate, somewhat wider above than below. A landmark found on its superior border in the form of a depression is called the **suprasternal** (jugular, presternal) **notch.** Lateral to this notch, on either side, is an oval articulatory facet which forms the point of articulation for the medial end of the clavicle (collarbone). On each lateral border of the manubrium, just beneath the sternoclavicular joint, is a depression for articulation with the costal cartilage of the first rib. The second costal cartilage joins the sternum at the level where the

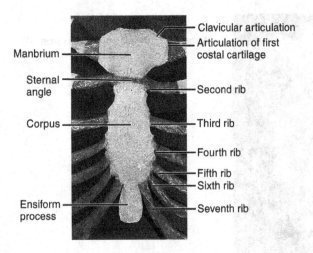

FIGURE 2-30

A sternum as seen from the front.

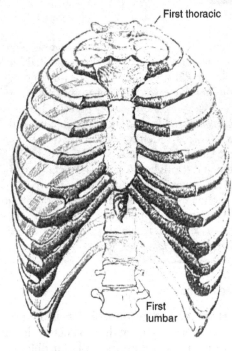

FIGURE 2-31

A rib cage as seen from the front.

manubrium and body are joined. A projection called the **sternal angle** indicates the junction of the manubrium and body of the sternum. Palpation of the sternal angle will also locate the level of articulation between the sternum and the second costal cartilage.

CLINICAL NOTE: The sternum is particularly vulnerable to fractures, in automobile accidents, for example, and the most frequent site of fracture is the **sternal angle.** Excessive displacement of the sternum may damage the trachea or the heart and great blood vessels.

The **body** (corpus) of the sternum is long and narrow, and is directed upward and somewhat backward, as shown in Figure 2-32. The lateral borders on the body of the sternum are marked by the articulatory facets for the cartilages of ribs 2 through 7. The inferior border of the body articulates with a small process that is cartilaginous in youth, but tends to ossify at its proximal part in the adult. It is called the **xiphoid** (Gk. *xiphos,* sword) or **ensiform** (L. *ensis,* sword) **process.**

CLINICAL NOTE: The **xiphoid process** is a useful landmark for measurement of chest excursion during breathing, and for hand placement during cardiopulmonary resuscitation (CPR).

The Ribs

The Rib Cage

Twelve pairs of ribs (L. *costae*) complete the rib cage. Like vertebrae, ribs are designated by numbers. Beginning above, the first seven ribs articulate posteriorly with the vertebral column, course obliquely downward, and *at their lowest point the osseous ribs abruptly give way to costal cartilages which course upward to articulate with the sternum.* In old age the costal cartilages tend to undergo superficial ossification, which reduces the compliance of the rib cage. Views of the rib cage are shown in Figures 2-31, 2-32, and 2-33.

The **rib cage** becomes progressively larger from the first through the seventh or eighth ribs, and then progressively smaller to the twelfth, so the thoracic framework takes on a barrel-like appearance. The course of the ribs also becomes progressively more oblique from ribs 1 through 8 or 9, and then the obliquity decreases. In addition, the costal cartilages vary in their direction and in their size. They increase in length from the first through the seventh, and at the same time their course becomes increasingly oblique.

CLINICAL NOTE: Extra ribs, especially on the seventh cervical vertebra, are not uncommon. They may cause a great deal of discomfort and pain. A rib on the first lumbar vertebra may occur and be the cause of back problems.

CLINICAL NOTE: **Rickets,** often the result of a dietary deficiency of vitamin D, especially in infancy and childhood, may result in deformities of the chest, such as "pigeon breast" with its greatly exaggerated sternal angle. A **rachitic** (pertaining to rickets) **rosary,** a condition characterized by enlargements at the bony and cartilaginous union in the ribs, may also result from malnutrition.

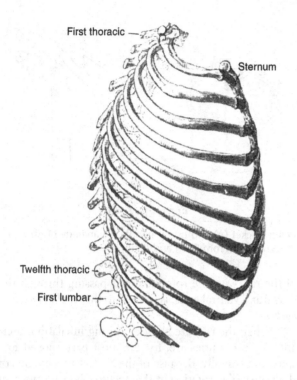

First thoracic —

Sternum

Twelfth thoracic —

First lumbar —

FIGURE 2-32

A rib cage as seen from the side (above). In the photograph at the right, the course of the ribs in an expiratory position is shown.

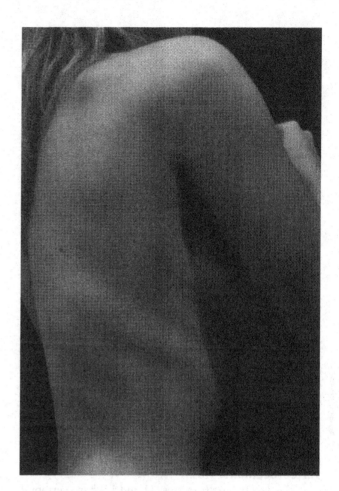

These conditions are noteworthy because, although they may be asymptomatic in and of themselves, malnutrition and mental retardation often go hand in hand.

The Anatomy of a Rib

The bulk of a typical rib is known as the **shaft,** and since it is somewhat flattened, it exhibits upper and lower borders and inner and outer surfaces. Posteriorly, the **head** of the rib is separated from the shaft by a short **neck.** At the junction of the neck and shaft, a tubercle on the posterior surface articulates with the tip of the transverse process of the numerically corresponding vertebra.

Beginning at the head, the course of the rib is at first posteriorly downward and lateral, until the rib abuts against the transverse process. A short distance from the tubercle, the shaft begins to course rather sharply in the anterior direction. The point where the rib abruptly changes direction is known as the **angle of the rib.** As the rib approaches the sternum, it reaches its lowest point; here there is a sharp demarcation between the osseous and cartilaginous portions of the rib.

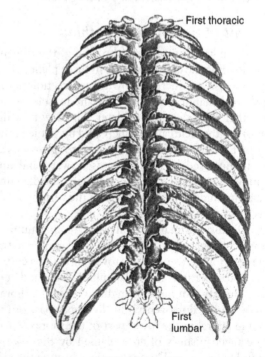

First thoracic

First lumbar

FIGURE 2-33

A rib cage as seen from behind.

The lower border of the shaft of a rib has a **costal groove** that accommodates and protects the intercostal blood vessels and nerves coursing along each rib.

As can be seen in Figures 2-31 and 2-32, the posterior end of the rib is generally higher than the anterior end. This is not nearly so true, however, in infants as in adults; *in infants the course of the ribs tends to be far more horizontal.*

Costal Articulations

All twelve pairs of ribs articulate with the vertebral column by means of arthrodial or gliding joints that are effected typically by two demiarticulations (Fr. *demi,* half). That is, *with the exception of the first rib and the last three pairs of ribs, the head of every rib articulates with the bodies of two adjacent vertebrae and their intervertebral discs.* The first, tenth, eleventh, and twelfth ribs join only with their numerically corresponding vertebrae.

Anteriorly, the costal cartilages of the first seven pairs of ribs join directly with the sternum; they are the **true ribs** or **vertebrosternal ribs.** Except for the first rib, which articulates with the sternum by means of a synchondrosis, the true ribs articulate with the sternum by means of a true synovial joint.

The next three pairs of ribs (ribs eight, nine, and ten) are indirectly connected to the sternum by means of long costal cartilages. They are called **false ribs** or **vertebrochondral ribs.**

The last two pairs of ribs (11 and 12) have vertebral attachments, but their anterior extremities are free. They are known as **vertebral** or **floating ribs.**

Movement of the Ribs in Breathing

During the inhalation phase of breathing, the dimensions of the thoracic cavity increase in three planes. The *vertical* dimension is increased by the contraction of the dome-shaped diaphragm, an important muscle of inhalation that will be considered later. The *transverse* diameter of the thoracic cavity is increased by virtue of the raising of the curved ribs, while the *anteroposterior* diameter is increased by simultaneous forward and upward movement of the sternum which, incidentally, maintains its angular relationship with the vertebral column as it is raised and lowered.

Two factors, primarily, contribute to the multidimensional changes that take place: the nature of the oblique rotational axis of the costovertebral (plus costotransvere) articulation, and the complex shape and curvature of the ribs. An increase in diameter of the thorax is predominantly dorsoventral in the upper part of the thorax and lateral in the lower part of the thorax.

The mechanism is often explained by the *analogy* shown in Figure 2-34. The rib rotating through the axis of its neck is likened to a *pump handle,* and the rotation

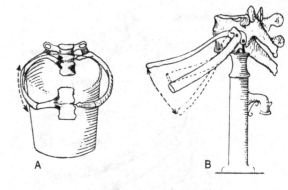

FIGURE 2-34

Water bucket (A) and pump handle (B) analogy of rib movements. (From Fenn and Rahn, 1964.)

of the rib, with the rotational axis passing through the dorsal and ventral ends, is likened to the *handle of a water bucket.*

When the ribs are elevated during inhalation, their anterior extremities are, for the most part, moved forward and laterally. Because of the sternal attachments of the upper ribs, rotation at the neck of the rib causes an upward and lateral movement. The net result is an increase in the anteroposterior as well as the lateral diameter of the chest. Muscles that tend to raise the ribs must be regarded as inspiratory, while those that lower the ribs are expiratory. We will soon learn, however, that this rule of thumb holds only during breathing for life purposes.

The Pelvic Girdle

The **coxal bone,** or **hip bone,** was known as *os innominatum* at one time, a term that means simply, "bone without a name." The paired coxal bones, shown in Figures 2-35 and 2-36, form the **pelvic** (L. basin) **girdle,** a supporting structure to which the lower limbs are attached. Each coxal bone is composed of three lesser bones. Together with the sacrum and coccyx, the hip bones form the **bony pelvis,** an extremely complex structure.

Probably the most distinctive landmark of the hip bone is the **acetabulum,** or "vinegar cup," which forms the socket for the reception of the head of the femur. The three individual bones that constitute the coxal bone meet at this point. They are the **ilium** (L. groin, flank), the **ischium** (Gk. *ischion,* hip), and the **pubis** (L. area of growth of pubic hair).

The great bulk of the hip bone is composed of the **ilium,** a roughly fan-shaped plate. Its upper margin forms the **iliac crest,** which is easily palpable from its anterior-superior spine to its posterior-superior spine. Just beneath each of these iliac spines is a corresponding inferior spine. The posterior part of the inner surface of each ilium is articulated, by means of a cartilaginous joint, with the lateral border of the sacrum. This union is known as the

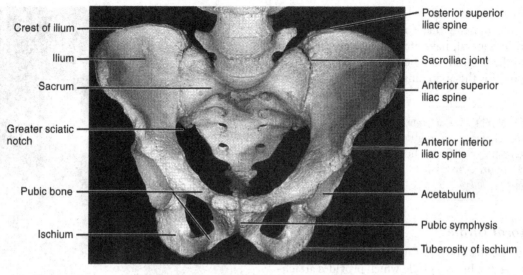

FIGURE 2-35

The coxal bones and adjacent structures (which comprise the pelvis) as viewed from the front.

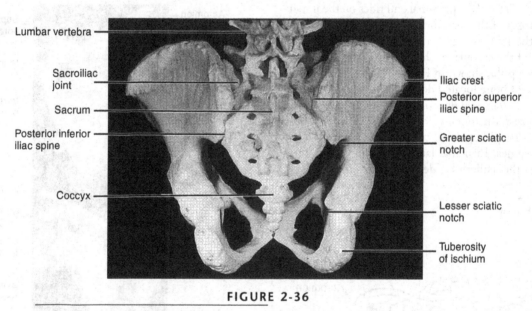

FIGURE 2-36

The coxal bones and adjacent structures (which comprise the pelvis) as viewed from behind.

sacroiliac joint, and just beneath it can be found a very prominent notch, the **greater sciatic notch,** through which passes the sciatic nerve. Just below the angle of the notch, the ilium articulates with the ischium.

The lower lateral portion of the acetabulum and a stout, triangular column of bone make up the **ischium.** It descends in a vertical direction to terminate as a rough and large **ischial tuberosity,** which absorbs the weight of the body when one sits up straight. The major muscle of the buttock (gluteus maximus muscle) conceals the ischial tuberosity, which is nevertheless easily palpated.

The anteromedial portion of the acetabulum belongs to the **pubis,** which is continued in a horizontal direction as a bony bar called the superior ramus. It expands to form the body of the pubis. The body meets its fellow from the opposite side at the midline to form the **pubic symphysis.**

Extending from the anterior-superior iliac spine to the pubic symphisis is the **inguinal ligament** (of Poupart), which marks the anatomical division between the lower abdomen and the leg. Between the palpable posterior iliac spines lies the rough posterior surface of the sacrum.

The contribution of the pelvis to speech production is through the muscles that constitute the abdominal wall. They, in general, have attachments on the ilium. In addition, the pelvis does function as a basin and provides a "floor" for the abdominal viscera.

CLINICAL NOTE: For many cerebral palsied individuals, proper positioning of the pelvis is crucial to the maintenance of adequate breath support for speech. Or, in other words, *speech therapy begins at the hips and goes to the lips.*[8]

The Pectoral Girdle

Two structures, the **clavicle** and the **scapula,** form the pectoral (L. *pectus,* breast) girdle which provides attachment of the upper limbs to the torso.

The **clavicle** (L. *clavicule,* small key) or **collarbone** serves to project the scapula (shoulder blade) sufficiently far laterally to clear the barrel-shaped chest wall. Shaped like the italic letter *f,* its proximal end rides on the upper-lateral margin of the manubrium of the scapula. Crossing over the first rib, its distal end articulates with the acromion of the scapula, as shown in Figure 2-37.

The **scapula,** shown in Figure 2-38, is a thin triangular plate of bone located dorsal to the upper seven or eight ribs. *It attaches to the axial skeleton only by way of the clavicle.* At rest, the longest side (vertebral border) of the scapula lies roughly parallel to and about 6 cm from the vertebral spines. Principal landmarks include the inferior angle; the axillary border; the **glenoid** (Gk. *glene,*

---

[8]Source unknown.

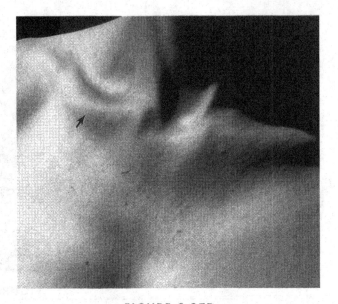

FIGURE 2-37B

Clavicle on young adult female (arrow points to clavicle).

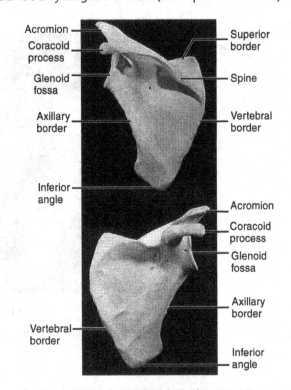

FIGURE 2-38

A scapula as seen from behind (top) and from the front (bottom).

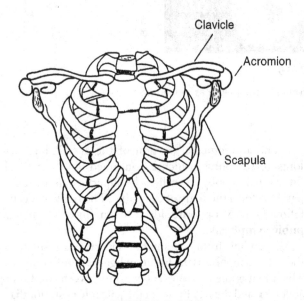

FIGURE 2-37A

A rib cage and pectoral girdle as seen from the front.

socket) **fossa,** which is the articular facet for the upper arm bone; the superior border; the hooked **coracoid** (Gk. *korakodes,* like the beak of a crow) **process;** the spine; and the **acromion** (Gk. *akron,* tip; *omos,* shoulder). The free upper (proximal) member of the arm is the **humerus.** It articulates with the glenoid fossa of the scapula, as illustrated in Figure 2-39.

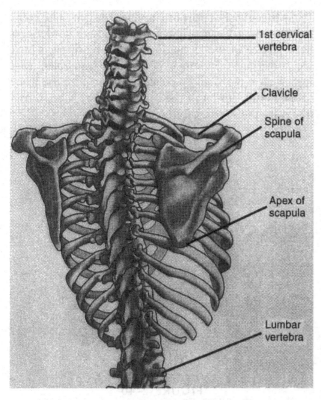

FIGURE 2-39

A scapula and clavicle as seen in perspective from behind. (Adapted from Eileen and W. Zemlin, *Study Guide/Workbook to Accompany Speech and Hearing Science,* 3rd ed., 1988, Stipes Publishing Co.)

THE MUSCULATURE OF THE BREATHING MECHANISM

Introduction

The mechanical events responsible for air exchange during quiet breathing can be stated quite simply. Through thoracic muscle contraction, all three dimensions of the chest are increased. That is, the anteroposterior, the lateral, and the vertical dimensions are all increased, and since the lungs are held bound to the thoracic wall by virtue of pleural linkage, they too are expanded. As a result, a negative pressure is momentarily generated within the pulmonary alveoli, and with the upper respiratory tract open, air rushes into the lungs until the intraalveolar pressure is the same as atmospheric. When this has happened, the muscles of inhalation cease to contract somewhat gradually, the dilated thorax-lung complex rebounds to generate a slightly positive intraalveolar (intrapulmonic) pressure, and the air is exhaled. The expiratory phase has taken place without the assistance of active muscle contraction. In other words, *quiet breathing requires active muscle contraction during the inspiratory phase, but the expiratory forces are passive, or nonmuscular.*

What we have just described takes place about 12 times a minute, for adults, with about 500 to 750 cc of air exchanged during each respiratory cycle.

When circumstances demand, however, and additional air needs to be exhaled beyond that exhaled by passive means, the *abdominal musculature may contract to facilitate forced exhalation.* These muscles may also become active in order to expel air at a very fast rate, for example, to blow out the flame of a candle. So, our seemingly simple process of breathing becomes suddenly complex when special demands are placed on the respiratory apparatus. This is especially true when breathing for speech or singing takes place.

The muscles for breathing may be divided on a **functional basis** into those responsible for inhalation and those responsible for exhalation. They may also be divided on an **anatomical basis** into muscles of the thorax and muscles of the abdomen. *Muscles of inhalation are confined largely to the thorax*, as might be expected, and the *muscles of exhalation primarily to the abdomen.* Accessory muscles of the neck also contribute to thoracic enlargement during inhalation.

Musculature associated with the **upper limb** and with the **back** has also been assigned a respiratory role, but supportive evidence is very meager. Under extreme conditions these muscles might possibly have some influence on the rib cage. Postural musculature, for example, can modify the secondary spinal curvature and total pulmonary compliance. Musculature of the upper limb and of the back will be briefly reviewed later in the chapter.

The Muscles of the Thorax

The eight muscles (or muscle groups) of the thorax are the **diaphragm,** the **internal intercostals,** the **external intercostals,** the **subcostals** and **transversus thoracis,** the **costal elevators,** the **serratus posterior superior** and the **serratus posterior inferior**—although the last two are sometimes described as muscles of the back (Woodburne, 1973).

The Diaphragm

The torso is divided into a thorax and an abdomen by a thin, but very *strong, musculotendinous septum* called the diaphragm (Gk. *diaphragma,* a partition, wall, barrier). We have seen that the thorax is almost completely filled by the lungs and heart, and by lesser structures located primarily within the mediastinum, while the abdomen is filled by the digestive tract, various glands, and other organs.

Many anatomists and physiologists consider the diaphragm to be the second most important muscle in the body, after the heart.

The diaphragm is often described as being dome-shaped, slightly higher on the right side than on the left; it is said to resemble an inverted bowl. The diaphragm *in situ* is shown in Figures 2-40 and 2-41. From these illustrations it can be seen that the diaphragm is indeed dome-shaped, and as a consequence, many important abdominal organs in contact with its lower surface enjoy the protection of the lower ribs. This is particularly true of the liver and spleen and to some extent the kidneys.

The periphery of the diaphragm consists of muscular fibers that take their origin from the margins at the outlet of the thorax. They course upward and inward and insert into the edges of the central tendon.

The Central Tendon Centrally, the diaphragm consists of an *aponeurosis* which is thin, but extremely strong. This aponeurosis, usually referred to as the central tendon, is located somewhat closer to the front than to the back of the thorax. In outline it is uneven, and is said to resemble a trifoliate leaf. Structurally, the central tendon is composed of several layers of fibers that intersect (indigitate) at different angles. This adds greatly to its strength. The muscular portion of the diaphragm is usually described as having three parts: **sternal, costal,** and **vertebral.**

The Muscular Portion of the Diaphragm The **sternal portion** takes it origin from the lower border and back surface of the xiphoid process. The fibers, which are sometimes tendinous rather than muscular, pass somewhat upward and medially to insert into the front of the middle leaflet of the central tendon. The sternal fibers are the shortest in the diaphragm.

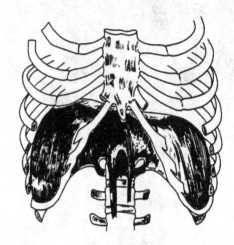

FIGURE 2-40

The diaphragm shown in relation to the rib cage and vertebral column.

FIGURE 2-41

Diaphragm *in situ*. The anterior portion of the rib cage and the abdominal wall have been removed.

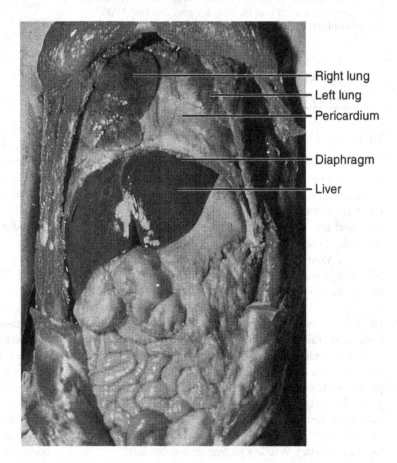

Right lung

Left lung

Pericardium

Diaphragm

Liver

The **costal portion** takes its origin, in the form of fleshy slips, from the lower border and inner surfaces of the cartilages of ribs 7 through 12. Some fibers may originate from the portion of the ribs adjacent to the costal cartilages. These slips of muscle fibers interdigitate with those of the transverse abdominis muscles (to be considered later). The fibers of the costal portion course at first sharply upward, and then medially to insert into the central tendon.

The **vertebral portion** takes its origin from the upper lumbar vertebrae by means of two stout pillars of muscle fibers known as **crura** (plural of L. *crus*, pertaining to a leglike part). The **right crus** is thicker and longer than the left. It arises from the upper three or four lumbar vertebrae and their intervertebral discs. Its fibers fan out as they course upward and medially. They decussate and encircle the esophagus before inserting into the central tendon. The **left crus** arises from the upper two lumbar vertebrae and their intervertebral disc. Its fibers course steeply upward and medially to insert into the central tendon. Figure 2-42 indicates that the diaphragm is pierced by three large apertures and several smaller ones.

Openings in the Diaphragm

The **aortic hiatus,** formed largely by the union of the crura, is located just at the level of the last thoracic vertebra. It permits the descending aorta to pass from the thorax into the abdomen.

The **esophageal hiatus** is located just posterior to the middle leaflet of the central tendon. It is nearly oval-shaped and is surrounded by a sphincter of muscle fibers. The esophagus and several small arteries pass through it.

The **foramen vena cava** is located at the level of the eighth thoracic vertebra, and it pierces the central tendon at the junction of the right and middle leaflets. The inferior vena cava,[9] several nerve bundles, and lymph vessels pass through it.

The Diaphragm and Associated Structures

Descriptions as well as illustrations suggest that, except for its muscular attachment at the thoracic outlet, the diaphragm has absolutely no continuity, functionally or anatomically, with the remainder of the torso. To fully appreciate the role of the diaphragm we should be aware of the relationships between it and associated structures, one of which is the pericardium, located in the mediastinum between the lungs, as illustrated in Figure 2-43.

The **pericardium** (Gk. *peri*, around + Gk. *kardia*, heart) is a membranous sac that encloses the heart. It is comprised of two distinctly different types of membranes, the **serous membrane** and the **fibrous sac.** The serous pericardium lines the fibrous sac and covers the outside of the heart.

The **fibrous pericardium** forms a flasklike sac surrounding the serous pericardium, in addition to the great blood vessels of the heart. It is an extremely tough membrane and quite thick. Its anterior surface is adherent to all the structures surrounding it. The sac attaches to the manubrium and xiphoid process of the sternum and to the vertebral column, and also securely attaches and blends into the central tendon and the muscular part of the left side of the diaphragm. In other words, *the fibrous pericardium becomes a part of the diaphragm.*

As shown schematically in Figure 2-44, the mediastinal surfaces of the pericardial sac are opposed by the mediastinal pleural membranes. According to Gray (1973) the membranes are adherent but not fused. The phrenic nerve and accompanying blood vessels are contained between them.

Thus, we see that the heart lies virtually unattached to its surroundings and is held in place primarily by the blood vessels that enter and leave the heart. *Because of the anatomical continuity between the thoracic surface of the diaphragm and the fibrous pericardium, the descent of the diaphragm will also cause the entire pericardium to follow,* just as the lungs follow movements of the diaphragm and thoracic walls. In addition, the viscera of the mediastinum (heart, blood and lymph vessels, esophagus, etc.) are all subjected to the same pressures that influence the lungs.

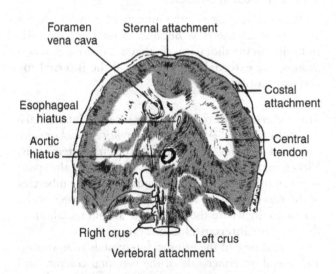

FIGURE 2-42

A diaphragm as seen from beneath. Blood vessels and the esophagus pass through it.

Foramen vena cava
Sternal attachment
Esophageal hiatus
Aortic hiatus
Costal attachment
Central tendon
Right crus
Left crus
Vertebral attachment

---

[9]The inferior vena cava is the venous trunk for the abdominal and pelvic viscera and for the lower extremities.

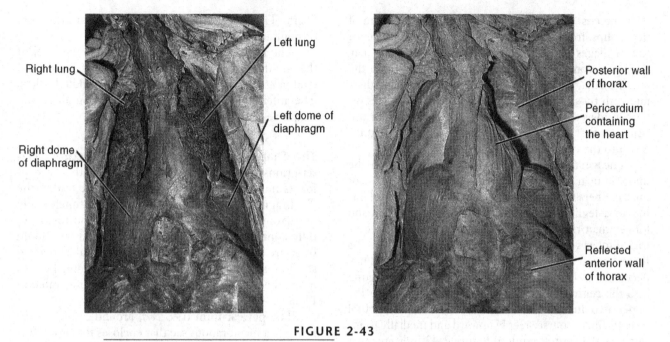

FIGURE 2-43

Diaphragm shown in relation to the lungs and pericardium (left). On the right, the thoracic cavity with lungs removed, to show relationship of diaphragm to pericardium.

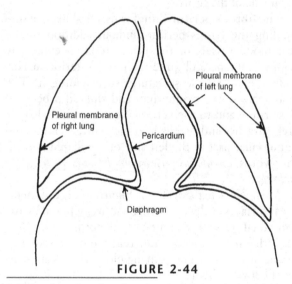

FIGURE 2-44

Relationship of pericardium to pleural membranes and to the diaphragm.

Inferiorly, the **liver,** which is almost totally invested with peritoneum, is suspended from the diaphragm by five ligaments formed by peritoneal folds. Similar ligaments also connect the liver to the anterior abdominal wall, the stomach, and the duodenum (a portion of the small intestine).

The diaphragm's anatomical continuity with structures of the thorax and abdomen necessitates functional continuity, as well. The diaphragm and its associated structures must always move in concert.

The **diaphragm** is unique in that it appears to be an *unpaired muscle.* It does, however, enjoy a *bilateral nerve and blood supply,* and so in a certain sense, it is a complex structure receiving muscular contributions from both sides of the body. With very few exceptions, all muscles in the body are paired. Unless stated otherwise, the remaining muscles described in the text should be so regarded.

The Intercostal Muscles

As their name suggests, the intercostal muscles are located between the ribs. Because of their surface relationships on the thoracic wall, they are divided into two groups, the **external intercostal** and the **internal intercostal muscles.**

The External Intercostals   The external intercostals, shown in Figure 2-45, are a *more prominent and stronger* group of muscles than are the internal intercostals. Eleven in number on either side, they occupy the space between the ribs in an area extending from the tubercles of the ribs dorsally to a region near the cartilages of the ribs ventrally where they terminate as thin membranes, the **anterior intercostal membranes.**

The course of the external intercostals is downward and lateral on either side of the vertebral column, and since the thorax is essentially circular, the course is downward and medially directed in front. As the muscles approach the ventral thoracic wall, they rapidly become less

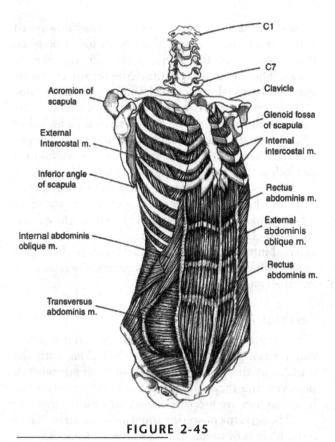

FIGURE 2-45

Principal muscles of respiration. (From Eileen and W. Zemlin, *Study Guide/Workbook to Accompany Speech and Hearing Science,* 3rd ed., 1988, Stipes Publishing Co.)

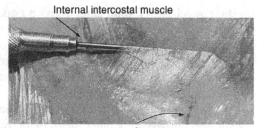

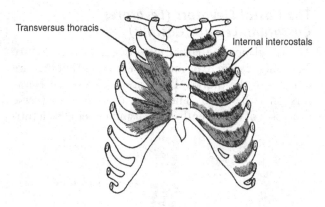

FIGURE 2-46

External intercostal muscle with probe under anterior intercostal membrane. The muscle fails to continue to the chondro-osseous union.

FIGURE 2-47

The rib cage as seen from within, showing transversus thoracis and internal intercostal muscles.

muscular and more aponeurotic in nature, and at distances 4 cm or more from the **chondro-osseous union,** the tissue is exclusively connective. The probe shown in Figure 2-46 is actually visible through the anterior intercostal membrane, which in this case terminates near the chondro-osseous union and is not continued to the sternum, as is often reported.

The Internal Intercostals The internal intercostal muscles, shown in Figure 2-47, lie just deep to the external intercostals and are also eleven in number. They occupy an area extending from the anterior limits of the intercostal spaces to the angle of the rib posteriorly, where they are continued to the vertebral column as thin aponeuroses, the **posterior intercostal membranes.** Thus, *the area just lateral to the vertebral column (paravertebral) is devoid of internal intercostal muscles,* while *the area immediately lateral to the sternum (parasternal) contains muscle fibers of just the internal intercostal muscles.* The significance of this muscle distribution will become apparent when we discuss the functions of the breathing musculature later in the chapter.

The internal intercostals take their origin from the lower borders of the upper eleven ribs and course from above to insert into the inner aspect of the ribs immediately below. Parasternally, the course of the fibers is downward and lateral. In other words, *the course of the fibers of the internal intercostals is just about at right angles to the course of the external intercostals.*

The Subcostals (Intracostals) Another group of muscles, the subcostals, is frequently recognized, although they are highly variable and are usually well developed only on the inner posterior surface of the lower thoracic wall. They form a *musculomembranous sheet that lines the back of the thorax,* lateral to the tubercles of the ribs. They have the same course as the internal intercostals and, in fact, can be distinguished from them only because they are not usually confined to just one intercostal space.

Transversus Thoracis (Triangularis Sterni)

The inner surface of the anterior thoracic wall contains the transversus thoracis muscles. Irregular muscles, they vary in their attachments, sometimes even on opposite sides of the same specimen. They are thin, fan-shaped muscles that originate from the posterior surface of the body of the sternum, from the posterior surface of the xiphoid process, and from the posterior surfaces of the chondral portion of ribs 5 through 7.

Their fibers course upward and outward to insert into the lower borders and inner surfaces of ribs 2 through 6. As shown in Figure 2-47, the uppermost fibers course almost vertically, while the lower fibers course horizontally. The lowermost fibers are usually continuous with those of the transversus abdominis, an abdominal muscle to be considered later.

The Costal Elevators (Levatores Costarum, Levator Costalis)

At first glance the costal elevators, shown in Figure 2-48, might seem to be muscles of the back, but they are muscles of the thorax. There are twelve costal elevators on either side. They arise from the transverse processes of the seventh cervical and upper eleven tho-

racic vertebrae. The fibers course obliquely downward and lateralward, diverging slightly, to insert between the tubercle and the angle of the rib immediately below. These muscles constitute the **levatores costaruman breves** (short costal elevators). The lower four muscles divide into two fasciculi, one of which is the same as the pars breves just described. The other passes over the rib immediately beneath their origin and continues to the outer surfaces of the second rib just below their point of origin. These fasciculi constitute the **levatores costarum longi** (long costal elevators) which, from a mechanical standpoint, are more efficient than the pars breves. Very well developed and stout muscles, they appear to be a continuation of the external intercostals. In fact, it is difficult to determine exactly where the external intercostals cease and the costal elevators begin.

Serratus Posterior Muscles

The serratus posterior superior and the serratus posterior inferior are sometimes described along with the muscles of the back. They are not postural muscles, however, and they are clearly not associated with the limbs, so they are properly associated with the thorax.

The **serratus posterior superior** is shown in Figure 2-48. It arises by means of a broad tendon from the spinous processes of the seventh cervical vertebra and of the first two or three thoracic vertebrae. The fibers, which are usually in the form of fleshy digitations, course downward and laterally to insert, just lateral to the angles, on ribs two through five.

The **serratus posterior inferior** muscle, shown in Figure 2-48, is an irregularly shaped, quadrilateral sheet of tissue which originates by means of aponeuroses from the spinous processes of thoracic vertebrae eleven and twelve, and from lumbar vertebrae one, two, and three. The fibers course upward and obliquely lateralward to insert, just beyond the angles, into the inferior borders of ribs eight through twelve. The serratus posterior muscles are largely aponeurotic and in many specimens appear to be very thin and poorly developed, and sometimes are entirely absent.

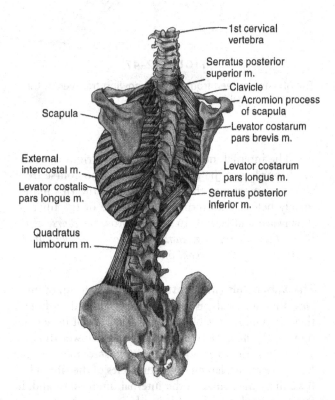

FIGURE 2-48

Costal elevators (levatores costarum), serratus posterior superior, serratus posterior inferior, and quadratus lumborum muscles. (From Eileen and W. Zemlin, *Study Guide/Workbook to Accompany Speech and Hearing Science*, 3rd ed., 1988, Stipes Publishing Co.)

Action of the Muscles of the Thorax

A complete description of the contributions of a muscle may be an arduous task. In addition to anatomical descriptions, the effects of contraction and the circumstances under which contraction occurs must be determined. **Electromyography** has proven valuable in understanding the functions of musculature, and **radiography** (x-ray) has contributed greatly to our knowledge of the action of the diaphragm.

Action of the Diaphragm

Contraction of the diaphragm pulls the central tendon downward and forward, thus increasing the vertical dimension of the thoracic cavity. Because of pleural linkage, the lungs are stretched, producing negative alveolar pressure. In addition, there is a decrease in volume and an increase in pressure within the abdominal cavity. The descending diaphragm acts like a piston, compressing the abdominal viscera and causing them to be displaced downward and forward against the abdominal wall. As a result, the abdominal wall may be distended during inhalation.

Research Findings Wade and Gilson (1951), using x-ray, found the *vertical excursion* of the diaphragm amounted to 1.5 cm during quiet breathing and 6 to 7 cm during deep breathing. In addition, Wade (1954), found that each centimeter of *diaphragmatic descent* accounts for an inhalation of about 350 cc of air. Inasmuch as diaphragm movement is about 1.5 cm during quiet breathing, it alone ought to be responsible for inhalation of 525 cc of air, which is about the amount of air many of us exchange during a cycle of quiet breathing.

In 1936 Bloomer pioneered in the use of x-ray for the study of the speech mechanism. He found that *diaphragmatic movement* was in a downward and forward direction and that it could account for anywhere from 29 to 63 percent of maximum inspiratory capacity. He noted that the upper ribs have movement similar to that of the other ribs but that the degree of *costal mobility* decreased from the second or third rib downward. He also found that the *sternum* moved upward and outward during inhalation and that it maintained its angle relative to the vertical axis of the thorax.

Electromyographic studies of diaphragm activity in conscious humans are few. Because of the location of the diaphragm in the body, exploration by means of surface electrodes has not been successful, and as Campbell (1958) has pointed out, "There are obvious ethical objections to the exploration of the diaphragm with needle electrodes in conscious human subjects." The ethical objections remain, but technological advances have circumvented many problems associated with early electrode designs, and although the data are limited in their usefulness, diaphragmatic activity patterns from anesthetized animals can provide some insight into the mechanics of the muscles of breathing.

We have obtained a number of electromyographic recordings from dogs and cats. In each instance, activity of the diaphragm was found throughout the inhalation phase, with its activity increasing progressively throughout the inspiration. In most cases the activity extended into the beginnings of the expiratory phase

and then decreased quickly. Because of the uncertain effects of the surgical opening of the abdomen in some instances, the results should be viewed with some caution.

The patterns of diaphragm activity have been studied using needle electrodes inserted through the body wall in the costal part of human subjects, and results very similar to those obtained from animals have emerged (Koepke, et al., 1955; Murphy, et al., 1959; and Taylor, 1960).

Electrode leads have also been introduced in the esophagus so that the vertebral portion of the diaphragm is measured. Draper et al., (1959) seem to have been successful in obtaining electromyographic recordings from conscious humans. *Their subjects swallowed a catheter (thin tube) that contained electrodes and electrode leads.* The tube was adjusted in height until the electrodes were at the point where the esophagus passes through the diaphragm. Thus, in effect, the electrodes were placed directly on the vertebral portion of the diaphragm. These subjects showed diaphragm activity throughout the inhalation phase, and in most cases the activity extended only slightly into the expiratory phase. Two of their subjects showed diaphragm activity throughout inhalation, during the initial phase of exhalation, and in addition, toward the end of exhalation when the quantity of air in the lungs was minimal.

Agostoni (1964) reports that the diaphragm contracts toward the very end of maximum expiration. Its activity increases progressively up to the very end, limiting a further collapse of the lungs. He also found that the diaphragm contracts strongly during expulsive efforts, probably in all efforts requiring the rigidity of the thoracic-abdominal system, especially when transmission of abdominal pressure to the thoracic cavity is necessary in coughing, sneezing, and laughing.

Mechanics of the Diaphragm The mechanics of the diaphragm are complex. We have seen that downward and forward movement of the central tendon results in an increase in the vertical dimensions of the thoracic cavity and a decrease in intrapulmonic pressure. This causes a simultaneous decrease in the volume of the abdominal cavity, and an increase in intraabdominal pressure. As can be seen from Figure 2-49, the course of the muscular fibers of the diaphragm is nearly vertical, while the tendinous or aponeurotic (nonmuscular) portion, which is continuous with the pericardium, is somewhat flattened. During inhalation the muscular portion of the diaphragm shortens and the diaphragm, in its entirety, descends but without any substantial change in its curvature.

The costal margin of the diaphragm is usually regarded as relatively fixed, both in position and in transverse dimensions. Under these conditions, contraction

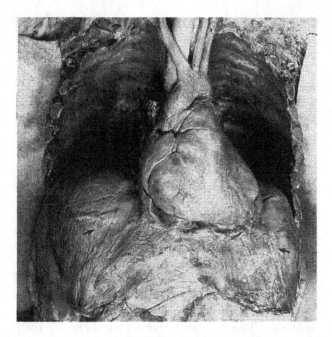

FIGURE 2-49

The heart shown in relation to the diaphragm, which is indicated by arrows.

of the diaphragm may compress the abdominal viscera and raise intraabdominal pressure to the extent there is an expansion of the abdominal wall. This is sometimes known as **abdominal** or **diaphragmatic breathing.**

A rather common result of contraction of the diaphragm is an expansion at the base of the thorax. The diaphragm is apparently responsible for thrusting the ribs upward and rotating them outward. The mechanism is as follows: When the diaphragm is in its normal, uncontracted state, it has a pronounced dome shape, and the direction of the costal fibers is almost vertical. *With the abdominal viscera in their normal spatial relation with the diaphragm, they may act as a fulcrum when the diaphragm contracts.* The result is a downward force against the viscera and an upward force against the costal margin of the diaphragm. This action, illustrated in Figure 2-50, is presumably what takes place during the so-called **costal breathing.** The base of the thorax expands with each inhalation, and the abdominal viscera may simply fill the space created in the abdomen. Very little protrusion of the abdominal wall takes place, and, in fact, it may actually be drawn in with each inhalation.

With progressively deeper breathing, however, expansion of the base of the thorax may diminish, and protrusion of the abdominal wall will increase proportionately. Near the very end of maximum inhalation the situation may be reversed; that is, the thorax may expand rapidly to the extent that the abdominal wall may actually be drawn inward.

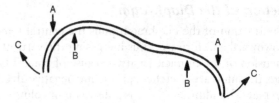

FIGURE 2-50

Schematic of the way in which a downward movement of the diaphragm is resolved into an upward movement of the costal margin. Contraction of the vertically directed diaphragmatic muscle fibers (A) would lower the dome of the diaphragm, as shown by arrows at (A). Resistance offered by abdominal viscera (B) prevents diaphragmatic descent, and the downward movement is resolved into an upward and outward movement at the costal margin (C).

Control of Diaphragmatic Action Although we seemingly have considerable voluntary control over the rate and depth of breathing, *there appears to be little if any voluntary control over diaphragmatic action,* according to Wade (1951, 1954) and Campbell and Jellife (1951, unpublished; reported by Campbell, 1958), who examined diaphragmatic movements in physiotherapists and singing teachers who believed they had voluntary control of their diaphragms. Although these subjects were able to control rib movements during breathing, there was no evidence of voluntary control over the regular muscles of inhalation, particularly the diaphragm.

On the other hand, we have considerable voluntary control over independent movement of the thoracic structures and the abdominal wall. Most of us, for example, have little difficulty inhaling, even forcefully, and compressing the abdominal wall simultaneously. As Hixon et al. (1973) state, "It is possible to move air both in and out of the lungs through a wide variety of relative displacements of the thoracic cage and diaphragm-abdomen."

Regardless of its significance in humans, *a functional diaphragm is not essential for breathing* (Agostoni, 1964), and there is considerable compensatory potential provided by other musculature. The most frequently cited accessory or auxiliary muscles of respiration seem to be the intercostal muscles of the thorax and the scalene and sternocleidomastoid muscles of the neck. Other muscles of the neck and torso may be involved in respiration, but to a lesser extent than the intercostals, and contributions of some of these muscles may be open to some question.

Action of the Intercostal Muscles

The functions of the intercostal musculature are not at all free from debate. Agostoni (1964) says, "The controversy on the action and function of the intercostal muscles has been such since the time of Galen that the historical aspect of the problem has overwhelmed the physiological one."

There seems to be general agreement, however, that as a group both the *external and internal intercostal muscles contribute to the rigidity of the thoracic wall* by preventing the intercostal spaces from bulging in and out during breathing. These muscles presumably *help control the degree of space between the ribs*, and in addition, they *couple the ribs*, one to the other, so that movement of any given rib will be transmitted to adjacent ribs and influence their position.

Probable Mechanical Effects of Contraction

It may be of value to examine the attachments and courses of the intercostals and to speculate as to the probable mechanical effects produced by their contraction. However, the best we can hope for in such an enterprise is to support someone who attempted much the same thing well over two hundred years ago.

External Intercostals. You will recall that the external intercostal muscles occupy the space between the ribs, in an area extending from the tubercle posteriorly to near the anterior extreme of the osseous portion of the rib. They are deficient in the chondral portion of the ribs. The fibers arise from the lower border of a rib and insert into the upper border of the rib immediately below. Anteriorly the fibers course obliquely down and forward (medially), and posteriorly they course downward and outward (laterally).

The course and probable effects of contraction of the external intercostals are shown schematically in Figure 2-51. The arrangements of the fibers are such that a Class III lever is formed with both the upper and lower ribs. Note, however, that the lever system of the lower rib is considerably more efficient than is that for the upper rib; that is, the force tending to raise the lower rib greatly exceeds the force tending to lower the upper rib. As a consequence, *contraction of each external intercostal muscle ought to elevate the lower rib to which it attaches.*

It is also important to note that this tendency to elevate the ribs would be minimized or negated if the external intercostals were to occupy the intercostal spaces in the chondral portion of the ribs. Fortunately for our mechanical model, this is not the case. Thus, on a mechanical basis, the *external intercostal muscles ought to act as muscles of inhalation*, or at least predispose the ribs to elevate.

Internal Intercostals. The internal intercostal muscles occupy an area extending from the anterior limits of the intercostal spaces to the angle of the ribs posteriorly. In front, the course of the fibers is downward and outward, while in the back, the course is downward and inward. The course and probable effects of contraction of the intercartilaginous portion of the internal intercostals are shown schematically in Figure 2-52. Note that the arrangement of the fibers is such that a Class III lever is formed with both the upper and lower rib, and, as in the case of the external intercostals, the elevating force applied to the lower rib exceeds the depressing force applied to the upper rib. On the basis of mechanics, the **intercartilaginous portion** of the internal intercostals should also be *inspiratory in function.*

The **interosseous portion** of the internal intercostals probably decreases the intercostal spaces and,

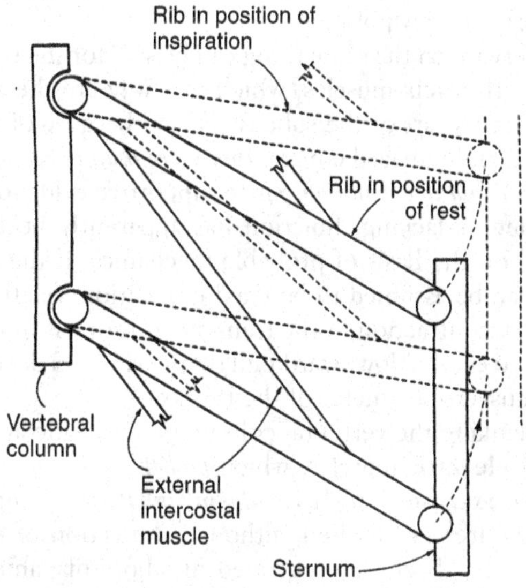

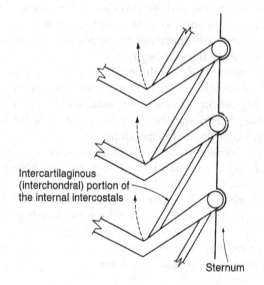

FIGURE 2-51

Schematic of the action of the external intercostal muscles. Muscle contraction exerts an upward force on the rib to enlarge the rib cage.

FIGURE 2-52

Schematic of the action of the intercartilaginous portion of the internal intercostal muscles. Contraction of the parasternal portion of the muscle elevates the ribs to enlarge the rib cage.

through the abdominal muscles, *depresses the ribs to aid in exhalation.*

Theory of Intercostal Muscle Function Probably the most widely accepted theory of intercostal muscle function is Hamberger's (Campbell, 1958), which states that *as the external intercostals and the intercartilaginous portion of the internal intercostals contract they elevate the ribs, and as the interosseous portion of the internal intercostals contract they depress the ribs.*

This theory was advanced in 1748, but for the most part Hamberger's conclusions have been substantiated by electromyographic findings. Campbell (1955) examined the intercostals in young male subjects and detected activity in the lower intercostal spaces (fifth through ninth) during inspiration. He also found that the muscular activity increased with progressively deeper inspiratory efforts. These same muscles were found to be inactive throughout expiration during quiet and rapid breathing. Draper et al. (1959), using needle electrodes, detected activity in the interosseous portion of the internal intercostals during speech production with a low expiratory reserve.

Checking Action After a deep inhalation preparatory to speech, the elastic recoil of the thorax may provide air pressure in excess of that required by the larynx for voice production. Researchers have found that under such circumstances *inspiratory muscles may continue to be active and thus counteract the elastic recoil of the inflated thorax.* During speech production, as the volume of air in the lungs decreases, the "relaxation pressure" becomes progressively less, and the checking action provided by the inspiratory muscles ceases; and, at some point, in order to maintain the necessary air pressure for speech, the expiratory muscles begin to contract with an ever-increasing vigor. Research suggests that the external intercostal muscles are largely responsible for providing checking action. This activity continues as long as relaxation pressure is in excess of that required by the larynx and articulators for speech production.

The inspiratory and expiratory muscles do not act completely as antagonists, with one set "switching on" while the other set quickly "switches off." Rather, they act in concert with both groups in a preparatory set disposed to complement the contributions of each group. As a consequence, the expiratory air flow is maintained under very precise control in order to meet the requirements of the larynx and articulators.

Summary of Intercostal Muscle Function The intercostal muscles are probably major contributors to inspiratory efforts. Campbell (1958) has shown that high levels of pulmonary ventilation can be produced with just the intercostal muscles, in the case of paralysis of the diaphragm, for example. In addition to producing rib movements during inhalation, the intercostal muscles contribute to the rigidity of the thoracic wall by preventing the intercostal spaces from bulging in and out during breathing. These muscles also help to control the amount of space between the ribs and, in addition, couple the ribs, one to the other, so that movements of any given rib will influence the position of adjacent ribs. This latter activity may be seen during expiratory efforts, when the lower ribs are drawn downward by contraction of the abdominal muscles.

It can be stated with reasonable certainty that the external intercostals and the intercartilaginous portion of the internal intercostals are major contributors to inspiratory efforts. These muscles are relatively inactive during expiration in quiet breathing, but they become very active during forced expiratory efforts. They also seem to remain in a contracted state after maximum inhalation and provide a checking action to counteract the relaxation pressure generated by the thorax-lung unit. And, finally, the interosseous portion of the internal intercostals is probably active during speech production, particularly on low expiratory reserve air.

Possible Contributions of Other Thoracic Muscles

Other muscles of the thorax have the potential to influence rib movement. Two of them are located on the inner surface of the thoracic wall. The **subcostals,** because of their location on the inner-posterior surface of the lower thoracic wall, *probably function in an expiratory role to depress the ribs,* but there is no direct evidence to support this viewpoint.

Very much the same thing can be said for the **transversus thoracis** muscles, which in a way are the anterior counterpart of the subcostals, and because of their upward and outward course, *they more than likely depress the ribs to aid in exhalation.* Since supportive evidence for this view is lacking, function has apparently been assigned on the basis of probable mechanics. If the sternum can be assumed to be fixed in position, relative to the ribs, contraction of the transversus thoracis muscles ought to exert a downward pull on the ribs and decrease the transverse diameter of the thorax.

Flanking the vertebral column on each side are the **costal elevator** muscles, which *probably play an important role as elevators of the ribs during inhalation.* Supportive data are very limited, although the action of these muscles has been demonstrated in laboratory animals. The costal elevators are also described as postural muscles; they extend the vertebral column, bend it laterally, and may even contribute to rotation of the torso.

Two additional muscles on the dorsum of the thorax should be mentioned, although their contribution to the respiratory process has yet to be verified. They are the **serratus posterior superior** and the **serratus posterior inferior.**

The fibers of the **serratus posterior superior** are so oriented as to enlarge the rib cage, so they may actively elevate ribs, or they may simply complement the action of other muscles, such as the intercostals and the costal elevators.

The **serratus posterior inferior** muscle may contribute to deep or forced inhalation; that is, during forced inhalation, it may anchor the lower four ribs and prevent them from being elevated as the diaphragm exerts pressure downward upon the abdominal viscera. On the other hand, with the lower ribs free to move, such a compression might simply maintain the diaphragm in the same position while the ribs move upward. Such action would result in little or no increase in the vertical diameter of the thoracic cavity, but its transverse dimensions would increase. The most probable action of the muscle is simply to exert a downward force on the lower ribs during forced exhalation.

Muscles of the Neck and Their Action

With the head in a fixed position, contraction of two neck muscles—the **sternocleidomastoid,** a lateral cervical muscle, and the **scalenes,** which are lateral vertebral muscles—may lift the sternum and the two uppermost ribs. They are often mentioned as muscles of inhalation.

Sternocleidomastoid (Sternomastoid)

The sternocleidomastoid, so named because of its attachments, is located on the anterolateral aspect of the neck. As shown in Figure 2-53, it is a prominent muscle that takes its origin in the form of sternal and clavicular heads, but this is quite variable. The **sternal head** arises from the anterior surface of the manubrium of the sternum. It courses upward, backward, and somewhat laterally. The **clavicular head** originates from the superior surface of the sternal end of the clavicle. The fibers course almost vertically upward. The clavicular and sternal heads unite, course upward and laterally across the side of the neck, and insert as a single muscle into the mastoid process of the temporal bone. A few fibers insert into an adjacent portion of the occipital bone known as the **superior nuchal line** (nape of the neck).

Upon *unilateral contraction* this muscle may draw the side of the head toward the shoulder and, at the same time, rotate it. We should note that because the insertion of this muscle is behind the rotational axis of the head, contraction of the right sternocleidomastoid will rotate the head toward the left. *Bilateral contraction* of the muscles tends to flex the neck toward the thorax.

When the head is held in a fixed position, this muscle may raise the sternum and clavicle to assist in inhala-

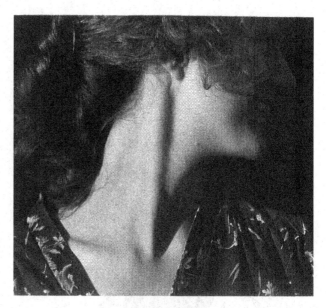

FIGURE 2-53

The sternocleidomastoid muscle is instrumental in turning the head. With the head fixed this muscle can assist in elevating the sternum during inspiration.

tion. Elevation of the sternum increases the anteroposterior diameter of the thorax.

The **sternocleidomastoid** is a highly variable muscle; much of its variability stems from the extent of its origin along the clavicle, and in its blending of the clavicular and sternal portions. In some instances the clavicular head may be a rounded bundle of muscle similar to the sternal head, and in other cases it may be a broad sheet of muscle, or a number of slips, distributed over 6–10 cm of the medial end of the clavicle.

The sternocleidomastoid is an important landmark muscle of the neck. It separates the anterior from the posterior cervical triangles, both of which can be further divided into triangles which are regions of approach to many important structures of the neck (see Figure 2-54).

Scalene (Lateral Vertebral) Muscles

The deep muscles of the anterolateral region of the neck are divided into an inner and an outer group, with the anterior tubercles of the cervical vertebrae forming the boundary line. The *inner group* is also known as the **prevertebral muscles,** and they flex the neck. The *outer group* constitutes the **lateral vertebral muscles,** which may at times serve as supplementary muscles of inhalation. This group, shown in Figure 2-55, consists of the scalene (Gk. *skalenos,* uneven) muscles, which course from their origin on the transverse processes of the cervical vertebrae to their insertion on the uppermost two ribs. (In some anatomy textbooks the ribs are given as the origin of the scaleni, and cervical vertebrae are given as the points of insertion.)

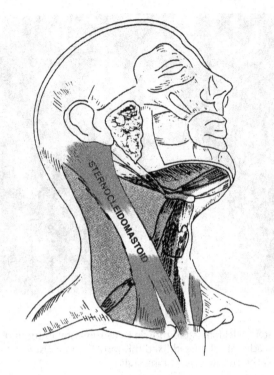

FIGURE 2-54

The anterior and posterior compartments of the neck (anterior and posterior cervical triangles) shown in relation to adjacent structures and the sternocleidomastoid muscle.

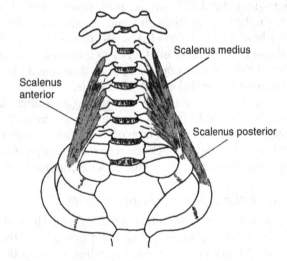

FIGURE 2-55

The scaleni facilitate flexion of the cervical column. With the head fixed, they elevate and fix the upper ribs.

The **anterior scalene** (scalenus anterior) muscle takes it origin, by means of four tendinous slips, from the transverse processes of cervical vertebrae 3 through 6. The fibers course almost vertically downward to insert into the scalene tubercle, which is located on the inner border of the upper surface of the first rib. The

anterior scalene is important for reference purposes in locating adjacent structures in the neck. In fact, Woodburne (1973) regards the anterior scalene as one of the "essential muscular landmarks of the neck."

The **middle scalene** (scalenus medius) is the *largest* and the *longest* muscle in the group. As the name implies, the middle scalene is located deep to the anterior scalene. It takes its origin, by means of five tendinous slips, from the transverse processes of cervical vertebrae 2 through 7. The fibers course vertically downward and insert into the upper surface of the first rib by means of a broad tendon.

The **posterior scalene** (scalenus posterior) is the *smallest* of the scalenes and the *deepest*. It takes its origin from the posterior tubercles of the lowest two or three cervical vertebrae. The fibers course down and laterally to insert into the outer surface of the second rib.

As a group the scalenes are inspiratory, acting to raise the first two ribs. Acting from below, the muscles on one side will bend the cervical column toward the side contracting, and when all scalene groups are active, they facilitate flexion of the cervical column.

> **CLINICAL NOTE:** Exaggerated use of the neck musculature is frequently seen in individuals with chronic lung disease. Pronounced use of the upper thoracic and neck muscles during inhalation is called **clavicular breathing**, and it is usually regarded as inefficient and undesirable. It may be seen, however, as a form of compensatory behavior in persons with paralysis of the principal breathing musculature.

Musculature of the Torso

Virtually all the musculature of the torso contributes either directly or indirectly to the respiratory process. Indeed, any structure or organ that contributes to the general well-being of an individual contributes to healthy function of systems in general, including the respiratory system. This tendency toward uniformity or stability in the normal body states of the organism is called **homeostasis.**

The assignment of specific respiratory functions, especially on the basis of muscle architecture, is probably hazardous. Nevertheless, the contributions of accessory musculature, be they real or potential, cannot be ignored, particularly from a clinical standpoint. We know, for example, that the diaphragm is not essential to sustain life, but very little is known regarding the potential contributions of compensatory musculature, in the event of diaphragmatic paralysis.

A detailed description of the deep muscles of the trunk is simply beyond the scope of this text and would probably contribute little if anything to an understanding of the respiratory process. And yet these muscles should not be completely ignored.

Muscles of the Upper Limb and Back

The superficial muscles of the back are all associated with connecting the upper limb to the vertebral column. They are the **trapezius, lattisimus dorsi, rhomboids** (major and minor), and the **levator scapulae** (Figure 2-56).

Trapezius. The most superficial muscle of the back is the trapezius. A flat triangular muscle, it covers the upper back, the neck, and shoulders. It has a broad origin, from the base of the skull to the twelfth thoracic vertebra. The muscle fibers converge to insert on the clavicle and the acromion and spine of the scapula. The trapezius rotates the scapula, raises the shoulder, helps to turn the head, and assists in tilting it backward. We also use these muscles to brace our shoulders and to shrug our shoulders to indicate "I don't know" or "I don't care."

Latissimus dorsi. The latissimus dorsi (L. *latus*, widest + L. *dorsum*, back), also a superficial muscle of the back, forms the second muscular layer. It arises from the spines of the lower thoracic, the lumbar vertebrae, and the sacrum, and from the posterior third of the iliac crest by means of a broad aponeurosis. Additional fibers originate from the outer surface of ribs 10, 11, and 12. The fibers converge rapidly and insert by means of a stout tendon into the upper humerus.

The principal function of this muscle is to extend, adduct, and rotate the arm medially, but because of its costal attachments, it may influence the lower three or four ribs. The latissimus dorsi has not been studied extensively, but the limited data fail to support a respiratory function. Tokizane, Kawamata, and Tokizane (1952) reported muscular activity during deep breathing.

Rhomboids. The thick and powerful rhomboids, shown in Figure 2-56, are divided into **major** and **minor** parts on the basis of their origins, but as a whole the muscle arises by tendinous slips from the spinous processes of the seventh cervical through the fifth thoracic vertebrae. It courses obliquely down and laterally to insert along the vertebral border of the scapula. Its action is to draw the scapula toward the vertebral column and to adduct the arm.

Levator scapulae. The levator scapulae are straplike muscles arising from the transverse processes of cervical vertebrae 1 through 4. As shown in Figure 2-56, their course is almost vertically downward where they insert into the vertebral border of the scapula. Their function, of course, is to elevate and steady the scapula.

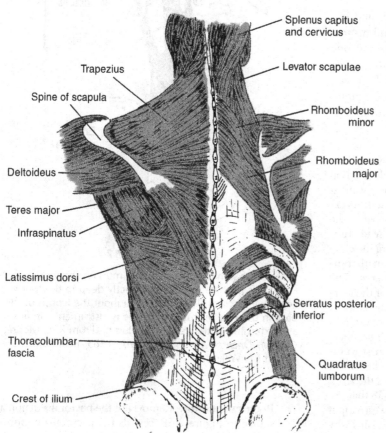

FIGURE 2-56

Muscles that connect the upper limb to the vertebral column (trapezius, lattissimus dorsi, rhomboids, and levator scapulae).

Splenus capitus and cervicus

Trapezius

Levator scapulae

Spine of scapula

Rhomboideus minor

Rhomboideus major

Deltoideus

Teres major

Infraspinatus

Latissimus dorsi

Serratus posterior inferior

Thoracolumbar fascia

Quadratus lumborum

Crest of ilium

Deep Muscles of the Back

Removal of the superficial muscles of the back reveals the **erector spinae** or **sacrospinalis** muscles, which, as a group, are postural in function. The erector spinae consists of vertically directed medial, intermediate, and lateral columns, and each of these columns is in turn divided into three components. The general plan of these muscles is shown in Figure 2-57 and listed below. Any respiratory function that may be assigned to these muscles is largely conjecture. Removal of the erector spinae reveals the **transversospinalis muscles.** They act directly on the vertebral column.

General Plan of the Deep Muscles of the Trunk

A. ERECTOR SPINAE or SACROSPINALIS (superficial stratum)
   1. Iliocostalis (dorsi, cervicis, lumborum)
   2. Longissimus (dorsi, cervicis, capitis)
   3. Spinalis (dorsi, cervicis, capitis)
B. TRANSVERSOSPINALIS (deep stratum)
   1. Rotatores (deepest)
   2. Semispinalis (thoracis, cervicis, capitis)
   3. Multifidus
   4. Suboccipital (rectus, oblique capitis)

Muscles of the Chest Wall and Shoulder

Four muscles connect the arm to the anterior and lateral thorax. They are the **pectoralis major** and **minor, subclavius,** and **serratus anterior.** All of them at one time or another have been assigned a respiratory role, and in particular, an inspiratory one. There is, however, virtually no supportive evidence for such an assignment, except for the fact that posture can influence total pulmonary compliance.

Pectoralis major. The pectoralis major, shown in Figure 2-58, is a prominent fan-shaped muscle located on the superficial surface of the anterior thoracic wall. It makes up most of the muscular bulk of the chest. Its extensive origin is usually considered in two parts, the clavicular and sternal heads. The **clavicular head** arises along the anterior surface of the medial half of the clavicle, and it forms a thick band of muscle fibers that inserts into the greater tubercle of the humerus. The **sternal head** arises from the entire length of the sternum, from the costal cartilages of ribs 1 through 6 or 7, and often from the aponeurosis of the oblique external abdominis muscle (to be considered later). The fibers converge rapidly as they course across the chest to insert in the greater tubercle of the humerus. The sternal head comprises the muscular mass that forms the front wall of the axilla (armpit). Note in Figure 2-58 that the fibers decussate, so that those with the lowest origin have the highest point of insertion, which explains why this muscle can aid in the rotation of the arm.

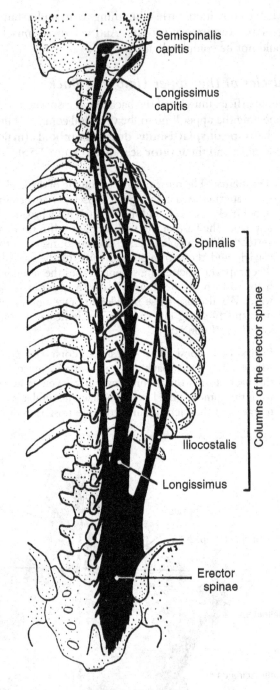

FIGURE 2-57

The erector spinae or sacrospinalis muscles shown schematically. This massive muscle lies directly deep to the thoracolumbar fascia and ascends throughout the length of the back in three columns. The muscle is instrumental in flexion and extension of the vertebral column. (From K. L. Moore, *Clinically Oriented Anatomy,* 2nd ed., 1985, Baltimore, Williams & Wilkins.)

Pectoralis minor. Removal of the pectoralis major, as shown in Figure 2-58, reveals the pectoralis minor as well as the subclavius muscle. Fibers of the pectoralis

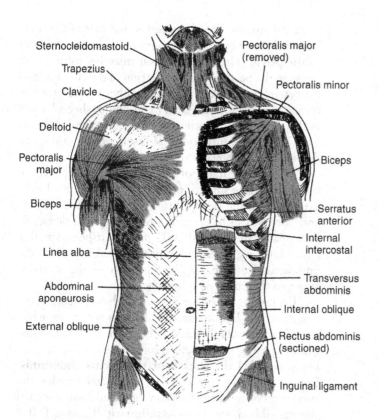

FIGURE 2-58

Muscles that connect the upper limb to the anterior and lateral thoracic walls (pectoralis major, pectoralis minor, and serratus anterior), along with some other muscles of the trunk.

Labels on figure:
Sternocleidomastoid
Trapezius
Clavicle
Deltoid
Pectoralis major
Biceps
Linea alba
Abdominal aponeurosis
External oblique
Pectoralis major (removed)
Pectoralis minor
Biceps
Serratus anterior
Internal intercostal
Transversus abdominis
Internal oblique
Rectus abdominis (sectioned)
Inguinal ligament

minor arise from the anterior ends of ribs 2 through 4 or 5. They course laterally and obliquely upward where they converge to insert on the coracoid process of the scapula. This muscle functions as a shoulder extensor when we reach for something but can't quite touch it.

Subclavius. The tiny subclavius originates at the junction of the first rib and its costal cartilage. It courses laterally to insert on the inferior surface of the clavicle, near the acromion of the scapula. It helps to draw the shoulder forward and slightly downward.

Serratus anterior (serratus magnum). The serratus (L. *serra*, saw) anterior is a thin muscle sheet located between the ribs and scapula. It overlies the lateral portion of the rib cage and the intercostal musculature (Figure 2-58). The fibers arise at the side from ribs 1 through 8 or 9 in the form of fleshy digitations, whose collective sawlike appearance gives the muscle its name. The fibers course between the outer surface of the ribs and inner surface of the scapula, inserting along its vertebral border. This muscle fixates and protracts the scapula.

Other Shoulder Muscles Some muscles of the shoulder are shown in Figure 2-59. They include the **deltoideus, subscapularis, supraspinatus, infraspinatus,** and the **teres major** and **minor.** As a group they abduct, flex, extend, and rotate the arm, functions that have little effect on fixation of the shoulder girdle, and so we need only acknowledge them.

Respiratory Functions of the Chest/Shoulder Muscles Any respiratory functions that might be attributed to these shoulder muscles are dependent upon fixation of the shoulder girdle, and in that event, from a mechanical standpoint, the **trapezius, latissimus dorsi,**[10] **pectoralis major** and **minor, subclavius,** and **serratus anterior** are all oriented in such a way as to function as supplemental (or compensatory) muscles of inhalation. Once again, we run the risk of incorrectly assigning function on the basis of architecture. For example, Campbell (1954) found activity (electromyographic) of the pectoralis muscles only at the very end of maximum inhalation. While Peterson (1964) found similar patterns, she also noted that activity did occur when, after maximum inhalation, the breath was held with an open airway.

On the basis of its attachments, the **subclavius** would appear to be a potential muscle of inhalation. There are no data on this muscle, and even if it were active, its contributions to inhalation would probably be inconsequential because it is so small.

Presumably the **serratus anterior muscle** can raise the ribs if the shoulder is fixed. Catton and Gray (1951) and Campbell (1954) examined this muscle

---

[10]The trapezius and latissimus dorsi muscles were described with the muscles of the upper limb and back.

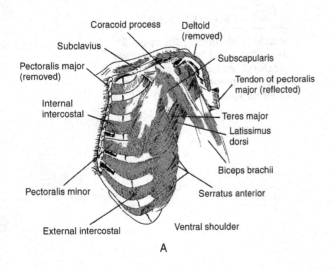

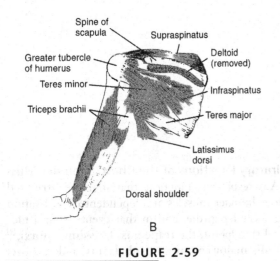

FIGURE 2-59

Muscles of the shoulder as seen from the front (A) and from behind (B).

electromyographically and failed to detect activity, even during very deep breathing. There is no evidence that the serratus anterior muscle contributes to breathing activity.

Abdominal Musculature and Its Role

Introduction

The muscles of the abdomen may be divided into an anterolateral group and a posterior group. The muscles of the *anterolateral group* are five in number: the **external oblique**, the **internal oblique**, the **transversus abdominis**, the **rectus abdominis**, and the **pyramidalis** muscles. The *posterior muscles* of the abdomen are four in number: the **quadratus lumborum**, the **iliacus**, and the **psoas major** and **minor.**

By definition the **abdomen** is that part of the body bounded above by the diaphragm and below by the inlet to the pelvis. The **anterolateral muscles** form a wall between the pelvis and lower margin of the rib cage, and they attach to the skeleton and to other musculature by means of an extensive system of tendinous sheets known as the **abdominal aponeurosis** on the ventral abdominal wall and the **lumbodorsal fascia** on the dorsal abdominal wall. They are complex.

The **abdominal aponeurosis**, a broad, flat sheet of tendinous tissue situated on the ventral abdominal wall, extends from the sternum to the pubis. At the midline anteriorly it can be seen in a dissection as a dense, fibrous band, the **linea alba** (L. *linea*, a stripe or streak + *alba*, white), which extends uninterrupted, except for the umbilicus, from the xiphoid process of the sternum above to the pubic symphysis below.

On either side of the linea alba, the aponeurosis divides into two layers, one of which passes deep to, while the other passes superficial to, the rectus abdominis muscle. In this way, the muscle becomes enclosed by an aponeurosis called the **sheath of the rectus abdominis.** Just lateral to the paired rectus abdominis muscles, the two layers of aponeurosis again meet and form a second vertical ribbon, the **linea semilunaris** (L. *semi*, half + *luna*, moon), a landmark far less identifiable than the linea alba. As shown in Figure 2-60, the linea semilunaris divides, giving rise to the three layers of aponeuroses into which the lateral abdominal muscles insert. The most superficial layer covers the entire ventral surface of the abdomen. It attaches superiorly to the lowermost fibers of the pectoralis major, to the xiphoid process of the sternum, and to adjacent costal cartilages. Inferiorly, it attaches to the pubic symphysis and to the anterior iliac spine. A prominent strand of thickened aponeurosis joins these two points and is known as the **inguinal** (L. *inguen*, groin) **ligament.** It is shown schematically in Figure 2-61. This ligament is often identified as a discrete structure, when it is really the rolled-over inferior margin of the aponeurosis of the external oblique muscle, and although it is called a ligament, it is tendinous in function. The inguinal ligament marks the separation in the groin between the abdominal wall and the lower limb. The ligament is most readily visualized by dropping one leg to the floor while lying on one's back (Woodburne, 1973).

A broad, two-layered sheet located on the dorsal aspect of the lower part of the vertebral column is called the **lumbodorsal fascia.** It has attachments on the spines of the lumbar vertebrae and on the posterior portion of the iliac crest. The fascia divides, as shown in Figure 2-60, giving rise to two layers of aponeurosis into which the fibers of the internal oblique and transversus abdominis attach.

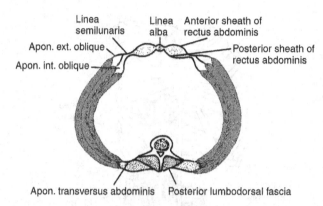

Linea semilunaris — Linea alba — Anterior sheath of rectus abdominis — Apon. ext. oblique — Posterior sheath of rectus abdominis — Apon. int. oblique — Apon. transversus abdominis — Posterior lumbodorsal fascia

FIGURE 2-60

Schematic of fasciae and aponeuroses of the abdominal wall as seen from above in a transverse section.

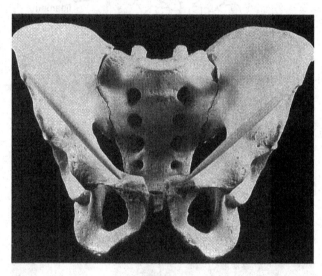

FIGURE 2-61

Reconstruction of inguinal (groin) ligament.

Anterolateral Abdominal Muscles

External Oblique The external obliques are the *largest*, the *strongest*, and the *most superficial* of the abdominal muscles. They are broad, thin, and roughly quadrilateral in shape. As shown in Figure 2-62, they take their origin by means of fleshy slips from the exterior surfaces and lower borders of ribs 5 through 12. Some of the fibers course downward and medially, where they terminate on the anterior half of the iliac crest, while the remaining fibers terminate along the extent of the external layer of the abdominal aponeurosis.

This muscle has various roles, one of them being to compress the abdominal contents. It is instrumental in raising intraabdominal and intrathoracic pressures; it assists in micturation (urination), defecation, emesis

(vomiting), parturition (L. *parturitio*, childbirth), and forced expiration. Acting together, the two sides flex the vertebral column, while one side acting alone bends the vertebral column laterally and rotates it.

Internal Oblique These muscles, also located on the lateral and ventral aspect of the abdominal wall, lie just deep to the external oblique muscles. Smaller and thinner, they form the *middle layer* of the abdominal musculature. As shown in Figure 2-63, *their course is just opposite to that of the external obliques, and for this reason they are sometimes called the ascending oblique muscles.* They arise from the lateral half of the inguinal ligament and from the anterior two-thirds of the iliac crest. The posterior fasciculi course almost vertically and insert, by means of fleshy slips, into the lower borders of the cartilages of the last three or four ribs.

The remainder of the fasciculi that arise from the iliac crest diverge as they spread over the lateral wall of the abdomen, and in the region of the linea semilunaris, they terminate in an aponeurosis that is fused to the aponeurosis of the external oblique and the transversus abdominis, at some variable distance from the midline. By means of this aponeurosis, however, the internal oblique makes its *final insertion* into the linea alba.

The fibers that arise from the inguinal ligament course downward and medially to terminate in a tendinous sheet that inserts into the pubis as a slip called the **falx** (L. sickle) **inguinalis.**

Action of the internal oblique muscle also compresses the abdominal contents, so it assists in those activities which tend to expel the contents of the abdominal viscera, as well as assisting in forced exhalation. The internal oblique muscles are also postural. Both sides acting together flex the vertebral column by drawing the costal cartilages toward the pubis and one side, acting alone, bends the vertebral column laterally and rotates it.

Transversus Abdominis The transversus abdominis muscles are the *deepest* of the abdominal muscles. As the name implies, *the course of their fibers is horizontal.* The muscle arises from the inner surfaces of ribs 6 through 12 by means of fleshy slips that interdigitate with the fibers of the diaphragm and the transversus thoracis. Fibers also arise from the lumbodorsal fascia, from the inner edge of the anterior three-fourths of the iliac crest, and from the lateral one-third of the inguinal ligament. The fibers course in a horizontal direction and insert into the deepest layer of the abdominal aponeurosis. A few of the inferiormost fibers course somewhat downward to insert into the pubis. The muscle is shown in Figure 2-64.

FIGURE 2-62

The external abdominal oblique and rectus abdominis muscles shown schematically in (A). In (B) a dissection of the rectus abdominis is shown and in (C) a dissection of the external abdominal oblique. (Dissections by Fang Ling Lu.)

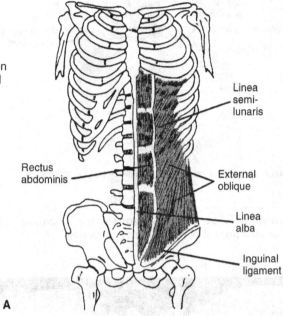

Linea semi-lunaris

Rectus abdominis

External oblique

Linea alba

Inguinal ligament

A

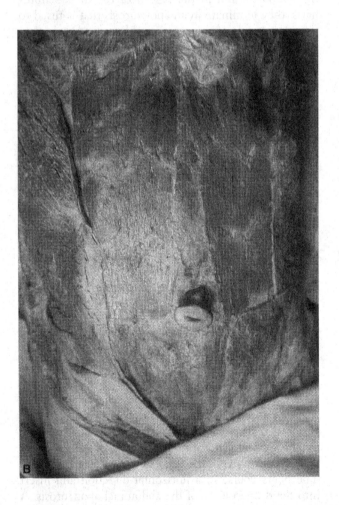

B

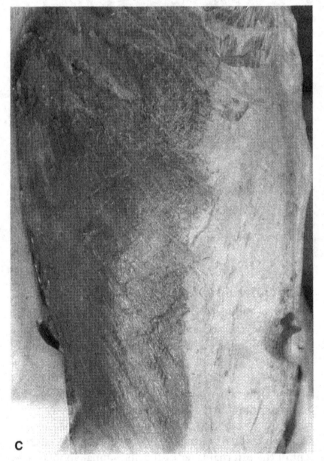

C

This muscle also constricts the abdomen, compressing its contents. It is not a postural muscle, but is probably instrumental in forced exhalation. In fact, on the basis of its architecture, the transversus abdominis might well be the most efficient or the most effective of the abdominal muscles.

FIGURE 2-63

Schematic (A) and dissection (B) of the internal oblique abdominis (IO) and external oblique (EO) abdominis muscles.

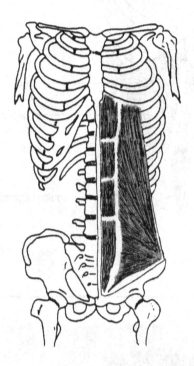

A

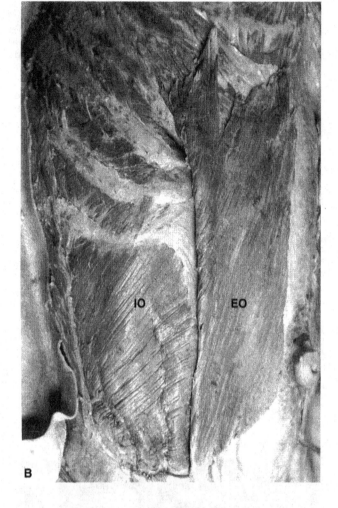

B

Rectus Abdominis As mentioned earlier, the rectus abdominis muscles are almost completely enclosed by an aponeurotic sheath which holds the muscles in position without offering restrictions to their movement. They lie parallel to the midline, just lateral to the linea alba. The muscle arises by means of tendons from the crest of the pubis, and by tendinous slips which interlace with their fellows from the opposite side. At first the muscle is narrow and thick, but it diverges somewhat as it courses vertically and becomes rather broad and thin in the upper abdominal region. The muscle is inserted into the cartilages of the fifth, sixth, and seventh ribs, although this is quite variable. Fibers also insert into the xiphoid process, as shown in Figures 2-62 and 2-64.

The rectus abdominis muscles are divided by transverse tendinous inscriptions which partially compartmentalize the muscle into four and sometimes five segments, each of which is capable of somewhat independent contraction.

As stated earlier, the **sheath of the rectus abdominis** is formed by the fusion and splitting of the abdominal aponeuroses. Above a level about midway between the umbilicus and the pubic symphysis, the aponeurosis of the internal oblique muscle fails to split, so all three layers of the aponeuroses pass ventral to the rectus abdominis muscle. The region where this change in the arrangement of the aponeuroses takes place is marked by an **arcuate line.**

The rectus abdominis flexes the vertebral column, especially in the lumbar region, by drawing the sternum toward the pubis. Its action also tenses the abdominal wall and assists in compression of the abdominal contents. Its role in respiration will be discussed when the group action of the abdominal muscles is considered.

> **Pyramidalis.** This muscle is frequently omitted in descriptions of the abdominal musculature. It is also omitted in about 10 percent of us. A small, extremely variable, and insignificant muscle, it is in the rectus sheath where it lies anterior to the lowermost part of the rectus abdominis muscle.

Group Actions of the Anterolateral Abdominal Musculature The actions of the abdominal musculature are

FIGURE 2-64

(A) Schematic of the transversus abdominis and rectus abdominis muscles. In (B) the internal abdominis muscle (IA) has been reflected to reveal the transversus abdominis (TA) muscle. In (C) windows in the anterolateral wall reveal the three layers of muscle. External abdominis (EA), internal abdominis (IA), and transversus abdominis (TA).

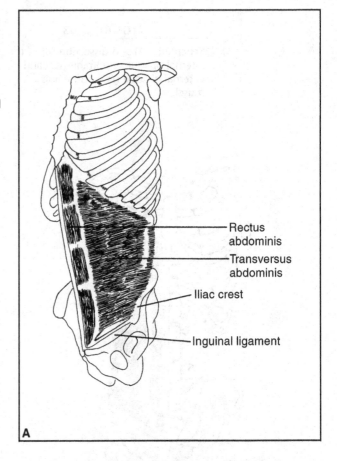

Rectus abdominis

Transversus abdominis

Iliac crest

Inguinal ligament

A

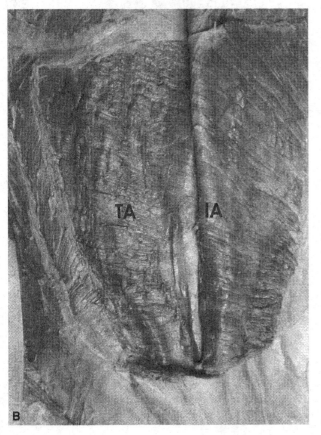

B

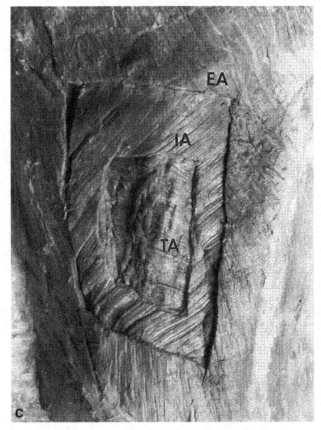

C

many and varied. A very important role of the antero-lateral abdominal muscles, and one often overlooked, is as *flexors of the vertebral column.* They are, in fact, the only muscles that can flex the thoracic and lumbar regions of the vertebral column. On the other hand, one quite obvious function is simply to *enclose and lend support to the abdominal contents.* This supportive function is facilitated by the varied courses of the three layers of the anterolateral abdominal muscles. Assuming that the muscles that fix the vertebral column are not especially active, we might examine the effects the abdominal muscles may produce.

If the abdominal muscles on both sides are contracted simultaneously, the vertebral column is flexed and the torso is bent forward. If the muscles on just one side are contracted, the body is bent laterally, and it is rotated toward the opposite side. With the vertebral column held rigid, contraction of the abdominal muscles *compresses the abdominal contents,* and, since these muscles have attachments on the rib cage, contraction also tends to *draw the ribs downward,* thus assisting in decreasing the size of the thoracic cavity. Because of their attachments and courses, the abdominal muscles probably do not all contribute to expiratory activity to the same degree. On mechanical grounds, the **oblique muscles** are probably the more effective in depressing the ribs, while the **transversus abdominis** muscles are more effective in compressing abdominal contents.

We have seen that with the laryngeal muscles contracted so as to prevent expulsion of air, as in the case of thoracic fixation, *the abdominal muscles function in those activities which require high intraabdominal and intrathoracic pressures.*

Because the external oblique and rectus abdominis muscles are superficial, they are the only abdominal muscles that have been studied rather extensively. For this reason the abdominal muscles are usually discussed as a group, but only the respiratory activity of the external oblique and the rectus abdominis muscles can be cited.

In one of his early studies, Campbell (1952) reported that there was no activity in the external oblique and rectus abdominis muscles of supine subjects breathing quietly, as one might easily suspect. Activity was detected, however, during maximum expiratory efforts. In addition, activity was detected at the height of maximum inspiration. On the basis of his data, Campbell concluded that *contraction of the abdominal muscles was a factor which limited the depth of inspiration,* and this is a very important function indeed. This limiting action was not detected in very rapid and deep breathing due to oxygen deprivation.

Davis and Zemlin (1965) examined the external obliques and the rectus abdominis muscles in a group of young adults. Activity was always detected during rapid forced expiration and during such activities as mild coughing. The external oblique was invariably found to be the more active of the two, and many subjects exhibited very little activity of the rectus abdominis, even at the end point of maximum expiration.

The postural role of abdominal muscles imposes constraints on electromyographic investigations, because some activity of the anterolateral abdominal muscles is almost always present in the standing and sitting positions. This activity can be minimized by careful postural adjustments, and, under these conditions, Campbell and Green (1955) reported that if activity remains and a respiratory rhythm is found, the activity decreases in inspiration and increases in expiration. In the supine position, no activity is detected during quiet breathing.

Campbell and Green also report that the abdominal muscles do not contract very forcefully either in the supine or the erect posture until ventilation reaches very high levels. In most normal subjects *contraction of the abdominal muscles occurs only when the expiratory pressure is very high* (10 cm H_2O) and the electrical activity during graded expiratory efforts is proportional to the magnitude of the effort, provided that lung volume is controlled. As lung volume increases, much of the expiratory pressure is generated by passive elastic forces.

Posterior Abdominal Muscles

The only posterior muscle of the abdomen we shall consider is the **quadratus lumborum.** The other three posterior muscles—the **iliacus** and the **psoas major** and **minor**—are often described with the muscles of the lower limb. They are active in flexion of the thigh and pelvis.

Quadratus Lumborum and Its Action   The quadratus lumborum (L. *lumbus,* loin), as its name suggests, is roughly quadrilateral in shape. It is a flat sheet of muscle located in the laterodorsal aspect of the abdominal wall. The muscle is shown in Figure 2-65. The fibers arise, by means of an aponeurosis, from the iliac crest and from a prominent ligament, the **iliolumbar ligament,** which attaches to the transverse processes of the fifth lumbar vertebra medially and the crest of the ilium laterally. The fibers course almost vertically upward, converge slightly, and insert by slips into the transverse processes of the lumbar vertebrae one through four and into the medial half and lower border of the last rib.

From the standpoint of mechanics, two functions may be attributed to this muscle. *Because of its costal attachments it may be regarded as an active muscle of exhalation.* In addition, the quadratus lumborum, along with

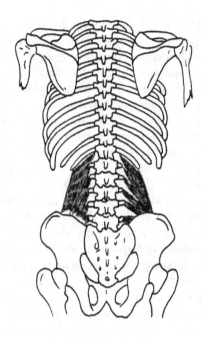

FIGURE 2-65

Schematic of the quadratus lumborum muscle.

the serratus posterior inferior, *may anchor the two lower ribs against the lifting force of the diaphragm when it presses downward on the viscera.*

Inasmuch as fixation of the lower ribs may be complementary to diaphragm action, the quadratus lumborum might well be considered an accessory to inhalation. There is little supportive evidence for this viewpoint, however. It is also a postural muscle that flexes the lumbar vertebrae laterally toward the side of the muscle acting.

THE MECHANICS OF BREATHING

Introduction

During quiet inhalation, contraction of the diaphragm, intercostals, and perhaps the scalene muscles increases the dimensions of the thorax in all three planes. Since the lungs closely follow the movements of the thoracic wall, they are expanded and air flows from the outside inward until the air pressure within the lungs is equal to that of the outside air. At the same time the abdominal viscera have been compressed by the descending diaphragm, and intraabdominal pressure is elevated.

The muscles of inhalation cease their activity somewhat gradually, once the lungs have become inflated, and restoring forces begin to play their role. Increased upward force against the diaphragm, provided by the

abdominal viscera and elevated intraabdominal pressure, is one of the restoring forces. The lung-thorax unit has also been subjected to expansive distortion, and as the inspiratory muscles cease their activity, additional restoring forces come into play. The ribs, which have been elevated and twisted in the inspiratory process, will "unwind" to provide a rotational restoration force called **torque.** It is illustrated in Figure 2-66.

The system is also acted upon by gravity, so **potential energy** (the energy of position) will be recovered in the form of **kinetic energy** (the energy of motion). And, finally, the lung tissue itself has considerable elasticity, and since the lungs are linked to the thoracic walls, they exert a progressive restoring force with increased stretch. This tends to restore the thorax to its undilated position; at the same time, the elasticity of the lungs provides the expiratory force necessary to expel air from the lungs.

We call the processes involved in this cycle of quiet breathing active inhalation and passive exhalation. In adult men and women it takes place about 12 times per minute. Between 500 and 750 cc of air are exchanged each time, for a total of between 6 and 9 liters per minute. This value, whatever it happens to be, is called **minute volume.**

There are frequent occasions in our day-to-day lives when this seemingly simple and straightforward process of quiet breathing is interrupted for one reason or another. This is especially true for the production of speech and may be even more dramatic for singing. Sooner or later we will have to examine the terms quiet inhalation and forced exhalation a little more closely, but we will find that the process demands a meaningful nomenclature.

Measurement of Pulmonary Subdivisions

Although the history of respiratory physiology dates to about 3000 B.C., it wasn't until 1950 that a standardized

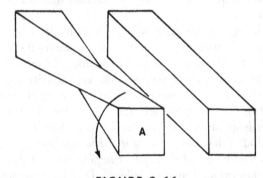

FIGURE 2-66

Schematic illustration of torque. An elastic rod, twisted as in A, will exert a rotational restoration force that is called torque.

system of definitions and symbols in respiratory physiology was adopted (Pappenheimer, et al., 1950).

Certain of the lung volumes and capacities are applicable primarily in the clinical environment, others in the laboratory setting, and, since some measures are dependent upon voluntary breathing behavior, they are clearly limited to humans. Some of the measures specify pulmonary capabilities for tasks in which we do not normally engage. They are, nonetheless, important in explaining and understanding how the respiratory system works.

Most of the pulmonary subdivisions and other values can be measured directly by means of a simple device known as a **wet spirometer.** As shown in Figure 2-67, it consists of one vessel inverted in a second vessel which is filled with water. The inverted vessel is either balanced by counterweights or it is spring loaded so that its effective mass is essentially zero. Air inhaled from and exhaled into

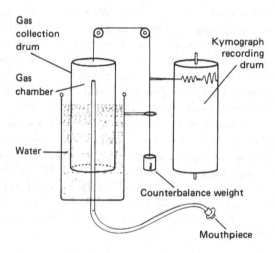

FIGURE 2-67

Schematic of a wet spirometer and a photograph of a commercial computerized spirometer.

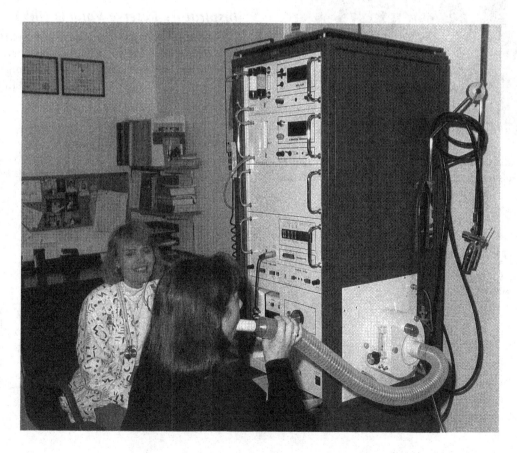

the inverted vessel causes it to descend and ascend, the extent of movement being dependent upon the quantity of air exchanged.

A commercial spirometer with an ink recording system is shown in Figure 2-67. Computerized systems now available can provide measurements of lung volumes and capacities far more rapidly. In the laboratory setting shown in Figure 2-68, associated apparatus includes a multichannel electromyograph and airflow recording equipment.

A graphic recording obtained with a spirometer is called a **spirogram.** A schematic example, along with some lung volumes and capacities, is shown in Figure 2-69.

Pulmonary subdivisions are specified in terms of lung volumes and lung capacities. **Lung volumes** are discrete values; no one volume includes another volume. There is no overlap between lung volumes. **Lung capacities,** however, include two or more lung volumes. Inspiratory and vital capacities can be measured directly with a spirometer, but functional residual and total lung capacities must be computed.

It is important to be aware that there is a considerable variation in lung volumes and capacities, even in a homogeneous group. As a consequence, deviations from a statistical norm must be large to be significant in diagnosis.

Lung Volumes

Tidal Volume (TV)

The volume of air inhaled and exhaled during any single expiratory cycle (an inhalation followed by an exhalation) is known as tidal volume. A frequently cited value of tidal volume for young adult males at rest is 750 cc. While engaged in light work, this same group has an average tidal volume of 1670 cc, and during heavy work, their tidal volumes average 2030 cc. This suggests that work demands an increased oxygen expenditure, which, in turn, will be reflected in the value of an individual's tidal volume.

In addition, wide variability in clinically normal individuals reduces the significance of tidal volume and complicates its interpretation. For example, the 95 percent range for adult males is from 675 to 895 cc, while the 95 percent range for adult females is from 285 to 393 cc, with a mean of 339. The mean tidal volume, then, for the adult population in general is about 500 cc, and this value is often cited.

Inspiratory Reserve Volume (IRV)

The quantity of air which can be inhaled beyond that inhaled in a tidal volume cycle is called inspiratory reserve volume. In a state of rest (quiet tidal breathing), inspiratory reserve volumes vary anywhere from about 1500 to about 2500 cc.

Expiratory Reserve Volume (ERV)

The amount of air that can be forcibly exhaled following a quiet or passive exhalation is known as expiratory reserve volume or **resting lung volume (RLV).** In the past, this

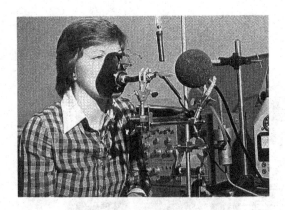

FIGURE 2-68

A laboratory setting for assessing respiratory functions and air flow.

FIGURE 2-69

A schematic spirogram showing pulmonary subdivisions.

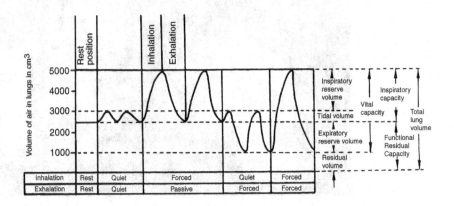

quantity has been known as *reserve air* or *supplemental air*, terms that are now archaic. Expiratory reserve volume usually amounts to about 1500 cc and may go as high as 2000 cc in a young adult.

Residual Volume (RV)

The quantity of air that remains in the lungs and airways even after a maximum exhalation is called residual volume. Lung tissue is subjected to considerable stretch, even after a maximum exhalation, because the lungs are bonded tightly against the walls of the thorax. For that reason a considerable quantity of air cannot be expelled, even with maximum effort. This air, called **residual air,** ranges in value from about 1000 to 1500 cc in young adult males. It remains in the lungs and upper airways even after death. *We cannot speak on residual air*, of course, and it is unfortunate that reference to "residual breathers" and "residual speakers" continues. Confusion between the terms residual volume and functional residual capacity, to be considered later, may account for the misuse of terms.

Since residual air cannot be voluntarily expelled from the lungs, it stands to reason it cannot be measured directly, but rather must be computed by specialized clinical tests (Mead and Milic-Emili, 1964).

If the lungs are removed from the thorax soon after death, the linkage between the lungs and thoracic walls is broken, and almost all the residual air is expelled by virtue of the inherent elasticity of the lungs. But a small quantity (about 500 cc) of minimal residual air remains. For this reason lungs have a specific gravity less than water and they will float. Lungs removed from a stillborn fetus, on the other hand, will sink.

Regardless of the depth of inhalation, approximately 150 cc of our residual air neither contributes oxygen to the blood nor receives carbon dioxide from it. It is called **dead air,** and remains in the nasal cavities, larynx, trachea, bronchi, and bronchioles, or collectively, the **dead-air spaces.** This air, which was the very last to be inhaled, is the first to be exhaled during the next cycle of respiration. The very last 150 cc of air which is forced from the alveoli during expiration remains in the dead-air spaces, and although it is laden with carbon dioxide, it is the first air to be drawn back into the alveoli at the beginning of the next inspiration. Therefore, about 150 cc of inspired air ought to be considered "nonfunctional" for purposes of internal respiration.

In the case of prolonged shallow breathing, where little more than dead air is exchanged, accumulations of excessive carbon dioxide may take place in the alveoli and bloodstream. When this happens, an automatic and involuntary deep inhalation may take place, and we say a person has just "yawned."

Lung Capacities

Inspiratory Capacity (IC)

The maximum volume of air that can be inhaled from the resting expiratory level[11] is called the inspiratory capacity. It can be measured directly with a spirometer and is equal to tidal volume plus inspiratory reserve volume.

Vital Capacity (VC)

The quantity of air that can be exhaled after as deep an inhalation as possible is known as vital capacity. It is the sum of tidal volume, inspiratory reserve volume, and expiratory reserve volume. In adult males it ranges from 3500 cc to 5000 cc. It is reasonable to expect a relationship between the relative size of individuals and their vital capacities. For example, five-year-old girls have a vital capacity of about 1.0 liters, while boys have a vital capacity of about 1.25 liters. Children at age nine have vital capacities of around 2 liters (both boys and girls). Seventeen-year-old males have vital capacities of about 4.5 liters, and females, a vital capacity of about 3.75 liters. These values reflect differences in general body size. In practice, vital capacity measurements are reduced to well-established standards that are based upon height and weight, or on body surface area.

Functional Residual Capacity (FRC)

The quantity of air in the lungs and airways at the resting expiratory level is known as functional residual capacity. It is computed by taking the sum of expiratory reserve volume and residual volume. In young adult males functional residual capacity amounts to about 2300 cc.

Total Lung Capacity (TLC)

The quantity of air the lungs are capable of holding at the height of a maximum inhalation is logically known as total lung capacity and is equal to the sum of all lung volumes.

Significance of Pulmonary Volumes and Capacities

Effects of Body Position

In normal, healthy persons, the volume of air in the lungs and the various lung capacities depend primarily on body size and build; however, position of the body will also influence pulmonary values.

---

[11]**Resting expiratory level** refers to a state of equilibrium in the respiratory system. The forces of compression of the lungs are balanced by the forces of expansion of the thorax.

Most of the volumes and capacities decrease when a person is lying down rather than standing. Two factors are primarily responsible for this change: first, there is a tendency for the abdominal viscera to press upward against the diaphragm when a person is lying down, and, second, the pulmonary blood volume increases in the lying position, which decreases the space available for pulmonary air.

As part of a comprehensive study of breathing, Hixon, Goldman, and Mead (1973) investigated the effects that various body positions had on respiratory behavior during oral reading. They found lung capacity at resting expiratory level to be about 20 percent of vital capacity lower in the supine than in the upright position and that speech was produced at a correspondingly lower level. In Figure 2-70 the functional residual capacity (FRC) levels for different body positions are shown along with the volumes of air expired during readings of a standard passage. The vertical lines represent expiratory volumes of breath groups during oral reading. **Breath group** denotes a group of syllables that are produced during the same expiratory movement. The ends of the breath groups represent short pauses for inspiratory purposes, and they have been found to coincide with sentence and phrase boundaries, particularly during oral reading.

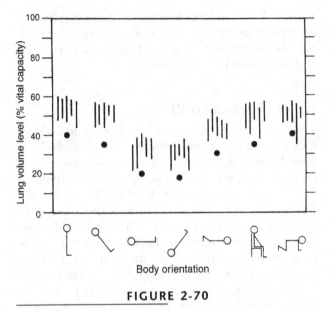

FIGURE 2-70

Functional residual capacity for different body positions. (From Hixon, T., M. Goldman, and J. Mead. *J. Sp. Hrng. Res.*, 16, 1973, with permission.)

CLINICAL NOTE: To experience the effects of body position on breathing, try slumping in a chair as if you were a cerebral palsied child confined to a wheel chair, and attempt to breathe deeply. You will probably find breathing difficult, but as the depth of breathing increases, your body tends to straighten and become upright.

Many cerebral palsied individuals, particularly those in wheel chairs, develop gradually worsening scoliosis (lateral curvature of the spine) which makes it increasingly difficult for them to "sit up straight."

The Role of Residual Volume

The word residual may call to mind something useless, or perhaps a necessary consequence of an important process. *Residual air has a very important role, because it provides air in the alveoli for aerating the blood, even though air exchange may not be taking place.* If it were not for residual air in the lungs, the concentration of oxygen and carbon dioxide in the bloodstream would rise and fall with each breath.

Because the lungs in newborn babies are proportionately quite large, they are not subjected to much stretch during the inspiratory process. The resting lung volume, also called expiratory reserve volume, is about the same as the nonaerated lung. In addition, the chest wall is so compliant it can provide virtually no expiratory force, and expiration is due to the elasticity of the

lung tissue. All this means that *newborn babies have virtually no expiratory reserve and residual volumes*, but their breathing rate is anywhere from 24 to 116 breaths per minute when they are asleep!

Factors Affecting Vital Capacity

Besides the anatomical build of a person, three other factors can affect vital capacity. First, the position of the body during the measurement, as we know, will influence vital capacity. The strength of the respiratory musculature is an important factor, as well as the distensibility of the thorax-lung unit or, in other words, **pulmonary compliance.** Pulmonary fibrotic diseases can strongly influence vital capacity measures, for example.

Subatmospheric pleural surface pressure is normally maintained throughout the lifetime of a person and only (momentarily) exceeds atmospheric pressure during extreme forced exhalation and during coughing or sneezing. No matter what the respiratory behavior is, inhaling, exhaling, or even not breathing at all, the *pleural surface pressure is always negative with respect to alveolar pressure.*

As shown in Figure 2-71, the difference between pleural surface and alveolar pressure does vary, and it is this difference in pressure that is responsible for the changes in the volume of the lungs during inhalation and exhalation.

The magnitude of the change in lung volume (ΔV) due to a change in the pressure difference across the lung wall (ΔP) defines **lung compliance.** The higher this ratio ($\Delta V/\Delta P$), the more compliant is the lung. Normally the compliance of the lungs and thorax combined is 0.13 liter per centimeter of water pressure. In other

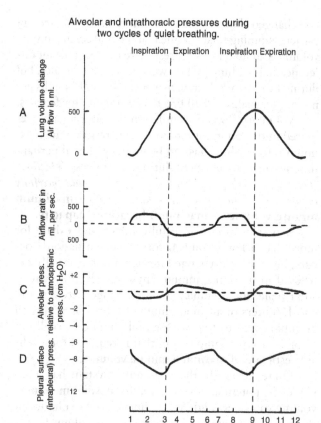

Alveolar and intrathoracic pressures during
two cycles of quiet breathing.

FIGURE 2-71

Alveolar pressure, air flow values, and pleural surface pressures during two cycles of quiet breathing. Lung volume change (A), air flow rate (B), alveolar pressure relative to atmospheric (C), and pleural surface pressure (D).

words, when the alveolar pressure is increased by 1 cm H_2O, the lungs expand 130 ml.

CLINICAL NOTE: Any disease or condition that destroys lung tissue, causes it to become fibrotic or edematous (Gk. *oidema*, swelling), obstructs the alveoli, or in some other way restricts lung expansion and contraction results in a decrease of lung compliance.

In **emphysema** the internal structure of the lung becomes excessively stretchable, which increases lung compliance. The result is an increase in the resting lung size because the alveolar-pleural surface pressure difference distends the lung more than usual. In addition, deformities of the chest wall such as **kyphosis** (hunchback), **poor posture, severe scoliosis,** or **fibrotic pleurisy** can reduce the expansibility of the lungs and reduce the total pulmonary compliance.

Young adult males can be expected to have a vital capacity of about 4.6 liters and young adult females about 3.1 liters; however, these values vary considerably depending upon body build, physical fitness, and other factors. A male athlete, for example, may have a vital capacity of 6 or 7 liters, which is 30 to 40 percent above normal.

In addition to the size and sex of an individual, lung volumes and capacities vary with age. Total lung capacities and vital capacities for both males and females from age 6 through 75 are shown graphically in Figure 2-72. The data are from Spector (1956, p. 267). In Figure 2-73, the residual volume, calculated on the basis of body surface area (BSA), is shown plotted from age 20 through 79

FIGURE 2-72

Graph of total lung and vital capacities as a function of age for males and females.

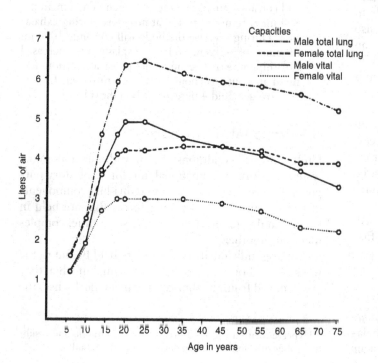

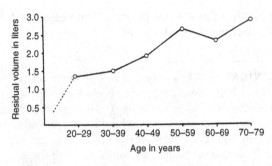

FIGURE 2-73

Graph of residual volume as a function of age for an adult male population.

years for a male population. Note that residual volume just about doubles during this period, reflecting changes in thorax-lung compliance.

Questions have arisen regarding the influence of sex and age on respiratory performance (Brody and Thurlbeck, 1986; Hoit, Hixon, Watson, and Morgan, 1990). In addition to changes in size and in tissue composition, overall pulmonary compliance changes with age and these all can be reflected in various respiratory functions (Agostoni and Hyatt, 1986; Agostoni and Mead, 1964; Gaultier and Zinman, 1983).

The relationship between age and breathing for speech has been investigated by Hoit and Hixon (1987). They found that total lung capacity does not change with age, while inspiratory capacity and functional residual capacities change slightly with age. Vital capacity was found to decrease, while residual volume increased.

Russell and Stathopoulas (1988) found that adults' percent of vital capacity increased from comfortable to loud conditions, whereas childrens' did not. Adults also went further into their functional residual capacity than did children. The results suggest that respiration in children is influenced primarily by articulatory demands and secondarily by intensity demands. Winkworth et al. (1995) found that, for spontaneous speech, lung volume varied between 42 and 63 percent of vital capacity. In addition, increases in speech intensity were not necessarily associated with increased lung volumes. Their results suggest that, in spontaneous speech (compared with reading tasks), neural planning influences respiratory behavior.

Research has suggested that, in children, speech breathing appears to be adultlike by the end of the first decade of life.

Air Exchange Rates

Minute volume is the *liters of air exchanged per minute during quiet breathing* (active inhalation, passive exhalation). We know that during quiet breathing and at rest air

is exchanged about 12 times a minute, and as pointed out earlier, assuming tidal volume is about 500 cc, the minute volume is about 6 liters. At rest there is no significant difference in breathing rate between males and females, but during heavy work the rate may increase to 21 breaths per minute for males and 30 breaths per minute for females.

Voluntary forced ventilation is occasionally required in the laboratory in order to determine the maximum rate at which gas can be exchanged, and perhaps the muscular involvement during the process. *The liters of air that would be exchanged if a person could forcefully inhale and exhale for a full minute* is called **maximum minute volume** or **maximum breathing capacity.**

A person cannot forcefully inhale and exhale for more than a few seconds before hyperventilation[12] occurs, but the air exchanged in such a task is usually expressed in liters per minute anyway. A healthy young adult male, for example, could exchange between 150 and 170 liters of air in a minute of forced breathing (if he could continue the task for a full minute). Usually an 8- or 10-second sample is all that is required for a reliable estimate of maximum minute volume.

Quite obviously the respiratory system has a remarkable potential for reserve. Its maximum minute volume can be as high as 25 times minute volume for short periods of time and 20 times minute volume for extended periods.

Atmospheric air is composed of about 79 percent nitrogen, 20 percent oxygen, and 0.04 percent carbon dioxide. At a normal ventilatory rate of 5 liters of air per minute, approximately 1 liter of oxygen is inhaled (5000 ml × .20 = 1000 ml), and of this, the body at rest will consume about 200 ml of oxygen. The remaining 800 ml is returned to the atmosphere during exhalation. During exercise the body will consume 1000 ml or more of oxygen, and this explains the increased breathing rate that accompanies physical exertion. Expired air contains about 75 percent nitrogen, 16 percent oxygen, and 4 percent carbon dioxide.

A Functional Unit Concept

Under normal conditions the lung-thorax-abdominal system constitutes a functional unit for respiratory purposes. In a resting position, the individual components of the system exhibit opposing forces that are held in balance and counteract and, at the same time, complement one another.

Acting individually the lungs are held bound to the walls of the thorax and to the diaphragm, but when they are removed from the thorax (only in an ideal sense) the

---

[12]Hyperventilation is caused by excessive respiration and results in an abnormal loss of carbon dioxide from the blood.

lungs will collapse, a clear indication that they are normally subjected to a stretching force. In a functional respiratory system, this will be manifested in the familiar **negative intrapleural pressure.**

The rebounding force of the lungs, on the other hand, tends to reduce the volume of the thorax, and when the lungs are removed the dimensions of the thorax will tend to increase while the volume of the abdominal cavity will decrease.

In Figure 2-74, the inherent elasticity of the lungs, represented by analogy as a stretched spring, tends to reduce the volume of the lungs. By similar analogy the thorax is represented by a compressed spring which tends to enlarge its dimensions. This means that the lung-thorax unit consists of two forces, not unlike vectors, acting in opposite directions. As a result, when the lungs are bound to the containing walls of the thorax by linkage of the pleural membrane, they are subjected to compression by the lung tissue.

At rest, then, these forces combined with the downward pull of the abdominal contents are just about balanced. We have seen that because of their spatial relationships, the gravitational effect of the abdominal contents exerts a downward force on the diaphragm, and since the lungs are also firmly bound to the diaphragm, they are also subjected to the same gravitational effects.

At the end of a normal expiration the intrapleural pressure is just about equal and opposite in direction, so the pressure beneath the dome of the diaphragm is approximately the same as the pressure on the surface of the dome. In other words, *transdiaphragmatic pressure is zero,* which means that a state of equilibrium exists among the elastic forces of the abdominal wall, the diaphragm, rib cage, lungs, and the force of gravity on the abdominal contents. This state of equilibrium is known as the **resting expiratory level.**

During normal respiration the equilibrium is only a transient condition because of the constant interplay between the abdominal and thoracic pressures.

While the role of direct mechanical coupling of the abdominal viscera should not be overlooked, the abdominal cavity, because it is a closed system, can also be regarded from the standpoint of mechanics as a *fluid-filled container.* In fact, the abdominal viscera float in the peritoneal fluid, and as a consequence a pressure difference exists between any two levels in the abdominal cavity. In an upright position, and with the respiratory muscles relaxed, the pressure in the upper part of the cavity is negative and since the abdominal wall is distensible, it tends to be drawn inward. Likewise, the top of the container (the diaphragm) is also distensible, and as stated earlier, it would be drawn downward were it not for the opposing intrapleural forces in the thorax. These effects are illustrated in Figure 2-75.

This abbreviated account of the role of the abdominal viscera in respiration should point out that a description of just the thorax and its role is incomplete and that the entire torso should be thought of as comprising the respiratory mechanism.

Returning to our spring analogy for a moment and keeping in mind that at rest the expansive forces of the thorax and the opposing recoil forces of the lungs are balanced or in equilibrium, we see that when the lung-thorax unit is expanded or compressed, the forces are no longer in a state of balance. As the thorax expands due to the forces of the muscles of inhalation, the lungs'

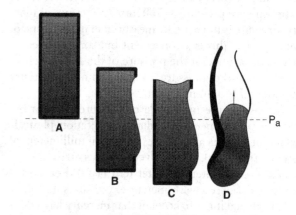

FIGURE 2-75

Model of diaphragm-abdomen unit. The abdominal cavity can be likened to a fluid-filled container with a flexible wall. In an inverted container (A) fluid pressure at the bottom is equal to atmospheric (Pa). With a flexible wall (B) atmospheric and fluid pressures are equal about midway, and with flexible top and walls (C, D) pressures are equalized nearer the top of the container. In the upright human body the elastic recoil of the lungs (arrow) resists downward force and atmospheric and fluid pressures are equal just beneath the dome of the diaphragm. (After Agostoni and Mead, 1964.)

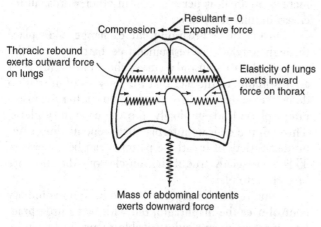

FIGURE 2-74

Schematic of lung-thorax unit in equilibrium.

springs are stretched beyond their normal equilibrium; consequently, they will exert a greater and greater rebounding force. When the expansive forces cease, the stretched springs will recoil until they are once again held in balance by the springs of the thorax. This is the equivalent of *passive exhalation*, when nonmuscular forces cause the pressure within the lungs to increase above atmospheric pressure.

On the other hand, when the thorax springs are compressed beyond their normal equilibrium by the active forces of the muscles of exhalation, they will exert a rebounding force that will tend to expand the dimensions of the thoracic cavity, along with the lung tissue, and the pressure within the lungs will momentarily drop below atmospheric pressure. Air will enter the lungs to account for **passive inhalation.**

Pressure Relationships in the Chest Cavity

Earlier we saw how pressures greater or less than atmospheric could be measured by means of a wet, open manometer, filled with either mercury or water.

The pressure within the lungs is called **pulmonic** or **alveolar pressure.** In either case, the reference is to atmospheric pressure. In addition, these pressures are usually expressed in centimeters of water (cm H_2O) or millimeters of mercury (mm Hg). **Atmospheric pressure,** for example, raises a column of mercury about 760 millimeters in the familiar evacuated glass tube we call a **mercury barometer.** It is common practice to speak of atmospheric pressure as 760 mm or 756 mm of mercury. Pressure is not actually measured in millimeters, of course, and so this is a convenient but somewhat cavalier way of saying that the pressure of the atmosphere is the same as the pressure of a column of mercury 760 mm or 756 mm in height.

Because of the magnitude of pressure changes between the pleural membranes during respiration, **pleural-surface pressures** are often expressed in millimeters of mercury (mm Hg), while **alveolar pressures** are expressed in centimeters of water (cm H_2O). For convenience, we can convert mercuric pressures to water pressures by taking into account that mercury has a density about 13.6 times that of water, so a pressure that will support a 1 cm column of mercury will also support a 13.6 cm column of water.

With the airway open and the muscles of respiration completely relaxed, there is relatively free and unrestricted communication between the interior of the lungs and the outside air, and the pressure within the lungs (alveolar pressure) is the same as atmospheric. From what we know about the behavior of gases, it is obvious that if alveolar pressure were anything but atmospheric, air would either be entering or leaving the

lungs. The moment inspiration begins and the lungs expand, however, the alveolar pressure falls below atmospheric, and at the height of inspiration the alveolar pressure is lowest, amounting to –1 to –2 cm H_2O. *Air, of course, enters the lungs with a flow proportional to the difference between alveolar and atmospheric pressures.*

As the inspiratory phase comes to an end with maximum lung expansion, the alveolar pressure rises once again, and at the very end of inspiration (with the airway open) alveolar pressure is the same as atmospheric. In the meantime, with progressive expansion of the lungs, pleural-surface pressure, which is about –3 to –5 cm H_2O at rest, begins to fall. It reaches a value of –8 to –10 cm H_2O at the height of inspiration. It is at this point, of course, that the lungs are subjected to maximum stretching force, and they exhibit maximum rebound.

As the expiratory phase begins, the lungs contract elastically as rapidly as the diminishing chest cavity permits, and the air within the lungs is compressed. Alveolar pressure exceeds atmospheric pressure by about 1 or 2 cm H_2O, and the air flows out of the lungs until once again the alveolar pressure reaches atmospheric. At the end of expiration the pleural-surface pressure has again returned to about –3 to –5 cm H_2O. During every cycle of respiration, then, *alveolar pressure is the same as atmospheric* at three points: at the *beginning of inspiration*, at the *end of inspiration*, and at the *end of expiration*.

The relationships among air flow, lung volume changes, and alveolar and pleural-surface (intrapleural) pressures during two cycles of quiet breathing are shown schematically in Figure 2-71. The shapes of the curves are idealistic, and they will vary depending upon a number of factors.

For example, if only breathing rate should increase, alveolar and pleural-surface pressure relationships and lung volume changes would remain the same. The time interval between successive breath cycles would naturally be decreased, and that would be reflected in an increase in air flow per second—in other words, an increase in minute volume.

During quiet breathing, air exchange takes place through a relatively resistance-free pathway, and the smooth, almost sinusoidal curves shown in Figure 2-71 are testimony to the fact that the muscles of inhalation do not cease their activity abruptly, but rather the inspiratory phase leads gradually into the expiratory phase. Through the delicate interplay between, an almost unlimited variety of breathing patterns can be generated. This is especially true if the muscles of exhalation are brought into play.

Some research suggests that we have no voluntary control over the diaphragm, but with just a little practice, most of us are quite capable of producing independent thoracic and abdominal movements during voluntary inhalation as well as exhalation. It isn't difficult, for example, to take a relatively deep breath, protrude the abdominal wall, and then voluntarily exhale a surprising quantity of air, while maintaining the protruded abdomen! Quite obviously a number of combinations of relative thoracic-diaphragmatic-abdominal movements can be effective in both inhalation and exhalation. This is just one more reason why dogmatic categorizations of musculature as either inspiratory or expiratory can be so hazardous, especially for speech and singing activities.

The curves shown in Figure 2-71 are quite symmetrical, but usually the expiratory phase is somewhat longer in duration than the inspiratory phase. In addition, there is a slight time lag between changes in alveolar pressure and air flow due to the effects of air friction. These effects can be maximized by the introduction of resistance to air flow.

Regulation of Alveolar Pressure

Forced Exhalation

During quiet breathing, expiratory forces are almost exclusively passive, as we have seen. When circumstances demand, however, active contraction of the abdominal musculature (primarily) can facilitate rapid ventilation, or in the event of increased airway resistance, forced expiration can provide the necessary compensatory increase in alveolar pressure.

In other words, forced expiration may complement passive expiration, or it may provide expiratory forces at lung volumes below resting level. Quite obviously, then, *forced expiration is possible at virtually any lung volume.* Suppose, for example, a person wished to blow out all the candles on a birthday cake. In my case three score and then some candles must be extinguished with one single respiratory maneuver. The challenge is not insurmountable, but it demands a very deep inhalation followed by immediate and prolonged forced exhalation. Loud speech, singing or shouting, or the playing of certain musical instruments may demand forced exhalation, even at very high lung volumes.

Elevated alveolar pressure can also be generated without active contraction of the muscles of expiration. This is especially true if airway resistance is introduced after a deep inhalation.

Relaxation Pressure

We know that as the lung-thorax unit is expanded during inhalation, passive forces of exhalation generate a rebounding force that tends to restore the system to an equilibrium position. Rebounding forces are also generated when the lung-thorax unit is compressed during forced expiration and the system tends to expand to its equilibrium position. In this instance, however, alveolar pressure is negative and air flow is into the lungs. *Pressures that are generated entirely by passive forces, be they positive (above atmospheric) or negative (subatmospheric), are called relaxation pressures.*

The magnitude of the restoring force can be measured directly in a simple experiment. A water manometer coupled to a flexible tube and a mouthpiece is all that is required. At resting lung volume, the respiratory system is at equilibrium, so no air exchange takes place. Since alveolar pressure is the same as atmospheric, the manometer will register "zero" pressure. At resting level, the lungs contain about 38 percent of the vital capacity in healthy persons. If the subject in the experiment were to inhale a small quantity of air beyond the resting level and *completely relax* (which can be a difficult task) with the mouthpiece in place, air flow is prevented by the column of water in the manometer, and the lung-thorax-manometer assembly becomes a closed system.

Under these conditions a small amount of positive alveolar pressure will be registered by the manometer. If the quantity of air inhaled or exhaled relative to resting lung volume is carefully measured using a spirometer, the relationship between lung volume and relaxation pressure can be shown graphically.

Relaxation-Pressure Curve A relaxation-pressure curve is shown in Figure 2-76. To permit comparisons between subjects, **lung volume** is expressed as percentage of vital capacity. **Alveolar pressure,** which is registered by the manometer, is expressed in cm H_2O. Air under pressure can do work, of course, and it is this compressed air which is the power source for the speech mechanism.

Note in Figure 2-76, the relatively linear relationship between lung volume and relaxation pressure in the midvolume range and the nonlinear relationship at the extremes of lung volume. This *nonlinearity* suggests that the limits of distensibility and compressibility are being approached and that the structures that constitute the breathing apparatus are beginning to resist further distortion. In the midvolume range, relaxation pressure changes at a rate of about 0.5 cm H_2O for each 1 percent of the vital capacity, but at the two extremes of lung volumes pressure changes take place more abruptly with changes in lung volume.

The **relaxation-pressure curve** represents the pressures generated by the total respiratory system, but the curve can be resolved into relaxation pressure generated by the lungs and by the chest wall (Agostoni and Mead, 1964; Konno and Mead, 1968). In Figure 2-77, the relaxation forces of the lungs and of the chest wall are pictured by arrows in the drawing of the thorax. They can be regarded as vectorlike, although the magnitude of the forces is not shown to scale. The dashed line on the left represents the relaxation curve of the

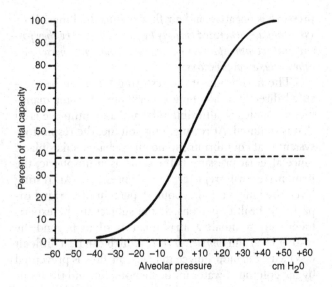

FIGURE 2-76

Relaxation-pressure curve showing relationship between passive pressures generated by the lung-thorax complex and the volume of air in the lungs.

chest wall. Its resting volume is at about 55 percent of vital capacity. The dashed line on the right represents the relaxation curve of the lungs. Note that its resting volume is not quite reached, even at zero percent of vital capacity. This implies that even after maximum expiratory efforts, the lungs are subjected to a certain amount of stretch. We have already seen how this accounts for the residual volume.

Influence of Lung Volumes At lung volumes *above 55 percent* vital capacity, both the lungs and thorax recoil inward, so both contribute to the relaxation pressure. At lung volumes *below 55 percent* vital capacity, the chest wall recoils outward, while the lungs recoil inward. At *mid-volume*, the lungs and chest wall contribute about equally to the change in relaxation pressure with changes in lung volume. The rapid changes in relaxation pressure that occur at the extremes of lung volumes can be attributed to the lungs at high volumes and to the chest wall at low volumes.

The relaxation-pressure curve of the total system also shows that at lung volumes *above 38 percent vital capacity, the inspiratory process is active*, requiring muscular efforts, while expiratory forces are passive. At lung volumes *below 38 percent vital capacity, the expiratory process is active*, requiring muscular efforts, while the inspiratory process is passive.

Implications of the Relaxation-Pressure Curve

Some of the implications of the relaxation-pressure curve may be easily overlooked. For example, the area between the relaxation-pressure curve and the zero axis above resting lung volume represents the force that the muscles of inspiration must exert to overcome the elastic forces of resistance. On the other hand, the area below the resting volume represents the force that must be exerted by the muscles of expiration during forced expiratory efforts. In other words, these areas represent the combined elastic forces of the lungs and thorax, or chest wall. The implications of the relaxation-pressure curve are discussed in much greater detail by Rahn et al. (1946), by Campbell (1958), and by Agostoni and Mead (1964).

Pressure-Volume Diagrams

Additional pressure curves may be obtained by measuring the active inspiratory and expiratory forces. When

FIGURE 2-77

Component forces contributing to the relaxation pressure curve. The resting volume of the chest wall is at 55 percent vital capacity, and the resting volume of the lungs is not reached, even at 0 percent vital capacity. Even after a maximum expiratory effort the lungs are subjected to a certain amount of stretch. This accounts for residual volume. (After Agostoni and Mead, 1964.)

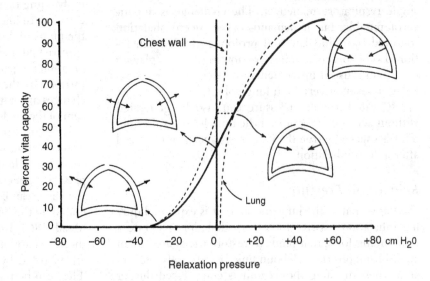

Pleural surface pressure at RLV = –5 cm H_2O
Resting volume of lung less than 0% vital capacity
Resting volume of chest wall 55% vital capacity
Arrows indicate direction and magnitude (approximately) of restoring forces.

maximum expiratory and maximum inspiratory pressures are graphed, along with the relaxation-pressure curve, the entire figure is known as a pressure-volume diagram. The one shown in Figure 2-78 represents three different conditions:

1. When the muscles of respiration are completely relaxed (R_p).

2. When the inspiratory muscles are maximally contracted (I_p).

3. When the expiratory muscles are maximally contracted (E_p).

The pressure-volume diagram shown in Figure 2-78 is based on data obtained by Rahn et al. Pressures are expressed in mm Hg.

In order to obtain the **inspiratory pressure curves,** the lungs are first voluntarily inflated to a given percentage of the vital capacity, after which the subject inhales through a manometer. The system is a closed one, of course, so no air can enter the lungs. Only a negative pressure is generated. *On mechanical grounds, the inspiratory pressure ought to be maximal with the lungs deflated, and ought to be minimal with the lungs completely inflated.* Values obtained by Rahn et al. are shown graphically as the I_p curve in Figure 2-78.

To obtain **expiratory pressure curves,** the subjects completely deflate their lungs voluntarily. When this has been accomplished, the only air in the lungs is residual. The subjects then inhale a given percentage of their vital capacity, after which they exhale maximally into the manometer. *Expiration forces ought to be minimal with almost deflated lungs and maximal with completely inflated lungs.* The expiratory pressure curve E_p is shown in Figure 2-78.

Interest in the ability of humans to generate very high and very low alveolar pressures seems to be historically related to the technological advances that have placed men and women in increasingly alien environments. Pressurized environments associated with underwater navigation and diving and rarefied environments associated with high altitude flying are among them. How deeply can a person descend into water, for example, breathing air at atmospheric pressure, before the thorax can no longer overcome the increasing water pressure?

In 1907, Jacquet in Basel, Switzerland, made use of a "pneumatic differentiation cabinet" in which a subject could sit, breathing through a tube to the outside. By using a bellows, he could vary the pressure within the chamber so that it was either below or above atmospheric. Jacquet measured the tidal volumes of a relaxed subject as pressure was varied, in this way obtaining the first **relaxation-pressure curve.**

In 1911, Bernoulli (descendant of the famed mathematician), using the same equipment, extended the experiment by measuring maximum inspired and expired volumes when different positive and negative pressures were generated within the cabinet. These maximum-effort curves, combined with the relaxation pressure curves of Jacquet, gave us the first **pressure-volume diagram.**

Then in 1919 Fritz Rohrer, a Swiss physiologist and physician, obtained relaxation and maximum-effort pressure curves, apparently unaware of the earlier work of Jacquet and Bernoulli. His experimental approach was unique, however, because he measured pressures at various lung volumes rather than lung volumes at various pressures. But, as Fenn and Rahn (1964) point out, although Rohrer's sophisticated analysis of the mechanics of breathing left little of fundamental importance to be discovered, his work never appeared in physiology textbooks. As a consequence, the entire pressure-volume problem was reinvestigated during World War II, again without knowledge of previous work!

This time, however, the world was receptive to the research because humans were flying high, diving deep, and dreaming of being catapulted free of the gravitational field of the Earth and into space.

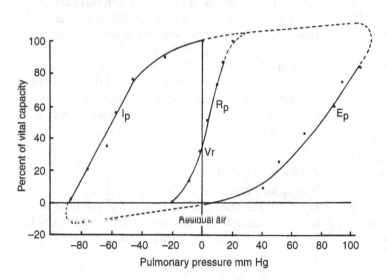

FIGURE 2-78

Pressure-volume diagram of breathing. Inspiratory pressures (I_p), relaxation pressures (R_p), and expiratory pressures (E_p) are based on data of Rahn et al., 1946.

Alveolar Pressure Requirements Very often in our day-to-day lives, alveolar pressures in excess of those generated passively are required. In addition, positive alveolar pressures over a wide range of lung volumes may be necessary in certain speech or singing tasks. In the following chapter on the larynx and phonation, we will learn that the pressure requirements for the speech mechanism are quite modest ones. A minimal value of alveolar pressure required to maintain laryngeal vibration, for example, is on the order of 3 cm H_2O, while values as high as 15 to 20 cm H_2O may be required for certain consonant production and for loud speech and singing.

The pressure-volume diagram in Figure 2-78 suggests that the respiratory system is indeed capable of generating rather high alveolar pressures, and from time to time they are required. During maximum expiratory efforts, in the case of a cough or a robust sneeze, for example, the alveolar pressure can be as high as 200 cm H_2O, and the explosively released air is expelled through the upper respiratory tract and out the mouth at velocities as high as 120 to 160 kilometers per hour! During maximum inspiratory efforts, alveolar pressures can be as low as –150 cm H_2O. This happens during hiccuping, which is a violent inspiratory act due to a sudden contraction of the diaphragm and interrupted by a sudden momentary closing of the vocal folds.

Implications of the Pressure-Volume Diagram One of the more interesting implications of the pressure-volume diagram can be seen by examination of the inspiratory and the expiratory pressure curves. The maximum inspiratory or expiratory pressures that can be generated at any given lung volume represent the algebraic sum of the relaxation and the muscular forces. Maximum expiratory pressures, with the lungs completely inflated, are the combined effects of relaxation plus muscular efforts. Surprisingly high expiratory pressures can also be generated at very low lung volumes. With the lungs inflated to just 10 percent vital capacity, for example, over 40 mm Hg pressure (55 cm H_2O) can be generated, but here the muscular effort is expended partly in overcoming the tendency of the thorax to recoil outward and partly in generating elevated alveolar pressure.

At resting level the expiratory pressure is due entirely to muscular efforts since relaxation pressure is zero at this lung volume. In other words, for the expiratory pressure curve, both the relaxation pressures and muscular pressures have positive signs at lung volumes above resting level, whereas relaxation pressures have negative signs at lung volumes below resting level where muscular pressures are positive. *Below resting level the relaxation pressures and the muscular pressures are in opposition to one another.*

For the inspiratory pressure curve the reciprocal is true. At lung volumes above resting level, the relaxation pres-

sures are positive while the muscular pressures are negative, and at lung volumes below resting level both the relaxation pressures and muscular pressures have negative signs.

Relationships such as these suggest that the respiratory apparatus is a versatile system and that almost unlimited combinations of positive and negative forces are possible to produce very precise regulation of alveolar pressures over a very wide range of lung volumes.

Inasmuch as inspiratory and expiratory forces can be generated simultaneously, very accurate specifications of the contributions of the respiratory musculature are necessary to fully account for any particular alveolar pressure. Alveolar pressure at a particular lung volume, which might be accounted for by relaxation pressure, could in fact be the consequence of opposing inspiratory and expiratory muscular forces and not of relaxation pressure at all.

We have been talking about production of alveolar pressures under relatively static conditions, when no actual air flow is taking place. To apply the mechanics of respiration to speech, we must consider dynamic conditions. And, to complicate matters further, we will need to account for very precise maintenance of specific alveolar pressures when resistances to air flow within the speech mechanism are continually changing due to articulation, pitch and voice intensity inflections, stress, and finally linguistic elements, The best we can hope for is an intuitive appreciation of the complexity of the problem. We also begin to see the hazards of trying to comprehend the complexities of speech production by studying only part of the system.

The Effects of Air Flow Resistance

The speech mechanism is an extraordinary sound-producing system. Think for a moment of the vast array of sounds that can be produced by this remarkable acoustical mechanism. The repertory is staggering, and yet, in spite of its versatility, the speech mechanism operates as nothing more than a variable resistance to the flow of air, and in that event the voice is hardly more than an epiphenomenon! To those of us who may be enamored of the beauty of the human voice, this attitude may be offensive. But an examination of the system from the standpoint of mechanics may help us to understand the functional relationships between the articulatory, phonatory, and respiratory systems, for example.

Airway Resistance

The speech mechanism is shown schematically in Figure 2-79. Resistance to air flow below the level of the larynx is relatively low and almost constant. The trachea and bronchi do yield somewhat to the influence of pres-

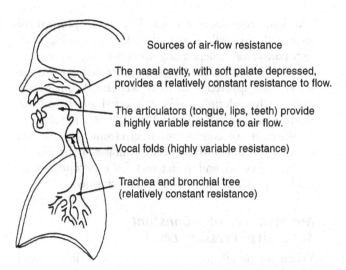

Sources of air-flow resistance

The nasal cavity, with soft palate depressed, provides a relatively constant resistance to flow.

The articulators (tongue, lips, teeth) provide a highly variable reistance to air flow.

Vocal folds (highly variable resistance)

Trachea and bronchial tree (relatively constant resistance)

FIGURE 2-79

Schematic of speech mechanism and simple electrical equivalent which relates air pressure, air flow, and air-flow resistance.

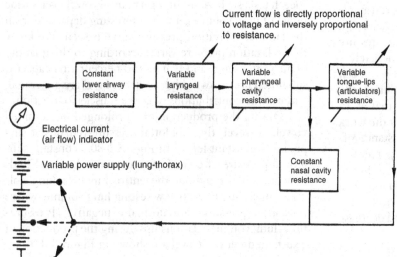

Current flow is directly proportional to voltage and inversely proportional to resistance.

| Constant lower airway resistance | Variable laryngeal resistance | Variable pharyngeal cavity resistance | Variable tongue-lips (articulators) resistance |

Electrical current (air flow) indicator

Variable power supply (lung-thorax)

Constant nasal cavity resistance

sures around them, but for our purposes air-flow resistance can be said to be low and invariant. The larynx, on the other hand, is a variable valve, and depending upon circumstances, its resistance varies from very low to absolute. During forced inhalation, for example, the vocal folds are separated widely, so the larynx offers little resistance to air flow. The vocal folds can also be brought tightly together at the midline to completely block the flow of air either into or out of the lungs. We can say that *laryngeal resistance is extremely variable, ranging from minimal to absolute.*

The structures that comprise the remainder of the vocal tract, such as the tongue, lips, and soft palate, are also capable of introducing a wide range of resistance to the flow of air. With the vocal tract in a neutral position, during the production of an "uh" vowel, for example, the articulators offer very little air-flow resistance. During the production of a continuant consonant they offer considerable resistance, and during the production of a stop or plosive they offer momentary absolute resistance to air flow.

As an air transmission system, then, the vocal tract is capable of almost countless adjustments, which result in varying degrees of flow resistance that can be represented on a continuum from minimal to absolute. Minimal air-flow resistance with an open airway represents one end of the continuum, and approximated vocal folds or lips (bilabial compression) represent the other end of the continuum. Resistance to air flow (somewhat less than absolute) is generated each time we speak, blow out a candle, or (when no one is watching) cool our soup by blowing on it.

Electrical Analog

If air flow is to be maintained under conditions of increasing flow resistance, a compensating increase in alveolar or pulmonic pressure will be required. The relationship between airway resistance and pressure requirements can be shown by an electrical analog in which the speech mechanism is likened to a simple electrical circuit such as the one shown in Figure 2-79. It consists of a battery (the lungs) and a series of electrical resistors (the airway). A meter in the circuit registers current (air) flow.

A very fundamental principle in electricity called **Ohm's law** states that electrical current flow is directly proportional to voltage and inversely proportional to the resistance offered by the circuit. By analogy, *air flow is directly proportional to alveolar pressure and inversely proportional to airway resistance.* In the circuit shown in Figure 2-79, the airway below the level of the larynx is represented by a single resistor, fixed in value. The laryngeal valve and the articulators are represented by a series of resistors that are variable.

In the electrical circuit, maintaining current flow with an increase in electrical resistance requires a proportional increase in the voltage source. Likewise, maintaining air flow with an increase in airway resistance requires an increase in alveolar or pulmonic pressure. On the other hand, if resistance is increased with pressure held constant, air flow will be reduced proportionately.

Although it has little direct bearing on speech production, air-flow resistance also occurs during the inspiratory process. Otis et al. (1950) found that at 15 inspirations per minute, about 28.5 percent of the work done in inhalation was to overcome the resistance offered by air movement. The remaining 71.5 percent of work done was to overcome the elastic forces of the rib cage and lung tissue. Notice, the next time you watch an athlete at the end of a strenuous run, how the neck is extended so as to straighten the upper airway and decrease air resistance.

Pressure and Air-Flow Regulation During Speech

Measurement of Subglottal (Alveolar) Pressure

Even in simple and ideal speech situations, the task of the respiratory system is a very complex one. During speech air flow is taking place, and the problem of measuring subglottal pressure—without introducing confounding resistance to air flow—becomes a very difficult one. The manometric technique for measuring static pressures cannot be employed where there is air flow.

One technique used to measure subglottal pressure is actually an *indirect* one. A catheter with a small rubber balloon attached to the end of it is passed into a subject's nostril, down the throat, and into the esophagus. With the balloon partially inflated, pressures in the trachea will be transmitted through the tracheal and esophageal walls to the balloon and then registered on a pressure-sensing device, such as an electronic manometer. The technique is not without its problems, however. Subjects, for one thing, don't like the procedure very much, and in addition, pressures as registered by the esophageal balloon will also reflect pleural-surface pressures, which vary considerably depending upon the lung volume.

Another technique for measuring subglottal pressure is *direct* and apparently far more accurate. A rather large-diameter hypodermic needle is inserted directly into the trachea just below the level of the larynx, and subglottal pressures are measured with an electronic pressure sensor that is coupled to the needle. Subjects don't like this procedure either, and in fact very few experiments using tracheal punctures have ever been performed.

Maintenance of a Constant Subglottal Pressure Level

When subglottal pressure is measured during a simple speech task, such as sustaining a neutral vowel over a wide range of lung volumes, a very interesting departure from the familiar relaxation-pressure curve is seen. We know that relaxation pressure varies according to the quantity of air in the lungs and that at 100 percent vital capacity, subglottal pressures as high as 40 cm H_2O are generated, without the contributions of active muscle contraction.

During the production of a prolonged or sustained vowel, however, the subglottal pressure remains at surprisingly constant levels. In Figure 2-80 a constant subglottal pressure of 6 cm H_2O maintains the vocal folds in vibration throughout the entire range of lung volumes, including those below resting lung volume, where relaxation pressures are normally negative. Pressure-flow–lung volume relationships during the production of a sustained neutral vowel are shown in Figure 2-80.

Somehow, the familiar relaxation-pressure–lung volume relationship is dramatically altered for even the simplest speech task. Air flow and subglottal pressure remain at a constant level throughout the entire utterance, and now the dimension of time begins to enter into the picture.

Probably the most obvious question confronting us is just how the respiratory system manages to regulate subglottal pressure at a *constant positive value*, both at high lung volumes where the relaxation pressure is in excess of the requirements of speech mechanism and at low lung volumes where the normal relaxation pressure is negative. Reexamination of the relaxation-pressure curve may provide us with some information.

In Figure 2-81, subglottal pressure of about 6 cm H_2O during phonation of the sustained neutral vowel [ə] has been superimposed on the relaxation-pressure curve. At high lung volumes, relaxation pressure is in excess of the demands of the speech mechanism. We learned earlier that regardless of the depth of inhalation, alveolar pressure is the same as atmospheric at the end of an inspiratory effort, provided airway resistance is negligible. You and I are perfectly capable of taking a very

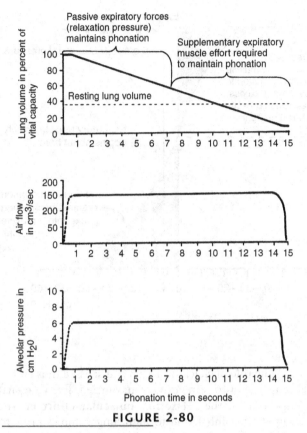

FIGURE 2-80

Air pressure, air flow, and lung volume relationships during the production of a sustained vowel.

deep breath (100 percent vital capacity) and maintaining this high lung volume with the respiratory tract completely open by simply maintaining the active contraction of the musculature of inhalation. Here, then, is an in-

stance where relaxation pressure has been defeated by the muscles of inhalation. Alveolar pressure is the same as atmospheric, of course, and would register zero on a manometer. Complete relaxation into a manometer would generate a subglottal or alveolar pressure of about 40 cm H_2O. Our simple speech task requires a compromise between maintaining zero alveolar pressure and the pressures generated by complete relaxation.

At 100 percent vital capacity, continued contraction of the inspiratory musculature during our simple speech task must overcome about 35 cm H_2O relaxation pressure, to leave a net of about 6 cm H_2O subglottal pressure for speech production. At 80 percent vital capacity, only about 15 cm H_2O pressure must be overcome by the musculature of inhalation, and *at about 55 percent vital capacity, relaxation pressure alone will maintain the speech utterance.*

Below 55 percent vital capacity, increasingly active contraction of the expiratory musculature is going to be required to overcome the negative relaxation pressure and to maintain subglottal pressure at 6 cm H_2O. We see, from inspection of Figure 2-81 that the relaxation pressure that must be overcome during speech is highest at maximum lung volume. It decreases gradually with continued air expenditure until, at about 55 percent vital capacity, subglottal and relaxation pressure are approximately equal in magnitude.

Checking Action

Muscular activity that prevents thorax-lung recoil from generating excessive subglottal pressure is called checking action. In Figure 2-82, the muscle action required to maintain a subglottal pressure of 6 cm H_2O during

FIGURE 2-81

Subglottal (alveolar) pressure superimposed on a relaxation pressure curve.

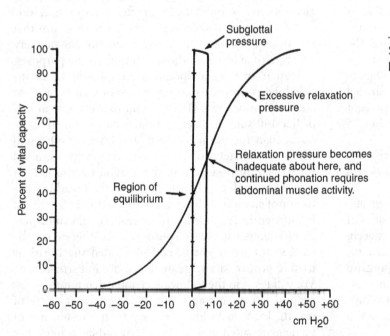

FIGURE 2-82

Illustration of muscle actions required to maintain a constant subglottal pressure during speech.

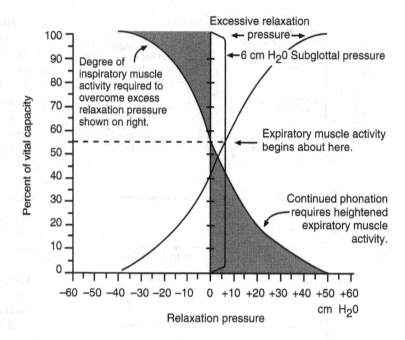

FIGURE 2-82

Illustration of muscle actions required to maintain a constant subglottal pressure during speech.

speech is shown as the shaded area to the left of the vertical pressure reference, above 55 percent vital capacity, and to the right of the pressure reference, below 55 percent vital capacity.

We might consider some additional speech activities—exploring the relationship between subglottal pressure demands and the need for checking action.

In the following chapter we will learn in some detail that subglottal requirements may vary from 3 cm H_2O during soft speech to about 20 cm H_2O for the production of intense speech. The fact that subglottal pressure increases for progressively more intense speech is an indication that increased resistance to air flow is being offered by the larynx. We ought to expect an inverse relationship between air-flow resistance and the need for checking action, as shown schematically in Figure 2-83. Muscular effort required to maintain subglottal pressure at 20 cm H_2O is again shown as the shaded area to the left at lung volumes above about 75 percent vital capacity and to the right at lung volumes below 75 percent vital capacity.

There is an inverse relationship between airway resistance and the degree of checking action required to maintain a given subglottal pressure.

When the complexities of airway resistance generated by the articulators, coupled with the complexities of the laryngeal resistance during conversational speech, are considered, the interactions between muscular effort, air flow, airway resistance, and subglottal pressure virtually defy description. The demands of conversational speech would require that the checking action turn on and off as airway resistances decrease and increase in the course of speaking.

The role of checking action as discussed thus far has been, at least to some extent, maximized. Even a casual inspection of the **relaxation–muscular-effort curves** suggests that inhalation to high lung volumes prior to speech is a very uneconomical practice from the standpoint of muscular activity.

Lung Volumes Required for Speech

Rahn et al. (1946) and others have shown that **resting lung volume** is equal to about 38 percent of vital capacity and that **tidal volume** amounts to about 15 percent of the vital capacity. In other words, about 53 percent of the vital capacity occupies the lungs after a quiet inhalation.

The results of at least two studies have shown that breath requirements for speech production are not very different (if at all) from those required for life purposes, at least from the standpoint of the quantity of air inhaled when expressed as percentage of vital capacity at end inspiration. Idol (1936) found that more than half of her 140 subjects breathed more deeply for life purposes than for normal speech. Hoshiko (1964) found that approximately 50 percent of vital capacity is inhaled for speech purposes. From these studies and others, it seems reasonable to conclude that if the breathing behavior of an individual is within normal broad limits and is sufficiently deep for life purposes, it ought to be perfectly adequate for speech purposes. And therein lies the clinker, for we ought to add—provided the breath is used to proper advantage by the larynx and articulators. We will learn in the following chapter that improper laryngeal behavior may result in a significant waste of breath. Inadequate loudness may be the result, not of inadequate subglottal pressure, but rather of improper

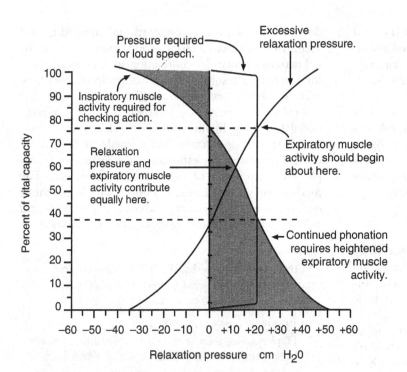

Pressure required for loud speech.

Excessive relaxation pressure.

Inspiratory muscle activity required for checking action.

Relaxation pressure and expiratory muscle activity contribute equally here.

Expiratory muscle activity should begin about here.

Continued phonation requires heightened expiratory muscle activity.

Percent of vital capacity

Relaxation pressure   cm H₂0

FIGURE 2-83

Relationship between airway resistance and the need for checking action. As airway resistance increases the inspiratory activity necessary required to overcome excess relaxation pressure decreases.

use of the larynx, the articulators, or the resonators. Studies have also shown that not everyone requires more breath for loud speech than for normal speech. Idol found that air expenditure for loud speech was less than for normal speech in about one-third of her 140 subjects. These results have been supported in a subsequent study by Ptacek and Sander (1963). This seemingly paradoxical state of affairs will be discussed again in the following chapter.

Hixon et al. (1973) have reported that "there are roughly defined lung volume limits within which certain types of utterances typically occur." They state that in the upright posture most conversational speech of normal loudness is produced within the midrange through volumes encompassing approximately 35 to 60 percent of the vital capacity. They also maintain that deeper breaths are taken during conversational speech than during normal quiet tidal breathing. During loud speech, which demands higher subglottal pressures, speech is initiated from higher lung volumes (60 to 80 percent vital capacity).

Russell and Stathopoulos (1988), in comparing childrens' and adults' respiratory behavior during speech tasks, found that, at loud intensity, adults used a higher percentage of their vital capacity than did the children. Adults also went further into their functional residual capacity at loud intensity whereas the children did not. Articulatory demands (consonants) have a greater effect on breathing for children than for adults.

The overall range of lung volumes in which speech can be expected to be produced is from about 35 to 70 percent of vital capacity, which is within the linear portion of the relaxation-pressure curve and which is not particularly demanding of the checking action phenomenon. Singing may generate far more demanding circumstances than speech.

Chest Wall Preparation for Speech

On the basis of their study of chest wall movements during speech, Hixon et al. (1973) suggest that there is a "speech-specific" posturing of the rib cage and abdomen. They suggest that the rib cage is relatively more expanded and the abdomen relatively less expanded for speech than they are in a relaxed state at the same lung volume. They further suggest that *this posturing places the chest wall in an optimum configuration for generating rapid pressure changes without further major changes in the shape of the system.*

Chest wall movements prior to the onset of phonation have also been investigated (Baken, et al., 1979; Wilder, 1980; Baken and Cavallo, 1981). In a study by Baken et al., subjects were required to produce the vowel [ɑ] as quickly as possible in response to stimuli delivered at varying lung volumes, regardless of respiratory phase within the tidal volume cycle. This meant that the signal to phonate was unexpected and served to deny the subject of the usual prephonatory inspiratory chest adjustment prior to phonation.

In their population of untrained young adult males, ongoing chest wall movements, wherever they happened to be at the time, continued for about 245 msec following the delivery of the stimulus to phonate. This latency was immediately followed by a well-defined chest wall adjustment just prior to the onset of phonation. The duration of this prephonatory adjustment was related to lung volume at the time of the delivery of the stimulus. Lung volume and adjustment times were found to be inversely related, with adjustment times of about 82 msec associated with lung volumes above 50 percent of quiet tidal volume and 100 msec associated with lung volumes below 50 percent of quiet tidal volume. *The typical prephonatory chest wall adjustment consisted of abdominal compression and rib cage expansion, although lung volume changes during the adjustment period were negligible.*

Variations in Breathing Patterns

It is well known that there are variations in breathing patterns. Some individuals exhibit a marked protrusion of the abdominal wall with each inhalation, while others exhibit a lateral expansion of the thorax, with little protrusion of the abdominal wall. In a few individuals, the expansion is predominantly in the extreme upper chest. These individuals seem to be "lifting" their rib cage by elevating their shoulders as they inhale. These differences have led to the use of popular descriptive terms such as **diaphragmatic** (or **abdominal**), **thoracic**, and **clavicular** breathing.

Campbell (1954) and Wade (1954) have shown that diaphragmatic breathing does not necessarily mean that an individual is selectively using the diaphragm as the principal muscle of inhalation. They also have shown that thoracic breathers do not demonstrate a marked increase over diaphragmatic breathers in the activity of the intercostal musculature.

It probably makes little or no difference in normal speech whether an individual uses diaphragmatic or thoracic breathing. Lindsley (1929) found a natural tendency for abdominal protrusion for both males and females, and in addition, he noted that females tended toward thoracic breathing. These results have been supported by those of Sallee (1936) and Gray (1936). In most persons, the abdomen and lower and upper thorax all expand during inhalation, but there is not much question that the region of predominant expansion may vary from individual to individual. Gray (1936) found that about 65 percent of men and women breathe diaphragmatically. He also found evidence that voice quality or audibility is unlikely to be affected by regional predominance.

Gray (1936) stresses that because clavicular breathing may result in excessive tension in the throat and an inadequate breath supply, it ought to be avoided. Pure clavicular breathers, however, are not encountered frequently. In fact, there is some question as to whether clavicular breathing ever occurs in isolation, that is, set apart from thoracic breathing.

Occasionally, however, a peculiar breathing pattern is encountered that seems to interfere with speech production. It is known as **oppositional breathing** and seems to result from a lack of control over the sequential pattern of muscular contraction, as in cerebral palsy, for example. Persons who use oppositional breathing seem to *simultaneously contract the muscles of inhalation and exhalation*. We all use a certain amount of oppositional breathing in the course of ordinary (conversational) speech production, but normally it is used for control purposes. Phonation can be arrested, for example, by contraction of inspiratory musculature. The mechanism is a subtle one, and difficult to document or quantify, but the *intercostal musculature is frequently cited as being capable of pulselike control over subglottal pressures.*

CLINICAL NOTE: In addition to regional predominance in breathing, other terms are frequently employed to describe types of breathing.

1. **Eupnea**—normal quiet breathing.
2. **Hyperpnea**—increased depth of breathing, usually increased tidal volume with or without an increased rate of breathing. When pulmonary ventilation approximates the volume of vital capacity, breathing becomes labored and is called **dyspnea** or air hunger.
3. **Apnea**—cessation of breathing at the end of a normal expiration. The condition sometimes occurs only during sleep, thus the term **sleep apnea.**
4. **Apneusis**—cessation of breathing in the inspiratory position.
5. **Cheyne-Stokes** respiration—a gradually increased tidal volume for several breaths, followed by several breaths with gradually decreasing tidal volume. The cycle repeats itself. Also called **periodic** breathing. The most common cause is cardiac failure.
6. **Biot's** respiration—a form of periodic breathing characterized by repeated sequences of deep gasps followed by apnea. Patients with very high cerebrospinal fluid pressure or with destructive disease of the brain often develop periodic breathing.

CLINICAL NOTE: The graph shown in Figure 2-84 illustrates some of the *consequences of lung disease.* Note that in **emphysema,** where lung compliance is increased and elastic recoil of the lungs is decreased, the depth of inhalation is increased, and forced exhalation is necessary in order to develop air pressures adequate for speech production. In **pulmonary fibrosis,** where lung compliance is reduced and the elastic recoil of the lung is increased, the quantity of air inhaled is minimal and frequent breath pauses can be expected. Both of these conditions can accompany old age, and both give an impression of what can be called "shortness of breath."

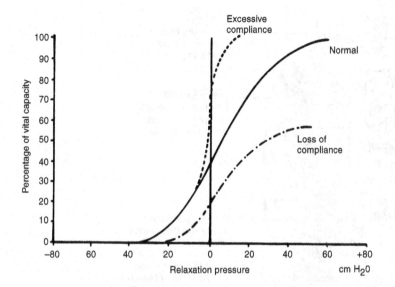

FIGURE 2-84

Relationship between lung compliance and pleural surface pressure in normal and diseased lungs.

Breathing is no simple process. Indeed, a complete and comprehensive integration of the vast body of knowledge accumulated to date would be, to say the least, a monumental task. The following concluding paragraphs are by no means intended to represent such an integration of information. Rather, they are intended to be a schematic account of a cycle of breathing for life purposes, of breathing for a simple speech utterance.

A Descriptive Account of a Cycle of Breathing

In a position of rest, the pressure within the lungs (alveolar pressure) is the same as atmospheric, and the diaphragm, which is the principal muscle of inhalation, presents the appearance of an inverted bowl. It separates the abdominal viscera from the thoracic viscera, and anatomically divides the torso into a thoracic and an abdominal cavity.

Upon initiation of inhalation, contraction of the posterior muscle fibers and, to a lesser extent, the anterior fibers draws the central tendon downward and somewhat forward to increase the vertical dimensions of the thorax, and at the same time compresses the abdominal contents to elevate intra-abdominal pressure. The diaphragm is apparently active in all healthy persons, but its action is almost always assisted by the intercostal muscles that evert the ribs, stiffen the intercostal spaces, and enlarge the anteroposterior and lateral dimensions of the thorax. The scaleni may also become active, especially toward the end of inhalation. They help raise the uppermost ribs. The respiratory musculature is summarized in Figure 2-85.

Subatmospheric pleural fluid pressure binds the lungs to the walls of the thorax, and so an increase in the dimensions of the thorax results in a negative alveolar pressure, which amounts to a modest -2 cm H_2O, relative to atmospheric pressure. Air flows inward until alveolar pressure is equalized to atmospheric. As the lungs inflate, the muscles of inhalation gradually cease their activity and the passive forces of exhalation begin to assume their role. Elevated intra-abdominal pressure tends to restore the diaphragm to its uncontracted state, the twisted ribs and distorted tissues resume their shape, and the overall dimensions of the thorax decrease so the lung tissue becomes subjected to less distortion. Alveolar pressure is momentarily elevated and air flows outward until once again alveolar and atmospheric pressures are equalized.

The muscles of inhalation slowly begin to contract and a new cycle of respirations begins. The normal respiratory rate is about 12 breaths per minute, with tidal volume between about 350 to 750 cc of air. Minute volume ranges from about 4 to 9 liters. With increased muscular effort, as much as 3 liters of air can be inhaled, starting from resting level.

If during exhalation airway resistance is introduced, greatly elevated alveolar pressures can be generated by the rebounding forces of the lung-thorax complex. Resistance can be the result of approximated vocal folds in the larynx, and in that event they may enter into vibration and phonation takes place. Additional resistances may be introduced by the tongue, the lips, etc., each of which calls for increased alveolar pressure, if air flow is to take place.

At high lung volumes the passive restoration force generated by the lung-thorax unit may produce alveolar pressures as high as 40 cm H_2O, and with supplemental muscular (abdominal) effort, alveolar pressures can be increased to levels as high as 200 cm H_2O. At very low lung volumes (0 to 38 percent VC), the passive restoration force generates a negative alveolar pressure, and

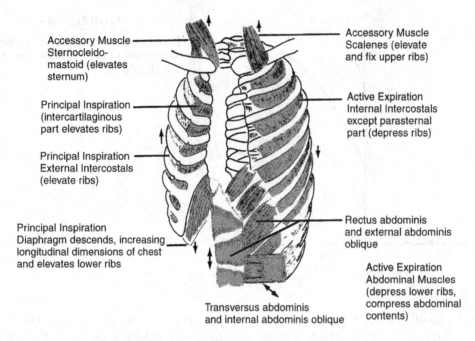

Accessory Muscle Sternocleido-mastoid (elevates sternum)

Accessory Muscle Scalenes (elevate and fix upper ribs)

Principal Inspiration (intercartilaginous part elevates ribs)

Active Expiration Internal Intercostals except parasternal part (depress ribs)

Principal Inspiration External Intercostals (elevate ribs)

Principal Inspiration Diaphragm descends, increasing longitudinal dimensions of chest and elevates lower ribs

Rectus abdominis and external abdominis oblique

Active Expiration Abdominal Muscles (depress lower ribs, compress abdominal contents)

Transversus abdominis and internal abdominis oblique

FIGURE 2-85

The principal muscles of respiration.

the pressure can be made increasingly negative through the contributions of the inspiratory musculature.

Speech production demands an alveolar or subglottal pressure in the range of 5 to 20 cm H_2O, and usually over a rather wide range of lung volumes. The range, of course, will depend upon the rate of air flow and the length of the speech utterance. At high lung volumes, the relaxation pressure generated by the thorax may be in excess of the demands of the speech mechanism. In that event, checking action provided by the inspiratory musculature can counteract excessive thoracic-lung rebound in order to regulate alveolar pressure. At midvolume, just the relaxation pressure may provide the necessary alveolar pressure for speech, and at low lung volumes (below resting level) positive alveolar pressure must be maintained by the muscles of exhalation. With proper interplay of checking action, relaxation pressures, and the expiratory muscles, the speech mechanism can be provided with precisely regulated subglottal pressures.

BIBLIOGRAPHY AND READING LIST

Agostoni, E., and R. Hyatt. "Static Behavior of the Respiratory System." In A. Fishman, P. Macklem, J. Mead, and S. Geiger, eds., *Handbook of Physiology, Vol. 3, Section 3, The Respiratory System*, Bethesda, MD: American Psychological Society, 1986, (113–130).

Agostoni, E., "Action of Respiratory Muscles," pp. 337–386, in W. Fenn and H. Rahn, eds., *Handbook of Physiology, Respiration 1*, Sect. 3. Washington, D.C.: Amer. Physiol. Soc., 1964. Baltimore: Williams & Wilkins.

———, and W. Fenn, "Velocity of Muscle Shortening as a Limiting Factor in Respiratory Air Flow," *J. Appl. Physiol.*, 15, 1960, 349–353.

———, and J. Mead, "Statics of the Respiratory System," pp. 387–409, in W. Fenn and H. Rahn, eds., *Handbook of Physiology, Respiration 1*, Sect. 3. Washington, D.C.: Amer. Physiol. Soc., 1964. Baltimore: Williams & Wilkins.

Adams, C., and R. Munro, "The Relationship between Internal Intercostal Muscle Activity and Pause Placement in the Connected Utterance of Native and Non-Native Speakers of English," *Phonetica*, 28, 1973, 227–250.

Altose, M., "The Physiological Basis of Pulmonary Function Testing," *Clinical Symposia*, 31, 1979.

Baken, R., and S. Cavallo, "Prephonatory Chest Wall Posturing," *Folia Phoniatrica*, 33, 1981, 193–202.

———, S. Cavallo, and K. Weissman, "Chest Wall Movements Prior to Phonation," *J. Sp. Hrng. Res.*, 22, 1979, 862–872.

Barnes, J., "Vital Capacity and Ability in Oral Reading," *Quart. J. Sp. Ed.*, 12, 1926, 76–181.

Basmajian, J., *Muscles Alive*. Baltimore: Williams & Wilkins, 1962.

Beckett, R., "The Respirometer as a Diagnostic and Clinical Tool in the Speech Clinic," *J. Sp. Hrng. Res.*, 36, 1971, 235–241.

Berg, Jw. van den., "An Electrical Analog of the Trachea, Lungs and Tissue," *Acta Physio. et. Pharmacol-Neer.*, 9, 1960, 361–385.

Berles, K., "Limitations of Surface Electromyography." Master's thesis, Champaign: University of Illinois, 1969.

———, and W. Zemlin, "Further Limitations of Surface Electromyography." Paper presented at ASHA Convention, Chicago, 1970.

Bloomer, H., "Roentgenographic Study of the Mechanics of Respiration," *Sp. Monog.*, 3, 1936, 118–124.

———, and H. Shohara, "The Study of Respiratory Movements by Roentgen Kymography," *Sp. Monog.*, 8, 1940, 91–102.

Bosma, J., H. Truby, and J. Lind, "Upper Respiratory Actions of the Infant." In *Proceedings of the Conference: Communicative Problems in Cleft Palate*. Washington, D.C.: ASHA Reports, No. 1, 35–49.

Bouhuys, A., D. Proctor, and J. Mead, "Kinetic Aspects of Singing," *J. Appl. Physiol.*, 21, 1966, 483–496.

Braun, N., N. S. Arora, and D. F. Rochester, "Force-length Relationship of the Normal Human Diaphragm," *J. of Appl. Physio: Environ. and Exercise Physio.*, 53, 1982, 405–412.

Brody, J. and W. Thurlbeck. "Development, Growth, and Aging of the Lung." In A. Fishman, P. Macklem, J. Mead, and S. Geiger, eds., *Handbook of Physiology, Vol. 3, Section 3. The Respiratory System*, Bethesda, MD: American Physiological Society, 1986, (179–191).

Campbell, E., "An Electromyographic Study of the Role of the Abdominal Muscles in Breathing," *J. Physiol.* (London), 117, 1952, 222–223.

———, "The Muscular Control of Breathing in Man," Ph.D. diss., University of London, 1954.

———, "An Electromyographic Examination of the Role of the Intercostal Muscles in Breathing in Man," *J. Physiol.* 129, 1955, 12–26.

———, *The Respiratory Muscles and the Mechanics of Breathing*. London: Lloyd-Luke Ltd., 1958.

———, *The Respiratory Muscles and the Mechanics of Breathing*. Chicago: Yearbook Medical Publishers, 1958.

———, "Motor Pathway," pp. 535–543, in W. Fenn and H. Rahn, eds., *Handbook of Physiology, Respiration* 1, Sect. 3. Washington, D.C.: Amer. Physiol. Soc., 1964. Baltimore: Williams & Wilkins.

———, "The Respiratory Muscles," pp. 135–140, in A. Bouhuys, ed., *Sound Production in Man, Annals of the N.Y. Acad. Sci.*, 155, 1968.

Campbell, E. J. M., and J. H. Green, "The Behavior of the Abdominal Muscles and the Intra-abdominal Pressure During Quiet Breathing and Increased Pulmonary Inhalation. A Study of Man," *J. Physiol.* (London), 127, 1955, 423–426.

Campbell, E., and Jellife, unpublished findings, 1951.

Catton, W., and J. Gray, "Electromyographic Study of the Action of the Serratus Anterior Muscle in Respiration," *J. Anat.* (London), 85, 1951, 412.

Caultier, C., and R. Zinman, "Maximal Static Pressures in Healthy Children." *Respiration Physiology*, 51, 45–61, 1983.

Cherniak, R., and L. Cherniak, *Respiration in Health and Disease*. Philadelphia: W. B. Saunders, 1961.

Comroe, J., *Physiology of Respiration*. Chicago: Yearbook Medical Publishers, 1965.

———, R. Forster, S. Dubois, W. Briscoe, and E. Carlson, *The Lung: Clinical Physiology and Pulmonary Function Tests*, 2nd ed. Chicago: Yearbook Medical Publishers, 1962.

Consolazio, C. F., H. Johnson, L. Matousch, R. Nelson, and G. Isaac, "Respiratory Function in Normal Young Adults at Sea Level and 4300 Meters," *Milit. Med.*, 133, 1968, 96–105. See also *DSH Abstracts*, 8, 1968, 223.

Constans, H., "An Objective Analysis of the Three Forms of Force in Speech," pp. 1–36, in G. W. Gray, ed., *Studies in Experimental Phonetics*, Louisiana University Studies, No. 27. Baton Rouge: Louisiana State University Press, 1936.

Crosjean, F., and M. Collins, "Breathing, Pausing and Reading," *Phonetica*, 36, 1979, 98–114.

Crouch, J., *Functional Human Anatomy*. Philadelphia: Lea & Febiger, 1979.

Dally, J., and F. Halls, "An Inquiry into the Physiological Mechanism of Respiration," *J. Anat. and Physiol.*, 53, 1908, 93–114.

Davis, S., and W. Zemlin, "An Electromyographic Study of Respiratory Musculature," 1965 (unpublished).

Demuth, G., W. Howatt, and B. Hill, "The Growth of Lung Function," *Pediatrics*, 35, Suppl. 1 (part II), 1965, 162–176.

Draper, M., P. Ladefoged, and D. Whitteridge, "Respiratory Muscles in Speech Breathing," *J. Sp. Hrng. Res.*, 2, 1959, 16–27.

Eblen, R., "Limitations on Use of Surface Electromyography in Studies of Speech Breathing," *J. Sp. Hrng. Res.*, 6, 1963, 3–18.

Felberbaum, R., "Upper Respiratory Tract Mechano-Receptors and Their Reflexes on Laryngeal Muscles" (Russian text) Fiziol. Zh. Schenov., 55, 1969, 783–744. Abstract in English found in *DSH Abstracts*, 10, 1970.

Fenn, W., "Mechanics of Respiration," *Amer. J. of Med.*, 10, 1951, 77–91.

———, "The Mechanics of Breathing," *Sci. American*, 203, Jan. 1960, 138–148.

———, and H. Rahn, eds. *Handbook of Physiology, Respiration*, 1, Sect. 3. Washington, D.C.: American Physiological Society, 1964. Baltimore: Williams & Wilkins.

Freud, E., "Voice and Breathing," *Arch Otolaryngol.*, 67, 1958, 1–7.

Gould, W., and H. Okamura, "Static Lung Volumes in Singers," *Ann. Otol. Rhinol. and Laryngol.*, 82, 1973, 89–95.

Gray, G., "Regional Predominance in Respiration in Relation to Certain Aspects of Voice," pp. 59–76, in G. W. Gray, ed., *Studies in Experimental Phonetics*, Louisiana University Studies, No. 27. Baton Rouge: Louisiana State University Press, 1936.

Gray, H., *The Anatomy of the Human Body*, 29th ed. (C. M. Coss ed.). Philadelphia: Lea & Febiger, 1973, 304–311.

Guyton, A., *Textbook of Medical Physiology*, 6th ed. Philadelphia: W. B. Saunders, 1981, Chaps. 5, 6, 7, 39.

Haldane, J., *Respiration*. New Haven, Conn.: Yale University Press, 1935.

Hart-Davis, A., *Scientific Eye: Exploring the marvels of science*. New York: Sterling Publishing Co., 1989.

Hanley, T., and R. Peters, "The Speech and Hearing Laboratory," in L. E. Travis, ed., *Handbook of Speech Pathology and Audiology*, 2nd ed. Englewood Cliffs, N.J.: Prentice-Hall, 1971.

Hardy, J., and T. Edmonds, "Electronic Integrator for Measurement of Partitions of the Lung Volume," *J. Sp. Hrng. Res.*, 11, 1968, 777–786.

Henderson, A., F. Goldman-Eisler, and A. Skarbek, "Temporal Patterns of Cognitive Activity and Breath Control in Speech," *Lang. Speech*, 8, 1965, 236–243.

Hirano, M., and J. Ohala, "Use of Hooked-Wire Electrodes for Electromyography of the Intrinsic Laryngeal Muscles," *J. Sp. Hrng. Res.*, 12, 1969, 362–373.

Hixon, T., and Collaborators, *Respiratory Function in Speech and Song*. Boston: College Hill Press, 1987.

Hixon, T., M. Goldman, and J. Mead, "Kinematics of the Chest Wall During Speech Production," *J. Sp. Hrng. Res.*, 16, 1973, 78–115.

Hixon, T., and G. Weismer, "Perspectives on the Edinburgh Study of Speech Breathing," *J. Sp. Hrng. Res.*, 38, 1995, 42–60.

Hoit, J., B. Plassman, R. Lansing, and T. Hixon, "Abdominal Muscle Activity During Speech Production," *J. of Appl. Physio.*, 65, 1988, 2656–2664.

Hoit, J., and T. Hixon, "Age and Speech Breathing," *J. Sp. Hrng. Res.*, 30, 1987, 351–366.

Hoit, J., T. Hixon, P. Watson, and W. Morgan, "Speech Breathing in Children and Adolescents," *J. Sp. Hrng. Res.*, 33, 1990, 51–69.

Hoover, G., "The Functions and Integrations of the Intercostal Muscles," *Arch. Int. Med.*, 30, 1922, 1–33.

Horii, Y., and P. Cooke, "Some Airflow, Volume, and Duration Characteristics of Oral Reading," *J. Sp. Hrng. Res.*, 21, 1978, 470–481.

Hoshiko, M., "Sequence of Action of Breathing Muscles During Speech," *J. Sp. Hrng. Res.*, 3, 1960, 291–297.

——, "Electromyographic Investigation of the Intercostal Muscles During Speech," *Arch. Physical. Med. Rehab.*, 43, 1962, 115–119.

——, (1964, unpublished findings.)

——, and K. Berger, "Sequence of Respiratory Muscle Activity During Varied Vocal Attack," *Sp. Monog.*, 32, 1965, 185–191.

Hoshiko, M., and V. Bolckcolsky, "A Respirometric Study of Lung Function During Utterance of Varying Speech Material," *Sp. Monog.*, 34, 1967, 74–79.

Huyck, M., and K. Allen, "Diaphragmatic Action in Good and Poor Speaking Voices," *Sp. Monog.*, 4, 1937, 101–109.

Idol, H. R., "A Statistical Study of Respiration in Relation to Speech Characteristics," pp. 79–98, in G. W. Gray, ed., *Studies in Experimental Phonetics*, Louisiana State Studies, No. 27. Baton Rouge: Louisiana State University Press, 1936.

Jaeger, M., and A. Otis, "Effects of the Compressibility of Alveolar Gas on the Dynamics and Work of Breathing," *USAF Sch. Aerospace Med.*, Rep. No. SAM-TDR-63-71, Conr. Mo. AF 41 (609)-1553, 1963, 15.

Jones, D., R. Beargie, and J. Pauly, "An Electromyographic Study of Some Muscles of Costal Respiration in Man," *Anatomical Record*, 117, 1953, 17–24.

Josephson, C., and M. Willens, "Physiology of the Singing Voice with Special Reference to the Relation of Respiration and Muscular Physiology," *Arch. Otol.*, 11, 1930.

Kalia, M., "Anatomical Organization of Central Respiratory Neurons," *Ann. Rev. of Physio.*, 43, 1981, 105–120.

Kent, R., B. Atal, and J. Miller eds., *Papers in Speech Communication*. Woodbury, N.Y.: Acoustical Society of America, 1991.

Koepke, G., A. Murphy, J. Rae, and E. Dickinson, "An Electromyographic Study of Some of the Muscles Used in Respiration," *Arch. Phys. Med. and Rehab.*, 36, 1955, 217–222.

Konno, K., and J. Mead, "Measurement of the Separate Volume Changes of Rib Cage and Abdomen During Breathing," *J. Appl. Physiol.*, 22, 1968, 407–422.

——, "Static Volume-Pressure Characteristics of the Rib Cage and Abdomen," *J. Appl. Physiol.*, 24, 1968, 544–548.

Kunze, L., "Evaluation of Methods of Estimating Sub-glottal Air Pressure," *J. Sp. Hrng. Res.*, 7, 1962, 151–164.

Ladefoged, P., "Linguistic Aspects of Respiratory Phenomena," pp. 177–181, in A. Bouheys, ed., *Sound Production in Man, Annals of the N.Y. Acad. Sci.*, 155, 1968.

Liljestrand, A., "Neural Control of Respiration," *Physiol. Rev.*, 38, 1958, 691–708.

Lindsley, C., "Objective Study of the Respiratory Processes Accompanying Speech," *Quart. J. Sp.*, 15, 1929, 42–48.

McFarland, D., and A. Smith, "Surface Recordings of Respiratory Muscle Activity During Speech: Some Preliminary Findings," *J. Sp. Hrng. Res.*, 32, 1989, 657–667.

McIlroy, M., R. Marshal, and R. Cristie, "The Work of Breathing in Normal Subjects," *Clinical Science*, 13, 1954, 125–136.

Mead, J., A. Bouhuys, and D. Proctor, "Mechanisms Generating Subglottic Pressure, pp. 177–181, in A. Bouheys, ed., *Sound Production in Man, Annals of the N.Y. Acad. Sci.*, 155, 1968.

——, and J. Marin, "Principles of Respiratory Mechanics," *J. Amer. Physical Therapy*, 48, 1968, 478–494.

——, and J. Milic-Emili, "Theory and Methodology in Respiratory Mechanics with Glossary of Symbols," pp. 363–376, in W. Fenn and H. Rahn, eds., *Handbook of Physiology, Respiration* 1, Sect. 3. Washington, D.C.: Amer. Physiol. Soc., 1964. Baltimore: Williams & Wilkins.

——, and J. Whittenberger, "Physical Properties of Human Lungs Measured During Spontaneous Respiration," *J. Appl. Physiol.*, 5, 1953, 779–796.

Minifie, F., T. Hixon, and F. Williams, eds., *Normal Aspects of Speech, Hearing, and Language*. Englewood Cliffs, N.J.: Prentice-Hall, 1973.

Müller, J., *The Physiology of the Senses, Voice, and Muscular Motion with the Mental Faculties*. Translated by W. Baly. London: Walton and Maberly, 1848.

Murphy, A., G. Koepke, E. Smith, and D. Dickenson, "Sequence of Action of the Diaphragm and Intercostal Muscles During Respiration, II Expiration," *Arch. Phys. Med. and Rehab.*, 40, 1959, 337–342.

Newsom Davis, J., T. Sears, D. Staff, and A. Taylor, "The Effects of Airway Obstructions on the Electrical Activity of Intercostal Muscles in Conscious Man," *J. Physiol.* (London), 185, 1966.

Otis, A., W. Fenn, and H. Rahn, "Mechanics of Breathing in Man," *J. Appl. Physiol.*, 2, 1950, 592–607.

Pappenheimer, J., J. Comroe, A. Cournand, J. Ferguson, G. Filley, W. Fowler, J. Gray, H. Helmholtz, Jr., A. Otis, H. Rahn, and R. Riley, "Standardization of Definitions and Symbols in Respiratory Physiology," *Fed. Proc.*, 9, 1950, 602–615.

Peterson, S., "An Electromyographic Study of the Respiratory Muscles in Man." Paper presented at ASHA Convention, Chicago, 1964.

Ptacek, P., and E. Sander, "Maximum Duration of Phonation," *J. Sp. Hrng. Res.*, 28, 1963, 171–182.

Radford, E., Jr., "Static Mechanical Properties of Mammalian Lungs," pp. 429–449, in W. Fenn and H. Rahn, eds., *Handbook of Physiology, Respiration* 1, Sect. 3. Washington, D.C.: Amer. Physiol. Soc., 1964. Baltimore: Williams & Wilkins.

Rahn, H., A. Otis, L. E. Chadwick, and W. Fenn, "The Pressure-Volume Diagram of the Thorax and Lung," *Amer. J. Physiol.*, 146, 1946, 161–178.

Russell, N., and E. Stathopoulos, "Lung Volume Changes in Children and Adults," *J. Sp. Hrng. Res.*, 31, 1988, 146–155.

Sallee, W., "An Objective Study of Respiration in Relation to Audibility in Connected Speech," pp. 52–58, in G. W. Gray, ed. *Studies in Experimental Phonetics*, Louisiana University Studies, No. 27. Baton Rouge: Louisiana State University Press, 1936.

Schilling, R., "Movements of the Diaphragm in Speaking and Singing," *Deutsche Medizinische Wochenschrift*, 58, 1922, 1551–1552.

Schiratzki, H., "Upper Airway Resistance in Normal Man During Mouth Breathing," *Acta Otolaryngol.*, 58, 1964, 535–554.

Sears, T., and J. Newsom Davis, "The Control of Respiratory Muscles During Voluntary Breathing," pp. 183–190, in A. Bouhuys, eds., *Sound Production in Man, Annals of the N.Y. Acad. Sci.*, 155, 1968.

Sieben, A., "The Mechanics of Breathing," in C. Best and N. Taylor, eds., *The Physical Basis of Medical Practice*, 8th ed. Baltimore: Williams & Wilkins, 1960.

Skarbek, Ã., "The Significance of Variations in Breathing Behaviour in Speech and at Rest," *Acta Psychiat. Scand.*, 45, 1969, 218–258.

Snidecor, J., "Temporal Aspects of Breathing in Superior Reading and Speaking Performances," *Sp. Monog.*, 22, 284–289.

Spector, W. S., *"Handbook of Biological Data,"* WADE Technical Report 56–273, ASTIA Document No. AD 110501, Aerospace Medical Research Laboratories, Wright-Patterson Air Force Base, Ohio, October 1956.

Steer, M. D., "Instruments in Speech Pathology," in L. E. Travis, ed., *Handbook of Speech Pathology*, 2nd ed., Englewood Cliffs, N.J.: Prentice-Hall, 1971.

Stetson, R., "The Breathing Movements in Speech," *Arch. Neer. de Phon. Exp.* 6, 1931, 113–164.

———, "The Breathing Movements in Speech," *Proc. Int. Cong. Phonetic Sciences*, 1932, 108–109.

———, "Speech Movements in Action," *Trans. Amer. Laryngol. Assn*, 1933, 29–42.

———, *"Motor Phonetics,"* 2nd ed. Amsterdam: North-Holland, 1951.

———, and C. Hudgins, "Functions of the Breathing Movements in the Mechanism of Speech," *Arch. Neer. Phon. Exper.*, 5, 1930, 1–30.

Taylor, A., "The Contribution of the Intercostal Muscles to the Effort of Respiration in Man," *J. Physiol.*, 151, 1960, 390–402.

Tokizane, T., K. Kawamata, and H. Tokizane, "Electromyographic Studies of the Human Respiratory Muscles," *Jap. J. Physiol.*, 2, 1952, 232–247.

Wade, O. L., "The Chest and Diaphragm in Respiration," M.D. thesis, University of Cambridge, 1951.

———, "Movements of the Thoracic Cage and Diaphragm in Respiration," *J. Physiol.* (London), 124, 1954, 193–212.

———, and J. C. Gilson, "The Effect of Posture on Diaphragmatic Movement and Vital Capacity in Normal Subjects with a Note on Spirometry as an Aid in Determining Radiological Chest Volumes," *Thorax*, 6, 1951, 103–126.

Weismer, G., "Speech Breathing: Contemporary Views and Findings," in R. Daniloff, ed., *Speech Science*. San Diego: College Hill Press, 1985.

Weismer, G., "Speech Production," in N. Lass, L. McReynolds, J. Northern, and D. Yoder, eds., *Handbook of Speech-Language Pathology and Audiology*. Toronto: D. C. Decker, 1988.

Wiksell, W. "An Experimental Analysis of Respiration in Relation to the Intensity of Vocal Tones in Speech," pp. 37–51, in G. W. Gray, ed., *Studies in Experimental Phonetics*, Louisiana University Studies, No. 27. Baton Rouge: Louisiana State University Press, 1936.

Wilder, C., "Chest Wall Preparation for Phonation in Trained Singers," in V. Lawrence, ed., *Transcripts of the Eighth Symposium Care of the Professional Voice, Part II: Respiratory and Phonatory Control Mechanisms*. New York: The Voice Foundation, 1980.

Wilder, C., *Chest Wall Preparation for Phonation in Female Speakers*, in D. Bless and J. Abbs, eds., *Vocal Fold Physiology*. San Diego: College-Hill Press, 1983.

Winkworth, A., P. Davis, R. Adams, and E. Ellis, "Breathing Patterns During Spontaneous Speech," *J. Sp. Hrng. Res.* 38, 1995, 124–144.

Woodburne, R. T., *Essentials of Human Anatomy*, 5th ed. New York: Oxford University Press, 1973.

Zemlin, W., "An Electromyographic Investigation of Certain Muscles of Respiration," unpublished.

Phonation

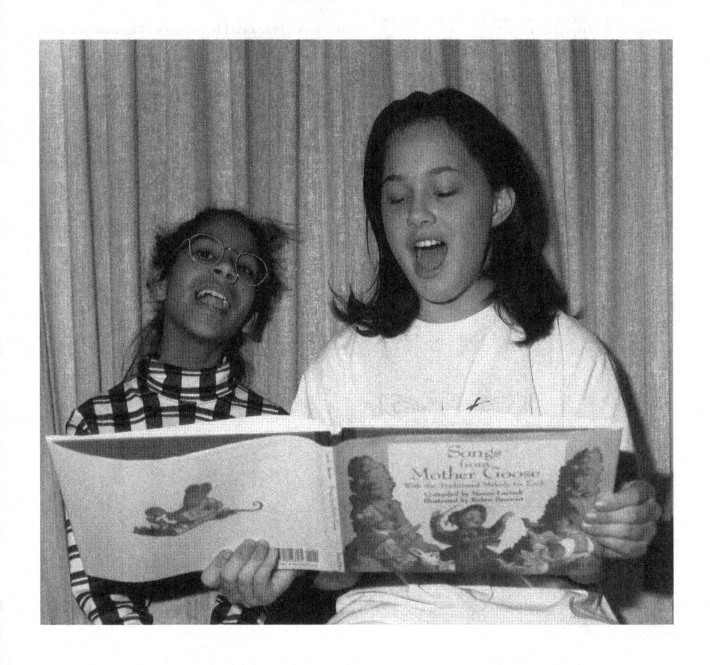

INTRODUCTION

In the previous chapter the speech mechanism was likened to a mechanical system consisting of a power supply, vibrating elements, and a system of valves and filters. Having accounted for the power supply, we should next examine the means by which vocal sounds are produced.

Energy, in the form of a relatively steady state or unmodulated stream of air from the lungs, passes into the trachea and finally into the larynx. The larynx is the principal structure for producing a vibrating air stream, and the **vocal folds,** which are part of the larynx, constitute the *vibrating elements*. Rapid opening and closing of the vocal folds periodically interrupt the air stream to produce a **vocal** or **glottal tone** within the pharyngeal, oral, and nasal cavities. Modifications of the configurations and, therefore, the acoustical properties of these cavities, which are known collectively as the **vocal tract,** transform the relatively undifferentiated glottal tone into meaningful speech sounds.

The **larynx,** which forms the superior terminal of the trachea, is an *unpaired, midline, musculocartilaginous* structure located in the anterior neck region, as shown in Figure 3-1. An anteriorly directed prominence of the larynx, located midway on the vertical axis, is easily palpated by placing the fingers on the midline of the neck, just beneath the chin. By exploring and pressing lightly, one may detect a rather definite notch. This is the **thyroid notch,** and it indicates the approximate anterior attachment of the vocal folds. With the index finger lightly in the thyroid notch, the fingernail will press up-

ward against the **hyoid bone,** the structure from which the larynx is often said to be "suspended."

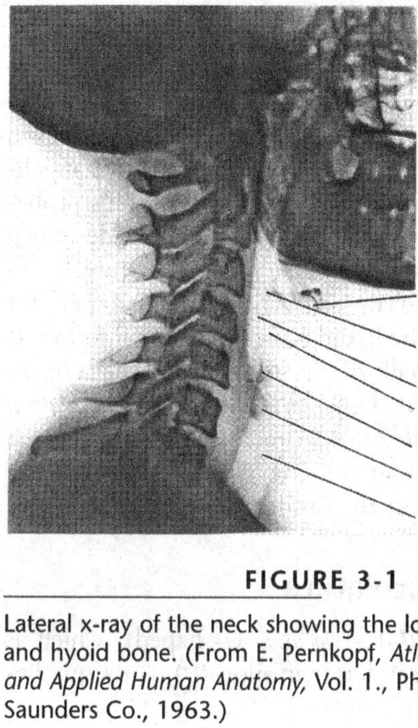

Thus, the larynx is located between the *trachea inferiorly* and the *hyoid bone superiorly*. Vertically, it is located at about the level of the third, fourth, fifth, and sixth cervical vertebrae, but this position may vary with age, sex, head position, and laryngeal activity. For example, the position of the larynx moves over a maximum range of 7 cm in extreme flexion and extension of the neck.

Production of an air stream for speech purposes has been referred to as a "nonrespiratory" function of the breathing mechanism; the production of sound by the larynx may be thought of as a nonbiological function. That is, we have seen how the breathing mechanism has biological and nonbiological functions; the larynx also has biological and nonbiological functions.

Biological Functions of the Larynx

Biologically the larynx may be regarded as an *instrinsic component of the respiratory system*, and as such it functions as a *protective device for the lower respiratory tract*. Acting as a valve, it (1) prevents air from escaping the lungs, (2) prevents foreign substances from entering the larynx, and (3) forcefully expels foreign substances which threaten to enter either the larynx or trachea.

Threatening substances and foreign bodies are prevented from entering the larynx by active closure of the **laryngeal valve.** Active closure also accompanies *thoracic fixation*, which was referred to in Chapter 2. Closure of the laryngeal valve prevents air escape and facilitates those activities demanding highly elevated abdominal pressures, such as forced bowel and bladder evacuation and heavy lifting. *For ordinary or normal biological functions, however, thoracic fixation is not necessary in order to generate adequately elevated intra-abdominal pressures* (Pressman, 1944).

The same mechanism responsible for thoracic fixation is active in forceful expulsion of foreign substances from the respiratory tract. Once elevated alveolar pressure has developed, a sudden, active dilation of the laryngeal valve results in a violent explosive emission of air to expel the foreign substance from the respiratory tract. This behavior, of course, is what we refer to as *coughing*.

Nonbiological Functions of the Larynx

As talking primates we are almost obligated to say that the principal nonbiological function of the larynx is sound production. Because speech is an integral part of human behavior, however, the notion that it is nonbiological may be open to criticism. It is largely through speech that we are able to communicate with others and

Body of hyoid bone
Major horn of hyoid bone
Aditus of larynx
Laryngeal part of pharynx
Arytenoid cartilage
Cricoid cartilage
Lumen of trachea

FIGURE 3-1

Lateral x-ray of the neck showing the location of the larynx and hyoid bone. (From E. Pernkopf, *Atlas of Topographical and Applied Human Anatomy,* Vol. 1., Philadelphia: W. B. Saunders Co., 1963.)

to make known our wants and needs. Indeed, speech is so much a part of human behavior, it might well be considered a biological function. Regardless of the stand one may take, there is no debating that the *larynx functions as a sound generator only when it is not fulfilling the vital biological functions* mentioned earlier.

The larynx is an extraordinarily versatile structure, capable of many rapid and subtle adjustments and capable of sound production over a very wide range of pitch and loudness. From the standpoint of mechanics, however, it can be regarded as *no more than a variable resistance to the flow of air in and out of the lungs*, and in that event the human voice becomes simply an epiphenomenon.

Regardless of the role assigned to the larynx, whether it be that of a biological valve, a mechanical variable resistance to the flow of air, or a beautiful and versatile sound-generating system, a full appreciation of its functions demands a thorough understanding of its unique structure. The human larynx is especially well equipped for sound production.

The **vocal folds** are long, smoothly rounded bands of muscle tissue that may be lengthened or shortened, tensed or relaxed, and abducted or adducted. Compared with those of less well-developed animals, the human arytenoid cartilages are quite small with respect to the total length of the valvular mechanism. This means that the muscular, vibrating portion of the vocal fold is quite long and well suited for sound production.

The Mechanics of the Sound Generator

During normal breathing, the vocal folds are spaced rather widely apart, and contrary to what is often stated, *their spacing is not somewhat less during exhalation than it is during inhalation.* At any rate, the air stream is unimpeded as it flows in and out of the lungs. Later, when the structural and behavioral characteristics of the larynx have been discussed, we will be in a position to examine closely how the unimpeded air stream may be set into vibration to produce the glottal tone. Very briefly, *the larynx produces glottal tones by generating a rapid series of short-duration air pulses, which excite the supralaryngeal air column so as to produce a complex tone.* Generation of the air pulses may be initiated as follows:

The vocal folds are adducted, either slightly less than completely or completely but rather loosely, to restrict the flow of air from the lungs. At the same time, the forces of exhalation produce an increasing amount of air pressure beneath the folds, and when it becomes sufficient, they are literally blown apart, thus releasing a puff of air into the vocal tract. This release of air results in an immediate decrease of pressure beneath the vocal folds, and the elasticity of the tissue, plus the reduction of air pressure, simply allows them to snap back into their adducted position, ready to be blown apart again once the air pressure has again built up. What has just been described is one cycle of **vocal fold vibration.** During normal vowel production such vibration occurs at a rate of about 125 complete vibrations per second for men, about 210 vibrations per second for women, and even higher for children.

Once sounds have been initiated, abrupt contraction of the adductor muscles in the larynx can forcibly approximate the vocal folds to arrest their vibrations. Such action is usually referred to as a **glottal stop.** Abrupt release of the adductor mechanism may also initiate vocal fold vibration suddenly in what is known as a **glottal attack** or **glottal stroke,** whereas a less abrupt release by the adductor mechanism may allow vocal fold vibration to be initiated gradually.

Glottal attacks and stops occur with great frequency in some languages other than English. In parts of Germany, for example, glottal attacks and stops are used with great regularity, but they do not enjoy *phonemic significance.* In Turkey, on the other hand, glottal attacks are used phonemically. In the English language, glottal arrests and releases are used far more often than one might suppose.

THE SUPPORTIVE FRAMEWORK OF THE LARYNX

The Hyoid Bone

The hyoid bone, which is part of the *axial skeleton,* is actually a supportive structure for the root of the tongue rather than an integral part of the laryngeal framework. The larynx is, nevertheless, suspended somewhat from the hyoid bone, which also serves as the superior attachment for some extrinsic laryngeal muscles. This probably explains why the hyoid bone is so often described (and illustrated) as an integral laryngeal structure.

In addition to serving as the point of attachment for laryngeal muscles, the hyoid bone forms the inferior attachment for the bulk of the tongue musculature. In German, the hyoid bone is called the *zungenbein* (tongue bone). In all, 22 or 23 muscles either take their origin from or insert into the hyoid bone. Many of them are very important for the production of speech.

The Hyoid Musculature

The **hyoid bone** (Gk. *hyoeides,* U-shaped), which is shaped like the Greek letter upsilon (U), is unique because it is *not directly attached to any other bone in the skeleton*; rather, it is bound in position by a complex system of muscles and ligaments that render it a highly mobile structure. Muscles from the tongue and chin approach the hyoid bone from above and in front, while muscles and ligaments from the temporal bone approach from above and behind. Extrinsic muscles from the larynx approach from below, as do the muscles from the sternum and clavicle. Muscles that attach to the hyoid bone and suspend it in position are sometimes called the **hyoid sling muscles** (see Table 3-1).

Anatomy of the Hyoid Bone

As shown in Figure 3-3, the hyoid bone is indeed somewhat U-shaped. It is located in the neck horizontally, at the level of the third cervical vertebra, with the limbs of the U directed backward and slightly upward.

The bulk of the hyoid bone consists of an unpaired ventral **body** or **corpus.** It is roughly quadrilateral in shape, presenting a convex anterior surface and a pronouncedly concave posterior surface, a feature that minimizes its weight without sacrificing strength. A vertical medial ridge divides the anterior surface into right and left halves, while a well-defined transverse ridge courses through the upper half.

Posteriorly directed limbs, one on either side of the body, are known as the **greater horns (cornua).** They are somewhat more flattened than the body and diminish in size from the body backward to terminate as tubercles, which articulate indirectly and loosely with the superior horns of the thyroid cartilage of the larynx. The junction of a greater horn with the body is characterized by a superiorly directed, cone-shaped prominence known as a **lesser horn (cornu).** The lesser horns are usually capped by small, cone-shaped elastic cartilages.

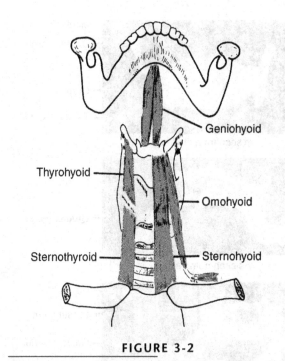

FIGURE 3-2

Schematic "dissection" of neck, showing some of the strap muscles.

A Note on Variability

The hyoid bone and the structures that constitute the cartilaginous framework of the larynx vary considerably from specimen to specimen. Variability is so frequently seen in *size, general morphology,* and *symmetry,* that generalizations are almost hazardous. The description of the larynx that follows is based primarily on the dissections of a small number of specimens, but variability will also be reported when the information is available.

TABLE 3-1

Hyoid sling muscles

Muscle	Origin	Insertion
1. Stylohyoid	styloid process	hyoid bone
2. Digastricus (posterior)	mastoid process	hyoid bone
3. Digastricus (anterior)	hyoid bone	mandible
*4. Geniohyoid	mandible	hyoid bone
*5. Thyrohyoid	thyroid cartilage	hyoid bone
*6. Sternohyoid	manubrium of sternum	hyoid bone
*7 Sternothyroid	manubrium of sternum	thyroid cartilage
*8 Omohyoid	superior border of scapula	hyoid bone

*These muscles, often known collectively as the "strap muscles" of the neck, are shown schematically in Figure 3-2.

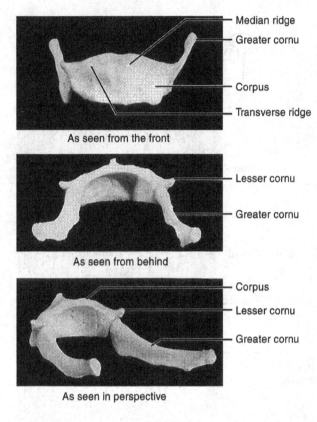

Median ridge
Greater cornu

Corpus

Transverse ridge

As seen from the front

Lesser cornu

Greater cornu

As seen from behind

Corpus

Lesser cornu

Greater cornu

As seen in perspective

FIGURE 3-3

Photographs of the hyoid bone from various angles.

THE CARTILAGINOUS FRAMEWORK OF THE LARYNX

The structural framework of the larynx consists of nine cartilages and their connecting membranes and ligaments. Three are unpaired, rather large cartilages, and three are paired, smaller cartilages, as follows:

1 Thyroid (hyaline)	2 Arytenoid (hyaline)
1 Cricoid (hyaline)	2 Corniculate (elastic)
1 Epiglottis (elastic)	2 Cuneiform (elastic)

As shown, the cartilages are composed of either *hyaline* or *elastic* cartilage. In young adulthood, after hyaline structures have achieved complete maturity and growth, they slowly begin to ossify.[1] This means that during the rough-and-tumble years of childhood and adolescence, the skeletal framework of the larynx is rather soft, pliable, flexible, and capable of interstitial growth, but later

---

[1]Calcification also occurs, a process quite different from ossification.

in life the cartilages gradually become bonelike and quite brittle.

The Thyroid Cartilage

The thyroid, illustrated in Figure 3-4, is the largest of the laryngeal cartilages. Although its name means shieldlike, the combining form *thyro-* denotes a relationship to the thyroid gland.

The thyroid cartilage is composed of two somewhat quadrilateral plates called the **thyroid laminae.** They are fused one with the other at the midline anteriorly and form most of the anterior and lateral walls of the larynx. The point of this junction is known as the **angle of the thyroid.** Incomplete fusion of the thyroid laminae superiorly results in the prominent V-shaped **thyroid notch.** It was identified earlier as a palpable depression just above the anterior projection of the larynx known as the **thyroid (laryngeal) prominence,** or **Adam's apple.**

When viewed from behind, as in Figure 3-4, the thyroid laminae may be seen to diverge to enclose a wedge-shaped space. The angle formed by the union of the thyroid laminae is about *80 degrees for adult males* and about *90 degrees for adult females.*

The posterior margin of each thyroid lamina is prolonged upward and downward as the **superior** and **inferior thyroid horns (cornua),** respectively. As shown in Figure 3-4, the **superior horns** are directed upward, backward, and medially. They are attached by means of a ligament to the corresponding major horn of the hyoid bone. The **inferior horns,** shorter and somewhat thicker than the superior, are directed down and slightly medially, and articulate with the cricoid cartilage by means of articular facets that are located on the medial surface of each horn tip. These facets are highly variable, from specimen to specimen, and may even be absent on one horn, or both.

Descriptions of the thyroid cartilage often include a "prominent landmark" called the *oblique line,* which courses across the face of each lamina, down and forward from the superior to the inferior tubercle. The tubercles are shown in Figure 3-4, and an oblique line is also identified, but its existence is somewhat questionable on this specimen. What we see is actually a tendon.

In dissections on a large number of specimens 90 percent have shown a fibrous band that bridges the superior and inferior tubercles and is placed obliquely across the thyroid plate (Zemlin and Angeline, 1984). This fibrous band was recognized by Beaunais and Bouchard (1868) and by Testut and Laterjet (1948). When this fibrous band is removed, the thyroid lamina is smooth, with no cartilaginous oblique line in about 90 percent of the specimens. Recent histological research has shown the fibrous arc to be a tendon.

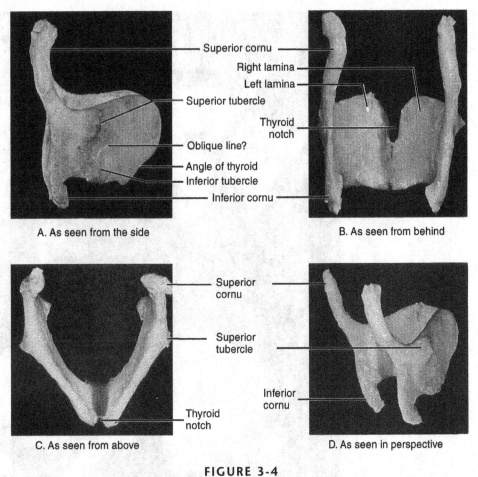

A. As seen from the side

Superior cornu
Right lamina
Left lamina
Thyroid notch

B. As seen from behind

Superior cornu
Superior tubercle
Oblique line?
Angle of thyroid
Inferior tubercle
Inferior cornu

Superior cornu

Superior tubercle

Inferior cornu

C. As seen from above

Thyroid notch

D. As seen in perspective

FIGURE 3-4

Various views of the thyroid cartilage.

An **oblique tendon** is shown in Figure 3-5. We will return to this topic in our description of extrinsic laryngeal musculature.

In addition, about one-third of the thyroid cartilages exhibit a **foramen** in the posterosuperior quadrant of the lamina, as shown in Figure 3-5. Extremely variable in dimensions, this foramen often provides blood vessels access to the interior of the larynx (Zemlin, Simmon, and Hammel, 1984).

And finally, the **superior horns** are extremely variable in size and shape, to the extent that a horn may be totally missing. The inferior horns are far less variable (Figure 3-5).

The Cricoid Cartilage

The cricoid cartilage (Gk. *krikos*, ring + *eidos*, form) is a hyaline structure which Vesalius compared to the ring used by Turkish archers. It is located immediately above the uppermost tracheal ring. It is smaller but stouter than the thyroid and forms the lower portion of the laryngeal framework. The cricoid cartilage consists of two parts: an **anterior arch** and a **posterior quadrate lamina.**

As shown in Figure 3-6, the **cricoid lamina** is a hexagonal plate, or nearly so, which is sometimes likened to the signet of a ring. It extends upward to occupy much of the space between the posterior margins of the thyroid cartilage. A prominent vertical ridge on the midline of the cricoid lamina separates two shallow depressions. The ridge serves as the point of attachment for the longitudinal muscle fibers of the upper esophaghus, while the shallow depressions are the sites of origin for the posterior cricoarytenoid muscles.

Laterally, on either side, the **arch** of the cricoid presents small oval articular facets for articulation with the inferior horns of the thyroid. The result is a diarthrodial pivot joint, *which permits either the thyroid or the cricoid to rotate about an axis through the joint*, as indicated by the dashed line in Figure 3-7. This rotational movement, a very important part of the pitch-changing mechanism, will be elaborated on later in the chapter.

The inferior border of the cricoid cartilage is smooth, usually a little asymmetrical, but otherwise has no important landmarks. It attaches to the first tracheal ring by means of the **cricotracheal membrane** or **ligament.**

Variations seen in the morphology of the thyroid cartilage. (A) Foramen thyroideum, which occurs in about one-third of the population. (B) An oblique tendon that provides attachments for the sternothyroid and thyrohyoid muscles. It is found in about 90 percent of the population. (C) Agenesis of a superior horn, which occurs in about 5 percent of the population. (D) Asymmetry of the thyroid cartilage.

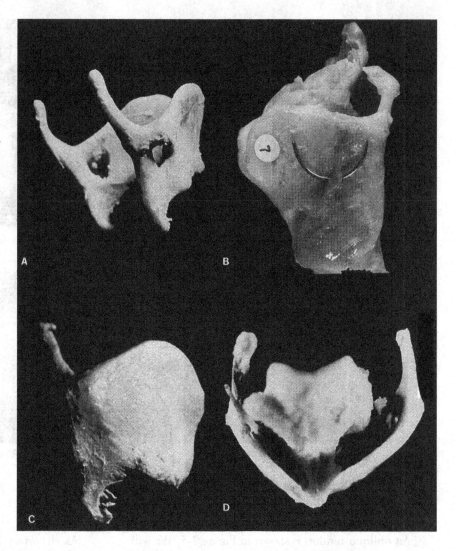

The Arytenoid Cartilages

The paired arytenoid cartilages (Gk. *arytaina,* ladle + *eidos,* form), shown in Figure 3-8, are located on the sloping border of the cricoid cartilage (Figure 3-7). Mainly hyaline and roughly resembling a three-sided pyramid (tetrahedral), each cartilage has a *base,* an *apex,* and *three surfaces.*

The anterolateral surface is the most extensive and complex. It presents two pits or foveae: a **triangular fovea** near the apex and a **fovea oblonga** near the base. The two foveae are separated by a horizontally directed **arcuate ridge.** The posterolateral angle of the arytenoid cartilage bears a laterally directed **muscular process** which presents a concave and rounded articular facet on its undersurface for articulation with the cricoid cartilage. This muscular process is also the point of attachment for some important laryngeal musculature. The anterior angle, near the base, is prolonged as a pointed projection called the **vocal process.** The **vocal liga-** **ment,** an important part of the vocal fold, inserts on the vocal process.

The Corniculate Cartilages

The apexes of the arytenoid cartilages are capped by a pair of conical elastic **corniculate cartilages,** a name that describes their hornlike shape. They are quite large in lower animals, but in humans they are probably vestigial[2] structures which once served an important protective function.

---

[2]The remnant of a structure that functioned in a previous stage of species or individual development. The term *vestigium* is used in the *Nomina Anatomica* to designate the degenerating remains of any structure that served as a functioning entity in the embryo or fetus. It should be contrasted with *rudiment* or *rudimentary,* a term that denotes a primitive structure, but they are sometimes used interchangeably.

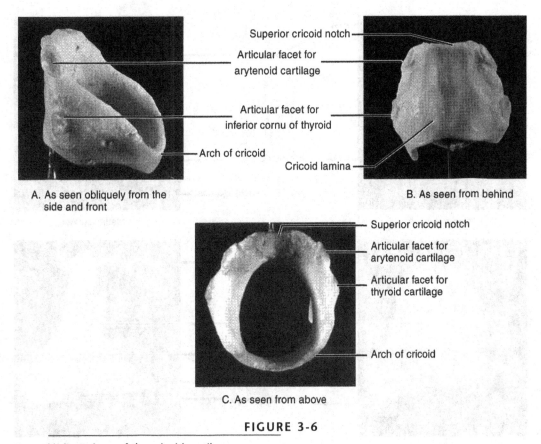

A. As seen obliquely from the side and front

Superior cricoid notch
Articular facet for arytenoid cartilage
Articular facet for inferior cornu of thyroid
Arch of cricoid

B. As seen from behind

Superior cricoid notch
Articular facet for arytenoid cartilage
Cricoid lamina

Superior cricoid notch
Articular facet for arytenoid cartilage
Articular facet for thyroid cartilage
Arch of cricoid

C. As seen from above

FIGURE 3-6

Various views of the cricoid cartilage.

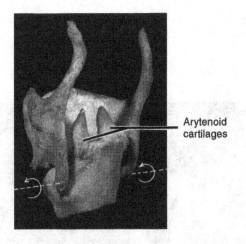

Arytenoid cartilages

FIGURE 3-7

Articulated laryngeal cartilages illustrating rotational axis at cricothyroid joint. Note the large superior thyroid horns.

The Epiglottis

Anatomy

The epiglottis is a flexible leaflike structure composed of elastic or fibroelastic cartilage. It is located just behind the hyoid bone and the root of the tongue. At its upper limits it is broad, rounded, and thin. Below, it narrows to a stalklike structure called the **petiolus** (L. little leg).

It is attached to the thyroid cartilage at the angle, just beneath the thyroid notch, by means of a **thyroepiglottic ligament.** Where the leaflike portion is broadest, it fastens to the hyoid bone by means of an elastic **hyoepiglottic ligament.** As shown in Figure 3-9, when viewed from the side the anterior (lingual) surface is curved forward, and when viewed from above, as in Figure 3-10, it appears sharply convex. The anterior surface is continued to the root of the tongue by a **median** and two **lateral glossoepiglottic ligaments** (or **folds**). Two pits or **valleculae** (L. small valleys) may be seen between the epiglottis and the root of the tongue, one on either side of the median glossoepiglottic fold.

A sizable **fat pad,** extending from the hyoid bone to the level of the thyroid notch, separates the epiglottis from the hyoid bone and the thyroid cartilage. The posterior or laryngeal surface is concave when viewed from the side. The lower portion is characterized by a tubercle that is easily seen during indirect laryngeal examination. The posterior surface is invested by closely adherent mucous membrane.

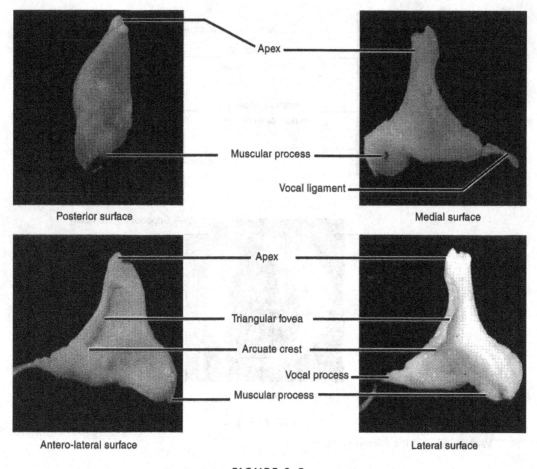

Apex

Apex

Muscular process

Vocal ligament

Posterior surface

Medial surface

Apex

Triangular fovea

Arcuate crest

Vocal process

Muscular process

Antero-lateral surface

Lateral surface

FIGURE 3-8

Various views of a left arytenoid cartilage.

FIGURE 3-9

The epiglottis *in situ,* as seen from the front and from the side. (E) epiglottis, (TH) thyroid cartilage, (CR) cricoid cartilage, (TR) trachea.

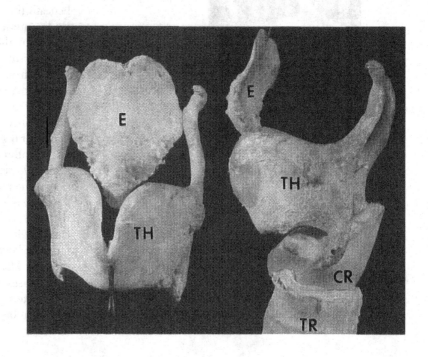

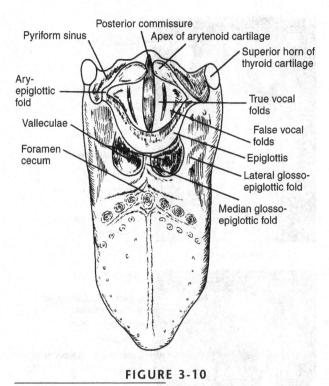

FIGURE 3-10

Schematic of epiglottis *in situ,* as seen from above, and its relationship to adjacent structures.

CLINICAL NOTE: The upper part of the epiglottis is easily seen during oral examinations of young children. It appears as a white or pink crescent just behind the back of the tongue. Later, when growth and changes in the configuration of the upper airway have taken place, the epiglottis becomes increasingly difficult to observe without the aid of a mirror.

Function

The human **epiglottis** is often said to function in preventing food from entering the larynx during deglutition (swallowing). The exact mechanism is open to some question.

One explanation is that the epiglottis acts as a sort of trapdoor, which by reflex snaps down over the entrance to the larynx while the bolus of food slides past on its way to the esophagus. Depression of the epiglottis is thought to be mediated through contraction of muscle fibers within the aryepiglottic fold.

Another viewpoint is that the tongue, in initiating deglutition, is pressed against the epiglottis while it simultaneously moves the bolus of food into the pharynx. Van Daele et al. (1995) have suggested that, during swallowing, as the larynx elevates and the hyoid bone moves anteriorly, the lateral hyoepiglottic ligaments act to depress the upper third of the epiglottis.

We can safely say that the *epiglottis contributes very little to the production of speech.* It may modify the laryngeal tone by producing changes in the size and shape of the laryngeal cavity. At low pitches the epiglottis virtually covers the entrance to the larynx and makes viewing of its interior difficult. As pitch is raised, the epiglottis "moves out of the way" to permit a full view of the vocal folds.

The epiglottis is often regarded as a vestigial structure in humans and as a structure with important biological functions in lower forms of life. *It is not a vital organ in humans.*

Negus (1949) noted that all mammals have an epiglottis, and that it is particularly well developed in those animals with a keen sense of smell. In Figure 3-11, note how the epiglottis rests on the soft palate. Negus supposed that the function of the epiglottis in lower animals is to isolate the oral cavity from the remainder of the respiratory tract, especially when the animals are feeding. Inhaled air must pass through the nasal cavities and past the olfactory sense organs. Thus, food in the mouth cannot contaminate the smell of the inhaled air, and furthermore, the animal has maximum olfaction, even when the mouth is open.

In a later work, Negus (1949) modified his viewpoint and stated that by the action of the tongue the epiglottis moves to a somewhat horizontal position, a movement that is of no importance.

The fact that the epiglottis moves down to cover the entrance to the larynx during swallowing has been verified by cineradiography (Ardran and Kemp, 1951, 1952, 1967; Saunders et al., 1951). The epiglottis is reported to make two distinct movements in covering the laryngeal aditus. The first movement occurs where the epiglottis attaches to the thyroid cartilage. The movement is from the vertical rest position to a horizontal position, followed by a second movement that takes place as the bolus passes through the pharynx. This brings the upper one-third of the epiglottis below the horizontal. These movements seem to be

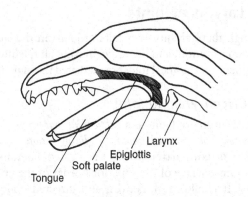

FIGURE 3-11

Schematic illustration of relationship between soft palate and epiglottis in the dog. Olfaction is preserved, even when the animal is eating.

the result of anterior displacement of the hyoid bone and of thyroid-hyoid approximation. VanDaele, Perlman, and Cassell (1995) propose that, as the larynx elevates during swallowing and the hyoid bone moves anteriorly, the paired lateral hyoepiglottic ligaments exert traction on the upper third of the epiglottis to bring it to a position below the horizontal.

In adult humans the shape of the epiglottis is markedly altered, and there is an unfilled gap between the epiglottis and soft palate. This is largely because humans are upright animals and their airway bends at almost a right angle in the region between the epiglottis and soft palate.

The Cuneiform Cartilages

Folds of mucous membrane, which enclose ligamentous and muscular fibers, extend from the sides of the epiglottis to the apexes of the arytenoid cartilages. Called the **aryepiglottic folds,** they form the entrance to the larynx. (They are shown schematically in Figure 3-26.) Imbedded within the aryepiglottic folds, just anterior and lateral to the corniculate cartilages described earlier, are paired, wedge-shaped rods of elastic cartilage appropriately called **cuneiform** (L. *cuneus*, wedge + *forma*, form).

Although these small cartilages are imbedded within the aryepiglottic folds and are covered by connective tissue, fat, and mucous membrane, they often appear as highlighted elevations or swellings (**cuneiform tubercles**) when the larynx is viewed from above. These cartilages may be absent in some specimens, however, for they are also vestigal structures, much more prominent in lower animals. *They lend support to the aryepiglottic folds and stiffen them to help maintain the opening to the larynx.*

The major laryngeal cartilages are shown in Figure 3-12, and a schematic of the cartilages and some associated structures as viewed from behind is illustrated in Figure 3-13.

The Laryngeal Joints

Although there are just two pairs of joints in the larynx, the **cricoarytenoid** and the **cricothyroid,** all the internal adjustments of the vocal folds are mediated through them.

The Cricoarytenoid Joint

The cricoarytenoid joint is a *saddle joint that permits rocking motion and a limited amount of gliding action.*

The **cricoid articular facet** is located, laterally, on the sloping surface of the superior border of the cricoid lamina. It is ellipitical, convex, and directed obliquely with its long axis directed from behind, laterally, anteriorly, and downward, by about 25 degrees or so. When the long axes of these facets are projected posteriorly, as in Figure 3-14, they intersect at an angle of about 50 to 60 degrees.

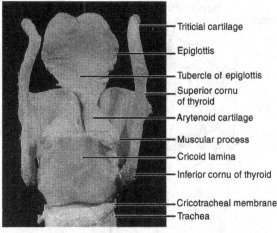

As viewed from behind

- Triticial cartilage
- Epiglottis
- Tubercle of epiglottis
- Superior cornu of thyroid
- Arytenoid cartilage
- Muscular process
- Cricoid lamina
- Inferior cornu of thyroid
- Cricotracheal membrane
- Trachea

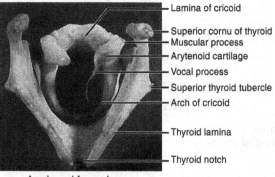

As viewed from above

- Lamina of cricoid
- Superior cornu of thyroid
- Muscular process
- Arytenoid cartilage
- Vocal process
- Superior thyroid tubercle
- Arch of cricoid
- Thyroid lamina
- Thyroid notch

FIGURE 3-12

Photographs of major laryngeal cartilages and trachea.

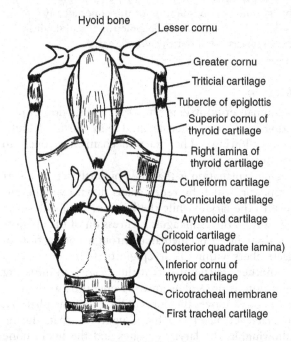

- Hyoid bone
- Lesser cornu
- Greater cornu
- Triticial cartilage
- Tubercle of epiglottis
- Superior cornu of thyroid cartilage
- Right lamina of thyroid cartilage
- Cuneiform cartilage
- Corniculate cartilage
- Arytenoid cartilage
- Cricoid cartilage (posterior quadrate lamina)
- Inferior cornu of thyroid cartilage
- Cricotracheal membrane
- First tracheal cartilage

FIGURE 3-13

Schematic of laryngeal cartilages and associated structures, as seen from behind.

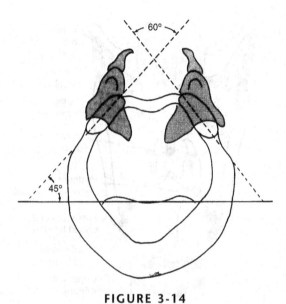

FIGURE 3-14

Angular orientation of the cricoid (cricoarytenoid) articular facets.

The **arytenoid articular facet,** mentioned earlier, is more nearly circular, but it is sharply concave. Located on the undersurface of the muscular process, the concave arytenoid facet neatly fits the convex cricoid facet; and when the muscular process is acted upon by the musculature that attaches to it, a rotary or rocking motion, at right angles to the long axis of the cricoid articulatory facet, takes place. However, since this facet slopes both downward and lateralward, the movement of the vocal process is upward and away from the midline, as illustrated in Figure 3-15. In other words, *rocking*

motion of the arytenoid cartilage produces an upward and outward swinging motion of the vocal process during abduction and an inward and downward swinging motion when the vocal processes are adducted.

Since the cricoarytenoid joint is a diarthrodial one, it permits a certain amount of gliding action in addition to a rocking motion, and this is illustrated in Figure 3-16. A third, very restricted pivot or rotary motion about a vertical axis is sometimes recognized. This controversial action is illustrated in Figure 3-17. A detailed description of this joint by Sonesson (1960) has been largely confirmed by means of a mathematical analysis by von Leden and Moore (1961).

A **posterior cricoarytenoid ligament** constitutes a large part of the cricoarytenoid articular capsule. It restricts and to a certain extent dictates the movements of the arytenoid cartilage. This well-developed and very important ligament extends from the posterior surface of the superior margin of the cricoid lamina to the base of the posterior surface of the arytenoid cartilage. Its course is obliquely upward and lateral as can be seen in Figures 3-18 and 3-19. *This ligament restricts the extent of the forward movement of the arytenoid cartilage, and probably imposes constraints on the extent of any gliding movements* (Sonesson, 1960).

A poorly developed and often absent **anterior cricoarytenoid ligament** extends from the cricoid cartilage to the anterolateral base of the arytenoid cartilage. When present, it may limit backward movement of the arytenoid cartilage.

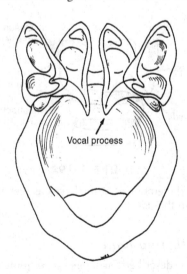

FIGURE 3-15

Movement at cricoarytenoid joint. Rocking motion of the arytenoid cartilage produces an upward and outward swinging motion of the vocal process during abduction, and an inward and downward swinging motion when the vocal processes are adducted.

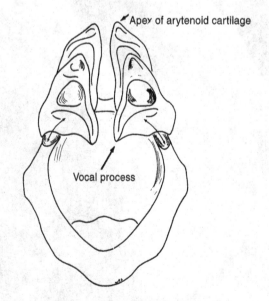

FIGURE 3-16

A limited amount of gliding action is permitted by the cricoarytenoid joint. Because of the orientation of the cricoid articular facet, movement of the arytenoid cartilage is a complex upward-inward, or downward-outward, gliding action. This can occur while rocking motion is also taking place.

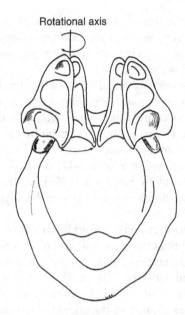

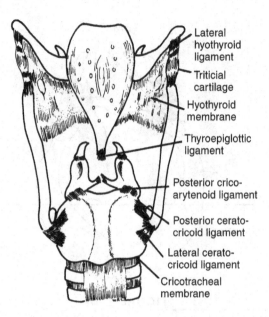

FIGURE 3-17

Controversial rotational action at the cricoarytenoid joint. Because of the nature of the joint, rotational action is negligible, and quite probably does not occur in the normal larynx.

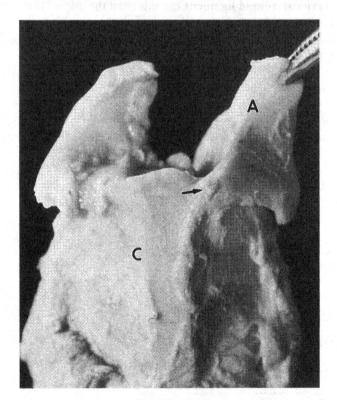

FIGURE 3-18

The posterior cricoarytenoid ligament is indicated by arrow. (C) cricoid cartilage, (A) arytenoid cartilage.

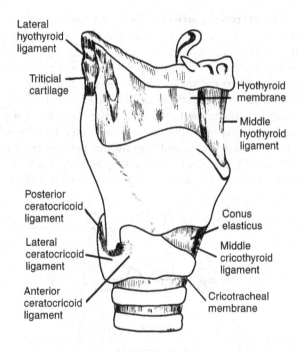

FIGURE 3-19

Ligaments and membranes of the larynx as seen from behind and from the side.

The Cricothyroid Joint

This joint was described earlier as a pivot joint and its rotational axis was illustrated in Figure 3-7. Small oval (or round) articular facets were described as being located laterally, on either side of the arch of the cricoid cartilage. These facets may be plano, slightly concave, slightly convex, or in some instances extremely rudimentary or even completely absent. The same holds true for the articular facets located on the medial surface of the lower limits of the inferior thyroid cornua. Usually, however, the joint is lined with a synovial membrane and is firmly bound by capsular ligaments which limit the movements at the joint. In those instances where the articular facets are very primitive or absent, the articulation is exclusively ligamentous.

Mayet and Muendnich (1958) identify **posterior, lateral,** and **anterior ceratocricoid** (Gk. *keras*, horn) **ligaments,** which together constitute the capsular ligament; they are shown in Figure 3-20. The architecture of the joint capsule largely determines the type of the movement that can take place.

The primary action is rotational about a horizontally directed axis through the joint, as was illustrated in Figure 3-7. Because this places the ligaments under tension, motion is confined to a rotational one. In a neutral position, however, the ligaments are somewhat slack, so a limited amount of gliding action along the sagittal plane can take place. *This rotational or gliding motion places the vocal folds under increased tension, thus causing an increase in the pitch of the voice.*

There is some controversy as to which of the cartilages actually engages in rotation. Mayet and Muendnich maintain that, since the thyroid cartilage is relatively fixed in position by muscles and other structures that attach to it, the rotational motion is executed by the **cricoid cartilage.** As shown in Figure 3-21, this action results in a decrease in the distance between the cricoid arch anteriorly and the thyroid cartilage. At the same time the distance between the vocal processes of the arytenoid cartilages and the angle of the thyroid cartilage is increased. Arnold (1961) and many others strongly support the view that the cricoid rather than the thyroid engages in this important rotational movement, and their supportive evidence is compelling.

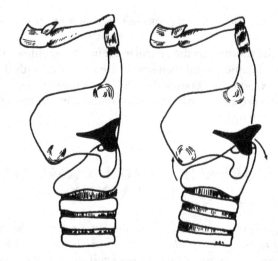

FIGURE 3-21

Rotational movement at the cricothyroid joint. Mayet and Muendnich (1958) suggest that the cricoid cartilage rotates to decrease the distance between the arch and the thyroid cartilage in front and, at the same time, increase the distance between the vocal processes of the arytenoid cartilage and the angle of the thyroid cartilage.

Cates and Basmajian (1955), Vennard (1967), Zemlin (1981), and others have suggested that the **thyroid cartilage** is actually the more mobile of the two. As illustrated in Figure 3-22, forward tilting of the thyroid cartilage accomplishes the same increase in the front-to-back distance of the larynx. In addition, Vennard suggests that *both the cricoid and thyroid yield to the*

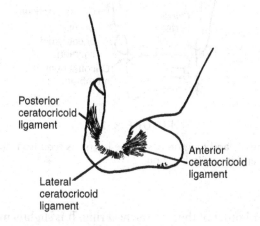

Posterior ceratocricoid ligament

Lateral ceratocricoid ligament

Anterior ceratocricoid ligament

FIGURE 3-20

Capsular ligaments of the cricothyroid joints.

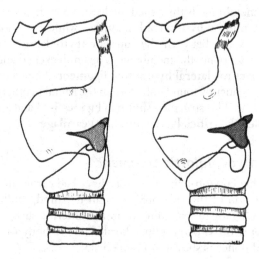

FIGURE 3-22

Rotational motion at the cricothyroid joint. Forward tilting of the thyroid cartilages increases the front-to-back distance of the larynx, and thus places the vocal folds under increased tension.

muscular forces, a compromise that is not at all unreasonable.

In addition to the articular ligaments, a number of other ligaments and membranes are associated with the larynx. Some are confined to the larynx (intrinsic) while others are associated with structures adjacent to the larynx (extrinsic).

MEMBRANES AND LIGAMENTS OF THE LARYNX

A group of ligaments and membranes *connects the laryngeal cartilages with adjacent structures.* They are called **extrinsic laryngeal membranes** and include the hyothyroid membrane (thyrohyoid), the paired lateral hyothyroid ligaments, the hyoepiglottic ligament, and the cricotracheal membrane.

Another group of ligaments and membranes *interconnects the various laryngeal cartilages* and *helps regulate the extent and direction of their movements.* They are the **intrinsic laryngeal membranes,** one of which (the conus elasticus) actually contributes to the composition of the vibrating portion of the vocal folds.

Extrinsic Laryngeal Membranes

The Hyothyroid Membrane and Ligaments

As shown in Figure 3-23, the *larynx seems to be suspended by the hyothyroid membrane.* It occupies the space between the hyoid bone and superior border of the thyroid cartilage. The membrane is thickened medially where it is known as the **middle hyothyroid ligament,** while posteriorly, in the space between the superior thyroid horns and the hyoid bone, the membrane is again thickened and is known as the **lateral hyothyroid ligament.** A small nodule is frequently found imbedded in the lateral hyothyroid ligament. This structure, shown in Figures 3-13 and 3-23, is called the **triticial** (grain of wheat) **cartilage.**

The Hyoepiglottic Ligament

The hyoepiglottic ligament was described earlier in the discussion of the epiglottis. It is an unpaired, midline, elastic ligament extending from the anterior surface of the epiglottis to the upper border of the body of the hyoid bone, as shown in Figure 3-23.

The Cricotracheal Membrane

The previously mentioned cricotracheal membrane connects the lower border of the cricoid cartilage with the

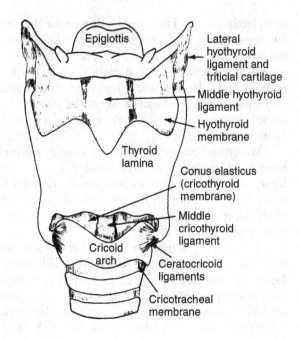

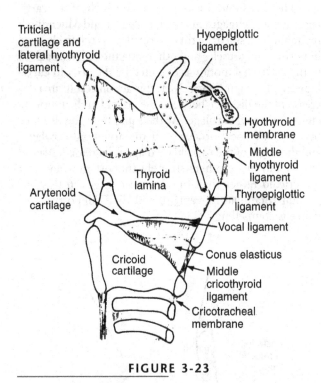

FIGURE 3-23

Ligaments and membranes of the larynx as seen from the front and in sagittal section.

upper border of the first tracheal ring. It is slightly more extensive than the membranes that connect the tracheal rings with each other.

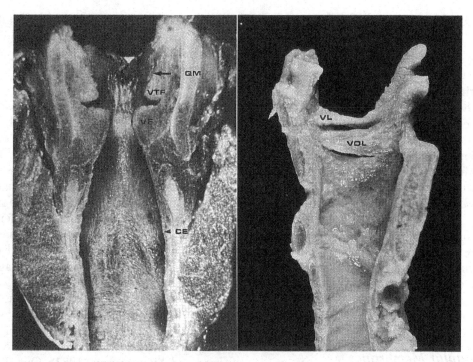

FIGURE 3-24

Left, frontal section of the larynx, illustrating the relationship of the quadrangular membrane (QM) with conus elasticus (CE). Right, conus elasticus and quadrangular membrane have been removed, leaving the vocal ligament (VOL) and ventricular ligament (VL) exposed. Also shown are the vocal fold (VF) and the ventricular fold (VTF).

Intrinsic Laryngeal Membranes and Ligaments

With the exception of the ligaments of the articular capsules, the **intrinsic laryngeal membranes** and **ligaments** stem from one broad sheet of connective tissue called the **elastic membrane** of the larynx. It is a *continuous fibroelastic sheet that, except for a small interval between the vocal and ventricular ligaments* (to be described later), *lines the entire larynx.* The *lower portion* of the elastic membrane is the most extensive and is well defined. It is known as the **conus elasticus.** The *upper portion*, less well defined, is called the **quadrangular membrane,** a term that describes its shape.

The Conus Elasticus (Cricovocal Membrane)

Figure 3-24 reveals the cavity below the vocal folds to be funnel- or cone-shaped, that explains the term **conus elasticus.** A continuous sheet of membrane that *connects the thyroid, cricoid, and arytenoid cartilages* with one another, it is divided into a **medial** (or **anterior**) **cricothyroid ligament** and two **lateral cricothyroid membranes.** Together they comprise the conus elasticus, which extends from the superior border of the arch and

lamina of the cricoid cartilage to the upper limits of the true vocal folds, as shown in Figures 3-23 and 3-25.

The Medial Cricothyroid Ligament This is a well-defined band of yellow elastic tissue. Figure 3-23 shows

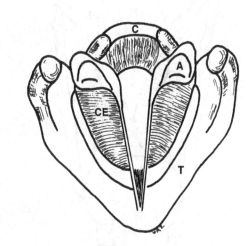

FIGURE 3-25

Top view schematic of relationship of conus elasticus (CE) to laryngeal cartilages. Thyroid (T), cricoid (C), arytenoid (A).

it as a midline structure extending from the superior border of the cricoid arch to the inferior border of the thyroid cartilage, at the angle.

The Lateral Cricothyroid Membranes These membranes are much *thinner* than the midline ligamentous portion just discussed. They originate from the superior border of the cricoid cartilage, course superiorly and medially, and terminate as free, thickened margins extending from the vocal processes of the arytenoid cartilages to the angle of the thyroid cartilage. These *free, thickened margins* are known as the **vocal ligaments.**

The vocal ligaments have a common point of attachment on the thyroid cartilage. It is called the **macula flava anterior** (L. *macula*, a region distinguished by color; L. *flava*, yellow). Each vocal ligament lies within the body of its corresponding vocal fold and forms the medial portion of the fold.

The Quadrangular Membranes

The paired quadrangular membranes arise from the lateral margins of the epiglottis and adjacent thyroid cartilage near the angle. The fibers course posteriorly downward and attach to the corniculate cartilages and the medial surfaces of the arytenoids. In Figure 3-26, each membrane appears roughly as a vertically directed sheet of membranous tissue. The membranes are *widely separated superiorly* and *converge as they descend.* Inferiorly they

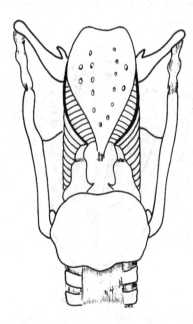

FIGURE 3-26

Schematic of quadrangular membrane and aryepiglottic folds (shown as heavy line).

terminate as *free, thickened borders* called the **ventricular ligaments.** Figure 3-24 shows the quadrangular membrane and its relationship with the conus elasticus and other laryngeal structures.

The Aryepiglottic Folds The *superior margins of the quadrangular membranes* are modified by submucous muscle tissue (the aryepiglottic muscles) to form the paired **aryepiglottic folds.** They are represented in Figure 3-26 by the heavy line that forms the upper limit of the quadrangular membranes. The poorly developed **aryepiglottic muscles** extend from the sides of the epiglottis near the rounded superior border, to the apexes of the arytenoid cartilages, where the fibers appear to be continuous with the oblique arytenoid muscles (to be described later). The **cuneiform cartilages** are embedded within the aryepiglottic folds.

Historically, the aryepiglottic muscles have been implicated in the mechanics of swallowing and have been said to exert an upward force on the arytenoid cartilages and a downward force on the epiglottis (Ekberg and Sigurjonsson, 1982). Our dissections have failed to consistently reveal muscle fibers in the aryepiglottic folds, and when found they were sparse. Van Daele et al. (1995) found aryepiglottic muscle fibers in just two out of twenty specimens. Muscle fibers that were found did not insert into the lateral edge of the epiglottis but rather they turned laterally and superiorly to become continuous with vertical fibers of the palatopharyngeus muscle. The aryepiglottic muscle has been a source of controversy. Testut and Laterjet (1948) described the aryepiglottic muscle, when found, as small and weak. Negus (1949) described the muscle fibers of the aryepiglottic folds as continuous with the interarytenoid muscle, findings that are consistent with our own.

Mucous Membrane of the Larynx

A **mucous membrane,** continuous above with the lining of the mouth and pharynx and below with the lining of the trachea, lines the whole of the cavity of the larynx. This membrane is particularly rich in mucous glands in the area between the vocal and ventricular ligaments.

It is closely adherent to the epiglottis, the aryepiglottic folds, and the vocal folds. Elsewhere it is loosely attached to a submucous basement membrane. The mucous membrane on the anterior surface and upper half of the posterior surface of the epiglottis, the upper portion of the aryepiglottic folds, and the medial surface of the ventricular and vocal folds is covered by stratified squamous epithelium. The remainder of the laryngeal mucous membrane is covered by columnar epithelium, as shown in Figure 3-27. The regions of the vocal folds that approximate during phonation are covered by squamous epithelium.

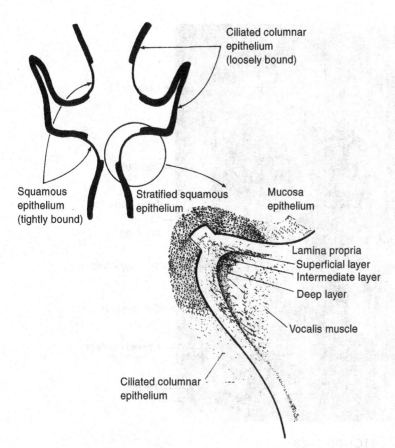

Ciliated columnar epithelium (loosely bound)

Squamous epithelium (tightly bound)

Stratified squamous epithelium

Mucosa epithelium

Lamina propria
Superficial layer
Intermediate layer
Deep layer

Vocalis muscle

Ciliated columnar epithelium

FIGURE 3-27

Schematic of distribution of laryngeal mucous membrane (top), and a diagrammatic representation of the structure of the human vocal fold, showing the relationship of epithelium to adjacent tissues, the lamina propria (three layers), and vocalis muscle, as reported by Hirano (1974).

THE INTERIOR OF THE LARYNX

The Cavity of the Larynx

The interior or cavity of the larynx extends from the **aditus** (L. entrance) **laryngis** to the inferior border of the cricoid cartilage. The aditus is a somewhat triangular opening, wider in front than behind, that slopes obliquely down and back. Its boundaries include the epiglottis in front, the aryepiglottic folds laterally, and the apexes of the arytenoid cartilages behind. Its shape is variable, depending on the position of the arytenoid cartilages and the epiglottis.

A deep depression, lateral to the aditus laryngis, is known as the **pyriform sinus.** As shown in Figure 3-10, it is bounded laterally by the thyroid cartilage and thyrohyoid membrane and medially by the aryepiglottic folds.

Note in Figure 3-28, how the true vocal folds project shelflike into the cavity of the larynx. The *space between the folds* is called the **rima glottidis,** or simply the **glottis.** With the vocal folds and glottis as a reference, the laryngeal cavity is divided into **supraglottal** and **subglottal spaces.**

The Supraglottal Region

The supraglottal region between the ventricular folds (false vocal folds) and the aditus is called the **vestibule** of the larynx, and a small supraglottal region located between the ventricular folds and the vocal folds is called the **ventricle.**

The Ventricle of the Larynx (Laryngeal Sinus)

The ventricle extends almost the entire length of the vocal folds, and anteriorly it is continued upward as the **laryngeal saccule.** The saccule is liberally supplied with mucous glands imbedded within submucous fatty tissue, a few muscle fibers, and the ventricular ligament.

CLINICAL NOTE: As can be seen in Figure 3-1, a well-defined shadow is cast by the **laryngeal ventricle** in a lateral x-ray of the neck. In a young person, especially, the hyaline structures of the larynx do not absorb x-rays very well, so the larynx is difficult to examine radiographically. The ventricle is a *valuable landmark* in locating and measuring the vocal folds and other laryngeal structures.

The Ventricular Folds

The ventricular folds present a soft and flaccid appearance and are *incapable of becoming tense.* They are most prominent anteriorly where they attach to the angle of the thyroid cartilage, just beneath the attachment of the

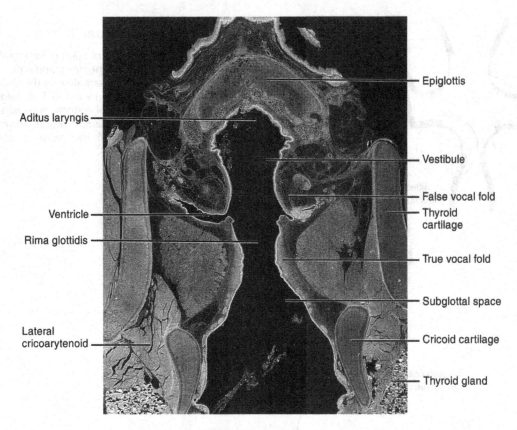

FIGURE 3-28

Frontal section through a fetal larynx, showing its divisions and landmarks.

epiglottis. Behind, the ventricular folds attach to the anterolateral surface of the arytenoid cartilages, in the area of the triangular fovea.

The ventricular folds move with the arytenoid cartilages, but they stand farther apart than the vocal folds. Under normal circumstances they do not vibrate during phonation. The space between the ventricular folds is called the **false glottis.**

CLINICAL NOTE: Sphincteric action of certain laryngeal muscles may approximate the ventricular folds, and in that event voice is either produced or significantly modified by their vibration. Every now and again a person is described clinically as having **ventricular dysphonia** or **hyperkinesia of the false vocal folds.**

The chief symptom is roughness of the voice, varying greatly in severity. The **ventricular folds,** which are normally widely separated, are adducted and may partially or completely cover the true vocal folds. This condition may be psychogenic, or it may be secondary to organic disease of the larynx.

Studies of the acoustics of the vocal mechanism have shown that the ventricle and ventricular folds may contribute to a modification of the laryngeal tone produced by the vibrating vocal folds.

The Subglottal Region

The subglottal portion of the laryngeal cavity is bounded above by the vocal folds and below by the inferior margin of the cricoid cartilage. When seen in a frontal section, as in Figure 3-28, it appears narrowest at the level of the vocal folds, becoming wider below, so it appears cone-shaped.

This portion of the larynx is lined with ciliated columnar epithelium which extends into the trachea and bronchi. The **cilia** in the larynx beat toward the pharynx, just as the cilia in the trachea beat toward the larynx, helping to remove accumulations of mucus and foreign matter from the lower respiratory tract.

The Vocal Folds (Plicae Vocales)

The true vocal folds lie parallel to, and just beneath, the ventricular folds, separated from them by the laryngeal ventricle. The paired vocal folds take their origin from the thyroid cartilage, near the angle and below the thyroid notch. This **anterior commissure** (anterior attachment) of the folds is common, but they diverge as they course posteriorly toward the **posterior commissure** (their attachments on the antero-lateral surface of the arytenoid cartilages). The medial borders of the vocal folds are free. Thus the vocal folds project shelflike into the cavity of the larynx (Figure 3-28).

Each vocal fold consists of a bundle of muscle tissue (**thyroarytenoid**) and a **vocal ligament** which is continuous with the conus elasticus. Depending upon their contractile state and other factors, the **vocal folds** may present anywhere from a sharp, well-defined medial border, as in a tense fold, to a rounded medial border, as in the relaxed fold.

Although the vocal folds are actually slightly pink, when viewed by conventional laryngoscopic techniques they appear glossy white. Due to the presence of elastic fibers and the vocal ligaments, the vocal folds appear yellowish at the anterior commisure. The vocal folds may also appear pink in heavy smokers and blood red in persons with laryngitis.

The Glottis (Rima Glottidis, Rima Glottis, Glottal Chink)

Although the term **glottis** is sometimes defined as the vocal folds and the opening between them, it usually refers to the *variable opening between the vocal folds*. In this text we shall use the latter definition.

The glottis extends from the anterior commissure to the vocal processes and bases of the arytenoid cartilages. The anterior portion, which is bounded by the vocal ligament, is called the **membranous** (or **intermembranous**) **glottis.** Extending from the anterior commissure to the vocal process, it comprises about three-fifths the total length of the glottis (Figure 3-29), and at rest is about 15 mm in adult males and 12 mm in females. The posterior two-fifths of the glottis is bounded by the vocal processes and the medial surfaces of the arytenoid cartilages and is known as the **cartilaginous** (or **intercartilaginous**) **glottis.** It measures about 8 mm in males, slightly less in females (Figures 3-29 and 3-30).

The dimensions and configurations of the glottis are highly variable, depending upon laryngeal activity and the adjustments of the arytenoid cartilages (Figure 3-31).

At rest, the width of the glottis, measured at the vocal processes, is about 8 mm in the male. During forced inhalation this value may almost double. In addition, the configuration of the glottis may vary anywhere from a thin slit to a wide, lozenge-shaped opening.

When studied by means of ultra-high-speed motion-picture photography, the *membranous portion of the vibrat-*

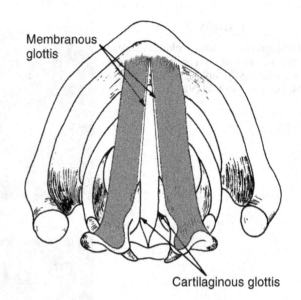

FIGURE 3-29

Schematic of larynx as seen from above, showing membranous or vocal glottis and the cartilaginous glottis.

ing vocal folds appears to be the most active, although the cartilaginous portion also enters into vibration. The configurations of the glottis during a single cycle of vocal fold vibration are shown in Figure 3-32. These pictures were

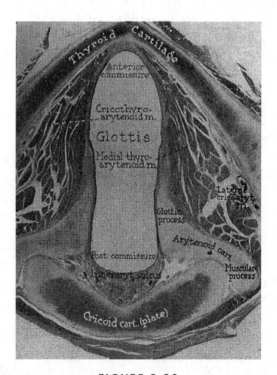

FIGURE 3-30

Transverse section of adult larynx at level of glottis illustrating the extent to which the vocal process projects into the vocal fold. (Courtesy F. L. Lederer, *Diseases of the Ear, Nose, and Throat.* Philadelphia: F. A. Davis Company, 1938.)

FIGURE 3-31A

Photographs of various glottal configurations. Apex of arytenoid cartilage (A), vocal fold (VF), epiglottis (E), ventricular (false vocal) fold (V).

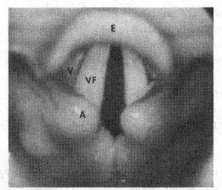
Quiet breathing

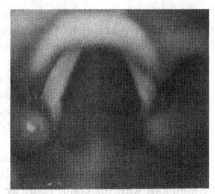
Forced inhalation

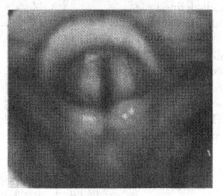
Normal phonation

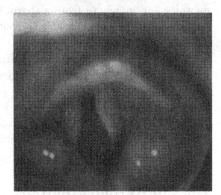
Whisper

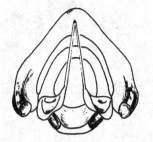
Quiet breathing

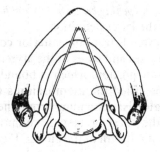
Forced inhalation

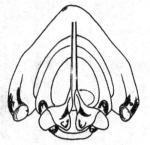
Normal phonation

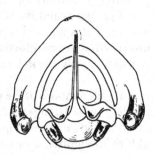
Whisper

FIGURE 3-31B

Schematic of various glottal configurations.

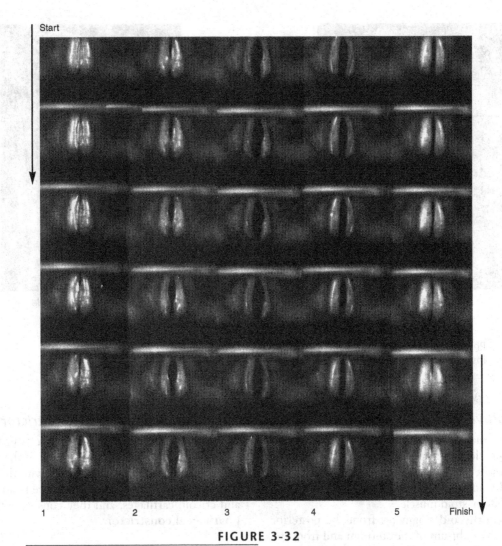

FIGURE 3-32

A single cycle of vocal fold vibration taken from a high-speed film exposed at 4,000 frames per second.

taken at an exposure rate of 4000 frames per second, and the entire vibratory cycle represents glottal activity during 1/140 second.

THE MUSCLES OF THE LARYNX

The musculature of the larynx is generally described as either extrinsic or intrinsic. **Extrinsic muscles** are those that have one attachment to structures outside the larynx, while **intrinsic muscles** have both attachments confined to the larynx. Although both extrinsic and intrinsic muscles influence laryngeal functions, *the extrinsic muscles are primarily responsible for the support of the larynx and for fixing it in position. The intrinsic muscles are largely responsible for the control of sound production.*

Other muscles (supplemental), which for the most part have one attachment on the hyoid bone, may also influence the larynx. They are divided into **suprahyoid** and **infrahyoid** muscles. Functionally they are classified as laryngeal **elevators** and **depressors.**[3]

The Extrinsic Muscles of the Larynx

The extrinsic muscles, which, as previously stated, position and support the larynx are the **sternothyroid muscles,** the **thyrohyoid muscles,** and the **inferior pharyngeal constrictor.**

---

[3]Two extrinsic muscles also function to elevate or depress the larynx. The sternothyroid is a depressor; the thyrohyoid is an elevator.

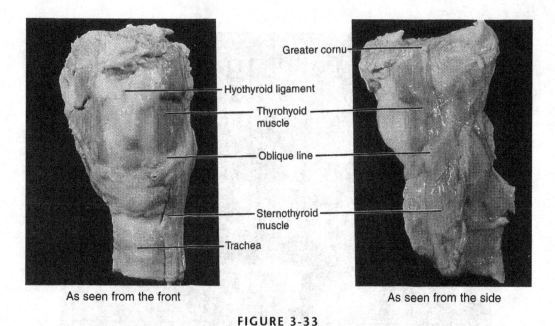

Greater cornu

Hyothyroid ligament

Thyrohyoid
muscle

Oblique line

Sternothyroid
muscle

Trachea

As seen from the front   As seen from the side

FIGURE 3-33

Photograph of a larynx showing the origin and insertion of the thyrohyoid muscle and insertion of the sternothyroid muscle.

The Sternothyroid Muscle

The sternothyroid muscle, shown in Figures 3-33 and 3-34, is a long slender muscle located in the anterior neck. It is almost completely covered by the sternohyoid and omohyoid muscles, as well as the lower third of the sternocleidomastoid muscle.

The **sternothyroid** originates from the posterior surface of the manubrium of the sternum and from the first costal cartilage. The fibers course upward and slightly laterally, and they insert on the oblique tendon or line of the thyroid cartilage.

The principal action of the sternothyroid muscle is to draw the thyroid cartilage downward. Some investigators claim that the sternothyroid muscle may enlarge the pharynx by drawing the larynx down and forward.

The Thyrohyoid Muscle

The thyrohyoid, also located in the anterior neck, is covered by the omohyoid and sternohyoid muscles. As shown in Figure 3-33, the muscle originates from the oblique tendon or line of the thyroid lamina. The fibers course vertically upward and insert into the lower border of the greater horn of the hyoid bone.

Contraction of this muscle decreases the distance between the thyroid cartilage and the hyoid bone. With the thyroid cartilage fixed, it depresses the hyoid bone, and with the hyoid bone fixed, it elevates the thyroid cartilage. The thyrohyoid muscle is also shown schematically in Figure 3-34.

The Inferior Pharyngeal Constrictor

A muscular tube called the **pharynx** extends from the base of the skull to the lower border of the cricoid cartilage, where it becomes continuous with the esophagus. Muscle fibers of the lower portion are from the thyroid and cricoid cartilages, and they constitute the **inferior pharyngeal constrictor.**

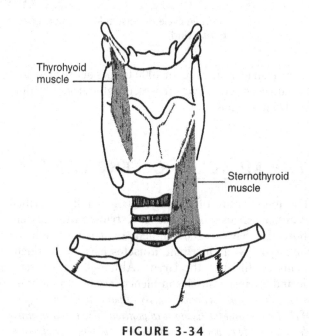

Thyrohyoid
muscle

Sternothyroid
muscle

FIGURE 3-34

Sternothyroid and thyrohyoid muscles shown schematically.

Fibers that arise from the cricoid cartilage have a horizontal course and are often known separately as the **cricopharyngeus muscle.** The fibers that arise from the thyroid cartilage have an oblique upward course. The fibers from each side meet at the midline so as to form a sphincteric-like tube. *The pharyngeal constrictors are active during deglutition, and they also form a principal resonating cavity of the vocal mechanism.*

The **sternothyroid, thyrohyoid,** and **inferior pharyngeal constrictor** muscles are far more complex than straightforward descriptions might suggest. The superficialmost fibers of the sternothyroid insert only in part on the oblique tendon or line of the thyroid cartilage. Some fibers continue uninterrupted and constitute part of the thyrohyoid muscle. When the sternothyroid is freed from its sternal attachments and is reflected forward to expose its deep surface (as in Figure 3-35), a large but variable proportion of the muscle fibers are seen to continue into the inferior pharyngeal constrictor.

Our assignments of laryngeal elevator-depressor functions to this muscle complex are probably simplistic. These muscles may well function primarily to stabilize the position of the larynx in the neck.

In addition, both the sternohyoid and thyrohyoid muscles often have the greater part of their origin on the **pericardium** (the fibrous sac that envelopes the heart).

The Suprahyoid Muscles (Laryngeal Elevators)

The **suprahyoid** muscles are the **digastric,** the **stylohyoid,** the **mylohyoid,** the **geniohyoid,** the **hyoglossus,** and the **genioglossus.** The latter two are muscles of the tongue that may influence the larynx indirectly. The thyrohyoid, an extrinsic muscle, also elevates the larynx.

The Digastric Muscle

As the name suggests, the digastric muscle, shown in Figure 3-36, consists of *two fleshy bellies.* The **anterior belly** takes its origin from the inside surface of the lower border of the mandible near the symphysis. It is separated from the skin only by a thin layer of fat, and the outlines of the muscle can be seen in emaciated persons. These fibers course downward and back to the region of the lesser horn of the hyoid bone. The **posterior belly** takes its origin from the mastoid process of the temporal bone. The fibers course down and forward, deep to the sternocleidomastoid muscle. The two bellies meet and are joined by an *intermediate tendon* which perforates the stylohyoid muscle. This tendon is attached to the junction of the body and greater horn of the hyoid bone by a fibrous loop, which is part of a more extensive suprahyoid aponeurosis.

Contraction of the digastric muscle raises the hyoid bone, or if the hyoid is in a fixed position, it may assist in depressing the lower jaw. Contraction of the anterior belly draws the hyoid up and forward, while contraction of the posterior belly draws the hyoid up and backward. Both actions are important in the early stages of deglutition.

The Stylohyoid Muscle

The stylohyoid, shown in Figure 3-37, is a long slender muscle placed just superficially to the posterior belly of the digastric muscle. It takes its origin from the posterior and lateral surface of the **styloid process** (L. *stilus,* a

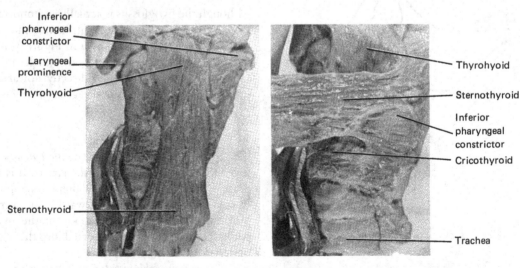

FIGURE 3-35

Reflected sternothyroid muscle (right) and the relationship of its deep fibers to the inferior constrictor of the pharynx.

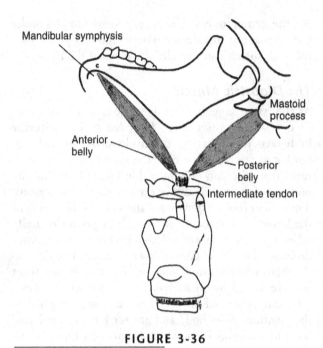

FIGURE 3-36

Schematic of the digastric muscle.

stake, pole; Gk. *stylos*, pillar) of the temporal bone. The fibers course down and forward, roughly parallel to the fibers of the posterior belly of the digastric muscle. Just prior to reaching the hyoid bone, the muscle splits into *two slips* that pass, one on either side of the intermediate tendon of the digastric, to insert into the body of the hyoid bone at its junction with the greater horn. *Contraction of this muscle draws the hyoid bone up and backward.*

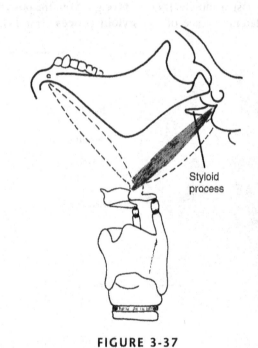

FIGURE 3-37

Schematic of the stylohyoid muscle. The digastric is shown in the dashed outline.

The Mylohyoid Muscle

The mylohyoid (Gk. *myle*, mill) is a thin, troughlike sheet of muscle that forms the *muscular floor of the mouth*. The fibers arise along the extent of the **mylohyoid line,** a well-defined bony ridge running along the inner surface of the body of the mandible, from the mental symphysis to the last molar (hence, *myle*, or mill). As shown in Figure 3-38, the fibers course medially and downward to join their fellows from the opposite side at a tendinous midline **raphe** (Gk. a seam), which extends from the mental symphysis to the hyoid bone. The posteriormost fibers attach directly to the body of the hyoid bone.

With the mandible fixed, contraction of the mylohyoid muscle *elevates the hyoid bone, the floor of the mouth, and the tongue.* This muscle is an *important contributor to the initial stages of deglutition.* With the hyoid bone in a fixed position, it *may assist in depressing the mandible.*

The Geniohyoid Muscle

The geniohyoid (Gk. *genion*, chin) is a paired cylindrical muscle located above the superior (buccal) surface of the mylohyoid muscle. It is shown in Figure 3-39. The two muscles often lie in direct contact with each other but on opposite sides of the midline, or they may be a single muscle.

The fibers take their origin, by means of a short tendon, from the lower part of the mental symphysis. They diverge slightly as they course back and downward to insert on the anterior surface of the body of the hyoid bone. *With the mandible in a fixed position, the geniohyoid muscles pull the hyoid bone up and forward.*

The Hyoglossus Muscle

Although the hyoglossus is actually an important *extrinsic muscle of the tongue*, it may influence the position of the larynx indirectly. As shown in Figure 3-40, it arises from the upper border of the body and greater horns of the hyoid bone and courses directly upward to insert into the posterior and lateral regions of the tongue.

The Genioglossus Muscle

The genioglossus is also an *extrinsic tongue muscle* that may influence the position of the larynx. It is a complex muscle that originates at the mental symphysis. The fibers fan out as they course toward their insertion. The lower fibers insert into the body of the hyoid bone, while the upper fibers are inserted into the whole of the under surface of the tongue.

Contraction of this muscle may elevate the hyoid bone and draw it forward. This muscle, along with the hyoglossus will be considered in more detail in Chapter 4. The extrinsic tongue muscles and their relation to the laryngeal structures are shown in Figure 3-40.

FIGURE 3-38

Muscles of the neck, some of which can influence the position and behavior of the larynx. They include the true extrinsic muscles and those that can be regarded as functionally extrinsic.

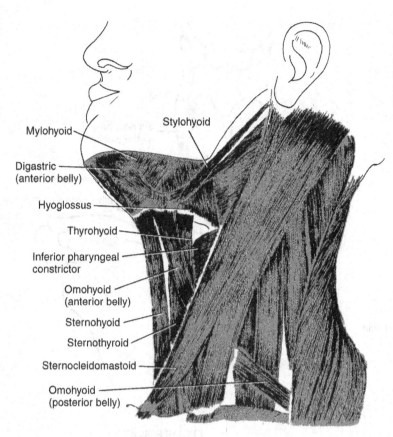

Stylohyoid

Mylohyoid

Digastric (anterior belly)

Hyoglossus

Thyrohyoid

Inferior pharyngeal constrictor

Omohyoid (anterior belly)

Sternohyoid

Sternothyroid

Sternocleidomastoid

Omohyoid (posterior belly)

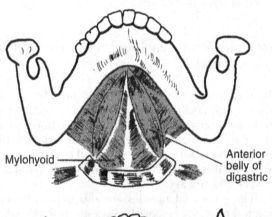

Mylohyoid

Anterior belly of digastric

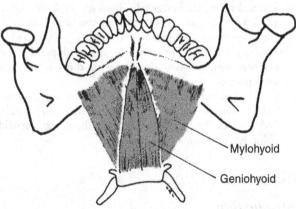

Mylohyoid

Geniohyoid

FIGURE 3-39

Schematic of the mylohyoid and geniohyoid muscles.

The Infrahyoid Muscles (Laryngeal Depressors)

Two muscles support the hyoid bone from below. They are the **sternohyoid** and the **omohyoid** muscles, both of which are "strap muscles" of the neck. The **sternothyroid**, an extrinsic muscle, is also considered a laryngeal depressor.

The Sternohyoid Muscle

The sternohyoid is a flat muscle lying on the anterior surface of the neck. It is shown schematically in Figure 3-41. It originates from the posterior surface of the manubrium of the sternum, from the medial end of the clavicle, and from adjacent ligamentous tissue. The fibers course vertically and insert on the lower border of the body of the hyoid bone. The muscles on either side come very near one another as they course upward toward their insertion, and they may even lie in direct contact with one another, or blend together and appear as a single muscle. *The sternohyoid acts to draw the hyoid bone downward and fixes the hyoid bone when the lower jaw is opened against resistance.*

The Omohyoid Muscle

The omohyoid is a long, narrow, two-bellied muscle located on the anterolateral surface of the neck. The **inferior (or posterior) belly** takes its origin from the upper

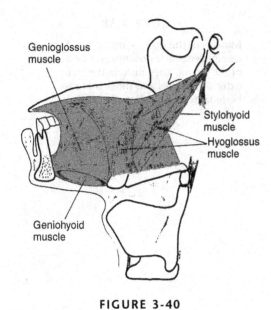

FIGURE 3-40

Schematic of extrinsic tongue muscles showing their relationship to the laryngeal structures.

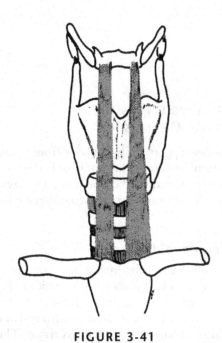

FIGURE 3-41

Schematic of sternohyoid muscles.

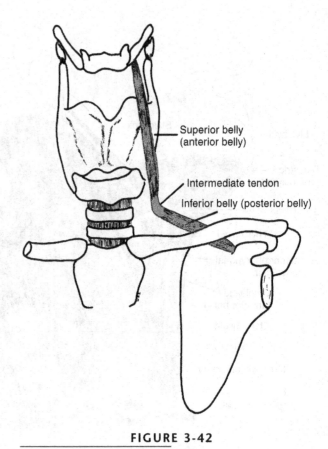

FIGURE 3-42

Schematic of omohyoid muscles.

horn of the hyoid bone, just lateral to the insertion of the sternohyoid muscle.

By their contraction the **omohyoid muscles** render the cervical fascia tense and prevent the neck region from collapsing during deep inspiratory efforts. Contraction of the omohyoid muscles also prevents the great blood vessels of the neck as well as the apexes of the lungs from being compressed during deep inspiration (see Figure 3-43).

The omohyoid muscles are also important anatomical reference landmarks, because, as shown schematically in Figures 3-44 and 3-45, the neck is divided, for descriptive and reference purposes, into triangles. The anterior and posterior triangles depend upon the sternocleidomastoid muscle for their anatomical recognition.

The **anterior triangle** is divided into three subsidiary triangles by means of the digastric and omohyoid muscles. They are known as the **digastric, carotid (bloody),** and **muscular triangles.**

The Intrinsic Muscles of the Larynx

Introduction

Socially adequate voice production, with appropriate pitch inflections and proper intensity changes, is a rather

border of the scapula, which accounts for the name of the muscle. *Omo* is a Greek word pertaining to shoulder. As shown in Figure 3-42, the fibers course almost horizontally forward to terminate at the *intermediate tendon*, which is held in position, just above the sternum, by tendinous slips that run to the sternum and to the first rib. These slips are part of the deep cervical fascia.

The **superior** (or **anterior**) **belly** originates from an intermediate tendon and courses vertically and slightly medially to insert along the lower border of the greater

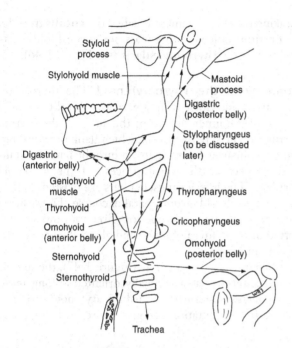

FIGURE 3-43

Schematic of the presumed actions of the extrinsic laryngeal and functionally related musculature.

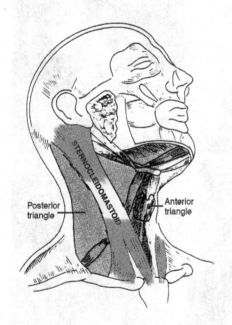

FIGURE 3-44

Schematic of the anterior and posterior triangles of the neck, shown in relation to the sternocleidomastoid muscle.

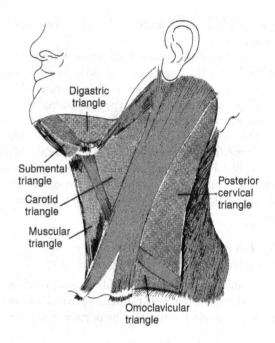

FIGURE 3-45

Schematic of the digastric, carotid, muscular, submental divisions of the anterior triangle of the neck, and the posterior cervical and omoclavicular divisions of the posterior triangle of the neck.

common event. Most of us are unimpressed by such things as voice quality in the speech of persons around us. Indeed, it is usually not until we are in the presence of someone with a voice disorder that we become aware of the quality or social adequacy of the voice. Students of speech and voice pathology are painfully aware of the

complexities of the speech mechanism and of the rapid sequences of subtle changes required of it during the production of everyday speech.

The **larynx** is one of the most complex structures in the entire speech and hearing mechanism. Despite its location in the neck, the larynx seems to be surprisingly vulnerable, but most of the insults suffered by it are due to abuse. It is subjected to the same diseases that affect the respiratory tract as a whole, and the fact we are talking animals means that we breathe through the mouth much of the time, subjecting the larynx to increased drying effects. In addition, alcohol, smoking, and vocal abuse, plus a lifetime of inhaling dirty, polluted air, must be included among the variety of abuses the larynx must endure.

A fairly intricate system of **intrinsic muscles** contributes to the complexity of the larynx. These muscles, by virtue of their unique structure and architecture, are able to accomplish the many and varied rapid changes that are required during ordinary speech production. *The intrinsic muscles of the larynx may be categorized according to their effects on the shape of the glottis and on the vibratory behavior of the vocal folds.* There are abductor, adductor, tensor, and relaxer muscles in the larynx. The **abductor** muscles, which separate the arytenoids and the vocal folds for respiratory activities, are opposed by the **adductors,** which approximate the arytenoid cartilages and the vocal folds for phonation and for protective purposes. The glottal **tensors** elongate and tighten the vocal folds. They are opposed by the **relaxers,** which shorten them.

The intrinsic laryngeal muscles always act in pairs. In a healthy larynx the muscles on one side do not contract independently of the muscles on the opposite side.

There are just two main types of internal laryngeal adjustments which take place. They are *the extent of force with which the vocal folds are brought together at the midline,* termed **medial compression,** and the *degree of stretching force,* called **longitudinal tension.** These two adjustments or combinations of them, plus a variable air supply, account for the astonishing versatility of the human voice.

The Thyroarytenoid Muscle (Adductor, Tensor, or Relaxer)

The main mass of the vocal folds is composed of the thyroarytenoid muscle. It is often described as consisting of two separate muscles. The portion of the muscle flanking the vocal ligament is called the **vocalis muscle.** It constitutes the vibrating mass of the vocal folds. Lateral to it is the **thyromuscularis** (see Figure 3-46).

Anatomy of the Thyroarytenoid The thyroarytenoid arises anteriorly from a narrow vertically oriented region of the inner surface of the angle of the thyroid cartilage. The superior fibers, which flank the vocal ligament, course backward to insert into the lateral and inferior aspect of the vocal process of the arytenoid cartilage. The inferior muscle fibers are twisted, so they depart considerably from a parallel course. They "swing off" in a lateroposterosuperior direction and are inserted into the fovea oblonga and along the base of the arytenoid cartilage.

When viewed as a whole (Figure 3-47), the muscle begins anteriorly as a vertically oriented oblong mass. As it courses posteriorly toward the arytenoid cartilage, this vertical orientation becomes more horizontal, and

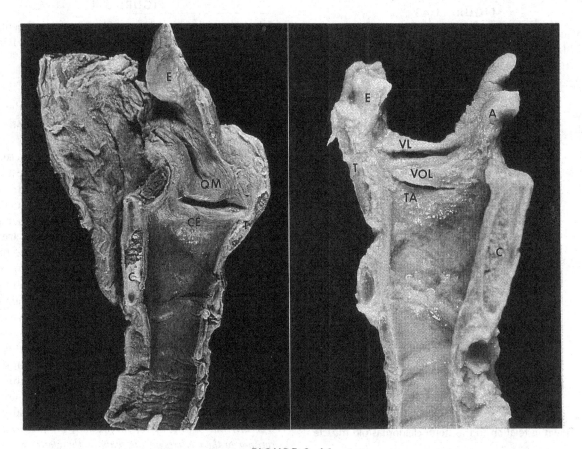

FIGURE 3-46

Photograph of vocal ligament and thyroarytenoid muscle as seen in a sagittal section. The epithelium and conus elasticus (CE) and the quadrangular membrane (QM) are shown on the left. These structures have been removed on the right to expose the thyroarytenoid muscle (TA), the arytenoid cartilage (A), the vocal ligament (VOL), and the ventricular ligament (VL). Other structures identified are the cricoid plate (C), the thyroid cartilage (T), and epiglottis (E).

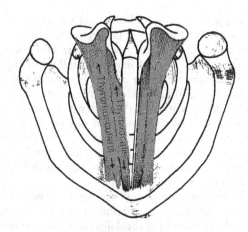

FIGURE 3-47

Schematic of vocal fold musculature and its primary action. Unopposed contraction of the medial portion (vocalis) will relax the vibrating mass of the vocal fold.

as a result, the muscle takes on a twisted appearance, as shown in Figure 3-48. This is the impression one gets when the vocal fold is in the *adducted* or cadaveric position. When the vocal folds are *abducted*, however, the vocal processes are raised and rotated laterally so the horizontal orientation is reduced. In other words, *when the vocal fold is abducted the twisted muscle "unwinds" to some extent*, as illustrated in Figure 3-48.

A few lateral fibers of the thyroarytenoid muscle depart from their anteroposterior course and are directed almost vertically upward from the angle of the thyroid cartilage. Some of them become lost in the aryepiglottic fold while others continue to the lateral

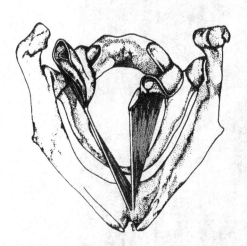

FIGURE 3-48

Vocal fold musculature in the adducted position, when seen from above has a twisted appearance (right). The abducted fold on the left seems to have "unwound." (From E. Zemlin and W. Zemlin, *Study-Guide/Workbook.* Champaign, Ill.: Stipes Publishing Company, 1988.)

margin of the epiglottis. This slip of muscle is identified as the **thyroepiglotticus.**

In addition, a few fibers course along the lateral margin of the ventricle and insert into the lateral margin of the epiglottis. They constitute the **ventricularis** muscle.

The Histology of the Vocal Fold Hirano (1974, 1981), has shown the vocal fold to be composed of five histologically distinct layers:

1. The **epithelium,** which is squamous. It can be regarded as a thin and stiff capsule that maintains the shape of the vocal fold.

2. The **superficial layer of the lamina propria** (Reinke's space), consisting of loose fibrous components and matrix, which can be regarded as a mass of soft gelatin.

3. The **intermediate layer of the lamina propria,** consisting chiefly of elastic fibers and likened to a bundle of soft rubber bands.

4. The **deep layer of the lamina propria,** consisting of collagenous fibers and somewhat like a bundle of cotton thread.

5. The **vocalis muscle,** which constitutes the main body of the vocal fold and is like a bundle of rather stiff rubber bands.

Physiology and Function of the Thyroarytenoid Hirano states that, from a mechanical point of view, the five layers can be reclassified into three sections: the **cover,** consisting of the epithelium and superficial layer of the lamina propria; the **transition,** consisting of intermediate and deep layers of the lamina propria (the vocal ligament); and the **body,** consisting of the vocalis muscle. *The mechanical properties of the outer four layers are controlled passively, while the mechanical properties of the body are regulated both passively and actively.*

During phonation, a wave traveling on the laryngeal mucosa from its inferior to superior surface can be seen during each cycle of vocal fold vibration, except when the vocal fold is very tense, as in falsetto. A soft and pliant superficial layer of the lamina propria is supposed to be essential for the occurrence of the **mucosal wave.** This wave will continue across the upper surface of the vocal fold, but is usually dissipated before the boundary of the thyroid cartilage is reached.

The principal function of the **thyroarytenoid muscle** is to act as a *regulator of longitudinal tension.* Acting unopposed by other intrinsic muscles, the thyroarytenoid will relax the vocal folds and will also assist in closing the glottis by pulling forward on the muscular process. When contraction of the thyroarytenoid is opposed by other intrinsic muscles, the result is an increase in vocal fold tension. Depending upon circumstances, then, this muscle may act as an *adductor*, a *tensor*, or a *relaxer* of the vocal folds.

The **thyroarytenoid muscle** has been the subject of considerable research and debate for well over a century. The debate centers on two fundamental questions: first, does the **vocalis muscle** exist as a discernably separate muscle, and second, do muscle fibers insert into the **vocal ligament?**

Wustrow (1952) identified the portion of the thyroarytenoid that inserts along the vocal process as the **thyrovocalis (vocalis)** muscle and the portion that inserts along the base of the arytenoid cartilage and the muscular process as the **thyromuscularis.** Wustrow also contended that the thyromuscularis functions to

approximate the vocal folds by exerting a forward pull on the muscular process of the arytenoid cartilage. The thyrovocalis, he said, functions to control the tension of the vocal folds. Van den Berg and Moll (1955) support this viewpoint, while our own dissections and those of Sonesson (1960) have failed to reveal any anatomical landmarks such as a fascial sheath within the thyroarytenoid muscle that will justify or support the thyrovocalis and thyromuscularis division. A frontal section through a human larynx is shown in Figure 3-49, and no evidence whatsoever of an anatomical division can be found.

To make matters even more complex, when the thyroarytenoid muscle is carefully removed, beginning from the region of the vocal ligament and working laterally toward the thyroid cartilage, a true demarcation

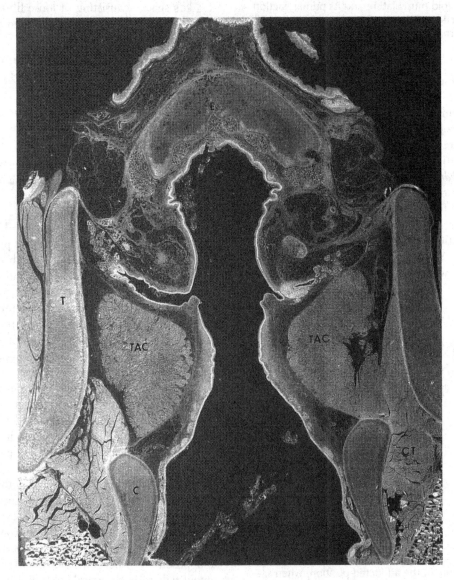

FIGURE 3-49

Frontal section through the larynx which reveals the vocal fold to consist of a single muscle mass. On the left side continuity between the thyroarytenoid and lateral cricoarytenoid muscles can be seen. Epiglottis (E), thyroid lamina (T), cricoid (C), thyroarytenoid-cricothyroid muscle mass (TAC), cricothyroid (CT).

between the musculature of the vocal fold and the lateral cricoarytenoid cannot be found. As Sonesson has reported,

"Anatomically the vocal muscle belongs to the cricothyro-arytenoid muscle mass, from which the muscle can only be partly dissected free (Cruveilhier, 1844; Ruhlmann, 1874; Cunningham, 1917; Elze, 1925). The thyroarytenoid and vocal muscles belonging to the muscle mass are fused along the major part of their length, and no fascia or connective tissue can be demonstrated between them (Elze, 1925; Mayet, 1955). At its insertion in the arytenoid cartilage, the third muscle in the muscle mass, the lateral cricoarytenoid muscle, is fused with the other two muscles. In the anterior and middle parts of the vocal fold, however, a connective tissue layer is generally found between the lateral cricoarytenoid muscle and the other two muscles (Mayet, 1955)."

The **lateral cricoarytenoid muscle** will be described later, along with the other adductors of the vocal folds.

Göerttler (1950) has contended that obliquely directed fibers of the thyroarytenoid muscles are inserted into the vocal ligament and that they contribute to opening of the glottis during phonation. These oblique fibers, according to Göerttler, are composed of an anterior and a posterior division. The anterior division is supposed to arise from the thyroid cartilage in front and course in a posteromedial direction to insert into the vocal ligament. It was identified as the thyrovocalis muscle. The posterior division, according to Göerttler, arises from the muscular process of the arytenoid cartilage and courses in an anteromedial direction to insert into the vocal ligament. This muscle, which he identified as the **aryvocalis muscle,** is shown schematically, along with the thyrovocalis muscle, in Figure 3-50.

Our findings, using microscopic dissection, reveal that the course of the muscle fibers immediately adjacent to the vocal ligament is parallel to the ligament, with no muscle fibers entering into it. Sonesson (1960), using low-power magnification and a differential staining technique, failed to find muscle fibers inserting into the vocal ligament. He did find some muscle fibers that seemed to insert into the conus elasticus, however.

Sonesson's findings, and ours, are consistent with those of Wustrow (1952), Mayet (1955), Van den Berg and Moll (1955), Schlossauer and Vosteen (1957, 1958), and Manjome (1959). These findings also have important implications with respect to theories of voice production, a topic we will encounter toward the end of this chapter.

The Superior Thyroarytenoid Muscle (Relaxer)

Very little is known about this muscle. Occurring in about half the human population, it might be regarded as a variation. This muscle can best be examined by removal of the thyroid laminae. This permits an unobstructed view of the lateral aspect of the thyroarytenoid, the superior thyroarytenoid, and the lateral cricoarytenoid muscles. As shown in Figure 3-51, the superior

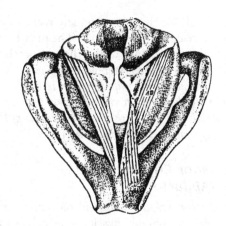

FIGURE 3-50

Schematic of the thyrovocalis and aryvocalis muscles as described by Göerttler (1950). The aryvocalis is shown on both the right and left sides, while the thyrovocalis is shown in the left. The drawing represents a horizontal section (transverse). The illustration also depicts the vocal folds and glottis as they appear from above. Subsequent research has failed to find support for the existence of the thyrovocalis and aryvocalis muscles (see text).

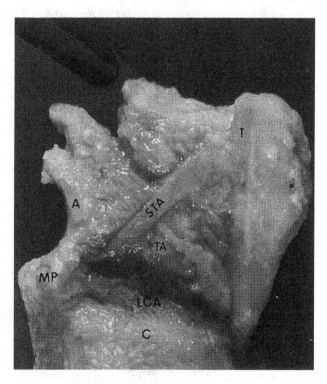

FIGURE 3-51

Photograph of a superior thyroarytenoid muscle (STA). It courses from the thyroid cartilage (T) in front, downward and back to the muscular process (MP) of the arytenoid cartilage (A). Also identified are the thyroarytenoid muscle (TA), and the lateral cricoarytenoid (LCA), which originates on the cricoid cartilage, courses up and back to the muscular process and lateral margin of the arytenoid cartilage. (From Zemlin, Elving, and Hull, 1984.)

thyroarytenoid muscle is an obliquely placed band on the lateral surface of the vocal fold. The muscle courses from near the upper limit of the thyroid notch to the muscular process of the arytenoid cartilage.

Upon contraction, the superior thyroarytenoid tilts the thyroid cartilage backward to relax the vocal folds and at the same time pulls forward on the muscular process of the arytenoid cartilage to assist in medial compression.

The Posterior Cricoarytenoid Muscle (Abductor)

There is just one abductor muscle in the larynx. It is the posterior cricoarytenoid muscle, a broad fan-shaped muscle that originates from a shallow depression of the posterior surface of the cricoid lamina.

Recent research findings (Zemlin, Davis, and Gaza, 1984) have shown this muscle to consist of *two parts,* a lateral vertically directed bundle which comprises most of the muscle mass and a medial fan-shaped part, as shown in Figure 3-52. The lateral bundle inserts on the upper surface of the muscular process of the arytenoid cartilage, while the medial part attaches by a short tendon on the posterior surface of the muscular process.

This muscle arrangement suggests that the lateral bundle is the abductor and that the remainder of the muscle stabilizes and fixes the arytenoid cartilage. Action of the lateral bundle produces a rotation of the arytenoid cartilage so that the vocal processes are abducted and, at the same time, elevated. This is easily observed when a person gasps for breath. The photograph of the abducted vocal folds in Figure 3-31A was taken while the subject was inhaling deeply.

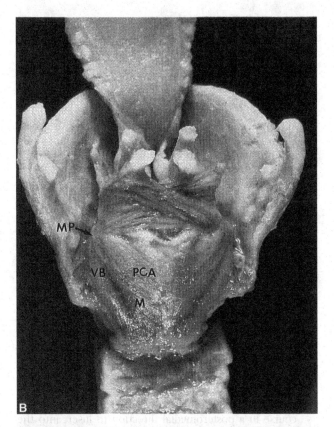

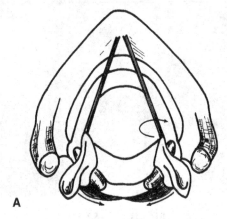

FIGURE 3-52

The posterior cricoarytenoid muscle (PCA). It consists of a vertically coursing bundle (VB), which is usually discrete and separate from the medial fan-shaped part (M). The muscle is shown enlarged in the lower right figure, and its action is shown schematically above. Muscular process (MP).

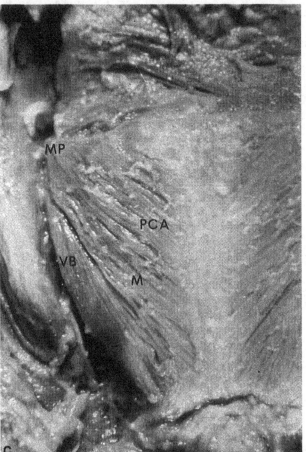

Two muscles act as *antagonists* to the posterior cricoarytenoid muscle. They are the **lateral cricoarytenoid** and the **arytenoid muscles.** Acting together, they rotate the arytenoid cartilage toward the midline to approximate the vocal processes and the vocal ligaments attached to them. Because of the complexity of this action, *approximation and depression are occurring simultaneously.*

The Lateral Cricoarytenoid Muscle (Adductor, Relaxer)

The lateral cricoarytenoid muscle is an important glottal adductor, which under certain circumstances may also function as a glottal relaxer. It is a slightly fan-shaped muscle, located deep to the thyroid cartilage. The muscle fibers originate along the upper border of the anterolateral arch of the cricoid cartilage. They course upward, back, and insert into the muscular process and anterior surface of the arytenoid cartilage, with some of their upper fibers blending with those of the thyroarytenoid muscle.

The principal action of the **lateral cricoarytenoid muscle** is to rotate the arytenoid cartilage to bring the vocal processes (and the vocal ligament) toward the midline. *This muscle is very instrumental in regulating medial compression of the vocal folds.* Acting unopposed this muscle will shape the glottis for the production of a whisper (see Figures 3-31A and 3-53).

The Arytenoid (Interarytenoid)[4] Muscles (Adductors)

The arytenoid is a muscle complex located on the posterior surfaces of the arytenoid cartilages. It is usually

---

[4]Although the term **interarytenoid,** which has been used in the previous editions of this text, seems more descriptive, **arytenoid** is now the more widely accepted name of the muscle.

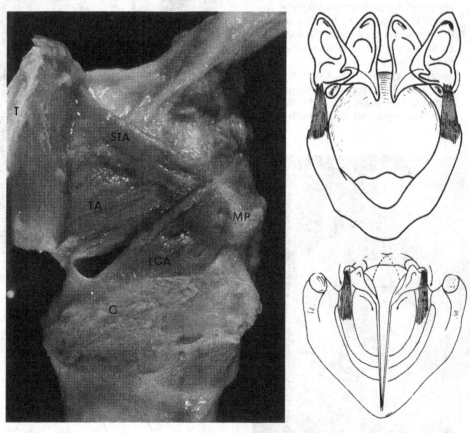

FIGURE 3-53

Photograph and schematic of lateral cricoarytenoid muscle (above left and top right) and an illustration of its action if unopposed. This muscle is one of the principal adductors of the vocal folds and so is responsible for regulating medial compression. Muscular process (MP), cricoid cartilage (C), thyroid cartilage (T), thyroarytenoid muscle (TA), superior thyroarytenoid muscle (STA), lateral cricoarytenoid muscle (LCA).

described in two parts, the **oblique arytenoid** and the **transverse arytenoid** muscles.

The Oblique Arytenoid Muscle The oblique arytenoid muscle is the more superficial of the two parts. It consists of a number of fasciculi that originate from the posterior surface of the muscular process and adjacent posterolateral surface of one arytenoid cartilage and insert near the apex of the opposite cartilage. When viewed from behind, as in Figure 3-54, the fasciculi can be seen to cross each other like the limbs of the letter X.

As shown in Figure 3-54, a few muscle fibers continue around the apex of the arytenoid cartilage laterally, angle upward and forward, and insert into the lateral borders of the epiglottis as the **aryepiglottic muscle.** This very small muscle, found buried within the aryepiglottic fold, is sometimes credited with depressing the epiglottis during the initial states of deglutition. *The oblique arytenoids function to approximate the arytenoid cartilages and are therefore regulators of medial compression.*

The Transverse Arytenoid Muscle The transverse arytenoid is a stout muscle, and anatomically it seems to be distinctly separate from the oblique part. As shown in Figure 3-55, the fibers arise from the lateral margin and posterior surface of one arytenoid cartilage, course in a horizontal direction, and insert into the lateral margin and posterior surface of the opposite arytenoid cartilage.

The deeper muscle fibers continue around the lateral margins of the arytenoid cartilage and blend with fibers of the thyroarytenoid muscle. *Contraction of this muscle approximates the arytenoid cartilages by causing them to slide along the long axis of the articular capsule toward the midline. The cartilages are elevated somewhat as they do so.*

FIGURE 3-54

Photograph of the oblique fibers of the arytenoid muscle (bottom left), enlarged (top right), and its action (right). Contraction approximates the arytenoid cartilages and the vocal ligaments. Also identified are the thyroid cartilage (T), epiglottis (E), posterior cricoarytenoid muscle (PCA), corniculate cartilages (C), cuneiform cartilages (∧), and muscular process of arytenoid cartilage (MP).

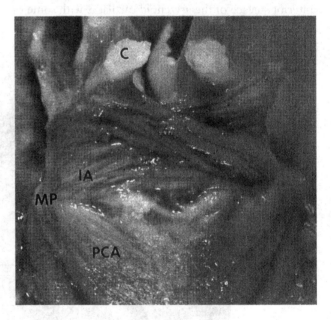

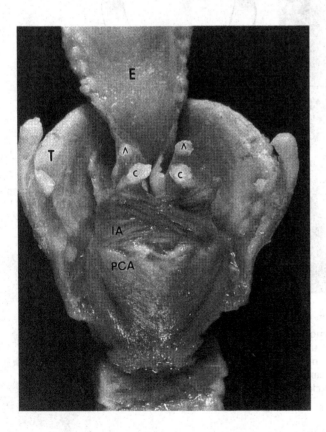

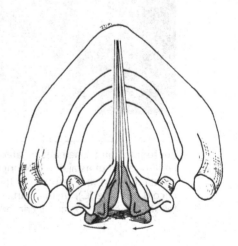

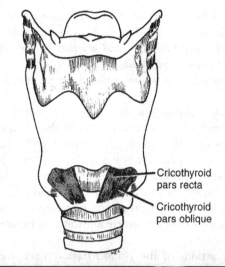

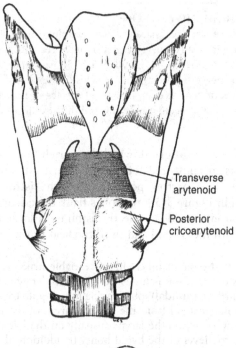

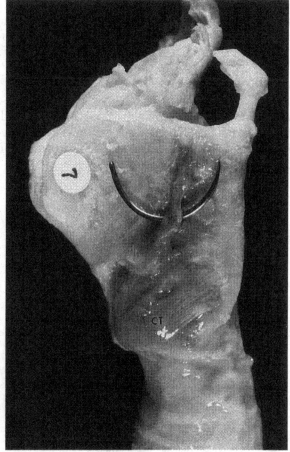

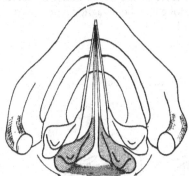

FIGURE 3-55

Schematic of transverse arytenoid muscle (top figure) and its action (bottom). Contraction approximates the arytenoid cartilages and vocal ligaments.

The Cricothyroid Muscle (Tensor)

Aside from the thyroarytenoid muscle, there is but one other muscle that can actively tense or elongate the vocal folds. It is the cricothyroid muscle. As shown in Figure 3-56, the cricothyroid is a fan-shaped muscle, broader above than below. It arises from the anterolateral arch of the cricoid cartilage. The fibers diverge and insert into the thyroid cartilage as two distinct parts.

The lower or oblique fibers (**pars oblique**) course upward and back to insert into the anterior margin of the inferior horn of the thyroid cartilage. The upper or anterior fibers (**pars recta**) course nearly vertically upward to insert along the inner aspect of the lower margin of the thyroid lamina (Figure 3-56).

FIGURE 3-56

Schematic and photograph of cricothyroid muscle and associated laryngeal structures.

Upon contraction of the anterior fibers, the distance between the cricoid arch and the thyroid cartilage is decreased. If the thyroid cartilage is fixed (by extrinsic laryngeal muscles), contraction of the cricothyroid muscle raises the cricoid; if the cricoid is fixed, the thyroid tilts downward like the visor of the helmet of a medieval knight. Either way *the distance between the thyroid cartilage (at the angle) and the vocal processes (of the arytenoid cartilages) is increased to elongate the vocal folds and place them under increased tension, action that is necessary for pitch changes.*

A slight sliding motion is also permitted by the cricothyroid joint, and contraction of the oblique portion of the cricothyroid muscle will produce such action; however, as Arnold (1961) notes, "When the cricothyroid distance is either distended or contracted, the sliding movements are prevented by the articular ligaments because they are then in a state of tension." Both the sliding and rocking actions are illustrated in Figures 3-53 and 3-55.

The actions of the *glottal tensors* (cricothyroid and thyroarytenoid), the *abductors* (posterior cricoarytenoid), the *adductors* (arytenoid and lateral cricoarytenoid), and the *glottal relaxers* (unopposed thyroarytenoid) are summarized in Figure 3-57.

The Thyroid Gland

A structure that is anatomically closely associated with the larynx, but is not directly involved in voice production, is the thyroid gland. Disease of this structure can markedly affect the laryngeal mechanism.

CLINICAL NOTE: One of the most common causes of laryngeal paralysis is **thyroidectomy,** which is the surgical removal of part or all of the thyroid gland (DeWeese and Saunders, 1977). An important motor nerve supplying the muscles of the larynx[5] courses under the deep or medial surface of the gland, and it may be accidentally severed during surgery.

The thyroid gland, which has a rich blood supply, consists of **right** and **left lobes** connected across the middle by a narrow portion called the **isthmus.** As shown in Figure 3-58, the lobes flank the cricoid cartilage on either side, while the isthmus is located on a level with the second and third tracheal rings.

The thyroid gland is a highly variable structure, to the extent that the isthmus may be completely absent. A third (**pyramidal**) lobe may be found quite frequently. It may extend from the upper margin of the isthmus upward across the larynx (usually on the left side) up to the level of the hyoid bone. In addition, the pyramidal lobe may be detached from the remainder of the thyroid gland.

---

[5]The recurrent laryngeal nerve.

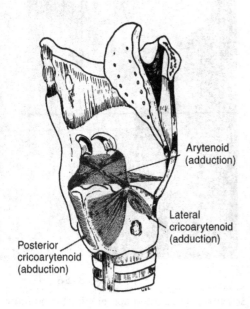
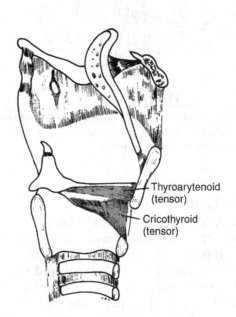

Arytenoid
(adduction)

Lateral
cricoarytenoid
(adduction)

Posterior
cricoarytenoid
(abduction)

Thyroarytenoid
(tensor)

Cricothyroid
(tensor)

FIGURE 3-57

Schematic summary of the actions of the intrinsic laryngeal muscles. Abduction of the vocal folds is due to the contraction of the posterior cricoarytenoid muscles, while partial adduction (medial compression) is due to the action of the lateral cricoarytenoid muscles. This adduction is complemented by the contraction of the arytenoid muscles. Longitudinal tension of the vocal folds is due primarily to the action of the cricothyroid and an opposing force due to the contraction of the thyroarytenoid musculature.

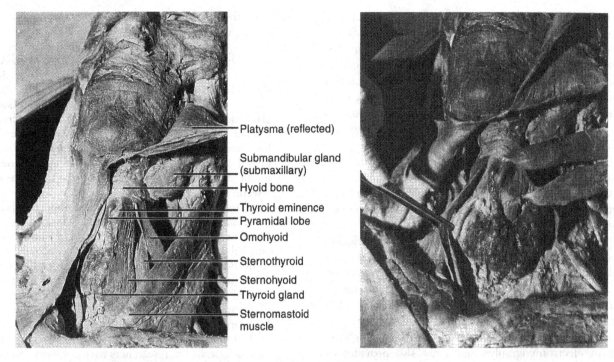

Platysma (reflected)

Submandibular gland
(submaxillary)

Hyoid bone

Thyroid eminence
Pyramidal lobe
Omohyoid

Sternothyroid

Sternohyoid

Thyroid gland

Sternomastoid
muscle

FIGURE 3-58

The thyroid gland in relation to the larynx. On the right the strap musculature has been reflected to reveal the thyroid gland.

The metabolic functions of the thyroid gland are discussed in Chapter 5.

METHODS OF INVESTIGATION OF LARYNGEAL PHYSIOLOGY

Researchers have been actively investigating the laryngeal mechanism for over a century and a half. There is good evidence, however, that speculations on the functions of the larynx took place long before any actual observations of the living internal larynx were ever made. Galen (A.D. 130–200), the famous physician and writer, was among the first to recognize the glottis as the source of vocal sounds. He supposed that vocal intensity was dependent upon the adjustment of the soft palate and uvula.

Much later, Andreas Vesalius, in his splendid *De Humani Corporis Fabrica*, which was published in 1543, shows the larynx, the hyoid bone, and the constrictor

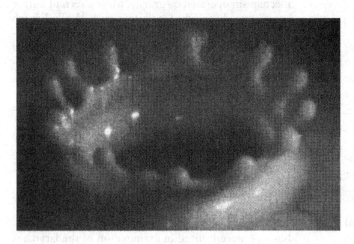

In the introduction to an early ultra-high speed film of the vocal folds, a drop of milk was photographed at 4000 frames per second as it fell into a saucer. The photographs demonstrated the resolving power of ultra-high speed photography. This image was extracted from the original motion picture film.

muscles of the pharynx with remarkable clarity. Another outstanding contribution to our understanding of the larynx was made in 1601 with the publication of *The Larynx, Organ of Voice* by Julius Casserius of Piacenza, and in the early 1700s Dodart described the relationship between glottal air stream and vocal intensity. He concluded that vocal sounds were produced by the impact of glottal air upon the relatively dormant supraglottal air column.

Since the first attempts at laryngoscopy in the early nineteenth century, many variations of several devices have been employed in an attempt to gain a better understanding of the nature of internal laryngeal activity during voice production.

Because function and structure are so inextricably bound to one another, the *basic anatomy of the larynx provides us with valuable information regarding the mechanics of voice production.* Much has yet to be learned—this is another instance in which anatomy is not a dead branch on the tree of learning. The contributions of laryngeal musculature can be assessed to some degree through the use of electromyography, and x-ray also provides us with some badly needed information.

Since the larynx is essentially an *aerodynamic system,* the air pressure and air volume requirements during voice production must be specified if we are to fully appreciate the mechanisms and functional interrelationship of the larynx and the respiratory system.

The internal larynx and the vibrating vocal folds can also be observed, either directly or indirectly by means of a mirror placed in the back of the throat—if the vocal folds can be seen, they can be photographed.

A major factor contributing to the accumulating body of knowledge has been the development of increasingly better techniques for examination of the larynx and for recording laryngeal activity. But, in spite of the number of significant technical advances in recent years, *differing opinions exist today on some very fundamental concepts of laryngeal physiology.*

The Development of Laryngoscopy

Laryngoscopy (examination of the interior of the larynx), for either clinical or research purposes, poses three very real problems that must be overcome before any success can be realized: (1) the larynx is located out of view, deep in the neck; (2) the interior of the larynx is dark, and it must be adequately illuminated to permit viewing; and (3) the movements of the vocal folds during phonation are much too rapid to be seen by any conventional optical system or by the unaided eye. The best one can hope for is a blurred image that only suggests what might be going on.

These problems (and others) have made successful laryngoscopy a formidable task indeed. Small wonder then that the development of satisfactory laryngoscopic techniques was 150 years in coming.

The Development of Indirect Laryngoscopy. Although a device intended for laryngoscopy was designed by Bozzini of Frankfort-am-Main in 1807 (see Moore, 1937a), it wasn't until 1855 that Manuel Garcia, a singing teacher in France, was able to describe internal laryngeal activity during voice production. A little mirror on a long handle (suitably bent) was placed in the throat of the person being examined. Sunlight was directed against the mirror by means of a second, hand-held mirror.

Garcia discovered several new and important facts concerning internal laryngeal behavior during singing. Many of his observations can be found in a little book entitled *Hints on Singing,* which has been translated from the French by Beata Garcia. It was published in 1894, and a great deal of subsequent research since the time of Garcia has done little more than confirm his observations. Manuel Garcia is to laryngoscopy what Herman Rohrer is to respiratory physiology.

Technique has not changed substantially since the time of Garcia, but researchers have not been content with observations of the unarmed eye, and with indirect laryngoscopy.

Transillumination. In 1860, Johann Czermak described a new technique called transillumination of the larynx. Rather than directing light down the throat, Czermak illuminated the interior of the larynx by directing a concentrated beam of light on the anterior surface of the neck, in the region of the cricoid cartilage. Inspection of the transilluminated larynx, by means of a laryngeal or "guttural" mirror, revealed it in "delicate shades of red," somewhat similar to the reddish hues of a hand held over the lens of a flashlight. Czermak suggested that transillumination might be a useful technique for measuring the vertical dimensions of the vocal folds.

Early Photography of the Larynx. In 1884, Dr. Thomas French published a report of a technique for laryngeal photography. French used a hand-held camera fastened to a laryngeal mirror. A simple shutter mechanism operated by gravity, while a second mirror concentrated sunlight for illumination. While French is often given credit for perfecting the process of laryngeal photography, Czermak published the results of his laryngeal photography in 1861, some 23 years before French (Moore, 1937a).

One shortcoming inherent in single-frame photography of the vibrating vocal folds is that it reveals little more than can be seen by conventional laryngoscopy. Information on gross glottal configurations during various phonatory and respiratory tasks, for example, is useful, but the folds themselves appear to be little more than a whitish blur.

Stroboscopy. Coincident with the development of motion-picture photography was the development of **strobolaryngoscopy,** in which the principles of stroboscopy were utilized in examination of the larynx. A stroboscope is an instrument that permits an observer to *view cyclical moving objects in such a manner that they appear to be stationary.*

A primitive form of stroboscope, such as the one built by Michael Faraday, consists of a revolving disc with holes or slots equally spaced around the periphery. A beam of light directed through the revolving disc will be interrupted periodically, and a moving object below will be illuminated for short, regular intervals. A cyclic movement, therefore, can be made to appear stationary if the speed of the disc is adjusted so that a hole is opposite the beam of light only when the moving object reaches the same point in each cycle; during the remainder of the cycle, the disc blocks out the light. Since the moving object is always viewed when it is exactly in the same position, the persistence of vision makes it appear to be standing still.

Contemporary stroboscopes utilize a brightly flashing light to illuminate the moving object periodically. Because a flash of light has an extremely short duration, the object being viewed moves a negligible distance while it is being illuminated and appears sharp and well defined. If the light is just a little out of synchrony with the cyclic rate of the moving object, the object will seem to be moving very slowly either in one direction or the other, depending upon whether the flashing light is slightly fast or slightly slow.

In 1930, Tiffin and Metfessel utilized an ingenious technique for firing a gaseous-discharge stroboscope. Their device used the output of an amplifier for the discharge voltage. The input of the amplifier was connected to a microphone, and as the subject phonated during strobolaryngoscopy, the flashing rate of the stroboscope lamp was determined by the basic rate of vibration of the vocal folds. When the rate was in synchrony with vibratory frequency of the vocal folds, they appeared motionless. By adjusting the flashing rate slightly out of synchrony, the vocal folds would have an apparent rate of vibration in the order of only one or two cycles per second. Examination of the vocal folds was accomplished as in the past, by directing the flashing light to a laryngeal mirror. For an excellent review of the history of strobolaryngoscopy, see Moore (1937a).

Today the "synchrostrobolaryngoscope" is sometimes used in laryngology clinics as a diagnostic instrument.

Motion-Picture Photograpy. As early as 1913, when cinematography was just beginning to be a reality, Chevroton and Vles took motion pictures of the larynx, and by combining the principles of stroboscopy and those of photography, Hegener and Panconcelli-Calzia were able to take stroboscopic motion pictures in 1913.

Numerous investigators modified and improved the cinematographic techniques, and although marked improvements in the quality of the results were realized, motion-picture films still revealed little more information than could be obtained by conventional, indirect laryngoscopy.

Contemporary Methods of Investigation

Endoscopy

Direct visualization of the larynx, trachea, bronchi, or esophagus is called **endoscopy** or **peroral endoscopy**. The term peroral pertains to something performed through or administered through the mouth. The specific examination is referred to by the structure endoscopy reveals, such as bronchoscopy, esophagoscopy, or **direct laryngoscopy.**

Although the instruments are available in a variety of sizes, they are all essentially a tube with a light source that illuminates the area just beyond the end of the instrument (Figure 3-59). In recent years, **fiber-optic endoscopes** have been used in clinical medicine and laryngeal research. The flexible laryngoscope or bronchoscope is inserted through the nose and is guided into the trachea (or esophagus with the gastroscope).

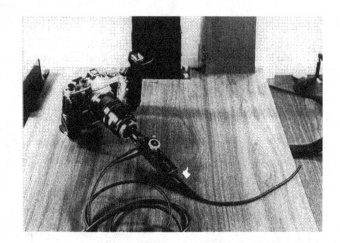

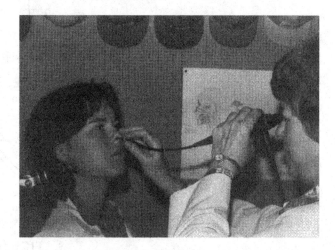

FIGURE 3-59

A fiber-optic endoscope used for viewing the larynx.

High-Speed Cinematography

In 1940, Farnsworth, at Bell Telephone Laboratories, used a high-speed motion-picture camera and a technique for taking high-speed motion pictures of the larynx at an exposure rate of 4000 frames per second (compared to 24 frames per second for conventional cinematography). The gratifying results stimulated considerable research, and much information regarding laryngeal functions has been accumulated by a number of subsequent high-speed motion-picture studies of the larynx.

To safely illuminate the larynx, the light emitted by a 5000-watt incandescent lamp was passed through a water-filled tank which absorbed the heat. Figure 3-60 shows a top view schematic drawing of an optical system very similar to that used by Bell Telephone Laboratories, Figure 3-61A shows a subject in position for laryngeal photography, and Figure 3-61B shows an experimenter prepared to fire a high-speed camera.[6] Figure 3-62 shows one complete cycle of vocal fold vibration taken out of a high-speed film exposed at 4000 frames per second (about 100 feet or 30.5 meters of film per second).

---

[6]In this installation at the University of Illinois, the camera is located inside a sound-treated room to help squelch its high-pitched whine, which may affect the subject's concentration.

A great deal of credit can be given Dr. Paul Moore, who pioneered in laryngeal cinematography and who was instrumental in developing high-speed laryngeal photography to the extent that it is a practical research tool. In fact, much of what we think we know about the larynx today has been seen through the "eyes" of a high-speed camera.

Although a great deal about laryngeal behavior has been learned through high-speed laryngeal photography, the technique has some serious drawbacks, not the least of which is the selection and training of subjects. Learning to be tolerant of a laryngeal (guttural) mirror and to produce for the experimenter an adequate view of the vocal folds can be time consuming and very demanding. As a result, subject participation is often very selective and is limited (generally) to adults. Laryngeal photography is one laboratory exercise that demands more motivation on the part of the subject than of the experimenter.

Glottography (Electroglottography)

A noninvasive technique for assessing some laryngeal functions makes use of a device called the *glottograph* or *laryngograph*. Electrodes, placed on either side of the neck directly over the thyroid cartilage, detect changes in conductance (the reciprocal of electrical resistance)

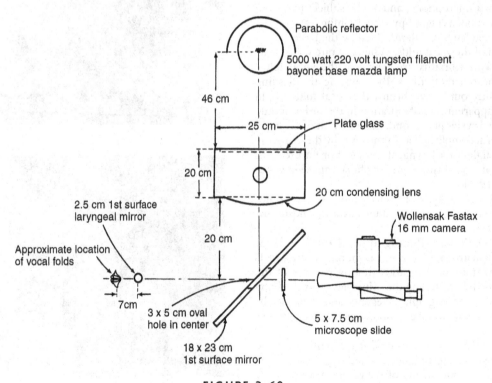

FIGURE 3-60

Top view schematic of high-speed photographic apparatus.

FIGURE 3-61

Subject in position for laryngeal photography (A) and experimenter prepared to photograph (B).

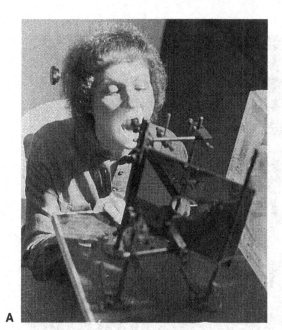

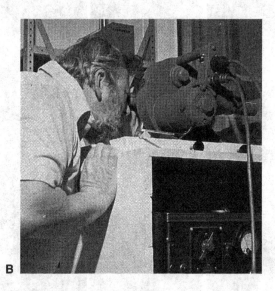

to a 4 megahertz (mhz) signal. The apparatus imposes virtually no constraints on speech production and, although it will not yield a graphic recording of glottal area as a function of time, it (ideally) measures vocal fold contact area as a function of time (Childers, et al., 1990).

Transillumination–Photoconduction

Because of the elaborate apparatus and quantities of film required, ultra-high-speed photography is an expensive process, and before the computer became an integral part of the research laboratory, analysis of the film was very time consuming. In 1959, Zemlin attempted to develop a less expensive and less time-consuming technique for investigation of the glottis during voice production. That same year, working independently, Sonesson published a preliminary report on a similar technique. Both are much like that used by Wullstein in 1936.

Sonesson and Zemlin subglottally transilluminated the larynx of a subject by directing a beam of light onto the anterior neck, just below the level of the cricoid cartilage. As the vocal folds opened and closed during voice production, they acted as a valve, permitting varying amounts of light to pass between them. The light excited a photoelectric cell which responded by passing electrical energy in amounts proportional to the amount of light striking it. Sonesson fed this voltage into a sensitive cathode-ray oscilloscope and photographed the image, while Zemlin fed the voltage to a variable area movie sound track.

Questions have been raised regarding the validity of the technique (Wendahl and Coleman, 1967; Coleman and Wendahl, 1968), but a later study by Harden (1975) suggests that "the photo-electric glottograph reveals essentially the same information on glottal area function as that provided by ultra high-speed photography."

Radiography

Because the framework of the larynx is composed of hyaline cartilage, it does not absorb x-rays well (especially in younger persons), so conventional x-ray procedures have sometimes been less than satisfactory. A newer technique called **sectional radiography** or **laminagraphy** has been employed with considerable success. It permits plane sections of structures to be made by showing considerable detail in a predetermined plane while blurring the images of structures in other planes.

These **radiographs** are produced by moving the film during exposure in a direction opposite and proportional to the simultaneous movement of the x-ray source, as shown schematically in Figure 3-63. In this way a frontal section through the larynx can be made, showing the positions and cross-sectional configurations of the vocal folds during various phonatory tasks.

A number of these x-ray laminagraphic studies have been reported, among them studies by Sonninen and Vaheri (1958); Zaliouk and Izkovitch (1958); Luchsinger and Dubois (1956); van den Berg (1955a);

Start

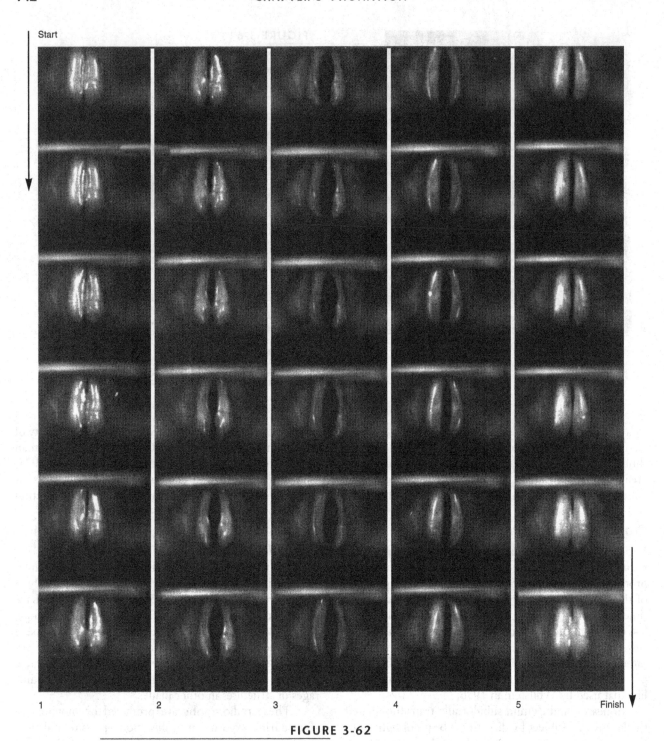

1   2   3   4   5   Finish

FIGURE 3-62

A single cycle of vocal fold vibration taken from a high-speed film exposed at 4,000 frames per second.

Hollien and Curtis (1960, 1962); Hollien (1964); and Hollien, Curtis, and Coleman (1968).

During voicing, however, the rapid movements of the vocal folds produce a blurred image, which limits the usefulness of laminagraphy. To overcome this difficulty,

Hollien has modified the conventional laminagraphic technique by combining the principles of stroboscopy and laminagraphy. The x-ray beam is pulsed at or near the vibratory rate of the vocal folds to produce a "slow-motion" film of the vibratory pattern of the vocal folds. The technique is called **strobolaminagraphy,** but more

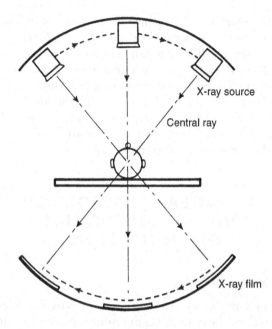

FIGURE 3-63

Schematic of principle of laminagraphy. The x-ray beam is pulsed at or near the vibratory rate of the vocal folds to produce a "slow-motion" film of the vibratory pattern of the vocal folds.

often is referred to by the less cumbersome **STROL.** The gratifying results obtained by Hollien and his co-workers have shed new light on the behavior of the internal larynx during voice production. For further details on the technique, see Hollien (1964) and Hollien and Coleman (1970).

Supplementary Diagnostic and Research Techniques

Some additional research and diagnostic techniques can provide useful information about the behavior and integrity of the larynx. Probably the most significant ones are electromyography (EMG) of the laryngeal musculature and techniques for measuring the air requirements of the larynx during various phonatory tasks.

Electromyography

The technique of recording the bioelectrical activity of muscles has been rewarding and at the same time very frustrating, especially in the area of laryngeal physiology. When compared to some muscles, such as the heart, the activity of laryngeal muscles is difficult to detect. Two properly placed electrodes located virtually anywhere on the surface of the body will detect cardiac muscle activity, in the case of the familiar EKG (ECG). Many muscles in the body can be "recorded" by simply placing electrodes on the surface of the skin, directly over the muscle.

Small or deep muscles demand a different technique. To minimize the contaminating effects of adjacent muscles, electrodes are best implanted directly into the muscle being investigated. **Hooked-wire electrodes** are very satisfactory. As shown in Figure 3-64, two very fine insulated wires are passed through a hypodermic needle and are then bent back to form a tiny hook. To record activity from a muscle, the needle is simply inserted and then withdrawn, leaving the two hooked wires implanted in the muscle tissue. Once implanted, these hooked-wire electrodes usually cannot be felt by the subject, and there is no pain associated with the procedure (or at least not much).

Regardless of the technique employed, however, *the only direct information that can be obtained from an EMG recording is that a particular muscle or group of muscles is active during a particular motor task.* An EMG tracing does not tell us what a muscle is doing; it can only report relative activity. This means that an EMG tracing requires interpretation, which very often entails supplementary information, not the least of which is *a clear understanding of the anatomy of a muscle and the probable consequences of its activity.* Techniques for implanting electrodes in the intrinsic laryngeal musculature have become refined to the extent that what seemed almost impossible just a few years ago can now be performed routinely.

The interested reader is urged to refer to Cooper (1965); Fromkin and Ladefoged (1966); Gay and Harris (1971); Hirano and Ohala (1969); Hirano et al. (1967); Hirano et al. (1969); and Hirose and Gay (1973).

Air-Flow and Subglottal Pressure Measures

An indication of the behavioral and structural integrity of the larynx, as well as information pertaining to basic laryngeal mechanics, can be obtained by the use of

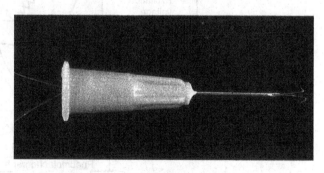

FIGURE 3-64

Photograph of hooked-wire electrode (three times natural size). The hairlike wires protruding from the end of the needle remain in the muscle when the hypodermic needle is withdrawn. Subjects are usually unaware of the presence of the wires.

"air-flow" apparatus. Usually just two important measures are necessary in the laboratory or clinic; the *air flow through the larynx* and *air-pressure requirements during various phonatory tests*. Specification of the intensity of the voice is also valuable.

Techniques vary somewhat, but usually some sort of a **pneumotachograph** is employed, and it is the "heart" of an air-flow recording system. Basically it is a device that offers an extremely slight resistance to the flow of air, and, as a consequence, a small pressure differential is generated. This pressure difference varies directly with the quantity of air flowing through the system. A block diagram of an air-flow recording system is shown in Figure 3-65. A face mask is coupled directly to the pneumotachograph. Note that the barrel of the "pneumotach" contains a grid system that offers a slight resistance to the air flowing through it. Flexible tubing couples the pneumotach to a pressure-sensing transducer,[7] and it responds by converting air-pressure differences into an electrical voltage, which in turn drives the pen of a strip-chart recorder. Air flow is usually expressed in cubic centimeters per second.

_____

[7]A **transducer** is a device that absorbs energy and emits energy either in the same form or in another form.

An important factor influencing the nature of the voice is the amount of resistance to air flow offered by the larynx; this resistance will be manifested in greater or less subglottal air pressure. It stands to reason that if a larynx is unable to offer appropriate resistance to air flow, something is wrong. Subglottal pressures will not build up to usual values, and the voice will suffer in terms of quality and intensity. Techniques for measuring subglottal (alveolar) pressure are described on page 90.

LARYNGEAL PHYSIOLOGY AND THE MECHANICS OF PHONATION

Introduction

Although the gross anatomy of the larynx has been known since the mid-sixteenth century, details of laryngeal structure are still being discovered. Researchers have been viewing and photographing the vibrating larynx for more than 100 years; electromyographic and air flow data are continually being published, and our constructs of structure and function are constantly being subjected to revision.

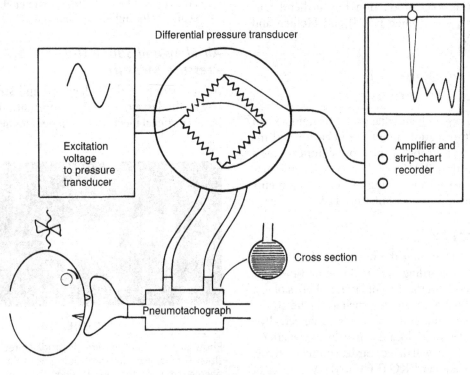

FIGURE 3-65

Block diagram of air flow recording system.

We have seen that there are just two basic internal laryngeal adjustments that can take place. They are the *force with which the vocal folds are brought together at the midline,* termed **medial compression,** and the *extent of the stretching force,* called **longitudinal tension.** These two adjustments, or combinations of them, plus a variable air supply account for the incredible versatility of the human voice.

In 1886, Stoker suggested that the larynx operated much like a simple stringed instrument. In 1892, Woods suggested that the larynx complies with the fundamental equation of vibrating strings, which states

$$n = \frac{1}{L}\sqrt{\frac{T}{M}}$$

n = frequency of vibration

L = length of folds

T = tension of folds

M = mass per unit length

The primary factors that determine the vibratory rate of a string are mass and tension in relation to length. Accordingly, a string's vibration may be doubled by halving its length or by increasing tension or decreasing mass by a factor of four. Strings behave in accordance with basic laws of physics, but the larynx is an aerodynamic structure and only partly complies. *The vocal folds should not be equated with vibrating strings.*

These problems have been recognized by Sonninen (1956), who stated that the relationship of the factors influencing the **pitch** of the voice can be represented by the following equation:

$$f = C\frac{K}{M}$$

f = frequency of vocal fold vibration

C = a constant

$K = K^1 + K^2$, where K^1 represents inner passive tension of the vocal fold (related to tissue elasticity) and K^2 represents an inner active tension (longitudinal tension related to muscle contraction and changes in length of the vocal fold).

M = mass of the vocal fold

Neither of the foregoing equations acknowledges the role of medial compression, but we should realize that the vocal folds must be approximated (or nearly so) at the midline before the issuing air stream can set them into vibration.

Both the pitch and spectral characteristics of the voice (voice quality) are dependent upon (1) the frequency of vocal fold vibration, (2) the pattern or mode of vocal fold vibration, and (3) the configuration of the vocal tract. For the remainder of the chapter, we will examine the mechanisms controlling the frequency and the mode of vocal fold vibration. But, first, a short discussion of the manner in which phonation is initiated.

The Onset of Phonation

The onset of phonation may be divided into two phases: the **prephonation phase** and the **attack phase.**

The Prephonation Phase

The prephonation phase is *the period during which the vocal folds move from an abducted to either an adducted or a partially adducted position.* When the vocal folds are viewed prior to the onset of phonation, they are usually seen to be in an abducted position; that is, the subject is breathing. During quiet breathing, the adult male glottis is about 13 mm wide at its broadest point, and according to Negus (1929), this value may almost double during forced exhalation. Figure 3-66 shows the larynx during forced inhalation, forced exhalation, and quiet breathing. Most persons maintain a rather constant glottal aperture during quiet breathing.

Vocal Fold Approximation The duration of the prephonation phase and the extent to which the vocal folds approximate are highly variable, depending largely upon the utterance to be emitted. If the forces of exhalation are released and the vocal folds approximate or nearly approximate, they begin to obstruct the outward flow of air from the lower respiratory tract, and *subglottal pressure, the pressure beneath the folds, begins to build up.* In addition, *the velocity of the air as it flows through the glottal constriction is raised sharply,* which is an important point to remember.

Photographs of a larynx during various stages of a prephonation phase are shown in Figure 3-67. These photographs are single-frame excerpts from a high-speed motion-picture film taken during the onset of phonation. For this subject the entire prephonation phase represents about 0.160 seconds. Figure 3-67A shows the vocal folds abducted, and B and C show the folds as they have moved toward the midline. Figure 3-67D shows the folds almost adducted. The extent to which the vocal folds are approximated is referred to as **medial compression,** which is *brought about by the action of the adductor muscles.*

Muscular Activity Responsible for Medial Compression Information regarding gross muscle function may be gained from knowledge of the muscle attachments and from the general architecture of the structures involved. It is crucial, however, that we weigh such information carefully, because *rarely do individual muscles*

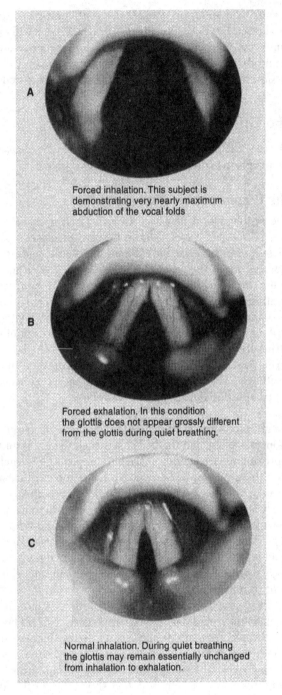

Forced inhalation. This subject is demonstrating very nearly maximum abduction of the vocal folds

Forced exhalation. In this condition the glottis does not appear grossly different from the glottis during quiet breathing.

Normal inhalation. During quiet breathing the glottis may remain essentially unchanged from inhalation to exhalation.

FIGURE 3-66

Glottal configurations for forced inhalation (A) and exhalation (B) and during quiet breathing (C).

act to execute movement. Rather, they work in pairs and groups, so that contraction of any one muscle is usually accompanied by contraction of companion muscles. A subtle, delicate interplay of the various muscle actions produces the appropriate movement.

A case in point is adduction of the vocal folds. We have called the **lateral cricoarytenoid** and **arytenoid**

muscles the adductors of the vocal folds. Figure 3-68 demonstrates what might happen if one or the other of these muscles should contract independently of the other. Note in A that contraction of the arytenoid muscles may draw the muscular processes posteriorly, thus toeing out the vocal processes. When just the lateral cricoarytenoid muscles are contracted, the arytenoid cartilages are rotated so that the muscular processes are pulled anteriorly and the vocal processes are toed inward to produce the glottal configuration often seen in the production of a whisper as in B. In C, simultaneous contraction of the lateral cricoarytenoid and the arytenoid muscles approximate the arytenoid cartilages and the vocal folds so that their medial borders are parallel. Such muscle action, however, may also tend to draw the arytenoid cartilages forward, a movement that is restricted by the posterior cricoarytenoid ligament and the antagonistic action of the posterior cricoarytenoid muscle, as illustrated by the arrows in Figure 3-68D. The result of the combined action of the three muscles is such that the vocal folds are tightly approximated, and if exhalation is initiated, the folds will be set into vibration to produce a laryngeal tone.

There is a direct relationship between the extent of medial compression and the magnitude of air pressure required to force the vocal folds apart and initiate phonation.

The Attack Phase

The attack phase begins with the vocal folds adducted, or nearly so, and extends through the initial vibratory cycles. This phase is also highly variable in its duration, depending primarily upon the extent to which the vocal folds are adducted during the prephonation phase and the manner in which the air stream is released.

Often the vocal folds are not completely adducted during the prephonation phase; *complete obstruction of the air passageway is not necessary to initiate phonation.* If the glottal chink is narrowed to about 3 mm, a minimal amount of air flow will set the vocal folds into vibration. Air-pressure requirements under these conditions will also be minimal. According to von Leden (1961b) a subglottic pressure equal to 20 to 40 mm of water is sufficient.

High-speed laryngeal photography shows that the *initial movement in incompletely adducted vocal folds is medialward.* This point will be emphasized later in the discussion of theories of vocal fold vibration. Medial movement can be adequately accounted for by the Bernoulli effect.

The Bernoulli Effect Daniel Bernoulli, a member of a family distinguished in scientific and mathematical history, formulated the following *aerodynamic law:*

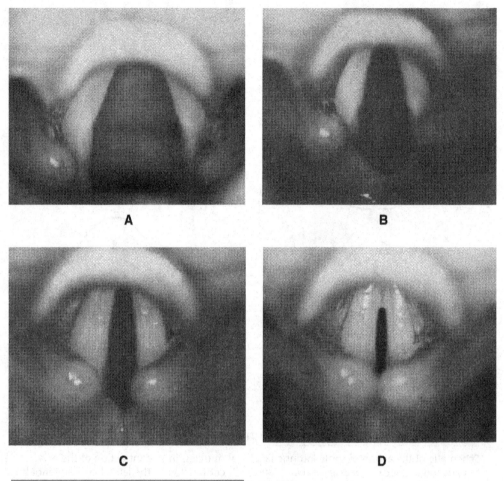

A   **B**

C   **D**

FIGURE 3-67

Four stages of prephonation phase.

$$d \times \tfrac{1}{2}(v^2 p) = c$$

d = density v = velocity

p = pressure c = a constant

Or, to put the Bernoulli effect another way, in the case of an ideal fluid, as velocity of fluid flow increases, pressure must decrease so long as total energy remains a constant. Pressure in this instance is perpendicular to the direction of the fluid flow. This means that *if volume fluid flow is constant, velocity of flow must increase at an area of constriction, but with a corresponding decrease of pressure at the constriction.*

Total energy as we are using the term pertains to **kinetic energy,** which is energy of motion, and **potential energy,** which is energy of position or stored energy.

In certain mechanical systems there is a constant exchange of kinetic and potential energies. In the case of a mass bobbing on a spring, for example, at the two extremes of movement the mass momentarily comes to

rest before its movement "changes direction." At the instant of rest, all the energy is potential, because no movement is taking place. The energy is stored! Halfway between the two extremes of displacement, all the energy is kinetic, because it is here that the velocity of the mass is maximum and the acceleration (the result of potential energy) is zero.

Total energy, once again, is the sum of kinetic and potential energies, and in the case of fluid flow, total energy is a constant. So

$$E = KE + PE = C$$

This means that as flowing fluid encounters a constriction, its velocity must increase, if the same amount of fluid that enters the system is to leave it.

If velocity increases, the energy of movement, or kinetic energy, must also increase, and if total energy is to be a constant, potential energy must decrease. In the case of our fluid flow, kinetic energy is equal to the product of one-half

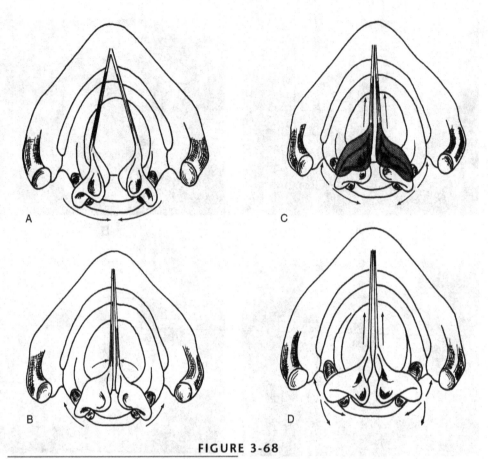

FIGURE 3-68

Schematic of the action of some intrinsic laryngeal muscles. In A, contraction of the arytenoids toe the vocal processes outward, and in B, contraction of the lateral cricoarytenoids partially adduct the vocal processes. In C, simultaneous contraction of the lateral cricoarytenoid and the arytenoid muscles completely adduct the vocal processes and vocal ligaments, although forward movement of the arytenoid cartilages may also take place. In D, forward movement is restricted by posterior cricoarytenoid ligament and the antagonistic action of the posterior cricoarytenoid muscle, and the combined action of the three muscles results in tightly approximated vocal ligaments and vocal folds.

the mass or density of the fluid and the velocity of fluid flow squared. The equation is very familiar

$$KE = \tfrac{1}{2}MV^2$$
$$M = \text{density or mass of fluid}$$
$$V = \text{velocity of flow}$$

Potential energy is pressure (force per unit area), so the total energy is equal to the sum of kinetic and potential energies, or

$$E = \tfrac{1}{2}MV^2 + P = C$$

As the velocity of fluid flow increases, kinetic energy must of necessity increase, and potential energy (pressure) must decrease accordingly. Atomizers, paint spray guns, and airplanes work on the principle of the Bernoulli effect.

A simple illustration of the Bernoulli effect is shown in Figure 3-69. The tube at the bottom of the illustration can be thought of as the trachea. The constriction represents the larynx and vocal folds, and the larger portion at top, the pharynx and oral cavity. Obviously the same amount of air that enters from beneath must leave through the top, so the velocity of air flow will be especially high at the constriction and low in the upper portion. Three manometers are shown, and they register the pressures along the tube.

The Bernoulli Effect Applied to Phonation To apply the Bernoulli effect to phonation, assume that the vocal folds are nearly approximated at the instant the air stream is released by the forces of exhalation. The air stream will have a constant velocity until it reaches the glottal constriction. Velocity will increase, however, as the air passes through the glottal chink. *The result is a*

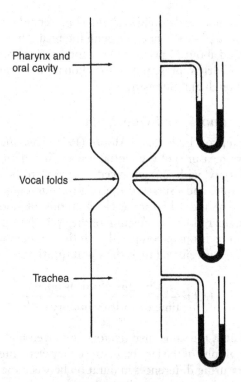

Pharynx and
oral cavity

Vocal folds

Trachea

FIGURE 3-69

Schematic illustration of the Bernoulli effect at the glottis. With increased air velocity at the constriction, the magnitude of negative pressure increases.

negative pressure between the medial edges of the vocal folds, and they will literally be sucked toward one another.

The Bernoulli effect is of major importance in understanding the vocal mechanism, especially as it applies to ordinary phonation (van den Berg, 1958a). Others such as Hiroto (1966) and Ishizaka and Matsudaira (1972) suggest that the role of the Bernoulli effect has been overemphasized.

Initiation of Phonation The movements of the vocal folds as they enter into vibration are shown graphically

in Figure 3-70. As glottal area reaches a certain critical value, the vocal folds begin to execute vibratory movement before they have actually approximated. *This initial movement results in a decrease in glottal area.* Also note that *the folds undergo a number of vibrations before they meet to completely obstruct the air stream.*

As long as subglottal pressure is adequate, the medial compression of the vocal folds will be overcome, and they will be blown apart to release a puff of air into the supraglottal area. This somewhat explosive release results in an immediate but short-duration decrease in subglottal pressure. The elasticity of the vocal fold tissue, along with the Bernoulli effect, causes the vocal folds to snap back again to the midline.

The nature of the initial vibratory cycles may be influenced by a host of variables, including the intensity of phonation, the linguistic environment of the sound to be emitted, the pitch of the voice, and vocal habits. The problem of identifying the manner in which phonation may be initiated was recognized by Moore in 1938. He suggested three ways in which the air stream might be released: the **simultaneous attack,** the **breathy attack,** and the **glottal attack.**

Vocal Attacks In the **simultaneous** attack there is a healthy balance between the respiratory and laryngeal mechanism, and the air stream is released just as the vocal folds meet at the midline.

In the **breathy** attack, the air stream is released before vocal fold adduction is completed, and a considerable quantity of air may be exhaled while the folds are being set into periodic vibration.

When phonation is initiated while the vocal folds are subjected to considerable medial compression, the voice exhibits an onset more sudden than during either the simultaneous or the breath attacks. The vocal tone is explosive in nature, and the initiation of phonation is called a **glottal attack, glottal shock,** or **stroke of the glottis (coup-de-glotte).**

FIGURE 3-70

Changes in glottal area during prephonation and attack phases.

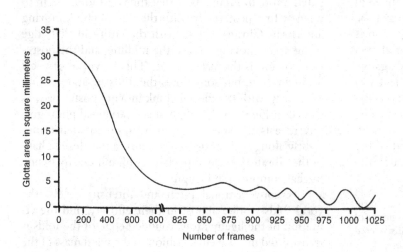

> **CLINICAL NOTE:** Most speech pathologists and laryngologists advocate the simultaneous attack, which they consider less abusive to the vocal mechanism than the glottal attack. A rough and unpleasant voice quality may be associated with abusive use of glottal attack. Most often, however, glottal attack is produced in such a manner as to be hardly, if at all, discernable from a simultaneous attack.
>
> Habitual use of breathy attack is simply an ineffective method of voice production. There are two reasons for this. Because of the unmodulated air that escapes from between the vocal folds during the attack, a fricative noise is often superimposed upon the vocal tone to produce what is known as a "breathy quality." In addition, since the vocal folds are not adducted when the air stream issues from the thorax, they are unable to afford appropriate resistance to air flow, and the voice will be weak.

We have identified just three "classes" or types of vocal attack, which are often thought of as discrete; in fact *they are regions along a continuum that represents laryngeal hypofunction at one extreme and hyperfunction at the other.* Somewhere in between lies the region we recognize as "normal."

Characteristics of a Vibratory Cycle

Glottal Area

One technique used to describe the characteristics of vocal fold vibration initially requires that the vibrating vocal folds be photographed at an exposure rate of about 4000 frames a second. One or more cycles of vibration are then projected, frame by frame, and the area that comprises the glottis is computed or measured. Graphs of glottal area as a function of time (or film frames) can then be constructed.

Much of what is known about the vibratory characteristics of the larynx has been learned through frame-by-frame analysis. A film of what might be thought of as a typical cycle of vocal fold vibration is shown in Figure 3-71. In Figure 3-72, the glottal area has been extracted from each frame and plotted against time. The *vibratory rate* for this particular subject was about 168 cycles per second (Hz),[8] and the film was exposed at a rate of about 4000 frames per second. The *opening phase* extended through the first 12 frames; in other words, it occupied one-half or 50 percent of the vibratory cycle. The *closing phase* extended through the

---

[8]The term *hertz*, abbreviated Hz, has generally replaced the term *cycles per second*, abbreviated cps. It is an eponym, used in honor of the nineteenth-century physicist, Heinrich Hertz, who discovered radio waves.

next 9 frames and occupied about 37 percent of the cycle. The *closed phase* extended through the final 3 frames and occupied about 13 percent of the total cycle. These values are fairly representative for phonation at conversational pitch and intensity.

Open and Speed Quotients

Timcke, von Leden, and Moore (1958) have made extensive measures of the glottal wave. They illuminated the larynx with an advanced "synchrostroboscopic" technique, and expressed the relative durations of the phases of the vibratory cycle in terms of quotients. Thus, the ratio of the fraction of the cycle during which the glottis is open, compared with the total duration of the cycle, is referred to as the **open quotient** (*OQ*).

$$OQ = \frac{\text{time the glottis is open}}{\text{time of entire vibratory cycle}}$$

Later, the same investigators employed high-speed photography of the larynx. Because they were interested in measuring differences in duration between the opening and closing phases, they selected the ratio between the two phases which they termed the **speed quotient** (*SQ*). So

$$SQ = \frac{\text{time of abduction or lateral excursion}}{\text{time of adduction or medial excursion}}$$

The advantage of using the speed quotient is that in some instances the glottis never completely closes, and the open quotient is therefore 1.0. The speed quotient provides additional descriptive information about the vibratory characteristics. For Figure 3-72, the open quotient = 0.85 and the speed quotient = 1.17.

The Mode of Vocal Fold Vibration

The mode of vocal fold vibration has also been investigated. Note in Figure 3-71 that the vocal folds begin to open at first posteriorly, with the glottal chink moving anteriorly. Closure begins with the entire medial edge of the folds moving toward the midline, and the posterior portion is the last to close. This is typical of vocal fold vibration, but sometimes the folds separate at first anteriorly, with the glottal chink moving posteriorly, as shown in Figure 3-73. High-speed laryngeal photography reveals the vocal folds to be approximated rather tightly along their entire length during the closed phase of the vibratory cycle, especially at high intensity (when medial compression is high).

At conversational pitch and intensity levels, the vocal folds vibrate almost in their entirety, and the vibration of the ligamentous rounded edge of the folds is transmitted in a wavelike fashion to the main mass of the

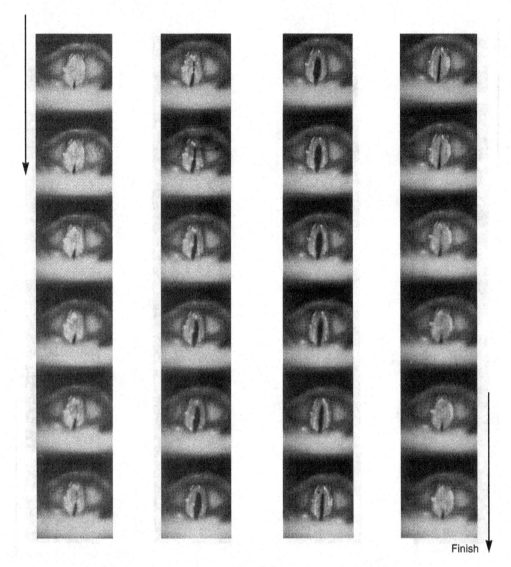

FIGURE 3-71

A typical cycle of normal vocal fold vibration taken from a high-speed motion picture film of the larynx.

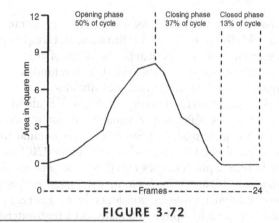

FIGURE 3-72

Curve of glottal area plotted as a function of frames in the cycle.

vocal folds. *The principal vibration is along the horizontal plane, but there is also a slight vertical displacement* (0.2 to 0.5 mm), *which increases slightly with loudness of the voice.*

High-speed motion pictures of the larynx reveal that the vocal folds begin to be forced open from beneath, with an upward progression of the opening in an undulating fashion. The lower edges of the vocal folds are the first, and the upper edges the last, to be blown apart. During the closing phase, however, the lower edges lead the upper edges. This produces what is known as a **vertical phase difference**, illustrated in schematic form in Figure 3-74. In addition, some single-frame excerpts from a vibratory cycle are shown in Figure 3-75. Evidence of a vertical phase difference is clearly seen.

Start

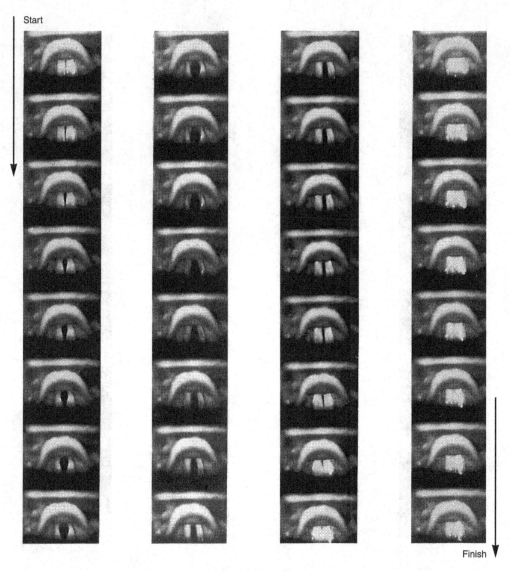

Finish

FIGURE 3-73

A cycle of normal vocal fold vibration demonstrating a mode of vibration that is different from that in Figure 3-72.

The larynx is a very versatile instrument, capable of producing tones over a wide range of pitches and intensities, and with different modes of vibration. A surprising amount of information can be conveyed by an individual's voice: it can tell us the sex of a speaker, perhaps something about the person's age, general state of health, and certainly the emotional status of the speaker. A voice may also tell us just who it is that is doing the talking.

The Pitch-Changing Mechanism

Introduction

A person engaged in normal conversation is liable to produce laryngeal tones that vary in pitch over a **range** of almost two octaves (Fairbanks, 1959). The average rate of vocal fold vibration is known as **fundamental frequency.** It determines to a large extent the pitch of the voice. There is a one-to-one relationship between fundamental frequency and the rate of vocal fold vibration.

The **pitch level** of young adult males is about C_3 on the musical scale, and of females, almost an octave higher. In other words, *males* have a fundamental frequency of about 130 Hz, and *females* about 220 Hz. A distribution of **pitch ranges** for adult males and females is shown in Figure 3-76. Note that the pitch ranges of males and females overlap considerably, so it is reasonable to expect a low-pitched female and a high-pitched male to have the same pitch.

In Figure 3-76, you can also see that the distribution extends somewhat farther below the mode than

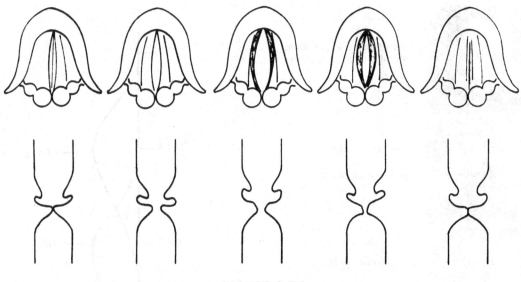

FIGURE 3-74

Schematic of vertical phase difference during a cycle of vocal fold vibration.

above the mode. This is because, during conversational speech, occasionally a pitch is used that is lower than any sustainable pitch. *These very low pitches tend to occur at the ends of sentences when the intensity of the speaking voice is decreasing rapidly* (Fairbanks, 1959).

There is a particularly suitable pitch level for each individual. Known as **natural level,** it is largely determined by the physical characteristics of the individual voice mechanism. The natural level is also known as the **optimum pitch level.** According to Fairbanks, the natural pitch is located about one-fourth of the way up the total singing range (including falsetto). The fraction one-fourth was derived from the work of Pronovost (1942), who studied superior male speakers.

The Pitch-Raising Mechanism

When measured in their abducted position, the vocal folds range in length from about 15 to 20 mm for males and from 9 to 13 mm for females. The vocal folds are probably near their maximum length in the abducted position and, contrary to popular opinion, are considerably shorter when adducted for phonation.

Vocal Fold Changes Accompanying Pitch Increases

The graph in Figure 3-77 illustrates **length** changes that accompany pitch change. *Note that the length of the vocal folds at various pitches never exceeds the length of the vocal folds in their abducted position.* Increases in length of the vocal folds result in a decrease in cross-sectional area (mass), which will result in an increase in pitch.

Mass per unit length must be decreased by a factor of four in order to double the frequency of vibration. From the data of Hollien and Curtis (1962), however, at high-pitch phonation vocal fold thickness (an index of

mass) was never reduced below one-half what it was during the lowest pitch of phonation. This means that increases in pitch cannot be accounted for solely by a reduction in mass and that the tension factor also plays an important role in the pitch-changing mechanism.

In fact, it is not at all unreasonable to suppose that an increase in tension of the vocal folds is the sole agent responsible for pitch increases and that the accompanying length and thickness change is simply the result of the elastic tissue of the vocal folds yielding to the marked increase in tension.

Modifications in the length (and tension) of the vocal folds necessary to produce an increase in pitch are mediated through the interplay of three intrinsic laryngeal muscles: the **cricothyroid,** the **thyroarytenoid,** and to a lesser extent the **posterior cricoarytenoid.**

Intrinsic Laryngeal Muscle Action and Pitch Increases The **cricothyroid muscle,** you will recall, arises from the anterolateral arch of the cricoid cartilage and inserts into the thyroid cartilage as an oblique and vertically directed rectus bundle. Contraction of the **rectus bundle** causes rotation about the cricothyroid joint which decreases the distance between the cricoid and thyroid cartilages anteriorly. This results in an increase in the distance between the arytenoid cartilages and the thyroid cartilage, at the angle, as illustrated in Figure 3-78. Since the vocal folds extend from the arytenoid to the thyroid cartilage, it follows that contraction of the rectus bundle of the cricothyroid muscles elongates the vocal folds and makes them thinner.

Contraction of the **oblique fibers** may slide the thyroid cartilage forward on the cricothyroid joint, as illustrated in Figure 3-79, and this action also elongates the vocal folds. This muscle action, if unopposed, will

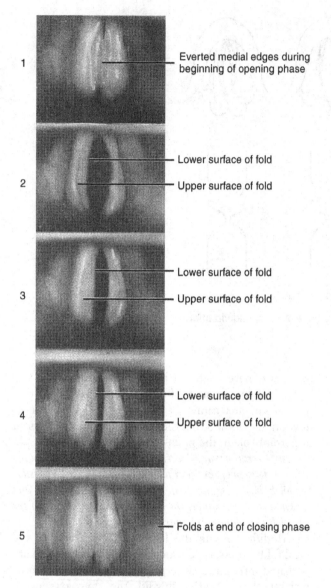

1 — Everted medial edges during beginning of opening phase

2 — Lower surface of fold
— Upper surface of fold

3 — Lower surface of fold
— Upper surface of fold

4 — Lower surface of fold
— Upper surface of fold

5 — Folds at end of closing phase

FIGURE 3-75

Single frame excerpts from a high-speed film showing vertical phase differences.

result in elongation of the vocal folds with a negligible increase in their tension (Greene, 1957).

With no opposing muscular forces acting upon the vocal folds, contraction of the cricothyroid muscle may simply enlongate them and make them thinner. In either case, little or no increase in tension (and pitch) will result.

Some additional mechanism is necessary to cause an increase in tension of the vocal folds. Anterior sliding movements of the arytenoid cartilages will be limited by the stout **posterior cricoarytenoid ligament** and by contraction of the **posterior cricoarytenoid muscle.** In our earlier discussion of the onset of phonation, we saw how the posterior cricoarytenoid muscle abducted

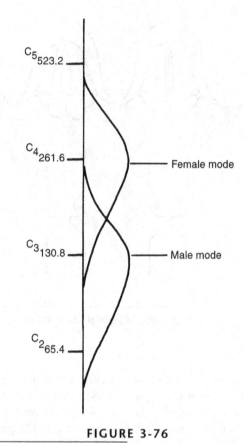

FIGURE 3-76

Schematic distribution of pitch ranges of adult males and females.

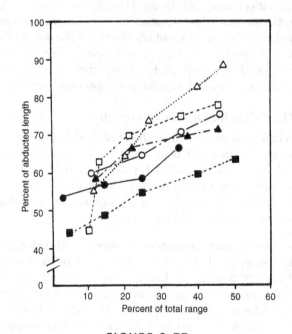

FIGURE 3-77

Variation in vocal fold length with changes in vocal pitch. (After Hollien and Moore, 1960.)

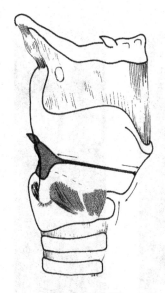

FIGURE 3-78

Rotation of the cricoid and thyroid cartilages to tense the vocal folds.

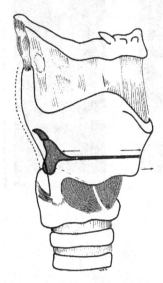

FIGURE 3-79

Sliding of the thyroid cartilage forward on the cricoid to increase the distance between the arytenoid and thyroid cartilages.

the vocal folds. We see how this very important muscle can also be active in producing pitch changes.

The **thyroarytenoid muscle,** acting without opposition, will simply decrease the distance between the arytenoid cartilages and the thyroid cartilage to produce a shortening (and relaxation) of the vocal folds. Pitch increases, therefore, are brought about by the antagonistic action of the cricothyroid and thyroarytenoid muscles (vocal fold tensors) with an assist from the pos-

terior cricoarytenoid muscle, which anchors the arytenoid cartilages.

Differential contraction of muscle bundles within the thyroarytenoid may result in increased tension, or, by a subtle balance of muscle forces, the folds may be tensed with no appreciable increase in length. Arnold (1961) states,

> It follows that the cricothyroid's primary function is that of crude or *external vocal cord tension*. Because this tension is achieved by increasing elongation of the cords with rising pitch, it is an isotonic tension. In contrast, the fine or *internal cord tension* from subsequent contraction of the internal thyroarytenoid (or vocalis) muscle occurs with equal cord length for a given pitch level and represents an isometric tension; consequently, the cricothyroid and vocalis are synergists with different modes and purposes of function.

Experimental evidence also supports the idea that the **cricothyroid muscle** functions to *"load" the vocal folds* and that the subtle, fine adjustments are mediated by contraction of the vocal fold musculature itself. In addition, there is evidence that the cricothyroid maintains a fairly constant level of activity over a limited pitch range, and when limits of this range are transcended, the cricothyroid suddenly bursts into a slightly higher level of activity. This *stairstep increment of muscle activity* supports the contention that the function of the cricothyroid is to load the vocal folds or to put them under tension in a gross manner. The finer adjustments are then mediated by the vocal fold musculature. In a twitch-response investigation of canine laryngeal muscles, Alipour-Haghighi et al. (1987) found the vocalis to be very fast, capable of performing rapid maneuvers in support of changes in fundamental frequency.

Research Findings on the Pitch-Raising Mechanism As the *vocal folds* are tensed and elongated for the production of higher-pitched tones, some predictable changes occur. The folds lengthen and change from round, thick lips to narrow bands, and whereas the vocal folds seem relaxed, almost flaccid during phonation at the natural pitch level, they appear stiff and rigid at higher pitches. The *glottis* appears as more of a variable slit, and only the medial edges of the folds seem to engage in vibration.

A single cycle from a high-speed film of phonation at natural pitch level is shown in Figure 3-80; for comparative purposes, a cycle of phonation at a pitch approximately one octave higher (twice the frequency) is shown in Figure 3-81. The relative durations of the opening, closing, and closed phases of the vibratory cycle remain about the same within the normal pitch range (Timcke, et al., 1958).

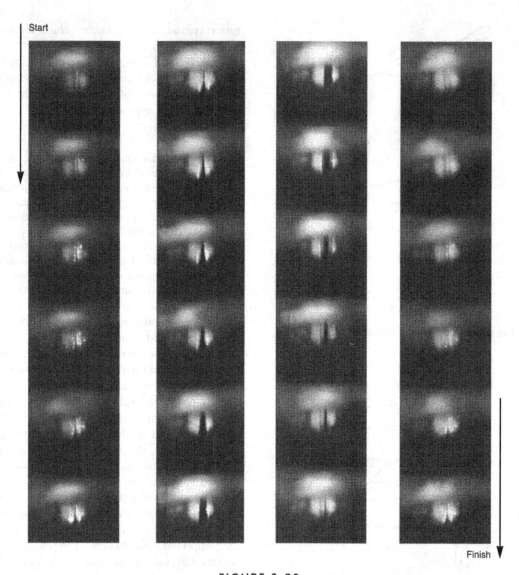

FIGURE 3-80

A cycle of normal vocal fold vibration (f_0 = 168 Hz).

At extremely high pitches, however, there is an increased tendency for failure of the vocal folds to approximate completely in the area of the vocal processes. This explains why voice quality tends to become breathy at the higher pitches.

We saw earlier that the length of the vocal folds increases systematically with increases in vocal pitch and that the degree of length increase is not significantly greater in any one portion of the pitch range (excluding falsetto). Hollien (1960a) also found a relationship between general vocal fold length and the natural frequency of phonation. Persons with large larynxes and long vocal folds tend to phonate at a lower pitch level than do persons with smaller larynxes and shorter vocal folds.

Hollien and Curtis (1960) employed x-ray laminagraphy in a study of the larynx during changes in vocal pitch. Results indicated that the folds became less massive and thinner as frequency was raised, with larger changes occurring in the low-frequency portion of the subjects' ranges.

In a subsequent x-ray study, Hollien and Curtis (1962) reported a tendency for the vocal folds to become progressively elevated as well as a tendency for **vocal fold tilt** (the superior borders slope upward toward the midline) to become progressively greater with increases in vocal pitch. These trends did not hold for falsetto, however.

Using electromyography (EMG) with bipolar electrodes inserted into the cricothyroid and thyroarytenoid muscles, Larson et al. (1987) were able to detect changes in fundamental frequency (f_0) associated with

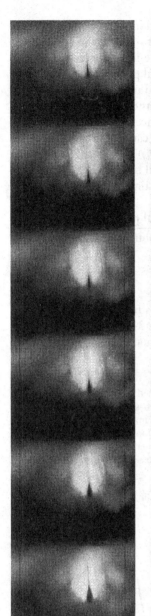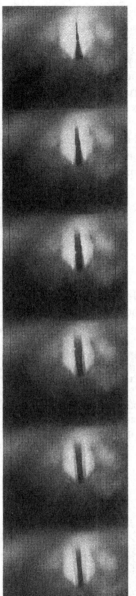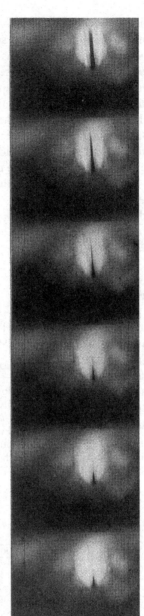

FIGURE 3-81

A cycle of high-pitch phonation (f_0 = 250 Hz).

single motor unit discharges (SMU). The time between the discharge of the SMU and the peak in change of the fundamental frequency (f_0 latency) was variable and ranged from 5 to 20 ms for the thyroarytenoid and 6 to 75 ms for the cricothyroid muscle. In addition, distinct oscillations in fundamental frequency were always present in recordings from the subjects when they phonated at higher than modal pitch levels.

Subglottal Pressure and Pitch The characteristics of air supply to the larynx have long been recognized as a factor that may influence pitch.

Early research on the relationship between subglottal pressure and pitch was conducted by the famous physiologist Johannes Müller (1843) and later by Liskovius (1846), both of whom concluded that pitch rose in response to increased air pressure. Negus, in 1929, also noted that in phonation, elastic tension of the vocal folds and air pressure are associated in such a way that a slight increase in air pressure causes a considerable rise in pitch. Wullstein (1936), using freshly excised human larynxes, found that fundamental frequency rose from 85 to 115 Hz when air pressure was doubled.

In evaluating these experiments relating subglottal pressure to pitch, we ought to be mindful of an important point. *Although rises in pitch may be accompanied by increases in subglottal pressure, increases in subglottal pressure need not produce rises in pitch.* We must be careful in interpreting the cause and effect relationship. Brodnitz (1959), for example, has noted that when a subject is singing an upward scale, the subglottic pressure increases because the greater stiffness of the stretched vocal folds offer increased resistance to air flow—so subglottal pressure must increase.

A number of animal experiments were conducted in the early to midpart of the century (Rubin, 1963a), and for the most part the conclusions reached were: *so long as vocal fold tension is held constant, increases in subglottal pressure do not result in increases in pitch.*

Timcke et al. (1958) and van den Berg (1957) report a simple experiment that may demonstrate the effect of subglottal pressure on pitch. A sudden push on the abdominal wall of a subject during the production of a sustained sound not only raises the intensity of the voice but also produces an increase in pitch. Rubin (1963a) notes, however: "If during sustained phonation at a constant pitch, a sharp push is given another part of the body . . . where applied pressure has no direct influence on the diaphragm or rib cage and cannot directly affect the air flow, the pitch also rises in the same manner." Rubin attributes the pitch increase to a **laryngeal reflex.**

Kunze, in 1962, measured intratracheal (subglottal) pressure directly as a group of subjects phonated at various pitch levels at a moderate intensity level. His purpose was to relate intratracheal pressure to fundamental frequency and to relate glottal resistance to fundamental frequency. **Glottal resistance or impedance** is an index of the amount of resistance the larynx is offering to the flow of air through it, and can be estimated from the ratio of subglottal pressure (P_{sg}) and volume velocity or the rate of air flow (U). Glottal resistance (P_g), expressed in dyne-second/cm^5, can be estimated as follows:[9]

$$P_g = \frac{\text{subglottal pressure}}{\text{flow rate (volume velocity)}}$$

$$= \frac{P_{sg}}{U} \text{ in dyne-sec/cm}^5$$

Intratracheal pressure as a function of fundamental frequency is shown in Figure 3-82A, and glottal resistance as a function of fundamental frequency is shown

---

[9]**Glottal resistance** is usually defined as the *complex ratio of the effective subglottal pressure* (root-mean-square-value) *to the effective air flow rate* (rms) according to Flanagan (1958), Isshiki (1964), and van den Berg, Zantema, and Doornenball (1957). Because of limitations in instrumentation, however, usually just mean values of these two parameters are used to *estimate* glottal resistance.

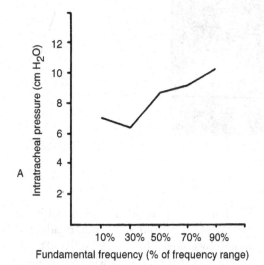

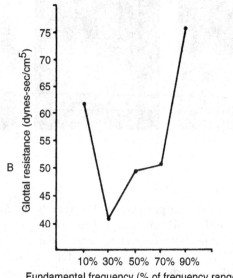

FIGURE 3-82

(A) Relationship between mean intratracheal pressure (expressed in cm H$_2$O) and fundamental frequency for ten adult males. (B) Relationship between glottal resistance (expressed in dyne-sec/cm^5) and fundamental frequency for ten adult males. The fundamental frequency levels are expressed in percentages of the total frequency range above the lowest sustainable frequency. (After Kunze, 1962.)

in Figure 3-82B. These data suggest that the larynx offers increased resistance to air flow as the vocal folds are placed under increased tension to raise the frequency of their vibration. They also illustrate that an increase in subglottal pressure is required to overcome the increase in glottal resistance. Note the profound drop in glottal resistance at 30 percent of the fundamental frequency range. This implies that the larynx operates most efficiently at the frequency of vibration that correlates closely with the **habitual pitch** of normal speakers.

All of this leads to the following conclusions: *Pitch changes are mediated primarily through modifications in glottic tension and mass; however, an increase in subglottal pressure, with laryngeal tension held constant, will produce a negligible rise in pitch.* This viewpoint is supported by Pressman and Keleman (1955) who state:

> Actually the variation produced in tone by pressure changes is relatively small, and if this were the primary mechanism involved, enormously impractical elevations of pressure would be required to cover the range of the human voice.

The Pitch-Lowering Mechanism

A person with a habitual pitch of about C_3 (131 Hz) can be expected to encompass a singing range that extends from D_2 (73.4 Hz) to about C_5 (523 Hz), not including falsetto, which may extend the range as high as C_6 (1047 Hz). In other words, *the habitual pitch is near the lower limits of the pitch range.*

We have seen that an increase in tension and a concomitant decrease in the mass of the vocal folds is primarily responsible for an increase in pitch. *This means that a decrease in vibratory rate must be accounted for by a decrease in tension and/or an increase in mass per unit length of the vocal folds.* Observations of laryngeal behavior suggest that reciprocity (to a degree) exists between vocal fold mass and tension; that is, one cannot be affected without influencing the other.

The glottal margins can be relaxed by two mechanisms. The first is the inherent elastic properties of tissue. Once the vocal folds have been placed under tension, they tend to resume their relaxation state solely by virtue of their inherent elasticity (once the stretching force has been removed). Tissue elasticity cannot satisfactorily explain how pitch can be lowered beyond the habitual pitch level. A further decrease in tension must be produced by active forces which shorten the vocal folds, thus relaxing and thickening them.

The logical contender for this task is the musculature of the vocal fold itself In this role, unopposed by other muscles, the **thyroarytenoid muscle** has one main action: to draw the arytenoid and thyroid cartilages toward one another, to shorten and relax the vocal

ligament. Medial compression at low pitches is probably facilitated by the **lateral cricoarytenoid muscle.** In a pitch-matching experiment (vocal shadowing) Leonard et al. (1988) found that for both men and women (in singing tasks) pitch lowering was faster than pitch raising.

The Extrinsic Muscles and the Pitch-Changing Mechanism

In order to produce tones near the extreme ends of the pitch range, and to facilitate rapid changes in pitch, some extrinsic and supplementary musculature may be called into play.

The larynx commonly rises and falls in position during phonation of high- and low-pitched tones, and much more so in some individuals than in others. These rapid changes in laryngeal position are brought about by laryngeal elevators and depressors, and by supplementary musculature that attaches to the hyoid bone.

These muscles and their probable actions were shown schematically in Figure 3-43. The exact contributions of this complex array of muscles are not well understood, and we know very little about the way the extrinsic musculature facilitates pitch changes. Electromyographic evidence, however, has shown heightened activity of the **sternothyroid muscle** when the larynx is depressed and of the **thyrohyoid muscle** when the larynx is elevated (Faaborg-Anderson and Sonninen, 1960).

The role of the **inferior pharyngeal constrictor** in changing laryngeal position is not well understood either. The inferior constrictor is a sphincteric muscle with loose attachments on the precervical fascia and, in spite of the obliquely upward course of its muscle fibers, contraction will not greatly influence laryngeal position. Zenker and Zenker (1960) identified the portion of the inferior pharyngeal constrictor which arises from the thyroid laminae as the **thyropharyngeus muscle** and they state,

> In lengthening the vocal cords the cricothyroid and the elastic ligamentum-conicum (conus elasticus) are important, besides also the *thyropharyngeal muscle, which approximates the plates of the thyroid cartilage, thus displacing the anterior origin of the vocal cords in a forward direction.*
>
> In tomograms taken on youthful individuals, we could see a considerable approximation of the two plates of the thyroid cartilage during the production of a high tone. Husson and DiJiab (1952) found that the plates of the thyroid moved toward each other during the progression from a soft to a loud tone, more specifically during the transition from falsetto to chest register. Moving together of the plates of the thyroid cartilage can lead to a considerable lengthening of the vocal cords (Figure 3-83). The narrowing of the laryngeal space must, in any event, be considered as the major function of the thyropharyngeus muscle.

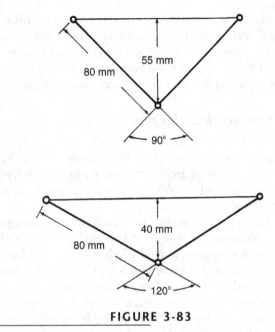

FIGURE 3-83

Changes in length of vocal folds due to approximation of thyroid laminae as proposed by Zenker and Zenker (1960).

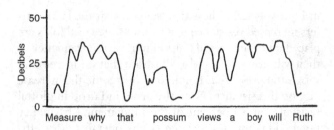

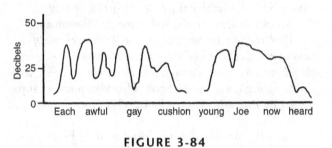

FIGURE 3-84

Intensity curve of nonsense sentence as spoken by author.

From what we have seen thus far, it ought to be evident that the laryngeal structures are complex and that muscles may complement each other's activities one moment and counteract them the next. In generating our constructs of laryngeal structure and function, we must realize that *any changes brought about in the larynx are the result of the algebraic (vector) sum of the various forces in action.*

The Intensity-Changing Mechanism

Intensity changes are an important part of our everyday verbal behavior, and the extremes in intensity of vocal tones span a considerable range, even during conversational speech. Figure 3-84 shows an intensity curve of a nonsense sentence spoken by the author. The sentence, devised by Fairbanks (1959), samples each phoneme of the general American dialect just once. From the curve it is evident that the range in intensity is in excess of 30 decibels. This represents a ratio of intensity in the order of 1000 to 1. The difference between the least and the most intense sounds a person can produce, from a faint sound to a genuine rebel yell, amounts to over 70 decibels.

Attempts to account for the mechanics of intensity changes can be traced back to Dodart in 1700; although a great deal of research has been conducted since that time, considerable disagreement existed well into the twentieth century.

Vocal Fold Movement and Intensity Changes

In one of his high-speed photographic studies, Farnsworth (1940) noted that as intensity is increased, the vocal folds remain closed for a proportionately longer time during the vibratory cycle. He also noted that maximum displacement of the folds increased, but not proportionately. Pressman (1942) stated that the amplitude of vibratory movement becomes greater as subglottal pressure is increased; the added excursion to the midline is more complete.

In another high-speed photographic study, Fletcher (1950) compared vocal fold vibration during phonation at moderate intensity and at 5 and 10 decibels above the moderate level. He also obtained high-speed films of the larynx during a crescendo (Italian for swelling, increasing in loudness). One finding stood out: the duration of the closed phase of the vibratory cycle increases with intensity. Figure 3-85 shows glottal area as a function of time with an intensity difference between phonations of 5 decibels. The dashed line is the high-intensity curve. Note the increase in the duration of the closed phase. These changes are also evident in high-speed films of crescendo. The total intensity change amounted to about 12 decibels at a frequency of 212 Hz. Two features are apparent: *the duration of the closed phase increases with intensity,* and *the maximum glottal area remains essentially constant.* These films do not support the contention that maximum lateral excursion of the vocal folds increases with vocal intensity (see Figure 3-86). This aspect of Fletcher's experiment has been replicated (Bernick, 1963), and the results are consistent with those of Fletcher.

Subglottal Pressure and Vocal Intensity

Measurements have also been made of the relationship between subglottal pressure and vocal intensity. Van den Berg (1956) and Ladefoged (1960) have demonstrated

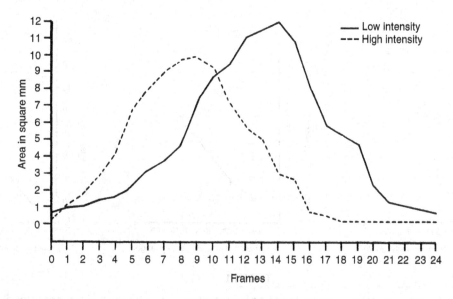

FIGURE 3-85

Glottal area as a function of time (time interval per frame = 0.25 msec) at low pitch (168 Hz). Intensity difference = 5 dB.

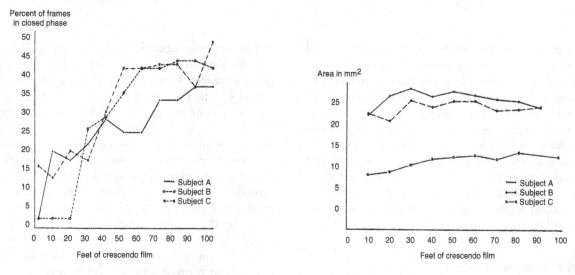

FIGURE 3-86

Percentage of frames in closed phase (left) and maximum glottal openings (right) of typical cycles at selected intervals from a high-speed crescendo (from W. Fletcher, 1950).

that the sound pressure level[10] of the voice is proportional to the square of the subglottal pressure. Ladefoged and McKinney (1963) found that peak subglottal pressure was proportional to the peak value of the effective sound pressure ($Sp^{0.6}$); that is, glottic pressure was proportional to the 0.6 power of the subglottic pressure.

Kunze (1962) has confirmed the positive relationship between subglottic pressure and the intensity of the voice, and a workable rule of thumb is that the *sound intensity level of the voice will increase by about 8 to 12 decibels when subglottic pressure is doubled.* Earlier we saw that a pressure of just 2 to 3 cm H_2O will sustain phonation at low intensities, but this value may go as high as 15 to 20 cm H_2O for loud speech, and even higher for shouting. The relationship between intratracheal (subglottal) pressure and vocal intensity is shown graphically in Figure 3-87B.

---

[10]**Sound pressure level (SPL)** is the difference in decibels between a particular pressure and the standard reference of .0002 dynes/cm^2.

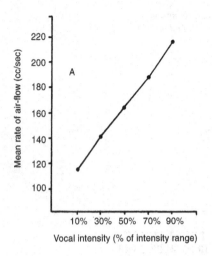
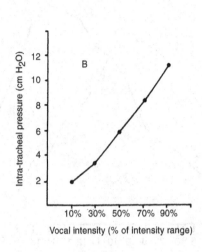
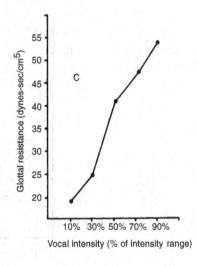

FIGURE 3-87

(A) Relationship between mean rate of air flow (expressed in cubic centimeters per second) and vocal intensity level, (B) relationship between intratracheal pressure (expressed in cm H_2O) and vocal intensity, and (C) relationship between glottal resistance (expressed in dyne-sec-cm^5) and vocal intensity for ten adult males. The vocal intensity levels are expressed in percentages of vocal intensity range above the lowest sustainable intensity. (After Kunze, 1962.)

To summarize thus far, the duration of the closed phase of the vibratory cycle increases with vocal intensity and subglottal pressure also increases with increases in intensity. The extent of the lateral excursion of the vocal folds increases with intensity for some subjects and remains unchanged for others, but the force with which the vocal folds meet at the midline increases for all subjects as voice intensity increases. *This means that medial compression is increased and that the larynx is offering increased resistance to air flow. The result is that subglottal pressure must be increased in order to overcome the increased glottal resistance.*

Glottal Resistance, Air Flow, and Vocal Intensity

Glottal resistance as it relates to vocal intensity is illustrated in the data of Kunze (1962). In Figure 3-87A, mean rate of air flow as a function of vocal intensity is shown, and in Figure 3-87B, intratracheal pressure is plotted against intensity. In Figure 3-87C, glottal resistance is shown plotted as a function of vocal intensity. Glottal resistance increases markedly as the intensity of the voice is increased, a condition reflected in the elevated subglottal pressures at high vocal intensities. Increased glottal resistance requires an increase in subglottal pressures. *Increased glottal resistance must be compensated for by increased subglottal pressure.*

In 1964, Isshiki investigated the relationship between vocal intensity, subglottal pressure, air flow rate, and glottal resistance. He found that *at low-pitch phonation, the intensity of the voice was raised by an increase in glottal resistance.* That is, the medial compression of the vocal folds and their tension are increased to provide increasing resistance to air flow, and that, in turn, requires elevated subglottal pressure. At high pitch, however, glottal resistance is already so high—nearly maximum—that resistance cannot be increased without affecting vocal pitch. Isshiki concluded that *intensity at high pitch is controlled, not by changes in glottal resistance, but by rate of air flow through the glottis.* This increased air flow is mediated by the forces of exhalation. At low and medium pitches, Isshiki found that air cost (volume velocity) was relatively constant over a wide intensity range, results that are inconsistent with those of Kunze.

In 1965 Charron attempted to test Isshiki's conclusions using high-speed photography of glottal activity during low- and high-pitch phonation at low and high intensities and electromyography of the musculature of exhalation. In general, Charron's data support those of Isshiki.

In some persons an increase in vocal intensity does not significantly affect the rate of expenditure of air (within limits). Although the amount of subglottal pressure required for phonation is elevated, the resistance of the larynx to air flow is also greater, and volume flow of air per unit time may actually be decreased. This is supported by the data of Isshiki and by Ptacek and Sander (1963B), who found that some of their subjects were able to maintain loud, low-frequency phonation longer than

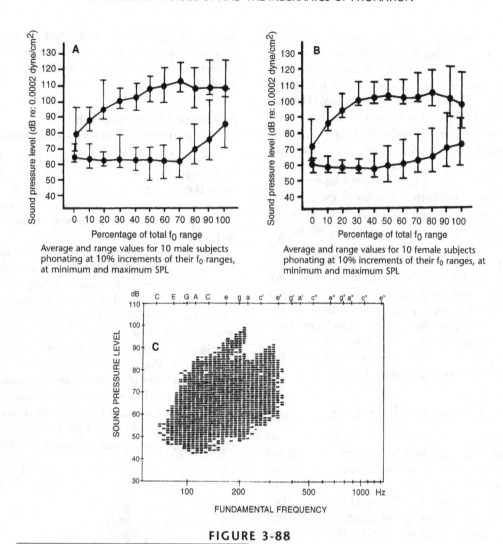

FIGURE 3-88

Fundamental frequency–SPL profiles for males (A) and females (B), (from Coleman, et al., 1977) and (C) an automatically recorded phonetogram (from Pabon & Plomp, 1988).

soft or moderately loud phonation. Because the vocal folds are in the closed phase for a greater proportion of the vibratory cycle in high-intensity than in low-intensity phonation, there is less time for air flow to occur. In other words, air flow (U) is directly related to subglottic pressure (P_{sg}) and inversely related to glottal resistance (P_g) or

$$U = \frac{P_{sg}}{P_g}$$

Musculature Responsible for Changes in Vocal Intensity

Three, and possibly four, laryngeal muscles, plus the forces of exhalation, are responsible for changes in vocal intensity. *Forceful adduction of the vocal folds* is accomplished by simultaneous contraction of the **lateral cricoarytenoid** and the **arytenoid muscles,** while an *increase in glottal tension* is mediated by the **thyroarytenoid muscles** or the **cricothyroid muscles,** or more likely both. The increases in pitch that often accompany increases in intensity of phonation can be accounted for by the greater tension of the vocal folds.

The Relationship of Pitch and Intensity

Although increases in vocal intensity are mediated by increased compression of the vocal folds and heightened activity of the respiratory mechanism, *intensity ranges are frequency (pitch) dependent* (Coleman, et al., 1977). Fundamental frequency-intensity profiles for males and females are shown in Figure 3-88. Relatively untrained singers were asked to produce tones at the lowest and highest intensity levels at selected intervals of their pitch range. *The intensity range is at a minimum at the low end of the fundamental frequency range, swells to a maximum in the 50 to 70 percent range, and diminishes again at the upper limits of the frequency range.* Fundamental frequency-intensity profiles are also known as *phonetograms* (Damste, 1970; Pabon and Plomp, 1988), *voice fields* (Rauhut, et al., 1979), or *voice profiles* (Bloothooft, 1982).

Pabon and Plomp (1988), by using a computer interface, have been able to display not only sound pressure level as a function of fundamental frequency, but also pitch perturbations (jitter), spectral shape as well as "noise" in the voice. An example of their automatically recorded phonetogram is shown in Figure 3-88C.

Titze (1992) offers an acoustic interpretation of the voice-range profile that explains why the intensity range is reduced at the low and high extremes of the voice range. He shows that the intensity of the voice depends on the spectral (harmonic energy) distribution of the voice source. He also suggests that at reduced intensity range at low fundamental frequency there is an inherent difficulty of keeping fundamental frequency from rising when subglottal pressure is increased.

Transglottal Pressure Differential

The relationship between air flow, frequency of vocal fold vibration, and vocal intensity is not a simple one. An important factor related to voice production is the *pressure differential across the glottis.* Earlier we learned that a subglottal pressure of from 2 to 3 cm H_2O will sustain phonation, and throughout all our discussions of pitch and intensity changes, we have assumed that the supraglottal part of the vocal tract offered little or no resistance to air flow. Thus, when supraglottal pressure is about the same as atmospheric pressure and subglottal pressure is above atmospheric, the transglottal pressure differential will be approximately equal to subglottal pressure.

If, however, a constriction in the supraglottal part of the vocal tract should cause intraoral and pharyngeal pressures to become elevated, as they are in the case of the production of a fricative consonant, the effective subglottal pressure will be diminished, and this will be reflected in a drop of the transglottal pressure differential. Transglottal pressure differential (*TPD*) is equal to subglottal pressure (P_{sg}) minus supraglottal pressure (P_o), or

$$TPD = P_{sg} - P_o$$

From this expression it is evident that if supraglottal pressure should approximate subglottal pressure, the pressure differential at the laryngeal level approaches zero and vocal fold vibration will be arrested. This is exactly what happens, for example, when a bilabial articulatory gesture "shuts off the larynx." Since the total pressure drop along the vocal tract is equal to subglottal pressure, we see that *articulatory constrictions during conversational speech are continually influencing the pressures available to the glottis.*

Influence of Articulation on Transglottal Pressure Differentials

Transglottal pressure differentials as influenced by oral airway opening are shown in Figure 3-89. Airway opening is the largest for vowel production, and supraglottal pressure is nearly atmospheric. A closed airway for voiced plosives results in approximately equal supra- and subglottal pressures.

Of particular interest is voicing that occurs during the stop phase of consonant production. If voicing is to occur, air displacement must be taking place, for example, by being shunted through the nasal cavity, or by pressurized expansion of the pharynx and walls of the oral cavity. A study by Lubker (1973) rejected nasal air flow in favor of an active mechanism for *dilating the supraglottal cavity.* Perkell (1969) and Kent and Moll (1969) have shown that *voiced stops are produced with larger supraglottal volumes than their voiceless cognates.* Supraglottal volume, for example, is larger for the production of [b] than it is for [p]. Kent and Moll found that *pharyngeal expansion was accompanied by depression of the hyoid bone, an*

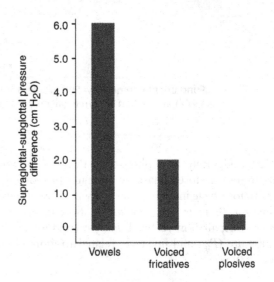

FIGURE 3-89

The transglottal pressure differential is influenced by the oral airway opening. Airway opening is largest for vowels and supraglottal pressure is nearly atmospheric under these conditions. A closed oral airway for voiced plosives results in a small pressure drop. Voiced fricatives fall between vowels and plosives. The slight opening of the oral port helps to maintain airway pressure. (From D. Warren, *Speech, Language, and Hearing,* Vol. 1, *Normal Processes,* Lass, McReynolds, Northern, and Yoder, eds. Philadelphia: W. B. Saunders Company, 1982.)

active process that would relax the walls of the pharynx. The pharyngeal walls may also expand passively due to muscle relaxation (Bell-Berti, 1975).

The total resistance (Z) to air flow in the speech mechanism is equal to the sum of the resistances offered by the component parts such as the larynx, tongue, the lips, etc., or

$$Z_{total} = Z_{glottic} + Z_{supraglottic}$$

Significance of Transglottal Pressure Differential

The significance of transglottal pressure should not be minimized. We have seen how the respiratory system may influence laryngeal behavior to modify pitch and intensity, and how the larynx and respiratory system work in concert during pitch and intensity changes. We must also bear in mind that the process of articulation imposes constraints upon laryngeal behavior. Unless there is respiratory compensation when intraoral pressures are elevated due to articulatory constrictions, the transglottal pressure differential must drop, and the consequence might be a decrease in pitch, intensity, or both. Here we see just an inkling of the subtle and exquisite interplay between the respiratory, laryngeal, and articulatory systems.

CLINICAL NOTE: An example of clinical application of the concept of transglottal pressure differential is seen in voice therapy where vocal abuse has resulted in vocal nodules or some other pathological condition. It is almost impossible to produce a sound at an excessively loud (abusive) level when the articulatory mechanism is constricted, as in the production of [m]. No matter how one tries, *there is a real limit to the loudness of a voiced consonant.* This technique will help the patient get the feel of nonabusive voice production.

Checking Action and Air-Flow Resistance

One more point should be mentioned before we leave the topic of transglottal pressure differential. In Chapter 2 we learned that pressures in excess of the requirements of the larynx can be generated by the inflated thorax unless sustained contraction of the inspiratory musculature checks the thoracic rebound. We should expect to find a certain reciprocity between the need for checking action and the resistance to air flow that is offered by the speech mechanism. The extreme case is complete blockage of air flow by the lips or tongue, or by the vocal folds, following a deep inhalation. The resistance or impedance is infinite; no air flow can take place, and so there is no need for checking action by the inspiratory musculature.

Phonating a neutral vowel, at conversational pitch and intensity following a deep inhalation, is quite a different matter. Except for the slight air flow resistance offered by the larynx, the vocal tract is an extremely low-impedance system, and if air flow is to be regulated, checking action is essential. The reciprocity between checking action and glottal resistance was investigated by Holstead (1972). She found that *checking action indeed decreased as laryngeal resistance increased.*

Much of the information in the following pages relates primarily to the singing voice. It is presented because an introduction to the full capabilities of the laryngeal mechanism should enhance our understanding of the complex process of phonation.

Voice Registers

By convention, the rate of vocal fold vibration is described either in terms of musical notes (pitch), or in terms of fundamental frequency (cycles per second or hertz). In either case the scale is on a continuum ranging from less than 60 Hz (B_1 on the musical scale) in the basso voice to over 1568 Hz (G_6 on the musical scale) in the soprano voice. Singers often describe phonation in terms of **registers,** and the term register means a portion of the vocal compass: as **high** or **low** register, **chest** or **head** register.

In 1841, Manuel Garcia defined the voice register as follows: "By the word register we mean a series of succeeding sounds of equal quality on a scale of from low to high, produced by the application of the same mechanical principle, the nature of which differs basically from another series of succeeding sounds of equal quality produced by another mechanical principle."

This definition is not very different from that given by Webster: "A particular series of tones, especially of the human voice, produced in the same way and having the same quality: the head register."

In his excellent little book *Traits complet de l'art du chant* (1841/1855), Garcia recognized three voice registers, which in English might be described as the **chest register,** the **middle register,** and the **head register.** Other voice register systems recognize as many as five registers within the compass of the voice; however, no one singer is expected to encompass all five registers.

Mörner et al. (1964), recognizing the problems of voice register terminology, state that music and voice specialists appear to agree reasonably well as to the average pitch of the boundaries between registers (i.e., the breaks or voice transitions). They have noted, for example, that the average boundary between the middle- and high-pitch levels varies little within the particular kind of voice. The boundary is located at C_4 (278 Hz) for a bass voice and at F_4 (349 Hz) for a soprano voice. The transition for low to midlevel occurs at D_3

(147 Hz) for a bass voice and at E₃ (165 Hz) for a tenor. Mörner et al. suggest: "The only secure common denominator for defining a register is by means of its range on the musical scale." They suggest five basic registers, referred to as the **deepest range, deep level, midlevel, high level,** and **highest range.** The approximate ranges and boundary limits of these registers are shown in Figure 3-90, and some synonyms for the registers are also given.

Voice Register and Mode of Vocal Fold Vibration

A particular mode or pattern of vocal fold vibration is usually confined within a given pitch range, and when phonation is attempted outside the limits of this range, the mode of vibration will be altered appropriately to accommodate the succeeding range. *This modification of the mode of vocal fold vibration may be regarded as an operational definition of voice register.*

Thus, as a person transcends the limits of a particular vocal register, the voice may undergo an abrupt modification of quality. This vocal quality is often the primary characteristic of voice register, and in fact, it serves as the criterion for register assignments. Voice specialists and singing teachers, in particular, seem to agree that one of the primary tasks in training for singing is to blend the registers (however many there may be) into a single functional unit so that even a trained listener may not be able to detect points of transition. In fact, this is ideal (Brodnitz, 1959).

Depending upon the extent of a singer's talent and particular type of voice, he or she may appear to have a "single register" that encompasses two or three "registers" of another singer. Some well-trained individuals are able to produce a gliding pitch (glissando) throughout their entire pitch range, which may be over three octaves, without a perceptible voice break or transition. Operationally, it is reasonable to regard such a person as having but a single register, but according to Mörner et al., such a singer would have produced vocal tones within a specified number of registers solely on the basis of the range of musical tones encompassed.

Voice Register Criteria

Much of the difficulty encountered in terminology stems from the fact that there are as yet no common grounds upon which to establish vocal register criteria. If we are to adhere to the definitions advanced by Garcia and others, registers ought to be defined from a physiological point of view. Our knowledge of the behavior of the internal larynx, however, is far from complete, and the boundaries that have been established from a subjective evaluation of the singing voice are

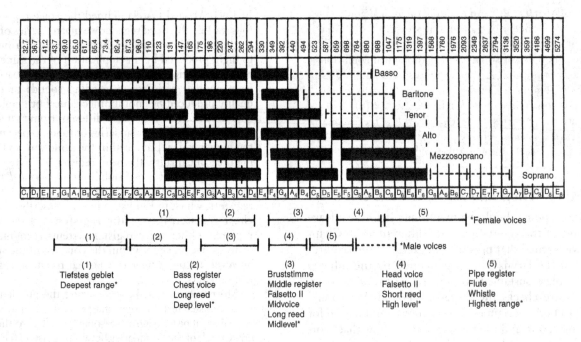

(1)	(2)	(3)	(4)	(5)
Tiefstes gebiet	Bass register	Brusstimme	Head voice	Pipe register
Deepest range*	Chest voice	Middle register	Falsetto II	Flute
	Long reed	Falsetto II	Short reed	Whistle
	Deep level*	Midvoice	High level*	Highest range*
		Long reed		
		Midlevel*		

*Terms and approximate boundaries of vocal registers as suggested by Mörner et al. (1964).

FIGURE 3-90

The physiological ranges of the singing voice according to Nadoleszny (1923), terms used to describe voice registers, and the approximate boundaries and terms for voice registers as suggested by Mörner et al. (1964).

probably just as valuable to singers as "objective boundaries" based on meager data might be.

Brodnitz (1959) has noted that the conventional classification of singing voices as bassos, baritones, tenors, contraltos, mezzo-sopranos, and sopranos has a practical value for the assignment of musical parts but does not stand up to anatomic physiologic criteria. Voice registration traditionally has been a scheme for the categorization of singing voices.

However, if we accept the general concept of the *voice quality criterion*, it becomes difficult to confine registration to the singing voice. It must be extended to include the voice during speech production as well. Nevertheless, as an individual approaches the limits of the normal pitch range, be it singing or speech, some interesting laryngeal adjustments may suddenly take place.

The Limits of the Pitch Range

When the upper limits of the **middle** or **modal pitch range** are reached, the manner of vocal fold vibration may suddenly be modified to produce a range of tones that is in the **falsetto** or **loft register.** Females with high soprano voices do not have a falsetto register, but may exhibit a **laryngeal whistle.** At the lower limits of the pitch range, laryngeal adjustments may result in what is called **glottal fry** or **pulse register.**

Falsetto

Although falsetto is confined to the extreme upper portion of the pitch range, *it is also a peculiar vocal quality that is a consequence of the manner, and not just the rate, of vocal fold vibration.* There is a considerable amount of overlap between the upper limits of the normal pitch range and the lower limits of the falsetto range. Most singers (and many of us who are definitely nonsingers) are capable of producing a high note that is recognized as being within the middle or modal register and of producing a note with exactly the same pitch that is recognized as being within the lower portion of the falsetto register. This is an instance where the falsetto assignment is made on the basis of vocal quality, but we have also been able to discover something about the internal laryngeal adjustments that accommodate this register.

High-speed motion pictures of the larynx during falsetto production reveal that the vocal folds vibrate and come into contact only at the free borders and that the other folds remain relatively firm and nonvibratory. Furthermore, the folds appear long, stiff, very thin along the edges, and often somewhat bow-shaped. A cycle of falsetto taken from a high-speed film is shown in Figure 3-91. This is the same subject that appears in Figures 3-80 and 3-81. The vibratory behavior suggests that the vocal fold musculature is tensed, and electromyography

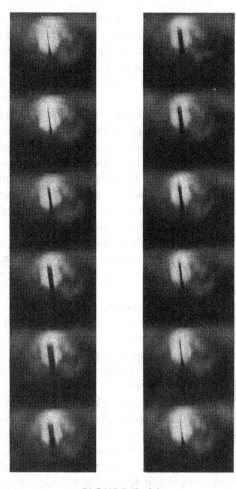

FIGURE 3-91

A cycle of falsetto (f_0 = 400 Hz) by the same subject as in Figure 3-81 and 3-82.

reveals heightened activity of the **cricothyroid muscle** as well. The mechanism of falsetto is not entirely free from debate, and there is a strong possibility that there is, in fact, more than one mechanism for producing it (Rubin and Hirt, 1960). An early description of falsetto by Aikin (1902) seems to have withstood the test of time:

> The [vocal] ligaments are pressed together so firmly by the strong contraction of the lateral crico-arytenoid muscles, as well as the other muscles of approximation, that their edges are in contact for a short distance in front of the vocal processes, leaving only a shortened length of ligament free to vibrate. It is possible to relax the arytenoid muscles a very little, and allow a slight opening of the valve, without disturbing the pitch.

Farnsworth (1940), Brodnitz (1959), Pressman (1942), and Pressman and Kelemen (1955) attribute falsetto to a similar mechanism. That is, when the folds have been tensed and lengthened as much as possible, further increases in pitch must be accomplished by a different mechanism, namely, **damping.** The posterior portions of the vocal folds, in the region of the vocal processes, are firmly approximated and do not enter into vibration. As a result, *the length of the vibrating glottis is shortened considerably.*

Rubin and Hirt (1960) employed high-speed photography and x-ray in a study of the falsetto mechanism as employed by singers. They too found that some singers (male) produced falsetto by means of the damping mechanism. They also found that falsetto is more frequently produced with the glottis assuming the shape of a tense, narrow slit, the edges of which vibrated during phonation, and not necessarily meeting at the midline. They called this the "open-chink" and "closed-chink" mechanism, and *the fact that the folds touch in one instance and not the other is a matter of intensity only* (Rubin, personal communication).

For comparative purposes, glottal configurations of a male subject during phonation at normal pitch, high pitch, and falsetto are shown in Figure 3-92. Note the bow-shaped leading edges of the vocal folds during falsetto, suggesting that vibration is confined to the anterior portion of the glottis.

The quality of the tone produced in the falsetto register is almost flutelike, partly due to the simple form of vibration executed by the vocal folds and partly to the high rate of vibration. As illustrated in Figure 3-93, when the fundamental frequency is very high, harmonically related overtones are widely separated in frequency; consequently, in any given frequency range, there are fewer components in the sound with a higher fundamental frequency than in a sound (or voice) with a lower fundamental frequency. This partly accounts for the rich quality of the bass voice when compared with the relatively thin quality of the tenor voice.

When the vocal folds are placed under extreme tension, they never completely approximate during the closed phase of the vibratory cycle. The posteriormost portion of the glottis seems to remain open. The result is a breathy quality that is overlaid on the vocal tone, in addition to a large expenditure of air.

Laryngeal Whistle

According to Brodnitz (1959), the falsetto lies above the head register (in accordance with the definition of register by Garcia). *High female voices do not exhibit a falsetto, but a laryngeal whistle, which does not seem to be produced by the vibration of the vocal folds but by the whistling escape of air from between them.*

Many children are able to produce a clear, flutelike laryngeal whistle. As can be seen in Figure 3-94, the vocal folds appear to be extremely tense and the glottis appears as a very narrow (about 1 mm) slit through which the air

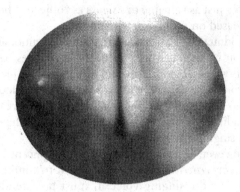

Falsetto

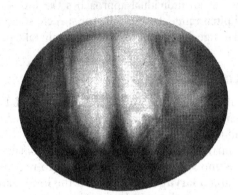

High pitch

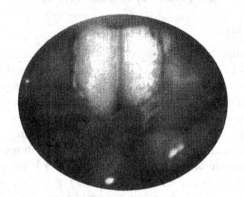

Normal pitch

FIGURE 3-92

General glottal configurations for phonation at normal pitch, high pitch, and falsetto.

flows. Subglottal pressure during whistle production is very high, amounting to 30 cm H_2O.

The location on the frequency scale of the falsetto and laryngeal whistle is shown in Figure 3-90. The range of the various singing voices is also shown. The interruptions of the black columns mark the points of transition from chest, to mixed, to head registers. The dashed areas above the columns of the male voices indicate the falsetto range; above the soprano, the whistle register. The horizontal black lines indicate the approx-

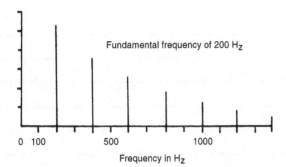

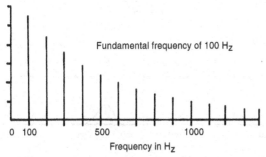

FIGURE 3-93

Schematic spectrum of laryngeal wave. When the fundamental frequency is very high, harmonics are widely spaced in frequency when compared to low fundamental frequency.

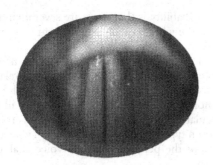

FIGURE 3-94

Photograph of a larynx during production of a laryngeal whistle.

imate average or habitual pitch of the speaking voice for each type.

Glottal Fry (Pulse Register)

Laryngeal adjustments at the lower limit of the pitch range may result in what is called glottal fry, or creaky voice. Moser (1942) says of glottal fry (pulse register): "It is very easy to demonstrate, but very difficult to describe. You may recognize it as the sound produced by many youngsters imitating a motor boat, but to me it more nearly resembles the sound of vigorously popping corn."

Glottal fry may be produced by attempting to phonate quietly at the lowest possible pitch, so that the

sound feels as if it is bubbling out of the larynx in discrete bursts. Indeed, that seems to be precisely what is happening. High-speed photography by the author has revealed that the folds are approximated tightly, but at the same time they appear flaccid along their free borders, and subglottal air simply bubbles up between them at about the junction of the anterior two-thirds of the glottis. The frequency of vocal fold vibration ranges from about 30 to 80 per second, with a mean of approximately 60 per second. *The closed phase occupies about 90 percent of the vibratory cycle, and the opening and closing phases combined occupy about 10 percent of the cycle.*

Moore and von Leden (1958) described vocal fold vibration during the production of glottal fry. *They found that the vocal folds opened and closed twice in rapid succession and then remained closed for a long period of time.* They termed this double vibration pattern "syncopated rhythm." Figure 3-95 illustrates the vibratory cycle as noted by the author and as described by Moore and von Leden. The mechanism of glottal fry is not well understood, and we are not even sure what the air-pressure requirements are for its production. Air flow is so minimal that it is difficult to measure, and our air-pressure measures show that *glottal fry is produced with a minimal (2 cm H_2O) amount of air pressure.* These results may be in conflict with other data, however (Murry and Brown, 1971b; Murry, 1971).

> **CLINICAL NOTE:** Glottal fry is often equated with or accompanies harsh or rough voice quality, and it has been classified as a clinical syndrome associated with "dicrotic dysphonia" (Gk. *dikrotos*, double beating).
>
> Because this type of vocal production is often heard at the very end of sentences, particularly when both pitch and vocal intensity are beginning to decay, it should be considered a normal part of our "vocal repertory." The production of glottal fry ought to be regarded as an extension of the lower limits of the normal or modal pitch range, and as a voice register in the true sense of the word. The use of glottal fry becomes objectionable when it is superimposed on voice production at places other than at the very end of sentences.

Vibrato

Thus far, we have limited our discussion to rather gross pitch changes that might occur with discrete vocal tasks and to the pitch and intensity changes that accompany inflection and other prosodies such as stress. A large body of literature is directed toward *small and rapid pitch and intensity changes that occur primarily during singing.* These pitch and intensity changes are referred to as vibrato, but when they are exaggerated the effect is known as **tremolo.**

FIGURE 3-95

Schematic representation of the vibratory cycle during glottal fry, as noted by Moore and von Leden (1958) above, and as seen by the author, below.

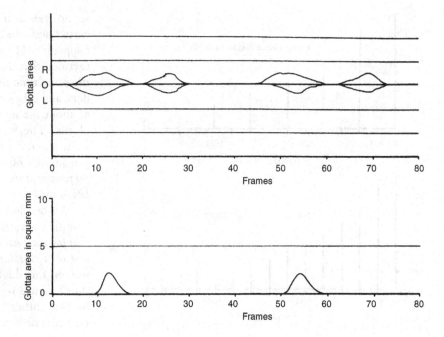

Vibrato is a vocal phenomenon that adds a peculiar "rich color" to the singing voice. Although almost anyone is capable of producing a vibrato of some sort, training is usually required to develop skillful control of the desired pitch and intensity variations. If pitch and intensity changes are extensive, the term trill is used. **Trill,** in music, pertains to a *rapid alternation of two consecutive tones,* and when applied to the singing voice, it means to sing in a manner of a trill.

Vocal vibrato is of interest to speech scientists because it represents such a fine control over fundamental frequency (F_0) adjustments. Horii (1989) has pointed out that the acoustic similarities between vocal vibrato in singing and the vocal tremor of neurologically impaired patients has stimulated interest among speech-language pathologists. Ramig and Shipp (1986), for example, found similar modulation frequencies and extent of F_0 modulation in vocal tremor and vibrato, but variability was greater in tremor than in vibrato.

Although vibrato has been the subject of considerable research, little is known about the physiological mechanism responsible for its production. Names such as Seashore (1923), Kwalwasser (1926), Metfessel (1932), Gray (1926), Tiffin (1932), and Schoen (1922) are frequently encountered in the literature describing and defining vibrato, but it was Schoen in 1922 who attempted a physiological account of its production.

Using indirect laryngoscopy, Schoen examined the larynxes of 14 subjects during vibrato production. In no case was the vibrato confined entirely within the larynx. All subjects had some definite muscle oscillation that could be felt either in the "region of the diaphragm" or just above the larynx. In some cases the back of the

tongue could be seen in oscillation at the vibrato rate. Schoen called these "supralaryngeal vibratos."

In 1932, Tiffin and Seashore commented upon the physiology of the vocal vibrato:

> The probability is that there are several kinds of control of the vibrato involving different sets or series of muscles.
>
> Much light has been thrown on the neurological problem by means of action current and related techniques. It seems probable that the vibrato is but one of the normal periodicities which occur in all the large musculatures in animal life. It also seems probable that a certain type of tension or instability favors the emergence of the periodicity in the voice analogous to a tremor.

Some of the questions raised by Tiffin and Seashore might be answered with contemporary laboratory instrumentation. In 1965, Mason studied the vibrato mechanism by means of simultaneous electromyography and high-speed photography. Laryngeal elevators, depressors, and some musculature of the tongue and of exhalation were studied by means of electromyography, while simultaneous high-speed motion pictures of the larynx producing a vibrato were made.

A summary of some typical data found by Mason is shown schematically in Figure 3-96. The upper two tracings are from voice recordings. The pitch and intensity changes, which took place at a rate of about five per second, were usually in phase with one another. Data indicate heightened activity of the **cricothyroid** muscle and, in some cases, increased activity of the muscles of exhalation during increases in pitch and intensity, and heightened activity of the **mylohyoid** muscle during decreases in pitch and intensity. The data further suggest that additional subglottal pressure may be provided in some subjects by increased activity of the muscles of exhalation. The additional subglottal air pressure may account for increases in intensity during vibrato, on the one hand, or the subtle changes in glottal resistance may result in changes in subglottal pressure.

The high-speed laryngeal photographs revealed little to differentiate vibrato from ordinary phonation. Apparently the changes in tension of the vocal folds are not accompanied by changes in length, or they are too subtle to be detected by ordinary visual means. Very slight modifications in vocal fold tension need not be accompanied by a change in length, as we have learned from Perkins and Yanigahara (1968).

In a comprehensive study of vocal vibrato, Horii (1989), like Mason, found a modulation frequency of about 5 per second. Although it is generally assumed that the predominant temporal pattern of frequency modulation in vocal vibrato is sinusoidal, Horii found that the prevalent pattern was linear (triangular or trapezoidal). Although singers (and speakers) can lower fundamental frequency faster than it can be raised, Horii found that in vibrato the fundamental frequency was increased faster than it was lowered. The mechanism responsible for this seemingly paradoxial behavior is not well understood.

Voice Quality
(The Semantic Merry-Go-Round)

We have seen repeatedly that the tension of the vocal folds and their mass per unit length will influence the mode and rate of vibration. Vocal folds act in pairs, however, and it is important that the tension and mass be exactly the same for both. A vocal fold slightly heavier than the other will vibrate at a lower rate, for example, and the perceptual consequences will be a rough-sounding voice. In addition, the vocal folds are influenced not only by the force with which they are approximated at the midline, but by the subglottal air pressure.

These factors, then—*longitudinal tension, mass per unit length, medial compression, subglottal pressure*, and *physical symmetry*—all have an important bearing on the quality of the voice. The larynx is an extremely sensitive aerodynamic organ, and the factors that influence the mode and rate of vibration must be held in delicate balance. Sometimes acute or chronic disease intervenes, and the laryngeal mechanism ceases to function properly. In other instances, local edema (Gk. *oidema*, swelling) due to allergic reactions or acute vocal abuse (tobacco, alcohol, yelling) will modify the physical characteristics of the vocal folds, and the voice will depart from its usual quality. The voice is a surprisingly good index of the general state of health of an individual, and that includes mental health.

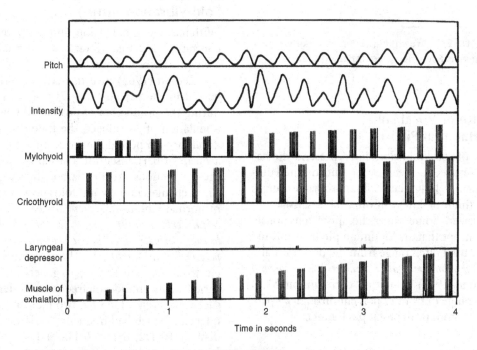

FIGURE 3-96

Schematic reproduction of acoustic and electromyographic recordings during the production of vibrato. (From Mason, 1965.)

Voice quality is a controversial issue, far from resolved, and terminology is the basis for much of the disagreement. The number of terms used to describe the human voice is limited only by the finite repertory of adjectives in our language.

A voice classification system, if it is to enjoy acceptance, should be based on the specifiable parameters of the voice, and that presupposes that the facts will support our images, which are often steeped in tradition.

Specifiable Parameters of Voice Production

Specifiable parameters of voice production are (1) maximum frequency (pitch) range, (2) mean rate of vocal fold vibration (habitual pitch), (3) air cost (maximum phonation time), (4) minimum-maximum intensity at various pitches, (5) periodicity of vocal fold vibration (jitter), (6) noise, and (7) resonance.

1. Maximum Frequency (Pitch) Range

The normal voice exhibits flexibility in pitch during casual conversation and speech sounds very monotonous without it. *An adult speaker can usually produce tones that extend over a frequency range of two octaves above the lowest sustainable tone.* (An octave is a two-to-one ratio in frequency.) By the use of a keyboard or pitchpipe, the lowest tone a person can sustain can be determined, and the highest tone should be at least two octaves above the lowest tone.

> **CLINICAL NOTE:** We should recognize that voice problems in general are often accompanied by a restricted range.

2. Mean Rate of Vocal Fold Vibration (Habitual Pitch)

The mean rate of vocal fold vibration represents the habitual pitch, but precise specification outside the laboratory is difficult. Judgments of appropriate versus inappropriate (high or low) can often be a satisfactory indicator, however. Some voice therapists tenaciously cling to the concept that an "optimum pitch" is located one-fourth the total pitch range from the bottom (Fairbanks, 1959), *a technique that is predicated on a normal pitch range.* Stone (1983) found the "optimum pitch" to be located in a range of from 17 percent through 29 percent from the bottom of the total pitch range.

> **CLINICAL NOTE:** Determining optimum pitch with the "um-hum" technique proposed by Cooper (1973) may be a useful clinical tool, and trial and error also has its place in the clinical environment (Boone, 1977).

3. Air Cost (Maximum Phonation Time)

A healthy larynx vibrating appropriately can be expected to utilize from about 100–200 cc of air per second. Although precise measures of air cost (volume velocity) are difficult outside the laboratory, *an adult speaker should be able to sustain comfortable phonation, for about 15–25 seconds.* Maximum phonation time (MPT) is commonly employed as a test of vocal efficiency. The test is fraught with obstacles to its validity, not the least of which is a practice effect (Stone, 1983).

> **CLINICAL NOTE:** Excessive air cost can usually be attributed to inadequate medial compression, to neoplasms (growths on the vocal cords), or to edema (swelling). The problem cannot be entirely separated from the noise factor in the voice.

4. Minimum-Maximum Intensity at Various Pitches

The test requires a sound pressure level (SPL) meter to determine the minimum and maximum sound pressure levels that can be produced by a speaker at various points along the frequency range. *At midrange, a minimum-maximum SPL of 50 dB is within the normal range* (Coleman, et al., 1977).

5. Periodicity of Vocal Fold Vibration (Jitter)

With mass, length, tension, and subglottal pressure held constant, vocal fold vibrations will recur with moderately precise regularity.

Zemlin (1962) investigated the variations that occurred in the period ($T = 1/f$) of vocal fold vibration during the production of prolonged vowel sounds. In a population of 33 subjects, he found that cycle-to-cycle differences in period ranged from 0.2 to 0.9 msec, with a mean of 0.41 msec for a sustained [ɑ] vowel. While these variations are not large, they suggest that very slight changes in the vocal folds occur during the course of normal vibration. *As long as the variations fall within certain critical limits, slight cycle-to-cycle differences in vibratory period (jitter) do not produce adverse effects in the perceived vocal quality.* In 1963, Wendahl employed an electronic laryngeal analog to generate vocal stimuli that varied in magnitude of frequency differences between successive cycles. He used two median fundamental frequencies, which had frequency variations about the median of 10 Hz, 8 Hz, 6 Hz, 4 Hz, 2 Hz, and 1 Hz. Listeners rated the stimuli for roughness of voice. *Wendahl found very slight frequency variations—as little as one cycle per second around the median—sounded rough,* and the magnitude of judged roughness was directly related to the frequency differences between successive cycles. He also found evidence to suggest that the degree of perceived roughness was related to median frequency, with frequency variation held constant. Thus, in the case of a male and a female voice, with equal frequency variations, the male would be judged to have the rougher voice. Vocal jitter can be detected on a sound spectrogram of the voice, as shown in Figure 3-97. Note the irregularity of the spacing of the vertical voice bars.[11] Karnell (1991) has shown that laryngeal perturbation measures depend on the sampling procedures employed. He found that as many as 190 cycles may be necessary before jitter asymptotes and as many as 130 cycles may be necessary before shimmer asymptotes. He suggests that pathological voices may require a longer "analysis window" for perturbation analysis than do nonpathological voices.

6. Noise

The term **noise** as used here pertains to *the quality of a voice as a consequence of aperiodicity or a random distribution of acoustical energy in the voice spectrum.* The term **vocal**

---

[11]The traditional means of specification of the distribution of acoustical energy, as a function of frequency, generates a graphic **spectrum,** where frequency is placed along the X axis and acoustical energy on the Y axis. In the production of a sound spectrogram, a short (2.4 second) sample of recorded sound is subjected to analysis by repeatedly playing the sample into a variable filter, the output of which drives a graphic recording system. The sample is examined first at low frequency (80 Hz) and with each successive repetition at a slightly high frequency, until an upper limit (8000 Hz) is reached. As the analysis takes place, a graphic representation of acoustical energy as a function of *time* is produced. Frequency is placed along the Y axis, time on the X axis, while the relative intensity of energy, whenever it exists in the sample, is represented by the darkness of the pattern (Z axis). Regularly spaced vertical striations as seen in the normal and nasal samples represent fairly periodic vocal fold vibrations. The other samples depict irregular or aperiodic vibrations with noise components superimposed.

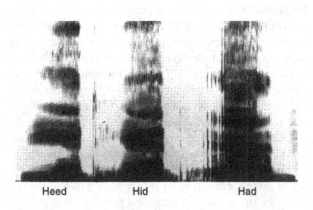

                        FIGURE 3-97

Aperiodic vocal fold vibration is clearly evident in this spectrogram by the irregularity of the spacing of the vertical voice bars, especially in the word *had.*

roughness refers to a voice quality that is detected, defined, and described on the basis of a listener's auditory impressions (Toner, et al., 1990). The authors employed psychophysical scaling to quantify vowel roughness. They compared Direct Estimates of Magnitude (DEM) and Equal Appearing Interval Scales (EAI) to obtain vowel roughness ratings. They found that either DEM or EAI scaling can validly be used to investigate the relationship between listener ratings of vowel roughness and spectral noise level (SNL).

Classification of Vocal Qualities We have seen that the vocal folds normally meet at the midline during the closed phase of the vibratory cycle to completely or nearly completely block the flow of air. When the folds fail to fully approximate, however, the result is a continuous flow of air during the entire vibratory cycle. Acoustic analysis of the voice reveals a broad-band noise superimposed on a tone that may or may not be periodic (Figures 3-98 and 3-99). Air leakage is generating a strong frictional component that accompanies the tone generated by the vibrating vocal folds. The resulting vocal quality is commonly referred to as breathy, or it may be called hoarse, or harsh, depending upon the periodicity of vocal fold vibration. These terms were assigned by Fairbanks (1959) on the basis of energy distribution and aperiodicity as revealed by spectrograms.

Spectrograms of the vowel [æ] produced deliberately with the different voice qualities are shown in Figure 3-99. The spectrograms are short segments taken from sustained vowels, and a normal sample is shown for reference purposes. Fairbanks stated that hoarseness combines the features of harshness and breathiness. He also pointed out that the harsh element may predominate in some hoarse voices, the breathy element in others, and variations of predominance may be heard within a given hoarse voice. These variations and differences in predominance probably contribute to the problem of identification or classification of deviant voice qualities and give rise to alternate terms such as husky, throaty, and so forth.

We should bear in mind that a voice that is judged to be harsh by one person may sound hoarse to another and breathy to yet a third judge. These assignments are based on perception, and the validity of the judgments cannot be questioned. You and I may disagree with one another only because we hear different aspects of a person's voice, and by the same token our judgments are very likely to be unreliable. This is because many factors besides the quality of the voice influence our judgments. For example, we tend to overlook the voice quality of a speaker who is eloquent and fluent and who has a well-chosen vocabulary, simply because we are listening to what is being said and not how it is being said. We attend to the message and not to the messenger.

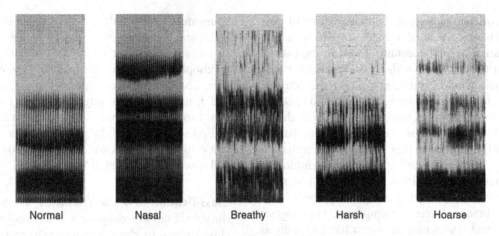

Normal   Nasal   Breathy   Harsh   Hoarse

FIGURE 3-98

Spectrograms of various voice qualities. (From Fairbanks, 1959.)

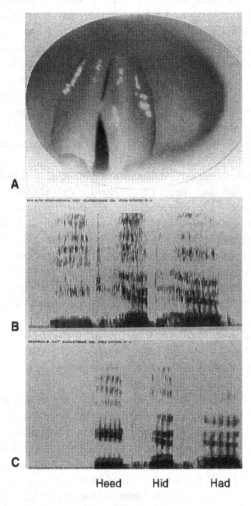

Heed   Hid   Had

FIGURE 3-99

A vocal nodule (A) and a spectrogram of the voice (B). Note the aperiodic vocal fold vibration and the noise component in the voice, compared to the voice six weeks after surgery (C).

CLINICAL NOTE: When dealing with any voice-quality problem, the acoustic end-product should not be regarded as the problem, but rather, as an epiphenomenon. Noisy and aperiodic voices and other vocal qualities are often symptoms of laryngeal disease or structural peculiarities, and *anyone troubled by such vocal problems must be advised to seek prompt and appropriate medical advice.* A common cause of a rough and noisy voice (hoarseness) is acute laryngitis, with its associated swelling and thickening of the vocal fold mucosa. As a result, vibration may be aperiodic and may occur with phase differences between the folds and incomplete glottal closure. Vocal abuse, allergy, or neoplasms may also produce hoarse or rough voices.

Fairbanks's classification system is clinically expedient and attractive, and it has been warmly embraced in spite of its questionable reliability and validity (Jensen, 1965).

Breathiness Breathiness or noisy voice is an inefficient form of phonation, usually resulting in a very limited intensity range. With inadequate medial compression of the vocal folds, subglottal pressure will not have to build up to very high values before the resistance offered by the vocal folds is overcome. *Low subglottic pressure means low vocal intensity. In addition, air cost is extremely high, often three to four times normal.*

The degree of noise in the voice may vary during the breathing cycle. It is usually most prominent at the beginning of the expiratory cycle. A noisy voice may be the result of poor vocal habits, or it may be organic in nature: it may be the result of a structural peculiarity in the larynx. The structural peculiarity, on the other hand, may be the result of chronic vocal abuse. A large **vocal nod-**

ule, the result of vocal abuse, is shown in Figure 3-99A, and a spectrogram of the voice is shown in Figure 3-99B. Voice production for this person required an air expenditure of 433 cc per second, about four times normal. *The severity of a noisy or breathy voice may also be dependent upon phonetic environment.* The vowel [æ] from the isolated word "apple," for example, is not likely to be nearly as breathy as the [æ] from the word "happy" where the vowel is preceded by an aspirate sound.

There seem to be two physiological correlates of a noisy or breathy voice, but whether the acoustic end-products are different is not known. *The most commonly cited correlate is a persistent chink in the posteriormost portion of the glottis* (Figure 3-100), undoubtedly the result of inadequate medial compression. High-speed films often reveal that persons with apparently healthy laryngeal structures and normal-sounding voices display a discernible chink in the posterior portion of the glottis. There is a critical value in the size of the glottal chink that will result in a noisy voice, but the relationship between size of glottal chink and vocal quality is not well understood. The presence of glottal chinks seems to be age related. Linville (1992) for example found that young female speakers demonstrated posterior chinks and incomplete closure more frequently than did older females. Young speakers rarely exhibited an anterior gap or "spindle" configuration. In contrast, anterior gap was the single most common type of gap in the elderly.

From a high-speed motion-picture study of glottal function in deliberate breathiness (and other vocal qualities), Fletcher (1947) concluded that *the distinctive difference between normal and breathy phonation was in the extent of the lateral excursion of the vocal folds.* As shown in Figure 3-101, glottal area during maximum lateral

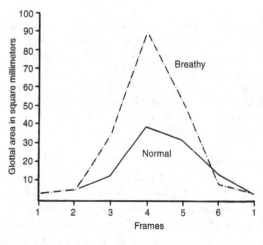

FIGURE 3-101

Comparison of vocal fold vibration in breathy and normal qualities.

excursion was equal to more than 130 percent of the normal area. Fletcher attributed the abnormal lateral excursion of the vocal folds to a relaxed thyroarytenoid muscle. He also pointed out that the *glottal closure may be complete, even during the production of an extremely breathy voice.*

7. Resonance

Voice quality problems associated with resonance of the vocal tract are often not included with various types of voice disorders. This is because the seat of the problem lies not in the larynx but in the transmission pathway between the larynx and the mouth opening.

The degree of **nasality** in the voice is dependent upon the extent of coupling of the nasal passages to the oral and pharyngeal cavities. The quality of the emitted sound can be noticeably affected by the presence (or absence) of the alternate or additional resonating nasal cavities. Nasality, then, can be placed on a continuum from **hyponasality** (e.g., when the nose is "stuffed-up") to **hypernasality** (e.g., when the soft palate is not closing off the nasal passages) with normal nasality occupying an ill-defined region between the extremes.

Nasal voice quality, or hypernasality, is not necessarily objectionable; in fact, a certain amount of nasality may be pleasant. And it is part of certain regional dialects. Hypernasality may be the result of insufficient palatal tissue to ensure proper isolation of the pharyngeal and nasal cavities; it may be the result of speaking habits, or it may be the result of an inability to control the musculature of the soft palate (because of brain-stem damage, for example). Hyponasality may be the result of excessive adenoid tissue, or it may be due to edema of the pharyngeal tissue secondary to allergic reactions.

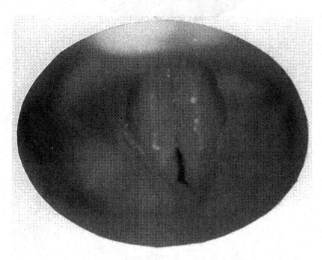

FIGURE 3-100

A persistent chink in the posteriormost portion of the glottis may result in a noisy voice.

While nasality is almost always regarded as a defect of the transmission pathway and not a true vocal problem, Fletcher (1947) has shown that vocal fold behavior is different from normal during the production of a nasalized vowel. He noted a peculiarity of vocal fold configuration that was consistent in all his subjects. As shown in Figure 3-102, the opening phase in hypernasality is quite different from the normal quality. Fletcher also noted that the degree of lateral movement was much greater for the right than for the left fold. *Asymmetrical vocal fold vibration was found only in the nasal quality.*

Earlier authors had also suggested that nasality may have its seat, at least in part, in the larynx. Curry (1910) postulated that nasality could be caused by insufficient velopharyngeal closure, by pharyngeal constriction, by excessive tension in the larynx, or by a combination of all these. Paget (1930), Russell and Tuttle (1930), Russell (1931), Travis et al. (1934), Warren (1936), and Curry (1959) have all suggested that nasality may be due in part to the vibratory pattern of the vocal folds.

Whisper

Most of us, at one time or another, have had occasion to supplant phonation by whispering, which is *nonvocal sound production.* The essential difference between vocal-

ization and whispering lies in the configuration of the nonvibrating vocal folds during exhalation and the resulting acoustic product. During normal phonation, the arytenoid cartilages are approximated so that their medial surfaces are in direct contact. The vocal folds lie parallel to one another. In whispering, however, the arytenoids are slightly abducted and "toed in," creating a small triangular chink in the region of the cartilaginous glottis. When the breath stream is released, turbulence occurs in the chink, and frictional sounds are generated. As shown in Figure 3-103, the glottis assumes a shape like that of an inverted Y, with the vocal folds somewhat abducted. This configuration is just one of a number that can be seen during whisper. At times the glottis looks much as it does during ordinary breathing. Air flow through the glottis plays a very important role in the production of a whisper, amounting to about 200 cm^3/sec for a forced whisper (Monoson and Zemlin, 1984).

Pressman and Keleman (1955) assert that in a low-volume whisper the folds assume a position a little more closely approximated than that for quiet respiration. They go on to state that when the vowel [ɑ] is produced, the margins of the glottis are straight, and that upon

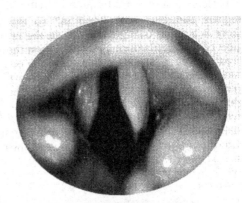

Whisper

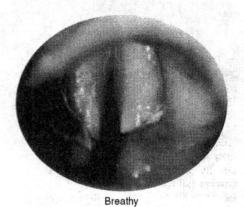

Breathy

FIGURE 3-103

Glottal configuration for whisper and for breathy phonation.

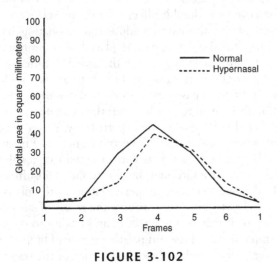

FIGURE 3-102

Schematic of the modes of vocal fold vibration during normal and hypernasal voice production. (From W. Fletcher, 1947.)

producing the [i], there is a toeing-in movement of the vocal processes of the arytenoids, but without a medial shift of the mass of their bodies. They account for such a glottal configuration by positing that the arytenoid muscles fail to contract during the production of an [i] vowel.

When the larynx is viewed by means of high-speed photography during a whisper, the vocal folds may be seen to move very slightly in some subjects, and not at all in others. In no case do they vibrate to any great extent or periodically as in conventional phonation. Although whispering places few demands upon the vocal mechanism, as a form of sound production it is, at best, second best. For example, *the intensity of a loud whisper is 20 dB less than the intensity of conversational speech. Whispering is also a very uneconomical way to use the breath supply.* Whereas a person can phonate for as long as 30 seconds during vocalization, the same person can whisper for only about 10 seconds before another breath must be taken.

Using procedures for making chest wall kinematic observations and pressure flow measures, Stathopoulos et al. (1991) found that whispering generally involves lower lung volumes, lower tracheal pressure, higher translaryngeal (air) flow, lower laryngeal airway resistance, and fewer syllables per breath group when compared with speaking. They also found that performance of the normal subjects studied does not resemble that of individuals with speech and voice disorders, in particular those characterized by low resistive (laryngeal) loads.

Frictional noises, such as those produced by whispering, are composed largely of aperiodic sounds which at any instant in time have a fairly unpredictable spectrum (energy distribution is nearly random). Whispered speech has no fundamental frequency and no harmonic structure. For this reason, whispered speech cannot easily be inflected. Only the bandwidth of the noise can be altered by slight changes in the vocal tract. These alterations may produce a subjective impression of an increase or decrease in pitch. Modifications of the volume velocity of the air stream through the glottis will also change the character of the noise that is being generated, but because the glottis offers virtually no resistance to air flow, only slight modifications in the intensity of whispered speech are possible.

CLINICAL NOTE: A thorough study of the characteristics of whisper has been conducted by Monoson (1976). Her data strongly support the contention that whisper cannot be regarded as abusive to the vocal folds and can thus be used as a substitute for conventional phonation in those instances where vocal rest is recommended as a therapeutic strategy.

Age and Sex Differences in the Larynx

The Infant Larynx

The infant larynx is not simply a miniature model of the adult larynx. It differs in shape, relative size, and position in the neck. At birth the lower border of the cricoid cartilage is located at a level between the second and third cervical vertebrae. The epiglottis lies in contact with the soft palate (Laitman and Crelin, 1976) which permits the infant to breathe while nursing. A drawing, based on a sagittal section of the head of a newborn is shown in Figure 3-104. It shows the relationship between the epiglottis and soft palate.

Infant and adult larynxes differ in shape and in their proximity to the hyoid bone. In the infant, the hyoid bone and thyroid cartilage are often in direct contact, with no space between them anteriorly. In Figure 3-105, the cartilaginous skeleton of an infant larynx is enlarged to approximately the same size as the adult larynx to illustrate the differences in proportionality of the various cartilages. Note the squat appearance of the infant structures in comparison to the adult and the proportionally large arytenoid cartilages in the infant.

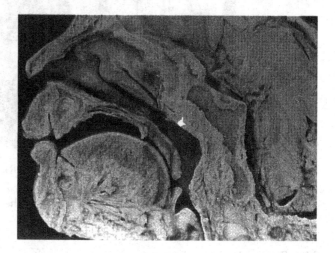

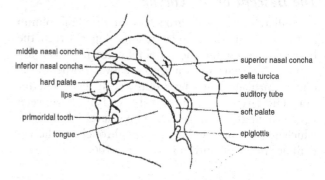

FIGURE 3-104

Schematic sagittal section through infant head, showing relationship of epiglottis to soft palate.

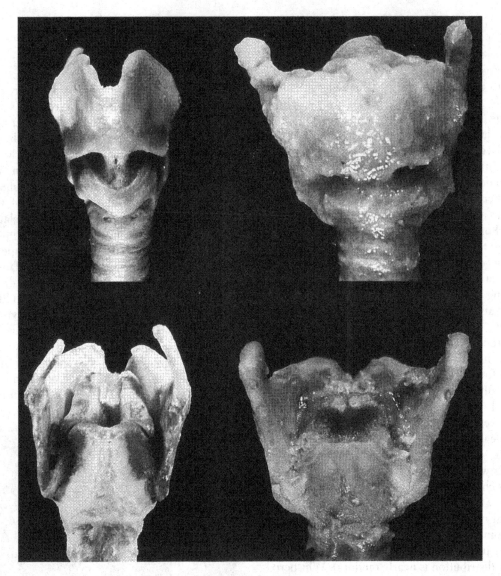

FIGURE 3-105

Adult (left) and infant (right) laryngeal cartilages shown approximately the same height to illustrate the proportionality of the sizes of the various cartilages.

The Descent of the Larynx

Immediately after birth, growth of the vertebral column and changes in the angular relationship between the base of the skull and the vertebral column cause a descent of the larynx, until at age 5 the lower border of the cricoid cartilage is at a level of the sixth cervical vertebra. The larynx continues to descend until, between ages 15 and 20, it reaches the upper level of C7, after which it continues a slow descent throughout the remainder of life, as shown in Figure 3-106.

The Young Larynx

There are no discernible sex differences in the infant's and children's larynx, and this is reflected in the similar-ity of their voices. Prior to the onset of puberty, there is very little difference in the pitch or pitch range between boys and girls (Fairbanks, Herbert, and Hammond, 1949; Fairbanks, Wiley, and Lassman, 1949). Wilson (1979), however, reported a decrease in fundamental frequency between ages 7 and 11 in both boys and girls. In girls the fundamental frequency decreased from 295 Hz (age 7) to 265 Hz (age 11), and in boys from 295 Hz (age 7) to 235 Hz (age 10).

The general shape of the laryngeal cartilages is fairly consistent in the prepubertal and pubertal specimens in each sex, but there is a marked difference between the prepubertal and adult male thyroid eminence (Kahane, 1975). During the pubertal period, the cartilaginous structure grows particularly rapidly. In males

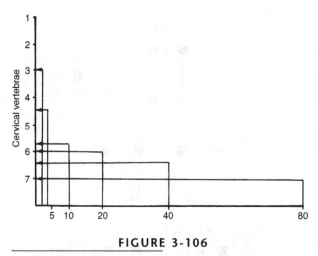

FIGURE 3-106

Vertical descent of larynx during life. Graph shows relationship of lower border of cricoid cartilage to cervical vertebrae at various ages. (Based on J. Wind, *On the Phylogeny and Ontogeny of the Human Larynx.* Groningen: Wolters-Noordhoff Publishing, 1970.)

the vocal folds not only increase in length by about 10 mm, but they also thicken and, as a result, the lower range of the voice drops by about a full octave. This change in the larynx is known as **mutation.**

The female larynx also grows during puberty, but at about the same rate as it does throughout childhood. The vocal folds increase in length by about 4 mm, and the lower range of the voice drops by about two or three musical tones.

The Vocal Folds

At birth, the vocal folds are about 2.5 to 3 mm in length, but they have increased to 5.5 mm at the end of the first year. There is little sex difference in vocal fold length up to the age of ten. For males, the onset of puberty marks a period of rapid growth, accelerated due to the influences of sex hormones. The postpubertal vocal folds are from 17 to 20 mm in length for the male and from about 12.5 to 17 mm in length for the female.

We have seen that the vocal folds have a layered structure consisting of the epithelium; the superficial, intermediate, and deep layers of the lamina propria; and finally the thyroarytenoid (vocalis) muscle. Hirano et al. (1981) group these layers into the cover (epithelium and superficial layer of lamina propria), the transition (intermediate and deep layers of the lamina propria), and the body, which consists of the vocalis muscle.

The **mucosa** of the vocal fold of a newborn is very thick, and the vocal ligament is not developed until about four years of age. By age 16 the inner structure is very similar to that of the adult. The layer structure of the vocal fold matures during adolescence. Hirano et al. state, "Thus, voice mutation is associated not only with

an increase in size of the vocal fold, but also with changes in the inner structure of the vocal fold mucosa."

In advanced age a variety of changes in the conus elasticus and in the elastic fibers of the lamina propria take place, especially in the male (Kahane, 1983). Elastic fibers become fragmented and the density of the vocal ligament decreases. There is also a loss of muscle tissue and an increase in connective tissue within the body of the vocal fold. These changes are not as well defined in the aging female larynx.

The Thyroid Angle

The thyroid laminae of the infant larynx form something of a semicircle, which during the growth process becomes increasingly angulated. Kahane (1975) found the angle formed by the union of the thyroid laminae was essentially the same for the male and female prepubertal population. In the adult population only slight differences were noted; the angle was 84.2 degrees for male adults and 92.5 degrees for the adult females. According to measurements of 200 larynxes (see Table 3-2), the angle of the thyroid is 78.5 degrees for adult males and 86.2 degrees for adult females. The angle tends to be more rounded in the female larynx (see Figure 3-107).

The assumed relationship between vocal fold length and the angular relationship of the thyroid laminae has been investigated. Since the anteroposterior dimension of the larynx decreases with increasingly divergent thyroid laminae, we might suspect that vocal fold length will decrease as well. However, we must remember that the thyroid cartilage only provides an anterior attachment for the vocal folds. Behind, the folds attach to the vocal processes of the arytenoid cartilages, and they in turn are anchored to the cricoid. This means that, from the standpoint of Euclidean geometry, there is no reason to suspect a relationship between the thyroid angle and vocal fold length. Smith (1978) found, in a detailed dissection

TABLE 3-2

Summary table comparing mean superior and inferior angle measurements for adult male and female thyroid laminae

Study	Mean Superior Angle		Mean Inferior Angle	
	Male	Female	Male	Female
Malinowski (1967)	85.30	91.10	71.00	79.00
Neiman (1971)	78.75	78.80	35.00	38.80
Maue (1970)	69.63	80.97	—	—
Kahane (1975)	84.20	92.50	—	—
Smith (1978)	74.57	87.58	91.05	104.38

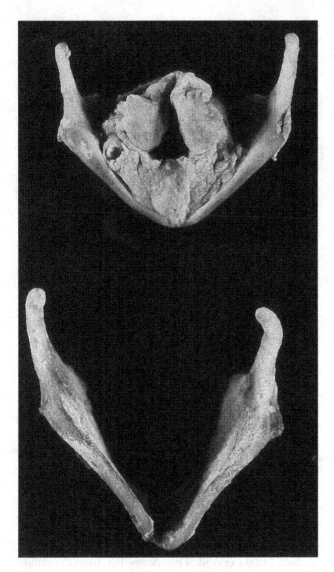

FIGURE 3-107

A male (bottom) and female (top) adult larynx as seen from above. Note the rounded configuration of the thyroid cartilage in the female as compared to the male.

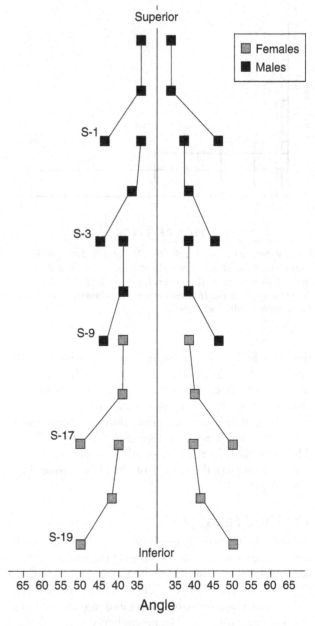

FIGURE 3-108A

Laryngeal specimens in this group (Type I) exhibit a slight increase in angularity from the superior to the middle angle and a very abrupt increase from middle to inferior angle. Five of twenty specimens (25%).

of 20 specimens, *no relationship between vocal fold length and thyroid angle.* Her results also shed light on the differences in thyroid angles as found in adult males and females. There seem to be three configurations that can be found in adults of both sexes. These configuration types are illustrated in Figure 3-108. Smith found that almost every specimen was slightly skewed at the superior border of the thyroid cartilage. Her results reinforce the notion that a certain amount of asymmetry is usually found in the thyroid cartilage. Her results, however, are at odds with the notion that the angle of the laminae is 90°–100° in males and 120°–130° in females, figures endorsed by a number of authors in the older literature. Her results are in keeping with those of Moore (1971), Kahane (1978), Neiman (1971), Malinowski (1967), and Zemlin (1981).

The Aging Larynx

Research has shown that changes in **pitch level** and **pitch range** accompany growth and the aging process. Results obtained by Fairbanks (1942), Fairbanks et al. (1949), and Mysak (1959) suggest that vocal pitch lowers at a rate roughly corresponding to laryngeal growth, and at middle age the pitch level begins to rise slightly. Changes in pitch range that may accompany increasing age are not well documented, but there seems to be a

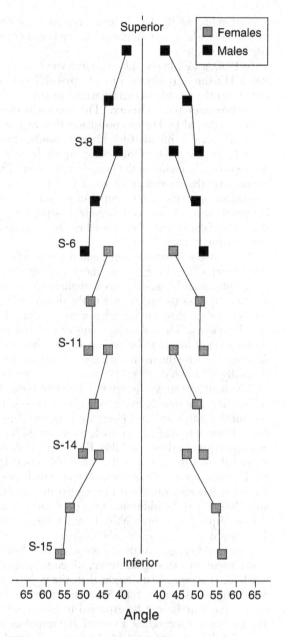

FIGURE 3-108B

Laryngeal specimens in this group (Type II) exhibited an abrupt increase from the superior to middle angle but very slight increase from middle to inferior angle. Five of twenty specimens (25%).

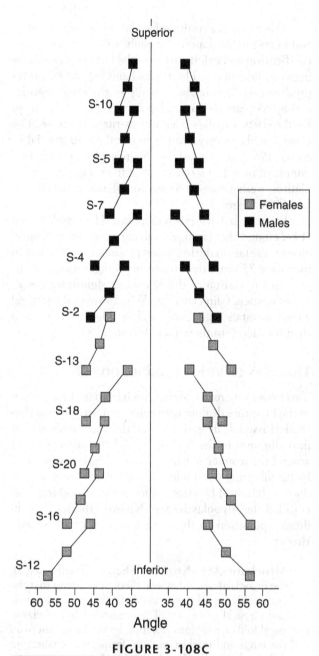

FIGURE 3-108C

Angular configurations (Type III) in this group had approximately equal increases in angularity from the superior to the middle to the inferior angles. Ten of twenty specimens (50%).

trend toward a decrease in range with increasing age. These changes are probably due to deterioration of muscle tissue and an increase in connective tissue in the vocal folds, along with the ossification of the thyroid and cricoid cartilages (Kahane, 1980; Hirano et al., 1981). Age-related changes (19 to 80 years) in the articular surfaces of the cricoarytenoid joint have been investigated by Kahn and Kahane (1986) using India ink pinprick patterns. They found that older articular surfaces exhibited

mechanical abrasions and ossification. These changes may result in functional consequences for voice production. A characteristic slit pattern was found on the articular surfaces on both the cricoid and arytenoid cartilages. In addition, the slits on the arytenoid cartilage were oriented at right angles to the slits on the cricoid cartilage. In a companion study, Kahane and Kahn (1986) found no age-related changes in collagen fibers in specimens ranging from three to 30 years.

The cartilages of the infant larynx are much softer and more pliable than in the adult; with increasing age, **ossification** and **calcification** of the laryngeal cartilages begin to take place. The thyroid and cricoid cartilages (hyaline cartilage) begin to ossify in the early twenties and by 65 years the entire laryngeal framework, except for the elastic cartilages, has usually turned to bone. The elastic cartilages may show signs of calcification (Malinowski, 1967), particularly in the muscular process. In a sample of over 190 larynxes taken from a geriatric population, we have never found completely calcified arytenoid cartilages.

From a behavioral standpoint, Hoit and Hixon (1992) found that laryngeal valving economy (laryngeal airway resistance) during vowel production was lower in men over 75 years than it was in younger men. Laryngeal airway resistance did not differ significantly with age in women. Clinicians should be aware that laryngeal airway resistance generally will be higher for women than for men (Smitheran and Hixon, 1981).

Theories of Voice Production

Two broad categories of theories have dominated much of the literature dealing with voice production. One theoretical issue deals with the way the vocal folds are set into vibration in the first place, and the other revolves around the manner in which the vocal tone is generated by the vibrating vocal folds. The classical theory of production (classical by virtue of longevity, if nothing else) is called the **myoelastic-aerodynamic theory.** It is in direct opposition to the more recent **neurochronaxic theory.**

Myoelastic-Aerodynamic Theory. Briefly stated, the myoelastic-aerodynamic theory postulates that the vocal folds are subject to well-established aerodynamic and physical principles. The compressible and elastic vocal folds are set into vibration by the air stream from the lungs and trachea, and the frequency of vibration is dependent upon their length in relation to their tension and mass. Properties of the mucus, mucous membrane, connective tissue (including the conus elasticus and vocal ligament), the muscle tissue, and the boundaries of the vocal folds all contribute to the mode and frequency of vibration. These properties are regulated primarily by the delicate interplay of the intrinsic laryngeal muscles.

The myoelastic-aerodynamic theory was first advanced by Johannes Muller in 1843 and has enjoyed popular acceptance ever since. Minor modifications of the theory have been suggested by Tonndorf (1925) and by Smith (1954), but its salient features have remained unchanged through the years. A very complete and quantitative interpretation of the myoelastic-aerodynamic theory can be found in van den Berg (1958a). In fact, van den Berg's contributions to our understanding of the larynx have been so significant that the myoelastic-aerodynamic theory is sometimes attributed to him.

In 1950, a well-known physicist and voice scientist, Raoul Husson, introduced a theory that differs radically from the myoelastic-aerodynamic theory.

Neurochronaxic Theory. The neurochronaxic theory advanced by Husson postulates that each new vibratory cycle is initiated by a nerve impulse transmitted from the brain to the vocalis muscle by way of the recurrent branches of the paired vagus nerve. This means that the frequency of vocal fold vibration is dependent upon the rate of impulses delivered to the laryngeal muscles and is relatively independent of those very factors which are crucial in the myoelastic-aerodynamic theory.

The myoelastic-aerodynamic and the neurochronaxic theories are divergent to the extent that they probably cannot be united into a single working theory. Shortly after the appearance of the theory of Husson, a number of research studies were conducted to test the theory. The following summary of research findings is not meant to be exhaustive, but the results demonstrate why the neurochronaxic theory has been generally discounted.

The neurochronaxic theory is dependent upon the supposition that muscle fibers in the vocal fold course obliquely medialward and insert into the vocal ligament. Contraction of these muscle fibers would result in a separation of the vocal folds. Research has shown repeatedly that the course of the vocal fold muscle fasciculi is anteroposterior and that oblique muscle fibers do not insert into the vocal ligament (van den Berg and Moll, 1955). In addition, high-speed films of initiation of phonation invariably show the initial vocal fold movement to be toward the midline.

Due to differences in their course, the left branch of the **recurrent laryngeal nerve,** which supplies the left fold, is about 10 cm longer than the right nerve which supplies the right fold. Since the highest velocity a nerve impulse can be expected to have is about 100 meters per second, at a rate of 500 impulses per second (which is unreasonably high) nerve impulses would arrive at the left vocal fold about 1 msec behind the impulse to the right fold, and so the vocal folds would be vibrating completely out of phase. One fold would be in the open position while the other would be in the midline position.

And finally, vocal folds simply cannot and do not vibrate in the absence of a pressurized air stream, as shown by van den Berg (1957) and Rubin (1960).

Whereas most normal laryngeal functions may be accounted for quite easily by the myoelastic-aerodynamic theory, very little conclusive evidence may be found to support the neurochronaxic theory of vocal fold vibration.

Cavity-Tone (Puff, Inharmonic, or Transient) Theory. Vocal tones and the way they are generated seem to have occupied curious minds for hundreds of years. One of the earliest major publications on the topic of vocal tones was by Willis (1830). After conducting a series of experiments with cavity resonators to determine the agents responsible for the production of vowel sounds, he concluded that the vowel was a cavity tone, the form of which was dependent upon the length of the resonating tube. He further supposed that the cavity tone had no relationship to the composition of the reed tone or to the fundamental frequency of the vibrating-reed sound source.

The theory of Willis, now considered the original "cavity-tone" theory of vowel production, stated that the sound identified as a vowel was dependent only upon the length of the resonating tube and was completely independent of the reed tone. In his experimentation he discovered that the vowels were heard in the following order as the length of the resonating tube was increased: *i, e, a, o,* and *u.* As the length of the tube reached multiples of the length of the wave of the reed tone, the pattern was repeated, but in reverse order. Willis felt that the larynx functioned simply to provide puffs of air that might excite the supraglottal resonating cavities.

Harmonic (Overtone, Steady State) Theory. Charles Wheatstone, in 1837, attempted to replicate the experiments of Willis. He noted that the reed tone was not simple, but rather complex, containing many harmonics of the fundamental frequency. He supposed that the vowel heard was the result of an augmentation of certain of the harmonic components of the reed tone. According to Wheatstone, the larynx functioned to generate a complex tone that would be acted upon by the supraglottal cavities.

In 1862, Helmholtz, a brilliant scholar who studied both speech and hearing, replicated Wheatstone's experiments and conducted further experiments. With the aid of a resonating device, since called a "Helmholtz resonator," he noted that the cavities of resonance acted upon all of the reed tone's harmonics that coincided or even closely approximated their natural frequencies. Although Helmholtz only refined Wheatstone's theory, he is sometimes given credit for originating the harmonic theory of vowel production. It seems, however, that Helmholtz was not a particular advocate of either the harmonic or the cavity-tone (inharmonic) theory. He suggested that they were simply different methods of representing the same mechanisms.

In 1890, Hermann illustrated the improbability of the harmonic theory on the basis of the overtone structure of a sound sung at 49 Hz, in which the frequency characteristics of a vowel were comparable to the twenty-eighth harmonic. He claimed such a harmonic would be too feeble to be heard, even if reinforced by a cavity resonator and concluded that the complex tone and the vowel tone were independent, one from the other. Hermann called the regions of prominent energy in vowels **formant bands,** a term that has persisted ever since.

In 1896, Rayleigh and Trendelenburg, after extensive analyses of vowel sounds, concluded both theories had merit, while Scripture, in 1904, claimed the vowel was solely a function of the natural resonance of the head cavities. In 1929 Fletcher reinforced the notion that the two theories were not incompatible. He stated: "The difference in the two theories is not, as some suppose, a difference in the conception of what is going on while the vowel sounds are being produced, but in the method of representing or describing the motions in definite physical terms."

He pointed out that the inharmonic (cavity-tone) theory enables one to visualize in a more direct way what is taking place, and is of value to the phonetician interested in the mechanism of speech production. The harmonic theory, on the other hand, is of use to the engineer who is interested in separating speech into its component frequencies.

The **mucoviscoelastic aerodynamic** theory of vocal fold vibration is presented in the following discussion of models of the larynx.

Models of the Larynx and Vocal Tract

Introduction

One technique for evaluating the contributions of the larynx to speech production, and for assessing the role of the various tissues, the influence of medial compression of the vocal folds and their longitudinal tension, is to make use of models. To be completely successful a model should manifest all the known properties of the structure or system it represents.

There have been at least two approaches to modeling the human speech mechanism. One approach, successfully employed by Sir Richard Paget (1930), was to construct a mechanical system consisting of rubber-like vocal folds, with a complex resonating cavity placed above it. Because, after a certain amount of trial and error, seemingly humanlike sounds could be produced, we can probably say that the models possessed some of the properties of the speech mechanism.

D. C. Miller, a contemporary of Paget, *analyzed* graphic recordings of vowel sounds, reducing the complex wave form to a series of simple (sinusoid) waves, each with a constant wavelength and amplitude. He then *synthesized* vowel sounds, as Paget says, "By combining together and simultaneously blowing a number of organ pipes—each of which was designed to give a sound comparable in wave form to *one* of the series of simple waves deduced by the analyser—Miller was able to reproduce to vowel the sound as originally intoned."

A fundamentally different approach is to construct a model of the larynx (and vocal tract) on the basis of some of the known properties of the system. If mass, elasticity, and compliance of the various tissues of the larynx are known, as well as tension factors, compression, subglottic pressure, volume velocity, and modes of vibration, to name a few, engineers might be able to design a self-oscillating system that has predictive value. That is, it will produce humanlike sounds. Mathematical models of the larynx for digital computer simulation of human speech have a number of virtues, one being that various parameters of vocal fold behavior can be varied, one at a time, to determine the effect on the acoustic product. Periodicity, vertical and longitudinal vocal fold phase differences, and other properties of laryngeal behavior can be systematically controlled and evaluated.

A Single-Degree-of-Freedom Model

A frequently cited example of a self-oscillating source for vocal tract synthesizers is a single-degree-of-freedom model, described by Flanagan and Landgraf (1967). In this model the vocal folds must move as a single mass toward and away from the midline, only. They have nowhere else to go. Flanagan and Landgraf note that the vocal folds operate as an aerodynamic oscillator and their motion is a self-determined function of physical parameters such as subglottal pressure, vocal fold tension, and vocal tract configuration. A realistic model for speech synthesis and articulatory studies ought to reflect these self-oscillating properties.

The model is shown in Figure 3-109. The folds are considered as a simple mechanical oscillator of *mass M*, which represents the mass of one of the paired vocal folds; a *spring constant K*, which represents vocal fold tension; and *viscous damping B*, which is due to a condition at the boundary where the vocal folds strike one another upon closure. That is, the opposing surface that the mass of the vocal fold strikes is relatively massless and mainly viscous or fluidlike. When the closing folds meet at the midline, they give up some of their momentum, but because of the internal properties of the folds, the tissue tends to be displaced toward the midline. As a result, the glottis is closed for a brief period of time, and at the same time the forces acting on the mass of the vocal folds are immediately in a direction to open the glottis. The vocal folds oscillate automatically.

The boundary may also be massive or hard, and in that case the folds give up their momentum instantaneously. The damping, of course, is quite different under these conditions. In the **viscous condition,** the folds

tend to mold into one another as they meet. At the **hard boundary condition,** they tend to rebound. *Viscous and hard boundary conditions can be thought of as representing low- and high-pitch phonation.*

In Figure 3-109 the symbol P_s denotes *subglottic pressure*, P_1 and P_2 represent *acoustical pressures at the inlet and outlet* of the glottal orifice, respectively, and U_g is the *acoustic volume velocity* through the glottal orifice. It should not be confused with the velocity of air flow through the glottis.

As stated earlier, the model shown in Figure 3-109 is described as a single-degree-of-freedom system. We have seen, however, that the vibrating vocal folds exhibit considerable vertical phase differences at low and moderate pitch levels and that they also manifest a certain amount of vertical displacement as they vibrate. The vocal folds do not move as a single mass toward and away from the midline, and this means that a more complex model is required if it is to exhibit "real larynx" behavior.

A Two-Degree-of-Freedom Model

These models have been proposed to account for vertical phase differences. As described by Ishizaka and Flanagan in 1972, the two-degree-of-freedom model shown in Figure 3-110 has several characteristics of oscillation in common with the vocal folds. The vocal folds are represented by *two masses*, M_1 and M_2, which are capable of purely horizontal motion independently.

Each mass can be thought of as a simple mechanical oscillator with a *mass M*, a *spring constant K*, and *viscous damping B*, as with the single-mass model. Note however, that the masses are coupled together by S_3, which acts to supply a force on M_1 and M_2 in the horizontal direction, by virtue of a difference in their *lateral displacements* x_1 and x_2, respectively. If we let L_g represent the *length of the glottis*, the *glottal area* A_1 and A_2, corresponding to the region of M_1 and M_2, for paired masses (as in the real larynx) becomes $A_1 = 2L_g^{-1}x_1$ and $A_2 = 2L_g^{-1}x_2$.

The *equilibrium position* of the masses is x_0, as shown in Figure 3-110. The *stiffness* exhibited by the spring S_1 and S_2 is due to the longitudinal tension of the vocal

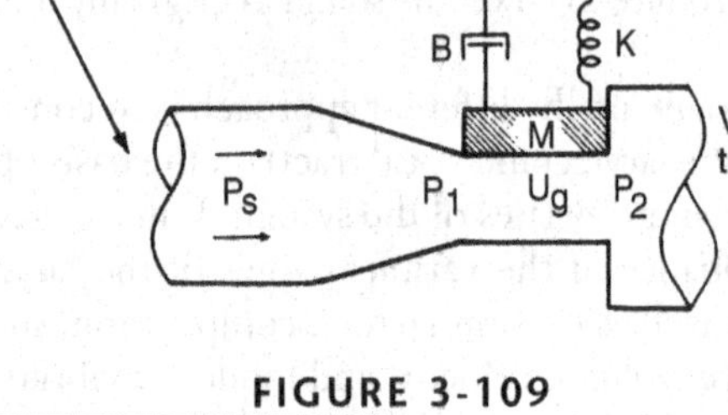

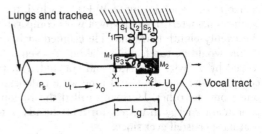

FIGURE 3-109

Schematic of a single-mass model of the vocal folds. (After Flanagan and Landgraf, 1967.)

FIGURE 3-110

Two-degree-of-freedom model of the vocal folds. (After Ishizaka and Flanagan, 1972.)

folds. If the masses are displaced from their equilibrium position x_0 by distances $x_1 - x_0$ and $x_2 - x_0$, the *restoration force* is equal to $S_1(x_1 - x_0)$ and $S_2(x_2 - x_0)$.

We should note, however, that (1) restoration forces are not linearly proportional to the displacement, (2) the vibratory pattern of the vocal folds is not sinusoid, and (3) under certain conditions the system can become unstable.

In Figure 3-110, the *resistances* r_1 and r_2 represent the viscous characteristics of the vocal fold tissues. The symbols for r_1 and r_2 represent **dashpots.** A common example of a dashpot is the familiar hydraulic piston-fluid-cylinder combination that is used to prevent opened doors from closing too quickly. In the larynx, the dashpots r_1 and r_2 function to decrease the velocities of the masses M_1 and M_2 due to the restoration forces of S_1 and S_2.

In this model, *air flow* through the trachea is shown as U_t. As the constriction at M_1 and M_2 is reached, the velocity increases, and so *the restoration forces are complemented by the important Bernoulli effect.*

The Sixteen-Mass Model

According to Matsushita (1975) and Hiroto (1966), the upheaval of the mucosa of the vibrating larynx is a very important factor, and so the viscous properties of the larynx should be given special emphasis. In fact, the term **mucoviscoelastic aerodynamic** is suggested as a theory of vocal fold vibration. This theory acknowledges the importance of the relatively loose coupling between the mucous membrane lining the larynx and the vocal ligament. If the coupling were rigid, vertical phase differences could not easily take place, and in fact, the larynx might not be capable of vibrating at all.

The vibrating vocal folds can be seen, by means of ultra-high-speed cinematography, to exhibit the familiar vertical phase differences as they are displaced back and forth horizontally. But their leading edges are also everted vertically somewhat, and undulating waves of disturbed mucus and mucosa occur along the upper surface of the vocal folds. This implies that the vocal folds actually have a number of degrees of freedom. If a model is to generate natural-sounding speech, it should reflect the properties of an actual vibrating human larynx.

A sixteen-mass model of the larynx was described by Titze in 1973 in an attempt to simulate humanlike speech that would (1) phonate in at least two distinct registers, (2) provide sufficient flexibility for pathological studies, (3) be capable of simulating transient responses of the folds, such as moderate coughs or voice breaks, (4) be regulated by parameters that have direct physiological correlates, and (5) increase the "naturalness" of utterances.

Titze's model attempts to simulate various observed vocal fold behaviors, including vertical and horizontal motion of the folds, and horizontal and vertical phase differences. Each vocal fold is conceived as consisting of two portions that behave differently during oscillation. They are the mucous membrane and the vocalis muscle, tightly coupled to the vocal ligament. While the two-mass systems are considered to be loosely coupled, their mass and tension differences as a whole count more heavily for the vertical phase differences between the mucous membrane and vocalis-vocal ligament masses. In addition, this coupling is not constant, but is altered during pitch changes that are accompanied by changes in tension and length.

The mucous membrane has been observed at high pitch phonation (that of a female singer) to collect in 8 nodal regions in a standing wave pattern. This pattern and some mathematical considerations led Titze to subdivide the mucous membrane and vocalis-vocal ligament masses each into 8 separate masses. The model then consists of 16 masses which are allowed to move in a direction perpendicular to air flow (in a lateral direction) and in the direction of this flow. No motion in a longitudinal direction is considered. The 16-mass model is shown in Figure 3-111.

Titze identifies three general categories of forces that act upon the vocal folds. They are **internal, external,** and **dissipative** forces in general. **Internal forces** refer to nearest neighbor forces only, with a maximum of four nearest neighbor forces acting on a given particle. They are *restoring forces*, which are space dependent and take the general form,

$$\text{stress} = k \times \text{strain (Hooke's law)}$$

Equations dealing with the restoring forces account for the position of the particle in space with respect to its position of equilibrium, and either the tension between

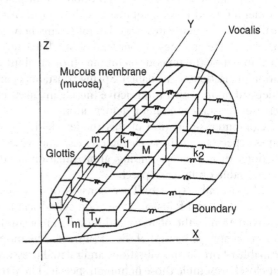

FIGURE 3-111

Sixteen-mass model of the vocal folds by Titze (1973).

the two neighboring particles in the case of the vocalis–vocal ligament mass particles, or the spring constant and lateral neighbor strains in the case of the nearest neighbor boundary or mucousal particles.

The two **external forces** are gravity and aerodynamic forces. **Dissipative forces** include losses associated with glottal flow, losses in the vocal tract, and losses in the vocal tissues. The *damping factor* of the system is variable, depending upon whether the vocal folds are abducted or adducted.

For quantitative inputs on elasticity to the model, Titze makes use of the following information from van den Berg (1960b):

1. The maximum strain exhibited by the vocal ligament is about 30 percent of the relaxed strength. To a first-order approximation, the stress-strain curve is exponential. After maximum strain, the ligament is indistensible and behaves like a conventional string.

2. Relaxed muscular tissue reaches this point at 50 percent of relaxed length.

3. Active stress supported by the vocalis varies continuously from zero to about 10 g/mm^2 (van den Berg, 1958a).

Titze assumes that **negative stresses** (compressions) are possible and that the negative stress characteristics are similar to the positive ones. In computing the total tension values for the ligament and the vocalis muscle, their depths, active stresses, and stress constants and strains are hypothesized. By varying the active muscular tension from zero to slight, we observe that *the tension supported by the ligaments decreases with muscle activity unless the strains are very high.*

The mucous membrane supports little tension when not engaged in vibration. In motion, it is displaced considerably, and it is out of phase with the rest of the vocal fold, so it generates large lateral strains between particles. Titze assumes exponential elastic behavior to be exhibited by the mucous membrane (no actual information of elasticity is available). Spring constants k_1 and k_2 depend upon registration; active muscle involvement increases resistance to lateral deformation.

Computer simulation of this model yields glottal shapes, spectra, air flow characteristics, and velocity functions that show promising approximation to the data available on human speech.

The overall system of Titze consists of a 16-mass model of the vocal folds, an 18-section cylindrical tube approximation of the pharynx and mouth, and a similar 12-section approximation of the nasal tract. The model is capable of producing vibrations and related pressures that closely resemble those of human speech. The parameters used to control the simulation have direct physiological correlates, for example, subglottic pressure, muscular tensions, and articulatory movements of the tongue and jaw. With this model, phonation is possible in at least two registers, transient responses of the vocal system can be simulated, and with it some pathologies can be studied.

In 1975, Titze and Strong treated the vocal fold as a *continuum* rather than a system of discrete masses and springs, and they applied viscoelastic properties of vocal fold tissue to their model. The effects of tissue viscosity and incompressibility were incorporated to account for coupling between horizontal and vertical motion when vertical phase differences occur, a limitation inherent in earlier finite-element models.

In 1979, Titze and Talkin were able to model the effects of various laryngeal configurations on phonation, taking into account the curved boundaries of the vocal folds and their viscoelastic properties. They found fundamental frequency to be affected primarily by vocal fold length. That is, *fundamental frequency is controlled through longitudinal stress in the muscle layers. They also found that subglottal pressure is not a major factor in the control of fundamental frequency.*

In 1984, Titze described parameters for glottal area, vocal fold contact area, and glottal volume flow. The parameters were an **abduction quotient**, a **shape quotient**, a **phase quotient**, and a **load quotient**, in addition to **fundamental frequency** and **vibrational amplitude**. Parameterization and computer modeling hold great promise in furthering our understanding of vocal fold behavior.

Having thus far in the text provided the speech mechanism with an air stream and a vibrating larynx, we shall move on to the structures responsible for modifying the laryngeal tone and producing additional speech sounds. These structures are called the **articulators**.

BIBLIOGRAPHY AND READING LIST

Abramson, A. S., L. Lisker, and F. Cooper, "Laryngeal Activity in Stop Consonants," *Haskins Labs. Status Rep. on Speech Res.*, SR-4, 1965, 6.1–6.13.

Aikin, W. A., "The Separate Functions of Different Parts of the Rima Glottidis," *J. Anat. and Physiol.*, 16, 1902, 253–256.

Alipour-Haqhiqi, F., I. Titze, and P. Durham. "Twitch Response in the Canine Vocalis Muscle." *J. Sp. Hrng. Res.*, 30, 1987, 290–294.

Allen, E. L., and H. Hollien, "A Laminagraphic Study of Pulse (Vocal Fry) Register Phonation," *Folia Phoniat.*, 25, 1973, 241–250.

Ardran, G., "The Mechanism of the Larynx, the Movements of the Arytenoid and Cricoid Cartilages," *Brit. J. Radiol.*, 39, 1966, 640–654.

Ardran, G., and F. Kemp, "The Mechanism of Swallowing," *Proc. Roy. Soc. Med.*, 1951, 1038–1040.

Ardran, G., and F. Kemp, "The Mechanism of Swallowing," *Dent. Pract.*, 5, 1955, 252–263.

Ardran, G., and F. Kemp, "The Mechanism of the Larynx I. The Movements of the Arytenoid and Cricoid Cartilages," *Brit. J. Radiol.*, 39, 1966, 641–654.

Ardran, G., and F. Kemp. "The Mechanism of the Larynx II. The Epiglottis and Closure of the Larynx.," *Brit. J. Radiol.*, 40, 1967, 372–389.

Arkebauer, H. J., T. Hixon, and J. Hardy, "Peak Intraoral Air Pressures During Speech," *J. Sp. Hrng. Res.*, 10, 1967, 196–208.

Arnold, G. E., "Physiology and Pathology of the Cricothyroid Muscle," *Laryngoscope*, 71, 1961, 687–753.

Babington, Benjamin, "Proceedings of the Humanitarian Society," *London Medical Gazette*, 10, 1829, 555.

Baisler, P. E., "A Study of Intra-laryngeal Activity of Voice in Normal and Falsetto Registers," Ph.D. diss, Northwestern Univ., 1950, Abstr., *Sp. Monog.*, 1951, 174.

Baken, R. J., "Neuromuscular Spindles in the Intrinsic Muscles of a Human Larynx," *Folia Phoniat.*, 23, 1971, 204–210.

———, and C. R. Noback, "Neuromuscular Spindles in Intrinsic Muscles of a Human Larynx," *JSHR*, 14, 1971, 513–518.

Barnes, J., "Vital Capacity and Ability in Oral Reading," *Quart. J. Sp.*, 12, 1926, 176–182.

Basmajian, J. V., and C. R. Dutta, "Electromyography of the Pharyngeal Constrictors and Levator Palati in Man," *Anat. Record*, 139, 1961a, 561–563.

———, "Electromyography of the Pharyngeal Constrictors and Soft Palate in Rabbits," *Anat. Record*, 139, 1961b, 443–449.

Beaunis, H., and A. Bouchard, *Nouveaux Elements d'Anatomie Descriptive*. Paris: J. B. Bailliere et fils, 1868.

Behringer, S., "Die Anordnung der Muskultur in der menschlichen Stimmlippe und im Gebiet des Connus elasticus," *Zeitschrift fur Anatomie und Enwicklungsgeschichte*, 117, 1955, 324–342.

Bell-Berti, F., "Control of Pharyngeal Cavity Size for English Voiced and Unvoiced Cognates," *J. Acoust. Soc. Amer.*, 57, 1975, 456–461.

Berg, Jw. van den, "Sur les theories myo-elastique et neurochronaxique de la phonation," *Rev. de Laryngol.*, (Bordeaux), 1954, 495–512.

———, "On the Role of the Laryngeal Ventricle in Voice Production," *Folia Phoniat.*, 7, 1955a, 57–69.

———, "Transmission of the Vocal Cavities," *J. Acoust. Soc. Amer.*, 27, 1955b, 161–168.

———, "Direct and Indirect Determination of Mean Subglottic Pressure," *Folia Phoniat.*, 8, 1956, 1–24.

———, "Subglottic Pressure and Vibrations of the Vocal Folds," *Folica Phoniat.*, 9, 1957, 65–71.

———, "Myo-elastic-aerodynamic Theory of Voice Production," *J. Sp. Hrng. Res.*, 1, 1958a, 227–244.

———, "On the Myoelastic-aerodynamic Theory of Voice Production," *Nat. Assoc. Teachers of Singing Bulletin (NATS)*, 14, 1958b, 6–12.

———, "Über die Regelung der Stimmlippenspannung durch von aussen eingreifende Mechanismen," *Folia Phoniat.*, 12, 1960a, 281–293.

———, "An Electrical Analogue of the Trachea, Lungs, and Tissues," *Acta Physiol. Pharmacol. Neerl*, 9, 1960b, 361–385.

———, "Vocal Ligaments versus Registers," *Current Problems in Phoniatrics and Logopedics*, 1, 1960c, 19–34.

———, "Sound Production in Isolated Human Larynges," *Ann. N.Y. Acad. Sci.*, 155, 1968, 18–27.

———, and J. Moll, "Zur Anatomie des menschlichen Musculus Vocalis," *Zeitschrift für Anatomie und Enwicklungsgeschichte*, 117, 1955, 465–470.

———, J. T. Zantema, and P. Doornenball, Jr., "On the Air Resistance and the Bernoulli Effect of the Human Larynx," *J. Acoust. Soc. Amer.*, 29, 1957, 626.

Bernick, H., "A Study of Internal Laryngeal Activities at Low and High Intensities," Master's thesis, University of Illinois, Champaign, Ill., 1963.

Black, J. W., "The Pressure Component in the Production of Consonants," *J. Sp. Hrng. Dis.*, 15, 1950, 207.

Bloothooft, G., "Nievwe ontwikkelingen in de fonetografie," *Logopedie en Foniatrie*, 54, 1982, 78–90.

———, "Some Physiological Accompaniments of Speaking," AD-622976. Springfield, Va.: Clearing House for Fed. Scientific and Tech. Inf., U.S. Dept. Commerce, 1965.

Boone, D., *The Voice and Voice Therapy*, 2nd ed. Englewood Cliffs, N.J.: Prentice-Hall, 1977.

Bordone-Sacerdote, C., and G. Sacerdote, "Investigations on the Movement of the Glottis by Ultrasounds," *Fifth Congress Inter. d'Acoustique*, Sept. 1965, paper A-42.

Brewer, D. W., and S. T. Dana, "Investigations in Laryngeal Physiology: The Canine Larynx," *Ann. of Otol. Rhinol. Laryngol.*, 72, 1963, 1060.

———, and K. Faaborg-Anderson, "Phonation: Clinical Testing Versus Electromyography," *Ann. Otol. Rhinol. Laryngol.*, 69, 1960, 781–804.

Broad, D. J., "Phonation," in F. D. Minifie, T. J. Hixon, and F. Williams, eds., *Normal Aspects of Speech, Hearing, and Language*. Englewood Cliffs, N.J.: Prentice-Hall, 1973.

———, and G. E. Peterson, "The Acoustics of Speech," in L. E. Travis, ed., *Handbook of Speech Pathology and Audiology*, Englewood Cliffs, N.J.: Prentice-Hall, 1971.

Brodnitz, F. S., *Vocal Rehabilitation*. Rochester, Minn.: Whiting Press, 1959.

Buchthal, F., "Electromyography of Intrinsic-Laryngeal Muscles," *Quart. J. Exp. Physiol.*, 44, 1959, 137–148.

———, and K. Faaborg-Anderson, "Electromyography of Laryngeal and Respiratory Muscles: Correlation with Phonation and Respiration," *Ann. Otol. Rhinol. Laryngol.*, 73, 1964, 118.

Carhart, R., "Infra-glottal Resonance and a Cushion Pipe," *Sp. Monog.*, 5, 1938, 65–97.

———, "The Spectra of Model Larynx Tones," *Sp. Monog.*, 8, 1941, 76–84.

Carr, P. B., and D. Trill, "Long-Term Larynx-Excitation Spectra," *J. Acoust. Soc. Amer.*, 36, 1964, 2033.

Casserius, Julius, "The Larynx, Organ of Voice," *Acta Oto-Laryng.*, Suppl., 261, 1969. Translated from the Latin by Malcolm Hast and Erling Holtsmark. Orig. Pub. 1601.

Cates, H. A., and J. V. Basmajian, *Primary Anatomy*, 3rd ed. Baltimore: Williams & Wilkins, 1955.

Cavagna, G. A., and R. Margaria, "An Analysis of the Mechanics of Phonation," *J. Appl. Physiol.*, 1965, 301–307.

Charron, R., "An Instrumental Study of the Mechanisms of Vocal Intensity," Master's thesis, University of Illinois, Champaign, Ill., 1965.

Chevroton, L., and F. Vles, "Cinematographie des Cordes Vocales et de Leurs Annexes Laryngienne," *Comptes Rendus Academie Science*, 156, 1913, 949–952.

Childers, D., D. Hicks, P. Moore, L. Eskenazi, and A. Lalwani, "Electroglottography and Vocal Fold Physiology," *J. Sp. Hrng. Res.*, 33, 1990, 245–254.

Clerf, Louis, "Photography of the Larynx," *Ann. Otol. Rhinol. Laryngol.*, 34, 1925, 101–121.

Coleman, R. F., "Decay Characteristics of Vocal Fry," *Folia Phoniat.*, 15, 1963, 256.

———, "Male and Female Voice Quality and Its Relation to Vowel Formant Frequencies," *J. Sp. Hrng. Res.*, 14, 1971, 565–577.

———, and R. Wendahl, "Vocal Roughness and Stimulus Duration," *Sp. Monog.*, 34, 1967, 85–92.

———, and R. Wendahl, "On the Validity of Laryngeal Photosensor Monitoring," *J. Acoust. Soc. Amer.*, 44, 1968, 1733–1735.

———, J. Mabis, and J. Hinson, "Fundamental Frequency-Sound Pressure Level Profiles of Adult Male and Female Voices," *J. Sp. Hrng. Res.*, 20, 1977, 197–204.

Collier, R., "Physiological Correlates of Intonation Patterns," *J. Acoust. Soc. Amer.*, 58, 1975, 249–255.

Colton, R. H., "Vocal Intensity in the Modal and Falsetto Registers," *Folia Phoniat.*, 25, 1973, 62–70.

———, and H. Hollien, "Phonational Range in the Modal and Falsetto Registers," *J. Sp. Hrng. Res.*, 15, 1972, 708–713.

———, and H. Hollien, "Perceptual Differentiation of the Modal and Falsetto Registers, *Folia Phoniat.*, 25, 1973, 270–280.

Cooper, F. S., "Research Techniques and Instrumentation: EMG," *Amer. Sp. Hrng. Assn. Reports*, No. 1, 1965, 153–168.

———, M. Sawashima, A. Abramson, and L. Lisker, "Looking at the Larynx During Running Speech," *Ann. Otol. Rhinol. Laryngol.*, 85, 1971, 678–682.

Cooper, M., *Modern Techniques of Vocal Rehabilitation.* Springfield, Ill.: Charles C Thomas, 1973.

Crystal, T. H., "Model of Larynx Activity During Phonation," *Mass. Inst. Tech. Quart. Rep.*, No. 78, 1966, 212–219.

Curry, R., *The Mechanism of the Human Voice.* New York: David McKay, 1959.

Curry, S. S., *Mind and Voice.* Boston: Expression Company, 1910.

Czermak, Johann, "Bemurkungen zur Lehr von Mechanismus des Larynx Verschlusses," *Wien Medizinische Wochenschrift*, 10, 1860a, 745–747.

———, *Der Kehlkopfspiegel.* Leipzig: Englemann, 1860b.

———, "Application de la Photographie à la Laryngoscopie et à la Rhinoscopie," *Comptes Rendus Academie Science*, 1861.

Damste, R. H., "The Phonetogram," *Practica Oto-Rhino-Laryng.*, 32, 1970.

Damste, P. H., and G. H. Wieneke, "Experiments on the Elasticity of the Vocal Cords," *J. S. African Speech Hrng. Assoc.*, 20, 1973, 14–21.

Dedo, H. H., "Electromyographic and Visual Evaluation of Recurrent Laryngeal Nerve Anastomosis in Dogs," *Ann. Otol. Rhinol. Laryngol.*, 85, 1971, 664–668.

DeWeese, D., and William Saunders, *Textbook of Otolatyngology*, 2nd ed. St. Louis: C. V. Mosby, 1977.

Dickson, D. R., J. C. Grant, H. Sicher, E. L. Debrul, and J. Paltan, "Status of Research in Cleft Lip and Palate: Anatomy and Physiology, Part 2," *Cleft Palate J.*, 12, 1975, 131–156.

Dodart, M., "Sur les Causes de la Voix de l'Homme, et de ses Differens Tons," *Memoires de l'Academie Royale des Sciences*, 1700, 256–266.

———, "Supplement au Memoire sur la Voix et les Tons," *Memoires de l'Acadamie Royale des Sciences*, 1707–1773.

Donovan, R., "Variables of Laryngeal Tone," *Folia Phoniat.*, 19, 1967, 281.

Draper, M. H., P. Ladefoged, and D. M. Whitteridge, "Expiratory Pressures and Air Flow During Speech," *British Medical J.*, 1, 1960, 1837–1843.

Duffy, R. J., "Fundamental Frequency Characteristics of Adolescent Females," *Lang. Speech*, 13, 1970, 14–24.

———, "Description and Perception of Frequency Breaks (Voice Breaks) in Adolescent Female Speakers," *Lang. Speech*, 13, 1970, 151–161.

Dunker, E., and B. Schlosshauer, "Klinische und experimentelle studien uber Stimmlippenschwingungen," *Archiv für Ohren-Nasen und Kehlkopfheilkunde*, 172, 1958, 363.

Ekberg, O., and S. Sigurjohsson, "Movement of the Epiglottis During Deglutition," *Gastrointestinal Radiology*, 7, 1982, 101–107.

Eskenazi, L., D. Childers, and D. Hicks, "Acoustic Correlates of Vocal Quality," *J. Sp. Hrng. Res.*, 33, 1990, 289–306.

Ewald, J. R., "Die physiologie des Kehlkopfes und der Luftrohre," in Paul Heymann, ed., *Handbuch der Laryngologie and Rhinologie*, Vienna, 1898.

Faaborg-Anderson, K., "Electromyographic Investigation of Intrinsic Laryngeal Muscles in Humans," *Acta Physiologica Scandinavica*, 41, Suppl. 140, 1957.

———, "Electromyography of Laryngeal Muscles in Humans: Techniques and Results," in F. Trojan, ed., *Current Problems in Phoniatrics and Logopedics*, Vol. III. Basel: S. Karger, 1965.

———, and A. Sonninen, "The Function of the Extrinsic Laryngeal Muscles at Different Pitch," *Acta Oto-Laryngol.*, Stockholm, 51, 1960, 89–93.

———, and William Vennard, "Electromyography of Extrinsic Laryngeal Muscles During Phonation of Different Vowels," *Ann. Otol. Rhinol. Laryngol.*, 73, 1964, 248.

Fairbanks, G., "An Acoustical Study of the Pitch of Infant Hunger Wails," *Child Development*, 13, 1942, 227–232.

———, *Voice and Articulation Drillbook*, 2nd ed. New York: Harper & Row, 1959.

———, E. L. Herbert, and J. M. Hammond, "An Acoustical Study of Vocal Pitch in Seven- and Eight-Year-Old Girls," *Child Development*, 20, 1949, 71–78.

———, J. H. Wiley, and F. M. Lassman, "An Acoustical Study of Vocal Pitch in Seven- and Eight-Year-Old-Boys," *Child Development*, 20, 1949, 63–69.

Fant, G., *Acoustic Theory of Speech Production.* The Hague: Mouton, 1960.

———, and B. Sonesson, "Indirect Studies of Glottal Cycles by Synchronous Inverse Filtering and Photo-electrical Glottography," *STL/QPR*, 4, 1962, 1–2.

Farnsworth, D. W., "High-Speed Motion Pictures of the Vocal Cords," *Bell Lab. Record*, 18, 1940, 203–208.

Ferguson, G. B., and W. J. Crowder, "A Simple Method of Laryngeal and Other Cavity Photography," *Arch. Otolaryngol.*, 92, 1970, 201–203.

Ferrein, A., "De la Formation de la Voix de l'Homme," *Historie de l'Academie Royale des Sciences de Paris.* Tome 51, 1741, 4–9.

Fessard, A., and B. Vallencien, "Données Electrophysiologiques sur le Fonctionnement de l'Appareil Phonatoire du Chien," *Folia Phoniat.*, 9, 1957, 152–163.

Fink, B. R., "Tensor Mechanism of the Vocal Folds," *Ann. Otol. Rhinol. Laryngol.*, 71, 1962, 591–600.

———, "Spring Mechanisms in the Human Larynx," *Acta Oto-Laryngol.*, 77, 1974a, 295–304.

———, "Folding Mechanisms of the Human Larynx," *Acta Oto-Laryngol.*, 78, 1974b, 124–128.

———, *The Human Larynx: A Functional Study.* New York: Raven Press, 1975.

———, and F. Kirschner, "Observations on the Acoustical and Mechanical Properties of the Vocal Folds," *Folia Phoniat.*, 11, 1959, 167.

Fischer-Jørgensen, E., and A. T. Hansen, "An Electrical Manometer and Its Use in Phonetic Research," *Phonetica*, 4, 1959, 43.

Fishman, B. V., R. E. McGlone, and T. Shipp, "The Effects of Certain Drugs on Phonation," *J. Sp. Hrng. Res.*, 14, 1971, 301–306.

Fitch, J. L., and A. Holbrook, "Modal Vocal Fundamental Frequency of Young Adults," *Arch. Otolaryngol.*, 92, 1970, 379–382.

Flanagan, J. L., "Some Properties of the Glottal Sound Source," *J. Sp. Hrng. Res.*, 1, 1958, 99–116.

———, "Estimates of Intraglottal Pressure During Phonation," *J. Sp. Hrng. Res.*, 2, 1959, 168–172.

———, *Speech Analysis, Synthesis, and Perception.* Berlin: Springer, 1972.

———, "Voices of Men and Machines," *J. Acoust. Soc. Amer.*, 51, 1972, 1375–1387.

———, and L. Landgraf, "Self-oscillating Source for Vocal Tract Synthesizers," *Conf. on Speech Communication and Professions*, M.I.T., 1967.

Fletcher, H., *Speech and Hearing.* Princeton, N.J.: D. Van Nostrand, 1929.

———, *Speech and Hearing in Communication.* Princeton, N.J.: D. Van Nostrand, 1953.

Fletcher, Wm. W., "A High-Speed Motion Picture Study of Vocal Fold Action in Certain Voice Qualities," Master's thesis, University of Washington, Seattle, Wash., 1947.

———, "A Study of Internal Laryngeal Activity in Relation to Vocal Intensity," Ph.D. diss., Northwestern University, Evanston, Ill., 1950.

Floyd, W. F., V. E. Negus, and E. Neil, "Observations on the Mechanism of Phonation," *Acta Otolaryngol.*, 48, 1957, 16–25.

Fourcin, A. J., "Laryngographic Examination of Vocal Fold Vibration," in B. Wyke, ed., *Ventilatory and Phonatory Control Systems.* London: Oxford University Press, 1974.

Fourcin, A. J., "Laryngographic Assessment of Phonatory Function," in C. L. Ludlow and M. O. Hart, eds., *Proceedings of the Conference of the Assessment of Vocal Fold Pathology.* ASHA Reports 11, 116–128. Rockville, MD: American Speech-Language-Hearing Association, 1982.

French, Thomas R., "On a Perfected Method of Photographing the Larynx," *N.Y. Med. J.*, 1884, 653.

———, "The Laryngeal Image Photographed During the Production of Tones in the Singing Voice," *Transactions of the American Laryngological Association*, 8, 1886, 107.

Freudenthal, Wolff, "On Transillumination of the Larynx and of the Sinus Maxillaris, with Special Reference to Voltolini's Work," *Amer. J. Medicine*, 23, 1917, 511–513.

Fromkin, V., and P. Ladefoged, "Electromyography in Speech Research," *Phonetica*, 15, 1966, 219–242.

Fry, D. L., W. W. Stead, R. V. Ebert, R. E. Lubin, and H. Wells, "The Measurement of Intraesophageal Pressure and Its Relationship to Intrathoracic Pressure," *J. Lab. and Clin. Med.*, 40, 1952, 664–673.

Fukuda, H., and J. A. Kirchner, "Changes in the Respiratory Activity of the Cricothyroid Muscle with Intrathoracic Interruption of the Vagus Nerve," *Ann. Otol. Rhinol. Laryngol.*, 81, 1972, 532–537.

Fukuda, H., C. T. Sasaki, and J. A. Kirchner, "Vagal Afferent Influences on the Phasic Activity of the Posterior Crioarytenoid Muscle," *Acta Oto-Laryngol.*, 75, 1973, 112–118.

Garcia, Manuel, "Observations on the Human voice," *London, Edinborough, and Dublin Philosophical Magazine and Journal of Science*, 10, 1855, 511–513.

———, *Hints on Singing.* New York: E. Schuberth, 1894.

Garel, J., "Nouvel Appareil Perfectionné pour la Photographie Stéréoscopique du Larynx sur le Vivant," *Review de Laryngologie*, 40, 1919, 249.

Gay, T., and K. S. Harris, "Some Recent Developments in the Use of Electromyography in Speech Research," *J. Sp. Hrng. Res.*, 14, 1971, 241–246.

———, M. Strome, H. Hirose, and M. Sawashima, "Electromyography of the Intrinsic Laryngeal Muscles During Phonation," *Ann. Otol. Rhinol. Laryngol.*, 81, 1972, 401–409.

Gilbert, H. R., C. Potter, and R. Hoodin, "Laryngograph as a Measure of Vocal Fold Contact Area, *J. Sp. Hrng. Res.*, 27, 1984, 173–178.

Gill, J. S., "Automatic Extraction of the Excitation Function of Speech with Particular Reference to the Use of Correlation Methods," *Proc. III Int. Congr. Acoust.*, Stuttgart, 1, 1959, 214–216.

———, "Recent Research on Methods for Automatic Estimation of Vocal Excitation," *Proc. Fourth Int. Congr. Phon. Sci.*, Helsinki, A. Souijarui and P. Aulto, eds. The Hague: Mouton & Co., 1962, 167–172.

———, "Estimation of Larynx-Pulse Timing During Speech," *Proc. Stockholm Speech Comm, Sem.*, 1, 1962.

Göerttler, K., "Die Anordnung, Histologie und Histogenese der quergestreiften Muskulatur in menschlichen Stimmband," *Zeitschrift für Anatomy und Enwicklungsgeschichte*, 115, 1950, 352–401.

Gottstein, J., "Die Durchleutung des Kehlkopfs," *Deutsche Medizinishe Wochenschrift*, 15, 1889, 140–141.

Gould, W. J., G. J. Jako, and M. Tanabe, "Advances in High-Speed Motion Picture Photography of the Larynx," *Trans. Amer. Acad. Ophthalmol. Otolaryngol.*, 78, 1974, 276–278.

Gray, G. W., "An Experimental Study of the Vibrato in Speech," *Quart. J. Speech Ed.*, 12, 1926, 296–333.

———, "Some Persistent Questions in Vocal Theory," *Quart. J. Sp.*, 2, 1934, 185–194.

Greene, M. C. L., *The Voice and Its Disorders.* New York: Macmillan, 1957.

Gross, W. B., "Voice Production by the Turkey," *Poultry Science*, 47, 1968, 1101–1105.

Grutzner, P., "Physiologie der Stimme und Sprache," *Handbuch der Physiologie*, 1, Berlin, 1879.

Gupta, V., and G. S. Beavers, "A Model for Vocal Cord Excitation," *J. Acoust. Soc. Amer.*, 54, 1973, 1607–1617.

Haglund, S., "The Normal Electromyogram in Human Cricothyroid Muscle," *Acta Oto-Laryngol.*, 75, 1973, 448–453.

Hamlet, S. L., "Vocal Compensation: An Ultrasonic Study of Vocal Fold Vibration in Normal and Nasal Vowels," *Cleft Palate J.*, 10, 267–285.

Hanson, D., B. Gerratt, and G. Berke, "Frequency, Intensity, and Target Matching Effects," *J. Sp. Hrng. Res.*, 33, 1990, 45–50.

Harden, J., "Comparison of Glottal Area Changes as Measured from Ultra High-Speed Photographs and Photoelectric Glottographs," *J. Sp. Hrng. Res.*, 18, 1975, 728–738.

Hardy, J. C., "Air Flow and Air Pressure Studies," *Amer. Sp. Hrng. Assoc. Reports No. 1*, 1965, 141–152.

———, "Techniques of Measuring Intraoral Air Pressure and Rate of Air flow," Letter to ed., *J. Sp. Hrng. Res.*, 10, 1967, 650.

Hast, M. H., "Subglottic Air Pressure and Neural Stimulation in Phonation," *J. Appl. Physiol.*, 16, 1961, 1142–1146.

———, "Physiological Mechanism of Phonation: Tension of the Vocal Fold Muscle," *Acta Oto-Laryngol.*, 62, 1966a, 309–318.

———, "Mechanical Properties of the Cricothyroid Muscle," *Laryngoscope*, 76, 1966b, 537–548.

———, "Mechanical Properties of the Vocal Fold Muscle," *Practica Oto-Rhino-Laryngol.*, 29, 1967, 53–56.

———, and S. Golbus, "Physiology of the Lateral Cricoarytenoid Muscle," *Practica Oto-Rhino-Laryngol.*, 33, 1971, 209–214.

———, and B. Milojevie, "The Response of the Vocal Folds to Electrical Stimulation of the Inferior Frontal Cortex of the Squirrel Monkey," *Acta Oto-Laryngol.*, 61, 1965, 196–204.

Hegener, J., and G. Panconcelli-Calzia, "Eine einfache Kinematographie und die Strobokinematographie der Stimmlippen bewegungen bein lebenden," *Vox*, 23, 1913, 81–82.

Heller, S. S., W. R. Hicks, and W. S. Root, "Lung Volumes of Singers," *J. Appl. Physiol.*, 15, 1960, 21–40.

Helmholtz, H. von, *On the Sensations of Tone*, trans. A. J. Ellis. New York: David McKay, 1912.

Hermann, J., "Photographische Untersuchungen," *Pflüger's Archiv für die Geschichte Physiologie*, 74, 1890, 380.

Hertz, C. H., K. Lindstrom, and B. Sonesson, "Ultrasonic Recording of the Vibrating Vocal Folds," *Acta Oto-Laryngol.*, 69, 1969, 223–230.

Hirano, M., "Intranasal Sound Pressure During Utterance of Speech Sounds," *Folia Phoniat.*, 18, 1966, 369–381.

———, "Morphological Structure of the Vocal Cord as a Vibrator and Its Variations," *Folia Phoniat.*, 26, 1974, 89–94.

———, *Phonosurgery*, Official Report of the 76th Annual Convention of the Oto-Rhino-Laryngological Society of Japan, May, 1975.

———, *Clinical Examination of Voice*. New York: Springer-Verlag, 1981.

———, Y. Koike, and H. von Leden, "The Sternohyoid Muscle During Phonation," *Acta Oto-Laryngol.*, 64, 1967, 500–507.

———, and J. Ohala, "Use of Hooked-Wire Electrodes for Electromyography of the Intrinsic Laryngeal Muscles," *J. Sp. Hrng. Res.*, 12, 1969, 362–373.

———, S. Kurita, and T. Nakashima, "Growth, Development and Aging of Human Vocal Folds." Paper presented at Vocal Fold Physiology Conference, Madison, Wisc., May 31, 1981.

———, J. Ohala, and William Vennard, "The Function of Laryngeal Muscles in Regulating Fundamental Frequency and Intensity of Phonation," *J. Sp. Hrng. Res.*, 12, 1969, 616–628.

Hirose, H., and T. Gay, "Laryngeal Control in Vocal Attack. An Electromographic Study," *Folia Phoniat.*, 25, 1973, 203–213.

Hiroto, I., "Pathophysiology of the Larynx from the Point of View of Vocal Mechanism," *Pract. Otol., Kyoto*, 59, 1966, 229–292 (Japanese text).

———, M. Hirano, Y. Toyozuma, and T. Shin, "Electromyographic Investigation of the Intrinsic Laryngeal Muscles Related to Speech Sounds," *Ann. Otol. Rhinol. Laryngol.*, 76, 1967, 861–872.

Hixon, T., "Turbulent Noise Sources for Speech," *Folia Phoniat.*, 18, 1966, 168–182.

Hoit, J., and T. Hixon, "Age and Airway Resistance During Vowel Production in Women," *J. Sp. Hrng. Res.*, 35, 1992, 309–313.

Holliday, J., "Light and Electron Microscopy of the Epithelium of the Human True Vocal Cord, *Laryngoscope*, 86, 1976, 1596–1601.

Hollien, H., "Some Laryngeal Correlates of Vocal Pitch," *J. Sp. Hrng. Res.*, 3, 1960a, 52–58.

———, "Vocal Pitch Variations Related to Changes in Vocal Fold Length," *J. Sp. Hrng. Res.*, 3, 1960b, 150–156.

———, "The Relationship of Vocal Fold Length to Vocal Pitch for Female Subjects," *Proc. XII Int. Speech and Voice Therapy Conf.*, Padua, 1962a.

———, "The Relationship of Vocal Fold Thickness to Absolute Fundamental Frequency of Phonation," *Proc. Fourth Int. Congr. Phon. Sci.* Helsinki, A. Sovigarvi and P. Aalto, eds. The Hague: Mouton, 1962b, 173–177.

———, "Vocal Fold Thickness and Fundamental Frequency of Phonation," *J. Sp. Hrng. Res.*, 5, 1962c, 237–243.

———, "Laryngeal Research By Means of Laminagraphy," *Archiv. of Otolaryngol.*, 80, 1964, 303–308.

———, and R. F. Coleman, "Laryngeal Correlates of Frequency Change: A STROL Study, *J. Sp. Hrng. Res.*, 13, 1970, 271–278.

———, and R. H. Colton, "Four Laminagraphic Studies of Vocal Fold Thickness," *Folia Phoniat.*, 21, 1969, 179–198.

———, and J. F. Curtis, "A Laminagraphic Study of Vocal Pitch," *J. Sp. Hrng. Res.*, 3, 1960, 361–371.

———, and J. F. Curtis, "Elevation and Tilting of Vocal Folds as a Function of Vocal Pitch," *Folia Phoniat.*, 14, 1962, 23–36.

———, and G. P. Moore, "Measurements of the Vocal Folds During Changes in Pitch," *J. Sp. Hrng. Res.*, 3, 1960, 157–165.

———, and P. Moore, "Stroboscopic Laminagraphy of the Larynx during Phonation," *Acta Oto-Laryngol.*, 65, 1968, 209–215.

———, and R. Wendahl, "Perceptual Study of Vocal Fry," *J. Acoust. Soc. Amer.*, 43, 1968, 506–509.

———, J. F. Curtis, and R. Coleman, "Investigation of Laryngeal Phenomena by Stroboscopic Laminagraphy," *Med. Res. Eng.*, 7, 1968, 24–27.

———, G. P. Moore, R. Wendahl, and J. Michel, "On the Nature of Vocal Fry," *J. Sp. Hrng. Res.*, 9, 1966, 245–247.

Holmes, J. N., "An Investigation of the Volume Velocity Waveform at the Larynx During Speech by Means of an Inverse Filter," *Proc. Stockholm Speech Comm. Sem.*, 1962.

Holstead, L., "Thoracic and Laryngeal Interaction in Regulating Subglottal Pressure During Phonation," Ph.D. diss., University of Illinois, Champaign, Ill., 1972.

Horii, Y., "Frequency Modulation Characteristics of Sustained /a/ Sung in Vocal Vibrato," *J. Sp. Hrng. Res.*, 32, 1989.

Hsu, Y.-H., Y.-H. Liu, and T.-C. Leng, "Anatomical Study of the Recurrent Laryngeal Nerve," *Chinese Med. J.*, 81, 1962, 481–484.

Husson, R., "Étude des Phenomemes Physiologiques et Acoustiques Foundamentaux de la Voix Chantee," Thesis, University of Paris, Paris, 1950.

———, "A New Look at Phonation," *Nat. Assoc. Teachers of Singing Bulletin (NATS)* 13, 1956, 12–13.

———, "Special Physiology in Singing Power," *Nat. Assoc. Teachers of Singing Bulletin (NATS)*, 14, 1957, 12–15.

———, "The Classification of Human Voices," *Nat. Assoc. Teachers of Singing Bulletin (NATS)*, 13, 1957, 671.

Husson, R., and A. DiJiab, "Tomographie et Phonation," *J. de Radiol. Electrol.*, 33, 1952, 127–135.

Ingelstedt, S., and N. G. Toremohm, "Aerodynamics Within the Larynx and Trachea," *Acta Otolaryngol., Suppl.* 158, 81–92.

Ishizaka, K., and J. L. Flanagan, "Acoustic Properties of a Two-Mass Model of the Vocal Cords," *J. Acoust. Soc. Amer.*, 51, 1972, 91.

———, and M. Matsudaira, "Fluid Mechanical Considerations of Vocal Cord Vibration," *SCRL Monograph No. 8*, Speech Communications Research Laboratory, Santa Barbara, 1972.

———, and M. Matsudaira, "What Makes the Vocal Cords Vibrate?" In Y. Kohasi, ed., *The 6th International Congress on Acoustics*, Vol. II. New York: Elsevier, B-9–B-12.

Isshiki, N., "Regulatory Mechanism of the Pitch and Volume of Voice," *Otorhinolaryngology Clinic*, Kyoto, 52, 1959, 1065.

———, "Voice and Subglottic Pressure," *Studia Phonologica*, 1, 1961, 86.

———, Regulatory Mechanisms of Voice Intensity Variation," *J. Sp. Hrng. Res.*, 1964, 17–29.

———, "Vocal Intensity and Air Flow Rate," *Folia Phoniat.*, 17, 1965, 92.

———, and R. Ringel, "Air Flow During the Production of Selected Consonants," *J. Sp. Hrng. Res.*, 7, 1964, 233–244.

Isshiki, N., and H. von Leden, "Laryngeal Movement During Coughing," *Studia Phonologica*, 3, 1963/4, 1.

Ito, H., "Histoanatomical Studies of the Intrinsic Laryngeal Muscles," *Studia Phonologica*, 1, 1961, 117.

Jensen, P., "Adequacy of Terminology for Clinical Judgment of Voice Quality Deviation," *Eye, Ear, Nose, and Throat Monthly*, 44, 1965, 77–82.

Judson, L. S., and A. T. Weaver, *Voice Science*, 2nd ed. New York: Appleton-Century-Crofts, 1965.

Kahane, J., "The Developmental Anatomy of the Human Prepubertal and Pubertal Larynx," Ph.D. diss., University of Pittsburgh, 1975.

———, "A Morphological Study of the Human Prepubertal and Pubertal Larynx," *Amer. J. of Anat.*, 151, 1978, 11–20.

———, "Age Related Histological Changes in the Human Male and Female Laryngeal Cartilages: Biological and Functional Implications," in V. Lawrence, ed., *Transcripts of the Ninth Symposium: Care of the Professional Voice*, Part I. New York: The Voice Foundation, 1980, 11–20.

———, "Postnatal Development and Aging of the Human Larynx," *Seminars in Speech and Language*, 4, 1983a, 189–203.

———, "A Survey of Age-Related Changes in the Connective Tissues of the Larynx," in D. Bless and J. Abbs, eds., *Vocal Fold Physiology*. San Diego: College-Hill Press, 1983.

Kahane, J., and A. Kahn, "India Pinprick Experiments on Surface Organization of Cricoarytenoid Joints," *J. Sp. Hrng. Res.*, 29, 1986, 544–548.

Kahn, A., and J. Kahane, "India Ink Pinprick Experiments on Surface Organization of Cricoarytenoid Joint (CAJ) Articular Surfaces," *J. Sp. Hrng. Res.*, 29, 1986, 536–543.

Kakita, Y., "Investigation of Laryngeal Control in Speech by Use of a Thyrometer. *J. Acoust. Soc. Amer.*, 59, 1976, 669–674.

Kaplan, H. L., *Anatomy and Physiology of Speech*. New York: McGraw-Hill, 1960.

Kaplan, M., and E. F. Kaplan, "Binary Recording of Vocalization and Gross Body Movement in Psychophysiological Study of Dogs. *J. Exper. Annals Behavior*, 6, 1963, 617–619.

Karnell, M., "Laryngeal Perturbation Analysis: Minimum Length of Analysis Window," *J. Sp. Hrng. Res.*, 34, 1991, 544–548.

Keenan, J. S., and G. C. Banett, "Intralaryngeal Relationships During Pitch and Intensity Changes," *J. Sp. Hrng. Res.*, 1962, 173–178.

Kelleher, R. E., R. C. Webster, R. J. Coffey, and L. Quigley, "Nasal and Oral Air Flow in Normal and Cleft Palate Speech: Velocity and Volume Studies, Using Warm Wire Meter and Two Channel Recorder," *Cleft Palate Bulletin*, 10, 1960, 1966.

Kempelen, W. von, *Mechanismus der menschlichen Sprache*. Wien: 1791.

Kent, R., and K. Moll, "Vocal-Tract Characteristics of the Stop Cognates," *J. Acoust. Soc. Amer.*, 46, 1969, 1549–1555.

Keros, P., and D. Nemanic, "The Terminal Branching of the Recurrent Laryngeal Nerve." *Pract. Oto-Rhino-Laryngol.*, 29, 1967, 5–10.

Kitzing, P., and B. Sonesson, "A Photoglottographical Study of the Female Vocal Folds During Phonation," *Folia Phoniat.*, 26, 1974, 138–149.

Koike, Y., and M. Hirano, "Glottal-Area Function and Subglottal-Pressure Variation," *J. Acoust. Soc. Amer.*, 54, 1973, 1618–1627.

Kotby, M. N., and L. K. Haugen, "The Mechanics of Laryngeal Function," *Acta Oto-laryngol.*, 70, 1970, 203–211.

———, "Critical Evaluation of the Action of the Posterior Cricoarytenoid Muscle Utilizing Direct EMG Study," *Acta Oto-laryngol.*, 70, 1970, 260–268.

Kovac, Akos, "Asymmetric Roentgenography of the Vocal Cords," *Acta Radiologica*, 53, 1960, 426–431.

Koyama, T., E. J. Harvey, and J. H. Ogura, "Mechanics of Voice Production, II. Regulation of Pitch.," *Laryngoscope*, 81, 1971, 47–65.

Kunze, L. H., An Investigation of the Ranges in Sub-glottal Air Pressure and Rate of Air Flow Accompanying Changes in Fundamental Frequency, Intensity, Vowels, and Voice Registers in Adult Male Speakers," Ph.D. diss., State University of Iowa, Iowa City, Iowa, 1962.

———, "Evaluation of Methods of Estimating Sub-glottal Air Pressure," *J. Sp. Hrng. Res.*, 7, 1964, 151–164.

Kwalwasser, J., "The Vibrato," *Psychological Monogr.*, 36, 1926, 84–108.

Ladefoged, P., "The Regulation of Sub-glottal Pressure," *Folia Phoniat.*, 12, 1960, 169–175.

———, "Physiological Studies of Speech," *Kungl. Tekniska Högskolan (KTH), Speech Transmission Laboratory (STL), Quarterly Progress Report (QPR)*, 3, 1961, 16–21.

———, "Subglottal Activity During Speech," in *Proc. of the Fourth Int'l Cong. of Phonetic Sciences*, Helsinki, 1961. The Hague: Mouton, 1962, 73–91.

———, "Some Physiological Parameters in Speech," *Lang. and Speech*, 6, 1963, 109–119.

———, M. H. Draper, and D. Whitteridge, "Syllables and Stress," *Miscellanea Phonetica*, 3, 1958, 1–14.

———, and V. Fromkin, "Electromyography in Speech Research," *UCLA Working Papers in Phonetics*, 2, 1965, 37–50.

———, and N. P. McKinney, "Loudness, Sound Pressure, and Subglottal Pressure in Speech," *J. Acoust. Soc. Amer.*, 35, 1963, 454–460.

Laitman, J., and E. Crelin, "Postnatal Development of the Basiocranium and Vocal Tract Region in Man," in J. Bosma, ed., *Symposium on Development of the Basiocranium.* Washington, D.C.: Department of Health, Education, and Welfare, 1976, 206–220.

Large, J., S. Iwata, and H. von Leden, "The Male Operatic Head Register Versus Falsetto," *Folia Phoniat.*, 24, 1972, 19–29.

Larson, C., G. Kempster, and M. Kistler, "Changes in Voice Fundamental Frequency Following Discharge of Single Motor Units in Cricothyroid and Thyroarytenoid Muscles," *J. Sp. Hrng. Res.*, 30, 1987, 552–558.

Lebrun, Y., "On the Activity of Thoraco-Abdominal Muscles During Phonation," *Folia Phoniat.*, 18, 1966, 354–368.

———, and J. Hasquin-Deleval, "On the So-called 'Dissociations' Between Electroglottogram and Phonogram," *Folia Phoniat.* 23, 1971, 225–227.

Leden, H. von, "The Peripheral Nervous System of the Human Larynx," *Arch. of Otolaryngol.*, 74, 1961a, 494–500.

———, "The Mechanism of Phonation" *Arch. of Otolaryngol.*, 74, 1961b, 660–676.

———, and N. Isshiki, "An Analysis of Cough at the Level of the Larynx," *Arch. of Otolaryngol.*, 81, 1965, 616–625.

———, and P. Moore, "The Mechanics of the Cricoarytenoid Joint," *Arch. of Otolaryngol.*, 73, 1961, 541–550.

———, M. Le Cover, R. L. Ringel, and N. Isshiki, "Improvements in Laryngeal Cinematography," *Arch. of Otolaryngol.*, 83, 1966, 482–487.

Lejune, F. E., R. H. Cox, and C. J. Haindel, "Review of the Available Literature on the Larynx for 1962," *The Laryngoscope*, 73, 1963, 1529–1588.

Lennox-Browne, "On Photography of the Larynx and Soft Palate," *British Medical Journal*, 2, 1883, 811–814.

Leonard, R., R. Ringel, Y. Horii, and R. Daniloff, "Vocal Shadowing in Singers and Non-singers," *J. Sp. Hrng. Res.*, 31, 1988.

Lieberman, P., "Pitch Perturbations of Normal and Pathological Larynxes," *Proc. Stockholm Speech Comm. Sem.*, 1, 1962.

———, R. Knudson, and J. Mead, "Determination of the Rate of Change of Fundamental Frequency with Respect to Subglottal Air Pressure During Sustained Phonation," *J. Acoust. Soc. Amer.*, 45, 1969, 1537–1543.

Lindqvist, J., "Inverse Filtering: Instrumentation and Techniques," *Kungl. Tekniska Högskolan (KTH), Speech Transmission Laboratory (STL), Quarterly Progress Report (QPR)*, 4, 1964, 1–4.

———, "Studies of the Voice Source by Means of Inverse Filtering," *Kungl. Tekniska Högskolan (KTH), Speech Transmission Laboratory (STL), Quarterly Progress Report (QPR)*, 2, 1965, 8–13.

Linville, S. E., "Glottal Gap Configuration in Two Age Groups of Women." *J. Sp. Hrng. Res.*, 35, 1992, 1209–1215.

Lisker, L., "Supraglottal Air Pressure in the Production of English Stops," *Haskins Labs. Status Rep. On Speech Res.*, SR-4, 1965, 3.1–3.15.

———, A. S. Abramson, F. S. Cooper, and M. H. Schvey, "Transillumination of the Larynx in Running Speech," *J. Acoust. Soc. Amer.*, 45, 1969, 1544–1546.

Liskovius, K. F., *Physiologie der menschichen Stimme.* Leipzig: 1846.

Lubker, J. F., "Simultaneous Oral-Nasal Air-Flow Measurements and Cinefluorographic Observations During Speech Production," Master's thesis, State University of Iowa, Iowa City, Iowa, 1962.

———, "A Consideration of Transglottal Airflow During Stop Consonant Production," *J. Acoust. Soc. Amer.*, 53, 1973, 212–215.

———, and K. L. Moll, "Simultaneous Oral-Nasal Air Flow Measurements and Cinefluorographic Observations During Speech Production," *Cleft Palate J.*, 2, 1965, 257–272.

Luchsinger, V. R., and C. Dubois, "Phonetische und Stroboskopische Untersuchungen on einem Stimmphenomen," *Folia Phoniat.*, 8, 1956, 201–210.

———, and K. Pfister, "Die messung der Stimmlippen ver langerung beim steigern der Tonhole" (The measurement of the lengthening of the vocal folds during pitch change), *Folia Phoniat.*, 13, 1961, 1–12.

Machida, J., "Air Flow Rate and Articulatory Movement During Speech," *Cleft Palate J.*, 4, 1967, 240–248.

Malannino, N., "Laryngeal Neuromuscular Spindles and Their Possible Function," *Folia Phoniat.*, 26, 1974, 291–292.

Malecot, A., "An Experimental Study of Force of Articulation," *Studia Linguistica*, 9, 1955, 35–43.

———, and K. Peebles, "An Optical Device for Recording Glottat Adduction-Abduction During Normal Speech," *Zeitschrift für Phonetik, Sprachwissenschaft und Kommunikationsforschung*, Band 18, Heft 6, 1965. Berlin: Akademie-Verlag, 545–550.

Malinowski, A., "Shape, Dimensions, and Process of Calcification of the Cartilagious Framework of the Larynx in Relation to Age and Sex in the Polish Population," *Folia Morphologica*, 26, 1967, 118–128.

Manjome, T., "The Anatomical Studies on the Laryngeal Muscles of the Japanese," *J. Oto-Rhino-Laryngol. Soc. Japan*, 62, 1959, 1890–1901.

Marinacci, A. A., *Applied Electromyography.* Philadelphia: Lea & Febiger, 1968, 298,

Martenson, A., and C. R. Sköglund, "Contraction Properties of Intrinsic Laryngeal Muscles," *Acta Physiol. Scand.*, 60, 1964, 318–336.

Martony, J., "On the Vowel Source Spectrum," *Kungl. Tekniska Högskolan (KTH), Speech Transmission Laboratory (STL), Quarterly Progress Report (QPR)*, 1, 1964, 3–4.

———, "Studies of the Voice Source," *Kungl. Tekniska Högskolan (KTH), Speech Transmission Laboratory (STL), Quarterly Progress Report (QPR)*, 1, 1965, 409.

Mason, R. M., "A Study of the Physiological Mechanisms of Vocal Vibrato," Ph.D. diss., University of Illinois, Champaign, Ill., 1965.

———, and W. R. Zemlin, "The Phenomenon of Vocal Vibrato," *Nat. Assoc. Teachers of Singing Bulletin (NATS)*, 22, 1969, 12–17.

Matsushita, H., "The Vibratory Mode of the Vocal Folds in the Excised Larynx," *Folia Phoniat.*, 27, 1975, 7–18.

Mathews, M. V., J. E. Miller, and E. E. David, Jr., "An Accurate Estimate of the Glottal Wave-Shape," *J. Acoust. Soc. Amer.*, 33, 1961, 843.

Maue, W., "Cartilages, Ligaments, and Articulations of the Adult Human Larynx." Ph.D. diss., University of Pittsburgh, 1970.

———, and D. R. Dickson, "Cartilages and Ligaments of the Adult Human Larynx," *Arch. Otolaryngol.*, 94, 1971, 432–439.

Mayet, A., "Zur functionellen Anatomie der menschlichen Stimmlippe," *Zeitschrift für Anatomy und Enwicklungsgeschichte*, 119, 1955, 87–111.

———, and K. Muendnich, "Beitrag zur Anatomie und zur function des M. Cricothyroideus und der Cricothyreiodgelenke," *Acta Anatomica*, 33, 1958, 273–288.

McGlone, R. E., W. R. Proffit, and R. L. Christiansen, "Lingual Pressures Associated with Alevolar Consonants," *J. Sp. Hrng. Res.*, 10, 1967, 606–615.

————, W. H. Richard, and J. F. Bosma, "A Physiological Model for Investigation of the Fundamental Frequency of Phonation," *Folia Phoniat.*, 18, 1966, 109–116.

Mead, J., M. B. McIlroy, N. J. Silverstone, and B. C. Kriete, "Measurement of Intraesophageal Pressure," *J. Appl. Physiol.*, 7, 1955, 491–495.

Meano, C., and A. Khoury, *The Human Voice in Speech and Song*. Springfield, Ill.: Charles C Thomas, 1967.

Megendie, F., *An Elementary Compendium of Physiology*. trans. E. Milligan. Philadelphia, 1824.

Merkel, C. L., *Der Kehlkopf*. Leipzig: 1873.

Mermelstein, P., "An Extension of Flanagan's Model of Vocal-Cord Oscillations," *J. Acoust. Soc. Amer.*, 50, 1971, 1208–1210.

Metfessel, M., "The Vibrato in Artistic Voices," *University of Iowa Studies in the Psychology of Music*, 1, 1932, 14–117.

Metzger, W., "How Do the Vocal Cords Vibrate?" *QJS*, 14, 1928, 29–39.

Meyer-Eppler, W., "Zum Erzeugungsmechanismus der Gerauschlaute," *Zeitschrift für Phonetic*, 7, 1953, 196–212.

Miller, D., *The Science of Musical Sounds*. New York: Macmillan, 1937.

Miller, R. L., "Nature of the Vocal Cord Wave," *J. Acoust. Soc. Amer.*, 31, 1959, 667–677.

Minifie, F. D., C. A. Kelsey, and T. J. Hixon, "Measurement of Vocal Fold Motion Using an Ultrasonic Droppler Velocity Monitor," *J. Acoust. Soc. Amer.*, 43, 1968, 1165.

Monoson, P., "A Quantitative Study of Whisper," Ph.D. diss., University of Illinois, Champaign, Ill., 1976.

————, and W. Zemlin, "Quantitative Study of Whisper," *Folia Phoniat.*, 36, 1984, 53–65.

Moore, P., "A Short History of Laryngeal Investigation," *Quart. J. Sp.*, 23, 1937a, 531–564.

————, "Vocal Fold Movement During Vocalization," *Sp. Monog.*, 4, 1937b, 44–55.

————, "Motion Picture Studies of the Vocal Folds and Vocal Attack," *J. Sp. Hrng. Dis.*, 3, 1938, 235–238.

————, and H. von Leden, "Dynamic Variations of the Vibratory Pattern in the Normal Larynx," *Folia Phoniat.*, 10, 1958, 205–238.

————, F. White, and H. von Leden, "Ultra-High-Speed Photography in Laryngeal Physiology," *J. Sp. Hrng. Dis.*, 27, 1962, 165–171.

Mörner, M., F. Fransson, and G. Fant, "Voice Registers," *Kungl. Tekniska Högskolan (KTH), Speech Transmission Laboratory (STL), Quarterly Progress Report (QPR)*, 4, 1964, 18–20.

Moser, H. M., "Symposium on Unique Cases of Speech Disorders: Presentation of a Case," *JSD*, 7, 1942, 102–114.

Moulonguet, A., P. Laget, and R. Husson, "Démonstration, chez l'Homme, de l'existence dans le nerf récurrent de potentiels d'action moteurs synchrones avec les vibrations des cordes vocales," *Bulletin de l'Academie Nationale Medicine*, 137, 1953, 475–482.

Müller, J., 1843: Cit. by Grutzner.

Murakami, Y., and J. A. Kirchner, "Reflex Tensor Mechanism of the Larynx by External Laryngeal Muscles," *Ann. Otol. Rhinol. Laryngol.*, 80, 1971a, 46–60.

————, "Vocal Cord Abduction by Regenerated Recurrent Laryngeal Nerve," *Arch. Oto-laryngol.*, 94, 1971b, 64–68.

Murry, T., "Subglottal Pressure and Airflow Measures During Vocal Fry Phonation," *J. Sp. Hrng. Res.*, 14, 1971b, 544–551.

————, and W. S. Brown, Jr., "Regulation of Vocal Intensity During Vocal Fry Phonation." *J. Acoust. Soc. Amer.*, 49, 1971a, 1905–1907.

————, and W. S. Brown, Jr., "Subglottal Air Pressure During Two Types of Vocal Activity," *Folia Phoniat.*, 23, 6, 1971b, 440–449.

Myerson, M., *The Human Larynx*. Springfield, Ill.: Charles C Thomas, 1964.

Mysak, E. D., "Pitch and Duration Characteristics of Older Males," *J. Sp. Hrng. Res.*, 2, 1959, 46–54.

Nadoleszny, Max, *Untersuchungen über den Kunstgesang*. Berlin: Springer, 1923.

Nauck, E., *Morphologisches Jarbuch*, 87, 1942, 536.

Negus, V. E., *The Mechanism of the Larynx*. London: Wm. Heinemann, 1929.

————, *The Mechanism of the Larynx*. St. Louis: C. V. Mosby, 1929.

————, *The Comparative Anatomy and Physiology of the Larynx*. New York: Grune and Stratton, 1949.

————, "The Mechanism of the Larynx," *Laryngoscope*, 67, 1957, 961–986.

Neiman, G. S., *Observations on the Anatomy of the Thyroid and Cricoid Cartilages of the Human Larynx*. Master's thesis, University of Illinois, Champaign, Ill., 1971.

Oertel, M., "Über eine neue Laryngostroboskopische Untersuchungsmethode," *Zentralbl.f.d med. Wissensch.* 16, 1878, 81–82.

Ohala, J., and R. Vanderslice, "Photography of States of the Glottis," *UCLA Working Papers in Phonetics*, 1, 1965, 58–59.

Öhman, S. E., "New Methods for Averaging EMG Records," *Kungl. Tekniska Högskolan (KTH), Speech Transmission Laboratory (STL), Quarterly Progress Report (QPR)*, 1, 1966, 5–8.

Ohyama, M., N. Ueda, J. E. Harvey, and J. Ogura, "Electrophysiologic Study of Reinnervated Laryngeal Motor Units," *Laryngoscope*, 82, 1972, 237–251.

Ondrackova, J., "Vocal-Cord Activity," *Folia Phoniat.*, 24, 1972, 405–419.

O'Rahilly, R., and J. A. Tucker, "The Early Development of the Larynx in Staged Human Embryos. Part 1: Embryos of the First Five Weeks (to Stage 15)," *Ann. Otol. Rhinol. Laryngol.*, 82, Suppl. 7, 1973.

Orlikoff, R., "Assessment of the Dynamics of Vocal Fold Contact from the Electroglottogram. Data from Normal Male Subjects," *J. Sp. Hrng. Res.*, 34, 1991, 1066–1072.

Pabon, J. P. H., and R. Plomp, "Automatic Phonetogram Recording Supplemented with Acoustic Voice Quality Parameters," *J. Sp. Hrng. Res.*, 31, 1988, 710–722.

Paget, R., *Human Speech*. New York: Harcourt, Brace, 1930.

————, "Artificial Vowels," *Proc. Roy. Soc. A.*, 102, 1923, 755.

Perkell, J., *Physiology of Speech Production: Results and Implications of a Quantitative Cinceradiographic Study*. Cambridge, Mass.: M.I.T. Press, 1969.

Perkins, W. H., and Y. Koike, "Patterns of Subglottal Pressure Variations During Phonation," *Folia Phoniat.*, 21, 1969, 1–8.

————, and N. Yanigahara, "Parameters of Voice Production: I. Some Mechanisms for the Regulation of Pitch," *J. Sp. Hrng. Res.*, 11, 1968, 246–267.

Perlman, A. L., I. R. Titze, and D. S. Cooper, "Elasticity of Canine Vocal Fold Tissue," *J. Sp. Hrng. Res.*, 27, 1984.

Pernkopf, E., *Atlas of Topographic and Applied Human Anatomy*, Vol. I. Philadelphia and London: W. B. Saunders, 1963.

Piquet, J., and G. Decroix, "Les Vibrations des Cordes Vocales," *Ann. Otol. Rhinol. Laryngol.*, 64, 1957a, 337–340.

———, C. Libersa, and J. Dujardin, "Die Stimmlippenschwingungen. Experimentelle Studien," *Archiv für Ohren-Nasen-Kehlkopf heilkunde*, 169, 1956, 297.

———, C. Libersa, and J. Dujardin, "Étude Experimentale Peroperatoire, chez l'Homme, des Vibrations des cordes Vocales sans Courant d'Air Sousglottique," *Revue de Laryngologie*, 77, 1957, 510–514.

Portmann, G., "The Physiology of Phonation," *J. of Laryngol. and Otol.*, 1957, 1–15.

———, R. Humbert, J. Robin, P. Laget, and R. Husson, "Étude Electromyographique des Cordes Vocales chez l'Homme," *Comptes Rendus Soc. Biol.*, 169, 1955, 296–300.

Pressman, J., "Physiology of the Vocal Cords in Phonation and Respiration," *Arch. Otolaryngol.*, 35, 1942, 355–398.

———, "Effect of Sphincteric Action of Larynx on Intraabdominal Pressure and on Muscular Action of Pectoral Girdle," *Arch. Otolaryngol*, 39, 1944, 14–42.

———, and G. Keleman, "Physiology of the Larynx," *Physiological Reviews*, 35, 1955, 506–554.

Pronovost, W., "An Experimental Study of Methods for Determining Natural and Habitual Pitch," *Sp. Monog.*, 9, 1942, 111–123.

Ptacek, P., and E. Sander, "Breathiness and Phonation Length," *J. Sp. Hrng. Dis.*, 28, 1963, 267–272.

———, "Maximum Duration of Phonation," *J. Sp. Hrng. Dis.*, 28, 1963, 171–182.

Quigley, L. F., Jr., R. C. Webster, R. J. Coffey, R. E. Kelleher, and H. P. Grant, "Velocity and Volume Measurements of Nasal and Oral Air Flow in Normal and Cleft-Palate Speech, Utilizing a Warm-Wire Flow Meter and a Two-Channel Recorder," *J. of Dental Res.*, 42, 1963, 1520–1527.

Rayleigh, Lord, and O. Trendelenburg, in Lord Rayleigh, *Theory of Sound*, 2 vols. 2 ed. London, 1896.

Ramig, L., and T. Shipp, "Comparative Measures of Vocal Tremor and Vocal Vibrato," *J. of Voice*, 1, 1986, 162–167.

Rauhut, A., E. Sturzebecher, H. Wagner, and W. Seidner, "Messung des Stimmfelder," *Folia Phoniat.*, 31, 1979.

Ringel, R., and N. Isshiki, "Intraoral Voice Recordings: An Aid to Laryngeal Photography," *Folia Phoniat.*, 16, 1964, 19–28.

Rothenberg, M., "A New Inverse-Filtering Technique for Deriving the Glottal Air Flow Wavework During Voicing," *J. Acoust. Soc. Amer.*, 53, 1971, 1632–1645.

Rubin, H. J., "Further Observations on the Neurochronaxic Theory of Voice Production," *Arch. Otolaryngol.*, 72, 1960, 207–211.

———, "Experimental Studies in Vocal Pitch and Intensity in Phonation," *Laryngoscope*, 72, 1963a, 973–1015.

———, "The Neurochronaxic Theory of Voice Production: A Refutation," *Arch. Otolaryngol.*, 28, 1963b, 267–272.

———, and C. C. Hirt, "The Falsetto. A High-Speed Cinematographic Study," *Laryngoscope*, 70, 1960, 1305–1324.

Rubin, H. J., M. LeCover, and W. Vennard, "Vocal Intensity, Subglottic Pressure, and Air Flow Relationships in Singers," *Folia Phoniat.*, 19, 1967, 393–413.

Rueger, R. S., "The Superior Laryngeal Nerve and the Interarytenoid Muscle in Humans: An Anatomical Study," *Laryngoscope*, 82, 11, 1972, 2008–2031.

Rumaswamy, S., "The Ganglion on the Internal Laryngeal Nerve," *Arch. Otolaryngol.*, 1, 1974, 28–31.

Russell, G. O., *Speech and Voice.* New York: Macmillan, 1931.

———, and C. H. Tuttle, "Some Experiments in Motion Photography of the Vocal Cords," *J. Soc. Motion Picture Eng.*, 15, 1930, 171–180.

Sasari, C. T., H. Fukuda, and J. A. Kirchner, "Laryngeal Abductor Activity in Response to Varying Ventilatory Resistance," *Trans. Amer. Acad. Ophthalmol. Otolaryngol.*, 77, 1973, 403–410.

Schlosshauer, B., and K. Vosteen, "Über die Anordnung und Wirkungsweise der im Conus elasticus ansetzended Fasern des Stimmuskels," *Laryngol. Zeitschrift.*, 36, 1957, 642–650.

Schoen, M., "The Pitch Factor in Artistic Singing," *Physiological Monog.*, 31, 1922, 230–259.

———, *The Vibrato*, University of Iowa Studies, Iowa City, Iowa, 1932.

Schwabe, F., and C. Siegert, "Bemerkungen zum Beitrag 'Vocal intensity, subglottic pressure and air flow relationships in singers,'" (Rubin, et al.), *Folia Phoniat.*, 25, 1973, 150–154.

Scripture, E. W., *Elements of Experimental Phonetics.* New York: Scribner, 1904.

Seashore, C., "Measurements on the Expression of Emotion in Music," *Proceedings of the National Academy of Science*, 1923, 323–325.

Shearer, W. T., H. F. Biller, J. H. Ogura, and D. Goldring, "Congenital Laryngeal Web and Interventricular Septal Defect," *Amer. J. Dis. Child.*, 123, 1972, 605–607.

Shin, T., and D. D. Rabuzzi, "Volume Conduction of Evoked Potentials in Adjacent Laryngeal Muscles," *Ann. Otol. Rhinol. Laryngol.*, 79, 1970, 290–299.

Shipp, T., and H. Hollien, "Perception of the Aging Male Voice," *J. Sp. Hrng. Res.*, 12, 1969, 703–710.

Smith, M., G. Berke, B. Garratt, and J. Kreiman, "Laryngeal Paralysis: Theoretical Considerations and Effects on Laryngeal Vibration," *J. Sp. Hrng. Res.*, 35, 1992, 545–554.

Smith, S., "Remarks on the Physiology of the Vibration of the Vocal Cords," *Folia Phoniat.*, 6, 1954, 166–178.

———, "Chest Register Versus Head Register in the Membrane Cushion Model of the Vocal Cords," *Folia Phoniat.*, 9, 1957, 32–36.

———, "On Pitch Variation," *Folia Phoniat.*, 11, 1959, 173.

Smith, S. B., "The Relationship between the Angle of the Thyroid Laminae and Vocal Fold Length." Masters thesis, University of Illinois, Champaign, Ill., 1978.

Smitheran, J., and T. Hixon, "A Clinical Method for Estimating Laryngeal Airway Resistance During Vowel Production," *J. Sp. Hrng. Dis.*, 46, 1981, 138–146.

Sondhi, M. M., "Measurement of the Glottal Waveform," *J. Acoust. Soc. Amer.*, 57, 1975, 228–232.

Sonesson, B., "Die Function elle Anatomie des Cricoarytenoidgelankes," *Z. Anat. entw.*, 121, 1959.

———, "A Method for Studying the Vibratory Movements of the Vocal Cords: A Preliminary Report," *J. Laryngol.*, 73, 1959, 732–727.

———, "On the Anatomy and Vibratory Pattern of the Human Vocal Folds," *Acta Oto-Laryngol.*, Suppl. 156, 1960.

Sonninen, A., "The Role of the External Laryngeal Muscles in Length-Adjustments of the Vocal Cords in Singing," *Acta Oto-Laryngol.*, Suppl. 130, 1956.

———, and E. Vaheri, "A Case of Voice Disorder Due to Laryngeal Asymmetry and Treated by Surgical Medioposition of the Vocal Cords," *Folia Phoniat.*, 10, 1958, 193–199.

Stathoopoulos, E., J. Hoit, T. Hixon, P. Watson, and N. Solomon, "Respiratory and Laryngeal Function During Whisper," *J. Sp. Hrng. Res.*, 34, 1991, 761–767.

Stevens, K., "Acoustical Aspects of Speech Production," Chap. 9, W. Fenn and O. Rahn, eds., *Handbook of Physiology, Respiration*, 3, Baltimore: Williams & Wilkins, 1965.

———, and A. House, "An Acoustical Theory of Vowel Production and Some of Its Implications," *J. Sp. Hrng. Res.*, 4, 1961, 303–320.

Stoker, G., "The Voice as a Stringed Instrument," *British Medical Journal*, 1, 1886, 641–642.

Stone, R., "Issues in Clinical Assessment of Laryngeal Function: Contraindications for Subscribing to Maximum Phonation Time and Optimum Fundamental Frequency," in D. Bless and J. Abbs, eds., *Vocal Fold Physiology*. San Diego: College-Hill Press, 1983.

Stone, R. E., Jr., and A. Nuttal, "Relative Movements of the Thyroid and Cricoid Cartilages Assessed by Neural Stimulation in Dogs," *Acta Oto-Laryngol.*, 78, 1974, 135–140.

Strenger, Folke, "Methods for Direct and Indirect Measurement of the Subglottic Air-Pressure in Phonation," *Studia Linguistica*, 14, 1960, 98–112.

Strube, H. W., "Determination of the Instant of Glottal Closure from the Speech Wave," *J. Acoust. Soc. Amer.*, 56, 1974, 1625–1629.

Sussman, H. M., R. J. Hanson, and P. F. MacNeilage, "Studies of Single Motor Units in the Speech Musculature: Methodology and Preliminary Findings," *J. Acoust. Soc. Amer.*, 51, 1972, 1372–1374.

Sutton, D., C. Larson, and D. Farrell, "Cricothyroid Motor Units," *Acta Oto-Laryngol*, 74, 1972, 145–151.

Svec, J. G., H. Schutte, and D. Miller, "A Subharminic Vibratory Pattern in Normal Vocal Folds," *J. Sp. Hrng. Res.*, 39, 1996.

Takase, S., "Studies on the Intrinsic Laryngeal Muscles of Mammals —Comparative Anatomy and Physiology (Japanese text), *Otol. Fukuoka.*, 10, 1964, 18–58. See also *disorders of speech and hearing Abstracts*, 6, 1966.

Tanabe, M., K. Kitajima, and W. J. Gould, "Laryngeal Phonatory Reflex. The Effect of Anesthetization of the Internal Branch of the Superior Laryngeal Nerve: Acoustic Aspects," *Ann. Otol. Rhinol. Laryngol.*, 84, 1975, 206–212.

Tarnoczy, T. H., "Opening Time and Opening Quotient of the Vocal Cords During Phonation," *J. Acoust. Soc. Amer.*, 23, 1951, 42–44.

Testut, L., and A. Laterjet, *Traite d'Anatomie Humaine*, 9th ed. Paris: G. Doin, 1948. Tome premier.

Tiffin, J., "The Role of Pitch and Intensity in the Vocal Vibrato of Students and Artists," *University of Iowa Studies in the Psychology of Music*, I, 1932, 134–165.

———, and M. Metfessel, "Use of the Neon Lamp in Phonophotography," *Amer. J. Psychol.*, 42, 1930, 638–639.

———, and H. Seashore, "Summary of the Established Facts in the Experimental Studies in the Vibrato up to 1932," *University of Iowa Studies in the Psychology of Music*, I, 1932, 344–376.

———, J. Saetveidt, and J. Snidecor, "An Approach to the Analysis of the Vibration of the Vocal Cords," *Quart. J. Sp.*, 24, 1938, 1–11.

Timcke, R., H. von Leden, and P. Moore, "Laryngeal Vibrations: Measurements of the Glottic Wave. Part I. The Normal Vibratory Cycle." *Arch. Otolaryngol.*, 68, 1958, 1–19.

———, H. von Leden, and P. Moore, "Laryngeal Vibrations: Measurements of the Glottic Wave. Part II. Physiologic Variations," *Arch. Otolaryngol.*, 69, 1959, 438–444.

———, H. von Leden, and P. Moore, "Laryngeal Vibrations: Measurements of the Glottic Wave. Part III. The Pathologic Larynx," 71, *Arch. Otolaryngol.*, 71, 1960, 16–35.

Titze, I., "The Human Vocal Cords: A Mathematical Model, Part I," *Phonetica*, 28, 1973, 129–170.

———, "The Human Vocal Cords: A Mathematical Model, Part II," *Phonetica*, 29, 1974, 1–21.

———, "Parameterization of the Glottal Area, Glottal Flow, and Vocal Fold Contact Area," *J. Acoust. Soc. Amer.*, 75, 1984, 570–580.

———, "Acoustic Interpretation of the Voice Range Profile (Phonetogram)," *J. Sp. Hrng. Res.*, 35, 1992, 21–34.

———, and W. Strong, "Normal Modes in Vocal Cord Tissues," *J. Acoust. Soc. Amer.*, 57, 1975, 736–744.

———, and D. Talkin, "A Theoretical Study of the Effects of Various Laryngeal Configurations on the Acoustics of Phonation," *J. Acoust. Soc. Amer.*, 66, 1979, 60–74.

Toner, M. A., F. Emanuel, and D. Parker, "Relationship of Spectral Noise Levels to Psychphysical Spacing of Vowel Roughness," *J. Sp. Hrng. Res.*, 33, 1990.

Tonndorf, W., "Die mechanik bei Stimmlippenschwingungen und beim Schnarchen," *Zeitschrift für Hals-Nasen und Ohrenheildunde*, 12, 1925, 241–245.

Töpler, A., "Das princip der Stroboskopischen scheiben," *Annals, d. Physik*, 128, 1886, 108–125.

Travis, E., R. Bender, and A. Buchanan, "Research Contributions to Vowel Theory," *Sp. Monogr.*, 1, 1934, 65–71.

Tschiassny, K., "Studies Concerning the Action of the Musculus Cricothyreoideus," *Laryngoscope*, 54, 1944, 589.

Tucker, G., Jr., W. Alonso, J. Tucker, M. Cowan, and N. Druck, "The Anterior Commissure Revisited," *Ann. Otol. Rhinol. Laryngol.*, 82, 1973, 625–636.

Tucker, J., and R. O'Rahilly, "Observations on the Embryology of the Human Larynx," *Ann. Otol. Rhinol. Laryngol.*, 81, 1972, 520–523.

———, and G. Tucker, "Some Aspects of Fetal Laryngeal Development," *Ann. Otol. Rhinol. Laryngol.*, 84, 1975, 49–55.

Van Daele, D., A. Perlman, and M. Cassell, "Intrinsic Fibre Architecture and Attachments of a Human Epiglottis and Their Contributions to the Mechanism of Deglutition, *J. Anat.*, 186, 1995, 1–15.

Van Hattum, R., and J. Worth, "Air Flow Rates in Normal Speakers," *Cleft Palate Jour.*, 4, 1967, 137–147.

Van Michel, C., "Phonatory Glottic Movements Without Emission of Sounds. An Electroglottographic Study," *Folia Phoniat.*, 18, 1966, 1–8.

Vennard, Wm., *Singing: The Mechanism and the Technic*, rev. ed., New York: Carl Fischer, 1967.

Verschuure, J., "The Electroglottography and Its Relation to Glottal Activity," *Folia Phoniat.*, 27, 1975, 215–224.

Vesalius, Andreas, *De Humani Corporis Fabrica*. Basel: Johannes Oporinus, June 1543a.

———, *Epitome*. Basel: Johannes Oporinus, June 1543b.

Voltolini, R., *Die Krankheiten der Nase*. Breslau: E. Morgenstern, 1888.

Walton, J. H., ed., "The Larynx," *Clinical Symposia*, CIBA, 1964.

Warden, Adem, "New Application of the Reflecting Prism," *London Medical Gazette*, 1844, 256.

Warren, N., "Vocal Cord Activity and Vowel Theory," *Quart. J. Sp.*, 1936, 651–655.

Wegel, R., "Theory of Vibration of the Larynx," *Bell Syst. Tech. J.*, 9, 1930, 207–227.

Weiss, D., "Discussion of the Neurochronaxic Theory," *Arch. Otolaryngol.*, 70, 1959, 607–618.

Wendahl, R., "Laryngeal Analog Synthesis of Harsh Voice Quality," *Folia Phoniat.*, 15, 1963, 241–250.

————, and R. Coleman, "Vocal-Cord Spectra Derived from Glottal Area Waveforms and Subglotta Photocell Monitoring," *J. Acoust. Soc. Amer.*, 41, 1967, 1613.

————, P. Moore, and H. Hollien, "Comments on Vocal Fry," *Folia Phoniat.*, 15, 1963, 251.

Werner-Kukuk, E., and H. von Leden, "Vocal Initiation," *Folia Phoniat.*, 22, 1970, 107–116.

West, R., "The Nature of Vocal Sounds," *Quart. J. Sp.*, 12, 1926, 244–295.

Wheatstone, C., *Westminister Review*, 1837, 27.

Whicker, J., and K. Devine, "The Commemoration of Great Men in Laryngology," *Arch. Otolaryngol.*, 95, 1972, 522–525.

Willis, W., "On Vowel Sounds, and on Reedorgan Pipes," *Transactions of the Cambridge Philosophical Society*, 3, 1830, 231.

Wilson, K., *Voice Disorders in Children*, Baltimore: Williams & Wilkins, 1979.

Winckel, F., "How to Measure the Effectiveness of Stage Singers' Voices," *Folia Phoniat.*, 23, 1971, 228–233.

Woods, R., "Law of Transverse Vibrations of Strings Applied to the Human Larynx," *J. Anat. and Physiology*, 27, 1892, 431–435.

Wright, J., "The Nose and Throat in Medical History," *Laryngoscope*, 12, 1902, 270–271.

Wullstein, Horst, "Der Bewegungsvorgang und den Stimmlippen warend der Stimmgebung," *Arch. für Ohren-Nasen-und-Kehlkopfheilkunde*, 142, 1936, 124.

Wustrow, F., "Bau und Funktion des menschliche Musculus Vocalis," *Zeitschrift für Anatomie und Enwicklungsgeschichte*, 116, 1952, 506–522.

Wyke, B., "Laryngeal Myotatic Reflexes and Phonation," *Folia Phoniat.*, 26, 1974, 249–264.

————, "Laryngeal Neuromuscular Control Systems in Singing. A Review of Current Concepts," *Folia Phoniat.*, 26, 1974, 295–306.

Yanagihara, N., "Aerodynamic Examination of the Laryngeal Function," *Stud. Phonol.*, 5, 1969–70, 45–51.

————, Y. Koike, and H. von Leden, "Phonation and Respiration Function Study in Normal Subjects," *Folia Phoniat.*, 18, 1966, 323–340.

————, and H. von Leden, "Respiration and Phonation," *Folia Phoniat.*, 19, 1967, 153–166.

Zaliouk, A., and I. Izkovitch, "Some Tomographic Aspects in Functional Voice Disorders," *Folia Phoniat.*, 10, 1958, 34–40.

Zboril, M., "Electromyographie der inneren Kehlkopfmuskelm bei verschiedenen Phonationstypen," *Arch. für Ohren-Nasen-und-Kehlkopfheilkunde*, 184, 1965, 443–449.

Zemlin, E., and W. Zemlin, *Study Guide/Workbook to Accompany Speech and Hearing Science. Anatomy and Physiology*. Stipes Publishing Co., Champaign, IL, 1988.

Zemlin, W. "A Comparison of a High-Speed Cinematographic and a Transillumination Photo-conductive Technique in the Study of the Glottis During Voice Production," Master's thesis, University of Minnesota, Minneapolis, Minn., 1959.

————, "A Comparison of the Periodic Function of Vocal-Fold Vibration in a Multiple Sclerosis and a Normal Population," Ph.D. diss., University of Minnesota, Minneapolis, Minn., 1962.

————, *Speech and Hearing Science: Anatomy and Physiology*, 2nd ed. Englewood Cliffs, N.J.: Prentice-Hall, 1981.

————, "Developing a Working Construct of the Structure and Function of the Speech Mechanism," *Amer. Sp. Hrng. Assn. (ASHA)* XXVI, 1984, 71.

————, and A. Angeline, "The Extrinsic Laryngeal Muscles in Relation to the Thyroid Cartilage," *Amer. Sp. Hrng. Assn. (ASHA)*, XXVI, 1984, 71.

————, P. Davis, and C. Gaza, "Fine Morphology of the Posterior Cricoarytenoid Muscle," *Folia Phoniat.*, 36, 1984, 233–240.

————, S. Elving, and L. Hull, "The Superior Thyroarytenoid Muscle in the Human Larynx," *Amer. Sp. Hrng. Assn.*, XXVI, 1984, 71.

————, R. Mason, and L. Holstead, "Notes on the Mechanics of Vocal Vibrato," *Nat. Assoc. Teachers of Singing Bulletin (NATS)*, 27, 1971, 22–26.

————, A. Simmon, and D. Hammel, "The Frequency of Occurrence of Foramen Thyroideum in the Human Larynx," *Folia Phoniat.*, 36, 1984, 296–300.

Zenker, W., and J. Glaniger, "Die Starke des Trachealzuges beim lebenden Menschen und seine Bedeutung für die Kehlkopfmechanick," *Zeitschrift fur Biol*, 11, 1959, 154–164.

————, and A. Zenker, "Uber die Regelung der Stimmlippenspannung durch von aussen eingreifende Mechanismen," *Folia Phoniat.*, 12, 1960, 1–36.

Articulation

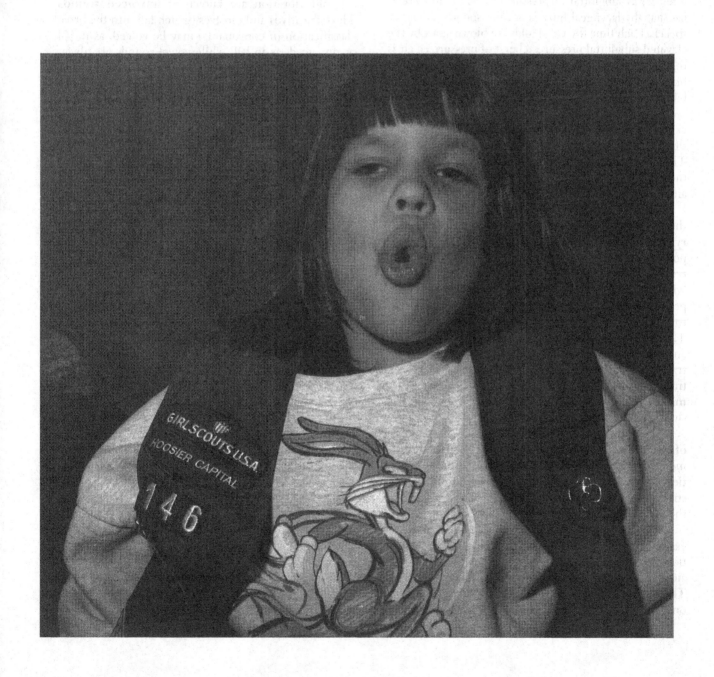

INTRODUCTION

Thus far in our account of the speech mechanism, we have described the power source and the vibrating elements. The power source, which consists of the lungs and associated skeletal and muscular structures, provides energy in the form of an inaudible stream of air. The vibrating vocal folds convert this breath stream into a rapid series of puffs.

If it were somehow possible to isolate the larynx from the remainder of the vocal tract, we would find that the output of the larynx consists simply of an unintelligible buzz that varies in frequency as the vocal folds vibrate at different rates. The output might also vary in intensity as subglottal air pressure varies. We must realize that the laryngeal buzz is not the sound we hear as speech. Each time the vocal folds are blown apart by the elevated subglottal pressure, a burst of pressurized air is released into the vocal tract. With the vocal folds vibrating at a rate of 200 times/sec, for example, a discrete burst of air is released into the vocal tract each 1/200 sec. The effect of these transient bursts of energy is to excite the dormant column of air above the larynx, and this column of air vibrates for a short period of time. The amplitude of each vibration dies away quickly, but the rapid succession of energy bursts serves to keep the air column vibrating.

These short-duration vibrations generated within the supraglottal air column constitute the **glottal** or **laryngeal tone.** This tone is acoustically rich, being composed of a number of **partials** that are harmonically related integral multiples of the fundamental frequency (vibratory rate of the vocal folds). The vocal tract, depending upon its configuration, is capable of resonating to or reinforcing some of the partials in the glottal tone. That is, the glottal tone is shaped by the configuration, and therefore the acoustical properties of the vocal tract, to produce our voiced speech sounds. The vocal tract has four or five prominent resonances called **formants,** and their frequencies are determined by the shape and length of the vocal tract.

Above the vocal folds, the vocal tract is composed of the pharyngeal, nasal, and mouth cavities. Adjustments of the shape and therefore the acoustical properties of the vocal tract are known as **articulation,** and the structures which mediate these adjustments are called the **articulators.**

The articulators may generate speech sounds. For example, when the air stream passes through a constriction somewhere along the vocal tract, friction causes the air to become turbulent, and **fricative noise** is generated. This is the sort of thing we do when we admonish someone to be quiet by producing a "sh-sh-sh-sh" sound.

Other speech sounds may be generated by momentarily blocking the outward flow of air through the vocal tract. Articulators such as the lips and tongue function as valves to block the vocal tract, and the sudden release of a valve produces an audible puff of air. Sounds generated by such manipulations are called **stops,** examples of which are the [p] and [t] sounds.

It is important to keep in mind that fricatives and stops may be generated rather independently of vocal fold vibration. If the vocal folds are active while stops and fricatives are being generated, the resultant speech sound consists of a noise superimposed upon the glottal tone. Speech elements that are produced with vocal fold vibration are referred to appropriately as **voiced sounds,** while those that are produced without vocal fold vibration are known as **unvoiced sounds.** Thus, fricatives and plosives (which fall into the broad classification of consonants) may be voiced, as in [ð], or unvoiced, as in [θ], while vowel sounds are always voiced.

The purposes of this chapter are to describe the articulatory mechanism and to relate the articulatory structures to speech production. As in the case with both the breathing and laryngeal mechanisms, the articulatory mechanism consists of a supportive framework and a muscular system. The supportive framework is formed primarily by facial skeleton, the lower jaw or mandible, and the cervical vertebrae.

THE SKULL

An Overview

The skull, which is the bony framework of the head, is composed of 22 irregular or flattened bones that, except for the mandible, are rigidly joined together by joints known as **sutures.** Sutures are immovable (fibrous) joints exclusive to the skull. Earlier we learned that the sagittal and coronal sutures form the lines of reference for the sagittal and frontal planes of the body. The principal sutures of the skull are shown in Figure 4-1A. They include the **sagittal** (L. arrow), the **coronal** (L. crown), the **lambdoidal** (the paired sutures form the Greek letter lambda), and the **occipitomastoid sutures,** a term that tells us where the suture is located. The arrowlike landmark which forms the basis for the term sagittal is best seen in an infant skull, viewed from above, as in Figure 4-1B.

Even though it is essentially one unified structure, the skull is divisible into the **cranium** (braincase), which houses and protects the brain, and the **facial skeleton,** which forms the framework for organs of mastication,

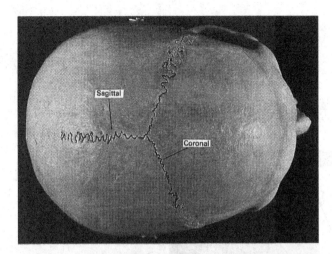

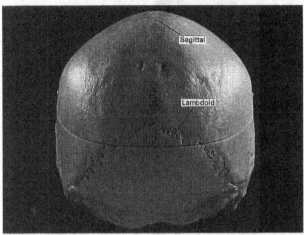

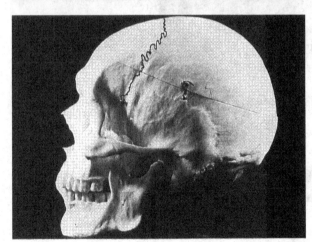

FIGURE 4-1A

(A) Principal sutures of the skull. Top view showing sagittal; back view showing lambdoid; side view showing coronal sutures.

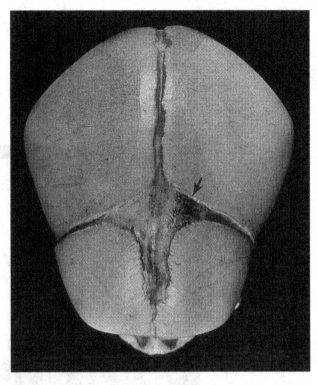

FIGURE 4-1B

(B) Infant skull from above showing the arrow-shaped anterior fontanelle for which the sagittal suture is named.*

Bones of the Facial Skeleton		Bones of the Cranial Skeleton	
Mandible	1	Ethmoid bone	1
Maxillae	2	Frontal bone	1
Nasal bones	2	Parietal bones	2
Palatine bones	2	Occipital bone	1
Lacrimal bones	2	Temporal bones	2
Zygomatic bones	2	Sphenoid bone	1
Inferior conchae	2		
Vomer	1		
Total	14	Total	8

In addition to the facial and cranial bones, the head possesses seven more bones, making a total of 29. They are the three pairs of **auditory** (middle ear) **ossicles**—the **incus** (2), **stapes** (2), and **malleus** (2), which are housed within the temporal bones—and the **hyoid bone,** a single, nonarticular bone that has no direct contact with any other bones of the skeleton.

speech production, respiration, special senses, and muscles for facial expression. The eight cranial bones and 14 facial bones are as follows:

*Sagittarius is a southern constellation represented as a centaur shooting an arrow (the archer). Also the ninth sign of the Zodiac in astrology.

Before discussing the individual bones of the head, let us examine the **articulated skull** presented in Figures 4-2, 4-3, and 4-4. These views show the individual bones and some of their major landmarks involving two or more bones, and they will serve as part of a general introduction.

As shown in Figure 4-2, the most obvious holes or depressions in the anterior view of the skull are the two

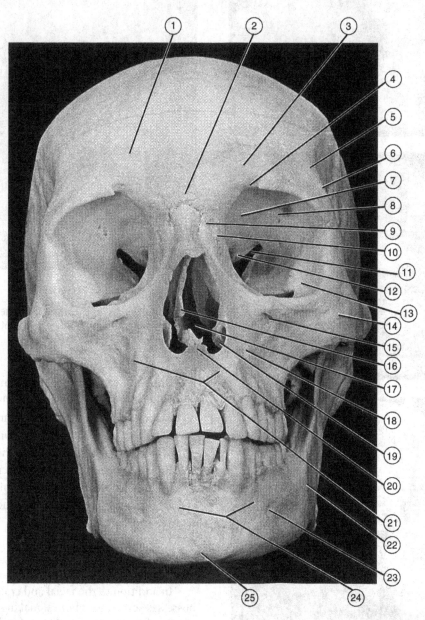

1. Frontal bone	10. Frontal process of maxilla	19. Inferior nasal concha
2. Glabella	11. Superior orbital fissure	20. Anterior nasal spine
3. Superciliary arch	12. Optic canal	21. Bodies of maxillae
4. Supraorbital notch	13. Orbital surface of zygomatic bone	22. Oblique line of mandible
5. Supraorbital margin	14. Zygomatic base	23. Mental foramen
6. Zygomatic process	15. Infraorbital foramen	24. Body of mandible
7. Orbital plate of frontal bone	16. Nasal septum	25. Mental protuberance
8. Orbital surface of sphenoid bone	17. Nasal cavity	
9. Nasal bone	18. Canine fossa of maxilla	

FIGURE 4-2

The skull as seen from the front. (From Zemlin and Stolpe, 1967.)

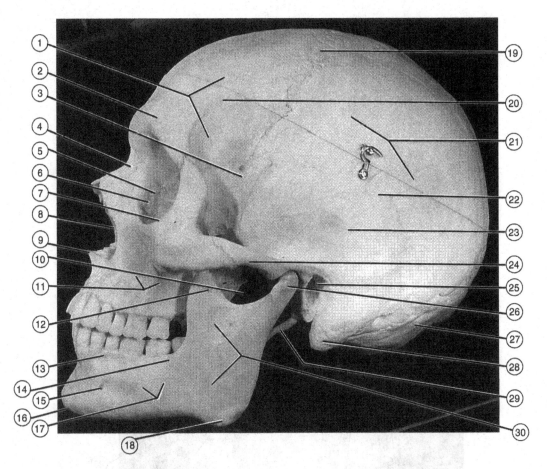

1. Frontal bone
2. Superciliary arch
3. Greater wing of sphenoid
4. Nasal bone
5. Lacrimal bone
6. Lacrimal groove
7. Zygomatic bone
8. Nasal notch
9. Anterior nasal spine
10. Mandibular notch
11. Body of maxilla
12. Coronoid process
13. Alveolar part (of mandible)
14. Oblique line of mandible
15. Mental foramen
16. Mental protuberance
17. Body of mandible
18. Angle of mandible
19. Coronal suture
20. Superior temporal line
21. Parietal bone
22. Squamosal surface
23. Temporal bone
24. Zygomatic arch
25. External auditory meatus
26. Condylar process
27. Occipital bone
28. Mastoid process
29. Styloid process
30. Ramus of mandible

FIGURE 4-3

The skull as seen from the side. (From Zemlin and Stolpe, 1967.)

orbits and the nasal cavity. Each **orbit** is a depression that, in life, contains an eye and associated tissues. The entrance to the orbit (*aditus orbitae*) is marked by **supraorbital** and **infraorbital margins,** and the cavity is bounded by superior, inferior, lateral, and medial walls. The lacrimal (tear) glands are, in life, located in the hollow in the upper, outer part of the orbit (in the frontal bone), but the tears drain down into a lacrimal sac located in the lacrimal fossa, which is found in the inferior medial part of the orbit (between the lacrimal and maxillary bones). In the back of the orbit are the diagonal superior and inferior orbital fissures, and the optic canal. In life, the optic canal carries the optic nerve (vision) and the ophthalmic artery. The superior orbital fissure transmits the motor nerve supply to the muscles of the eye (oculomotor, trochlear, and abducent). The inferior orbital fissure carries the sensory nerve to the eye region (ophthalmic), and the ophthalmic vein.

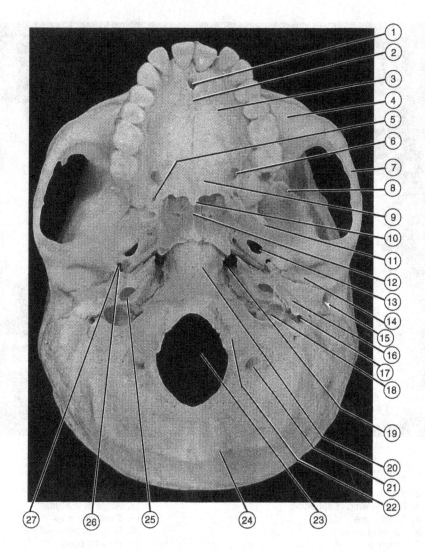

1. Incisive foramen
2. Median palatine (Intermaxillary) suture
3. Palatine process of maxilla
4. Zygomatic process of maxilla
5. Lesser palatine foramen
6. Greater palatine foramen
7. Zygomatic arch
8. Greater wing of sphenoid
9. Horizontal part of palatine bone
10. Posterior nasal spine
11. Lateral pterygoid plate
12. Vomer
13. Foramen ovale
14. Mandibular fossa
15. External auditory meatus
16. Styloid process
17. Stylomastoid foramen
18. Jugular fossa
19. Foramen lacerum
20. Basilar part of sphenoid bone
21. Condylar fossa
22. Occipital condyle
23. Foramen magnum
24. Inferior nuchal line
25. Carotid canal
26. Spine of sphenoid
27. Foramen spinosum

FIGURE 4-4

The skull as seen from beneath. (From Zemlin and Stolpe, 1967.)

The **nasal cavity,** which traverses the depth of the facial skeleton, is divided into right and left halves by the bony **nasal septum.** In Figure 4-2, it is not located exactly in the midline, so the cavity is divided into unequal parts. The septum characteristically exhibits some deviation, which reflects effects of the vicissitudes of life (a blow to the nose) rather than the result of normal ontogenesis. The septum will be described in some detail later in the chapter, but for now we might mention the scrolls of bone on the lateral walls. These scrolls project medially to divide the passageway into **meatuses,** channels for air, and they are called the **conchae** or **turbinated bones.**

Certain landmarks used primarily in anthropometry will sometimes be used as references in describing individual specimens. They include the tempora, vertex, frons, and occiput. The **temporae** (temples) are the lateral sides of the skull, the most superior point of the skull is the **vertex,** the **frons** is the forehead, and the **occiput** is the back of the skull.

The word **skull** originally meant bowl, but now refers to the 22 articulated bones of the cranium and facial skeleton. The term **calvaria** refers to the bowl that comprises the skullcap. When the calvaria is removed, as in Figure 4-5, the three major divisions of the floor of the cranium can be seen. They are the **anterior, middle,** and **posterior cranial fossae** which are shaped to accommodate the frontal and temporal lobes of the cerebrum and the cerebellum, respectively.

Some obvious bony markings are located on individual bones, for example, the **foramen magnum** of the occipital bone and the **mastoid** and **styloid processes** of the temporal bones. Other prominent parts of the skull are associated with more than one bone, and two of these are (1) the **zygomatic arch,** which curves over the concavity known as the **temporal fossa,** and (2) the **hard palate** (Figure 4-4), which is composed of part of the maxillary and palatine bones.

Higher-order mammals, including humans, are provided with two sets of teeth. The first set is well developed in utero and appears in infancy and early childhood. They are the **milk** or **deciduous teeth,** and as the word deciduous implies, they are temporary. The second set, however, is **permanent.** They erupt at an early age and, unless disease or trauma intervene, remain for life. The integrity of the dentition has a profound influence on the growth patterns of the facial skeleton, and the loss of teeth, especially at an early age, can have marked effects on the configurations of the bones of the facial skeleton.

A word of encouragement: The skull is an extraordinarily complex structure, and a full appreciation of its organization and architecture can be attained only with deliberate and disciplined study. It will take two, three, or perhaps more exposures before an integrated picture begins to form. Although the illustrations and brief text may be useful in themselves, nothing is quite so useful as an actual skull to study. Structural differences among people are to be expected, and they help us to recognize one another as individuals. Because these individual structural differences also occur in the skull, you should not be surprised if specimens you study are not exactly the same as illustrations in anatomy books.

Bones of the Facial Skeleton

The Mandible

The adult mandible, shown in Figure 4-6, is regarded as a single bone. At birth, however, its mirrored halves are joined by a fibrous symphysis, which usually ossifies during the first year of life. When viewed from above, as in Figure 4-7A, the mandible appears to be U-shaped. That portion making up the arch is called the **body** (or corpus), and the point where the two halves are joined is called the **mental** (L. *mentum,* chin) **symphysis.** When viewed from the front as in Figure 4-7B, the mental symphysis appears as a vertically directed midline ridge that bifurcates near the lower border to form a triangular projection called the **mental protuberance** (point of the chin). It is usually depressed in the center, thus giving rise to two anterior projections called **mental tubercles.**

The inner surface of the mandible, near the symphysis, presents two small posteriorly directed ridges, one placed just above the other. They are known as **mental spines,** and they vary in size from ill-defined ridges to prominent double spines. The mandible as seen from behind is shown in Figure 4-7C.

The upper surface of a tooth-bearing mandible is known as the **alveolar arch.** It contains a **dental alveolus** (tooth socket) for each tooth. The alveoli are separated from each other by **interalveolar septa.**

The arch of the mandible is continued in a posterior and somewhat lateral direction until it joins the **mandibular ramus** (literally, branch from the body), at which point the two halves of the jaw have become widely separated. When viewed from the side, as in Figure 4-7D, the posterior border of a ramus meets the inferior border of the corpus to form the **angle of the mandible,** which approximates a right angle (90°) in the adult. Each ramus

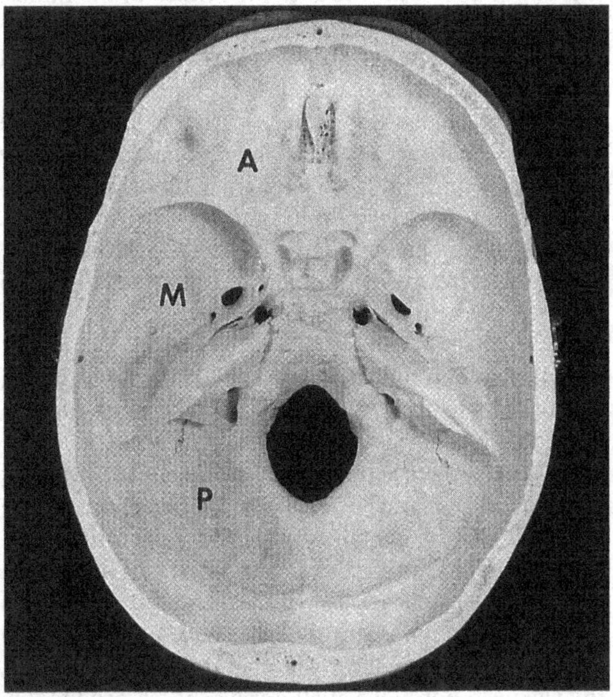

FIGURE 4-5

The floor of the cranium showing the anterior (A), middle (M), and posterior (P) cranial fossae.

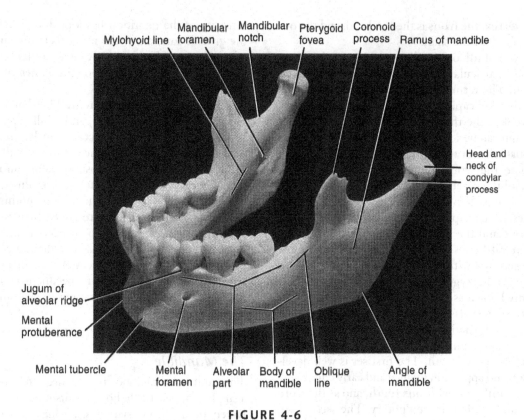

Mylohyoid line · Mandibular foramen · Mandibular notch · Pterygoid fovea · Coronoid process · Ramus of mandible

Head and neck of condylar process

Jugum of alveolar ridge

Mental protuberance

Mental tubercle · Mental foramen · Alveolar part · Body of mandible · Oblique line · Angle of mandible

FIGURE 4-6

The mandible as seen in perspective. (From Zemlin and Stolpe, 1967.)

is a quadrilateral and perpendicularly directed plate extending upward from the posterior portion of the body of the mandible. The superior border of each ramus contains two prominent and important landmarks, the **coronoid** and the **condylar processes,** which are separated by the **mandibular** (or semilunar) **notch.**

The **coronoid process,** the anterior of the two, is a beaklike projection directed somewhat posteriorly and is therefore convex forward and concave behind. It serves as the point of attachment for the temporalis muscle (to be described later). The **condylar process** is composed of a head and neck. The **head** of the mandibular condyle articulates with the cranium at the temporal bone on each side in the only freely movable joints of the skull. The **pterygoid fovea,** a depression for the attachment of the lateral pterygoid muscle, is also located on the condylar process. The medial surface of the ramus contains an easily identifiable landmark, the **mandibular foramen,** which permits entrance of nerves and blood vessels. Anterior and superior to the mandibular foramen is the **lingula** (L. small tongue), which serves as the point of attachment for the sphenomandibular ligament.

The **body** of the mandible also presents some worthwhile landmarks. Beginning from each mental tubercle, running posteriorly and upward, is an indistinct ridge called the **oblique line.** As shown in Figure 4-7D,

it is continuous with the anterior surface of the ramus. A prominent landmark may be seen just above the oblique line, lateral to the symphysis. It is the **mental foramen,** a perforation in the bone that permits the mental nerve and blood vessels to pass from within the bone to the external surface. Outstanding landmarks on the medial surface of the body of the mandible are the **mylohyoid line** (Gk. *myle,* mill)[1] and **mylohyoid groove.** The mylohyoid line marks the site of the mandibular attachment of the mylohyoid muscle which contributes to the floor of the mouth.

Articulatory Function The mandible is a large, dense, and extremely strong bone. Its major contribution to speech production is probably that it houses the lower teeth and forms the points of attachment for much of the tongue and other musculature. Movements of the mandible and its contained tongue result in modifications of the size and acoustic characteristics of the oral cavity. The extent of jaw movement during normal speech production is surprisingly small, amounting to a few millimeters when measured at the incisors. In fact, the jaw need not move at all during speech production.

_____

[1]Pertaining to the molar (*grinding*) teeth.

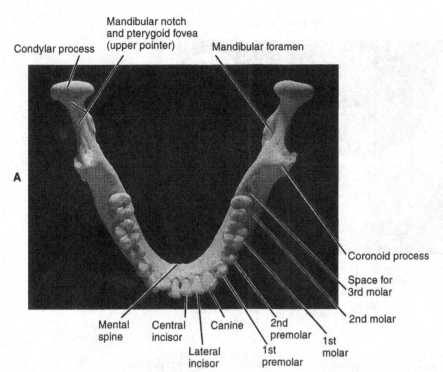

Condylar process

Mandibular notch
and pterygoid fovea
(upper pointer)

Mandibular foramen

A

Coronoid process

Space for
3rd molar

2nd molar

Mental
spine

Central
incisor

Canine

2nd
premolar

1st
molar

Lateral
incisor

1st
premolar

FIGURE 4-7

(A) The mandible as seen from above.
(B) The mandible as seen from the front.

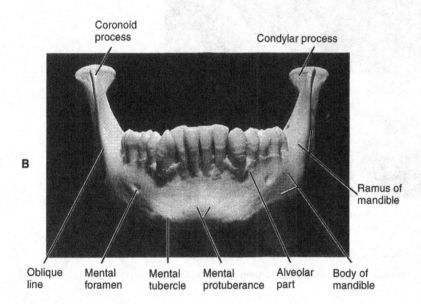

Coronoid
process

Condylar process

B

Ramus of
mandible

Oblique
line

Mental
foramen

Mental
tubercle

Mental
protuberance

Alveolar
part

Body of
mandible

Testimony to this may be seen in the cigar and pipe smokers who seem to have no trouble at all producing perfectly adequate speech with their oral pacifiers clenched firmly between their teeth.

Anomalies *Hypoplasia of the Mandible (Pierre Robin Syndrome).* This syndrome consists of **micrognathia** (unusually small jaw) with an associated **pseudomacroglossia.** (The tongue is usually normal in size, but the floor of the mouth is shortened and the buccal cavity reduced in size. One consequence is obstruction of air flow during inhalation.) Other characteristics are **glossoptosis** (downward displacement of the tongue) and **high-arched** or **cleft palate.** A postalveolar cleft of the hard and soft palates is common but not necessarily a feature of the syndrome. Often growth of the mandible will progress so that a normal or near-normal facial profile develops within four to six years. Because of the mandibular hypoplasia (incomplete development), a variety of **dental anomalies** accompanies the syndrome.

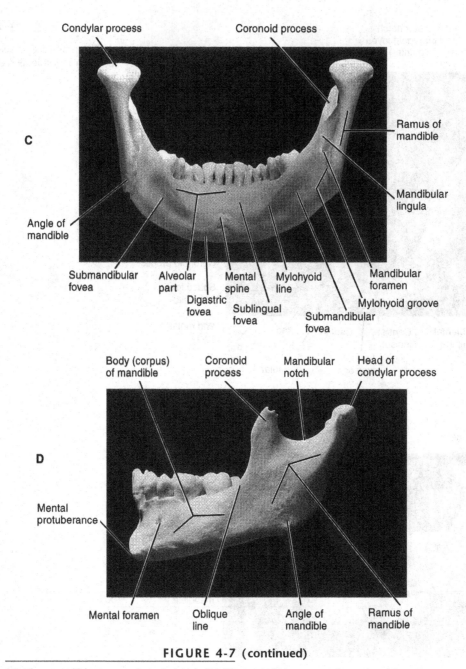

FIGURE 4-7 (continued)

(C) The mandible as seen from behind. (D) The mandible as seen from the side.

Mandibulofacial Dysostosis (Treacher Collins Syndrome or Francescetti-Zwahlen-Klein Syndrome). There is good evidence that this syndrome is inherited as a dominant trait, but its expression is often incomplete. It is characterized by **micrognathia** (less severe than in Pierre Robin syndrome) and **palpebral** (L. eyelid) **fissures** sloping downward toward the outer canthi (the angles at the corners of the eye), which give the eyes an antimongoloid obliquity. **Colobomas** (an absence or defect of some ocular tissue) of the lower eyelids,

sunken cheekbones, **blind fissures**[2] opening between the angles of the mouth and the ears, deformed pinnas, receding chin, and large mouth complete the facial description. In about one out of four affected persons, a finger of hair growth extends toward the cheeks.

The palatal vault may be very high or, in about 40 percent of the cases, cleft. As might be expected, dental

---

[2]Fissures that are concealed or closed at one end.

malocclusions are common and frequently very severe. The deformity of the pinna is often accompanied by absence of the external auditory canal, part or all of the middle ear, and deafness.

The incidence of mental retardation is not known for certain. This is a syndrome that, once seen, is unforgettable, and one that is made far more understandable when considered in light of the embryonic development of the face and hearing mechanism. For illustrative purposes, an example of mandibular hypoplasia and of mandibulofacial dysostosis is shown in Figure 4-8.

The Maxillae

Except for the mandible, the maxillae are the largest bones in the face. These paired bones, which form the entire upper jaw and contribute to the formation of the roof of the mouth, the floor and lateral walls of the nasal cavity, and the floor of the orbital cavity, play an important role in speech production.

Each bone consists of a **body,** roughly pyramidal in shape, and the **zygomatic, frontal, alveolar,** and **palatine processes.** Since the body of the maxilla is tetrahedral, it presents four surfaces for inspection: the anterior, posterior (infratemporal), superior (orbital), and medial (nasal) surfaces.

The *anterior surface* presents a number of landmarks, some of which are shown in Figure 4-9. Those worth noting include the **canine eminence,** the **infraorbital foramen,** and the **anterior nasal spine.** The significance of some of these landmarks may become apparent as we progress through the chapter. The *posterior surface* forms part of the **infratemporal fossa.** The anterior and posterior surfaces would be continuous were it not for the zygomatic process, which forms a dividing boundary. The posterior surface contains two landmarks: (1) the **alveolar canals,** which carry the posterior-superior blood vessels and nerves, and (2) the **maxillary tuberosity,** which articulates with the palatine bone. The *superior surface* of the maxilla is triangular in shape, and it forms most of the floor of the orbital cavity. The *medial border* articulates with the lacrimal, ethmoid, and palatine bones. The outstanding landmark of the superior surface is the **infraorbital groove,** which carries infraorbital blood vessels and nerves. The *medial surface* is broken by an opening into the maxillary sinus. As shown in Figure 4-10, this opening is best seen in a disarticulated skull. In the articulated specimen, the medial surfaces are all but hidden by the nasal conchae.

Buttresses The maxillae are not the massive bones their size might indicate. This is because they are not solid masses, but rather each contains an extensive **maxillary sinus** (antrum of Highmore). Thus, the maxillae in the adult skull are but hollow shells that might easily

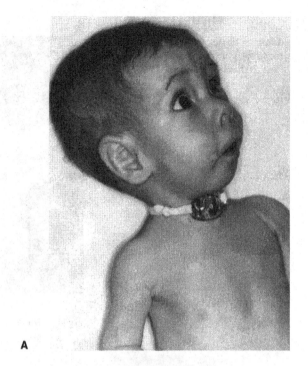

A

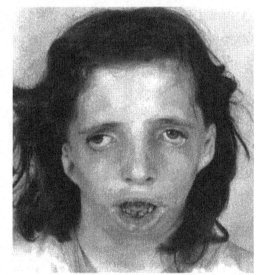

B

FIGURE 4-8

An example of (A) mandibular hypoplasia (Pierre Robin Syndrome) and (B) mandibulofacial dysostosis (Treacher Collins or Francescetti-Zwahlen-Klein Syndrome). (Courtesy Center for Craniofacial Anomalies, Univ. of Illinois Medical Center, Chicago, Ill.)

yield to the pressures of biting and chewing, were it not for three buttresses of bone which course upward obliquely from the alveolar arch. These buttresses are shown in schematic form in Figure 4-11. One runs up the medial side of the orbit, while another runs up the lateral side and divides into an upper and lower limb, one of which courses horizontally back as the **zygoma,** to be

FIGURE 4-9

Juxtaposed maxillae as seen from the front (top) and a maxilla as seen from the side (bottom).

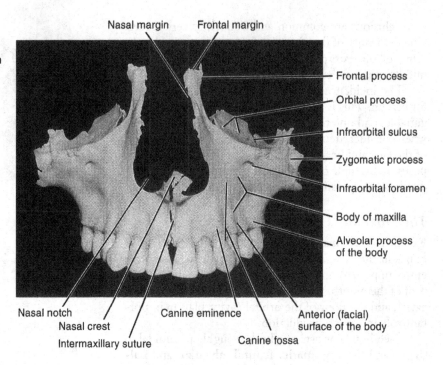

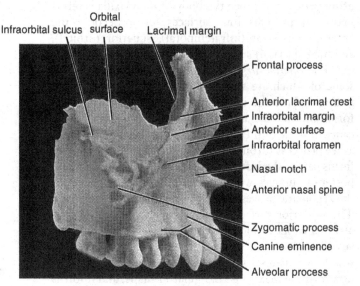

discussed later. The other (upper limb) forms the lateral boundary and wall of the orbital cavity and ultimately reaches the frontal bone. The third buttress is formed by the pterygoid processes of the sphenoid bone (also to be discussed later). It extends from the last upper molar to the base of the skull, as shown in Figure 4-11. It is apparent that the processes of the maxillae contribute to the strength of the facial skeleton.

Processes The triangular **zygomatic process** is directed laterally. It articulates with the zygomatic bone. The **frontal process** is a very strong bony plate that is directed upward, medially, and slightly posteriorly. It forms

the lateral bony framework of the nose, while its medial surface contributes to the lateral wall of the nasal cavity. The **alveolar process** is the thick, spongy part of the maxilla that houses the teeth. The adult alveolar process is divided into eight cavities, each of which contains a tooth. In some specimens the canine tooth may perforate the alveolar process and extend into the maxillary sinus. In the articulated, tooth-bearing skull, the alveolar processes of the maxillae form the alveolar arch or ridge.

The **palatine process** is a thick, horizontal, medially directed projection, which articulates with its fellow from the opposite side at the midline to form most (three-fourths) of the floor of the nasal cavity and bony

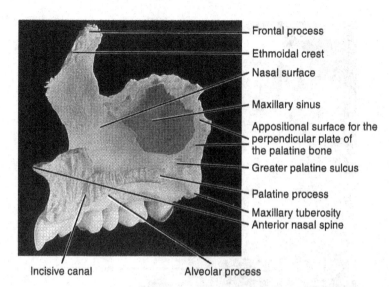

— Frontal process
— Ethmoidal crest
— Nasal surface
— Maxillary sinus
— Appositional surface for the perpendicular plate of the palatine bone
— Greater palatine sulcus
— Palatine process
— Maxillary tuberosity
— Anterior nasal spine

Incisive canal   Alveolar process

FIGURE 4-10

A right maxilla as seen in medial view showing opening of sinus.

roof of the mouth. As shown in Figure 4-10, it is considerably thicker in front than behind. When viewed from beneath, as in Figure 4-12B, the concave, rough surface presents some noteworthy landmarks. A midline **intermaxillary** suture courses anteriorly and terminates at the **incisive foramen.**

In the very young, and in lower animals, a fine suture may be seen extending from the incisive foramen to the space between the lateral incisors and the canine or cuspid teeth. The small triangular part in front of this fine suture forms the **premaxilla** (or intermaxillary bone), which in most vertebrates is a separate bone. In humans the fine sutures that form the boundary lines of the premaxilla disappear at a very early age, and often no trace of them can be found in the adult skull. In Fig-

ure 4-12, the bony palate of an ape and of an adult human are shown for comparative purposes. Note the fine sutures extending laterally from the incisive foramen in the ape palate and the absence of such sutures in the human palate.

When seen in a frontal section, as in Figure 4-13, the medial border of the palatine process presents a raised ridge known as the **nasal crest,** which, together with the crest from the opposite side, forms a longitudinal groove that accommodates the perpendicular vomer bone. Anteriorly, the nasal crest is continued forward as a sharp process called the **anterior nasal spine,** an important landmark in x-ray studies of the skull.

Articulations   Each maxilla articulates with nine bones: the frontal and ethmoid bones of the cranium; the nasal, lacrimal, zygomatic, palatine, vomer, and inferior nasal concha of the facial skeleton; and the maxilla from the opposite side.

The Nasal Bones

Two small oblong plates of bones, placed side by side, form the bridge of the nose. They are the nasal bones shown in Figures 4-3 and 4-14. Situated medial to the frontal processes of the maxillae, they articulate with the frontal bone above, with the perpendicular plate of the ethmoid bone, and with the nasal base from the opposite side. They also articulate with the septal cartilage of the nose.

The Palatine Bones

Although the palatine bones are relatively small, they are extremely important and equally complex (Figure 4-15). As shown schematically in Figure 4-16, they are located

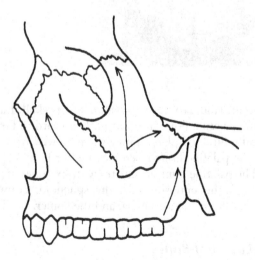

FIGURE 4-11

Schematic of buttresses that lend support to the facial skeleton.

FIGURE 4-12

Photograph of the palate of an ape (A)
and of an adult human (B).

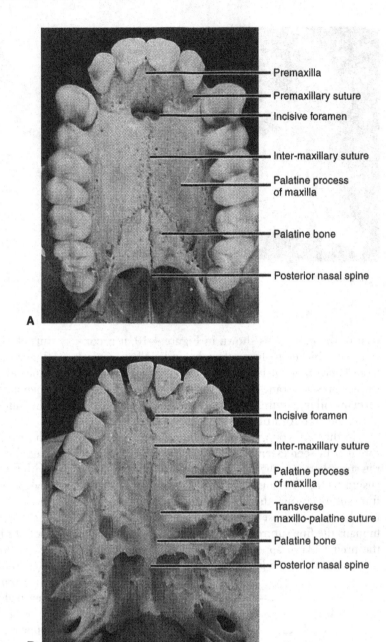

A

- Premaxilla
- Premaxillary suture
- Incisive foramen
- Inter-maxillary suture
- Palatine process of maxilla
- Palatine bone
- Posterior nasal spine

B

- Incisive foramen
- Inter-maxillary suture
- Palatine process of maxilla
- Transverse maxillo-palatine suture
- Palatine bone
- Posterior nasal spine

at the back of the nasal cavity and, like the maxillae with which they are so closely associated, the palatine bones contribute to the formation of three cavities: the floor and lateral wall of the nasal cavity, the roof of the mouth, and the floor of the orbital cavity.

Of particular interest to us is the horizontal part of the palatine bone. It is quadrilateral in shape and has two surfaces: a concave superior surface, which forms part of the floor of the nasal cavity, and a concave inferior surface, which forms the posterior one-fourth of the bony palate. Its anterior border is serrated for articulation with the palatine process of the maxilla, while the posterior border is free. Medially, the bone is continued posteriorly and, when united with its fellow from the opposite side, forms the **posterior nasal spine,** an

important landmark for x-ray study of the skull. Laterally, the palatine bone turns abruptly upward to form a vertically directed plate. Thus, when viewed from behind, the palatine bone resembles a letter L.

The palatine bone articulates with six bones: its fellow from the opposite side, the sphenoid, ethmoid, maxilla, inferior nasal concha, and the vomer.

The Lacrimal Bones

The lacrimal bones, the smallest of the facial bones, form part of the medial walls of the orbital cavities. Each has an orbital and nasal surface and articulates with four bones: the frontal, ethmoid, maxilla, and inferior nasal concha. A lacrimal bone is shown in Figure 4-3.

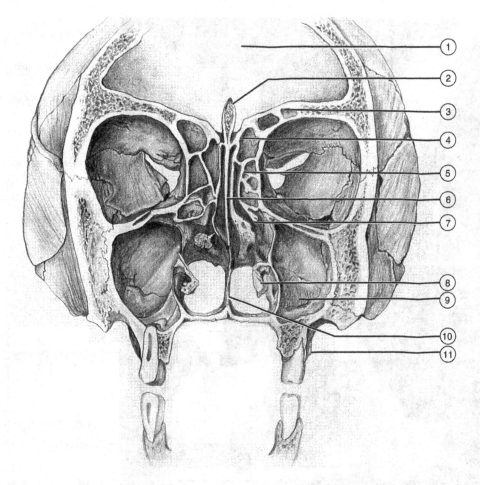

1. Anterior cranial cavity
2. Crista galli of the ethmoid
3. Frontal sinus
4. Cribriform plate of ethmoid
5. Ethmoid sinus
6. Perpendicular plate of ethmoid
7. Middle nasal concha
8. Inferior nasal concha
9. Antrum of maxilla
10. Vomer bone
11. Alveolar process of maxilla

FIGURE 4-13

A frontal section through the skull (drawing by Adrienne Warren).

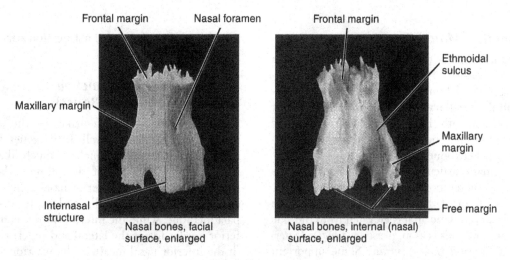

Frontal margin   Nasal foramen

Maxillary margin

Internasal
structure

Nasal bones, facial
surface, enlarged

Frontal margin

Ethmoidal
sulcus

Maxillary
margin

Free margin

Nasal bones, internal (nasal)
surface, enlarged

FIGURE 4-14

Juxtaposed nasal bones as seen from the front and behind. (From Zemlin and Stolpe, 1967.)

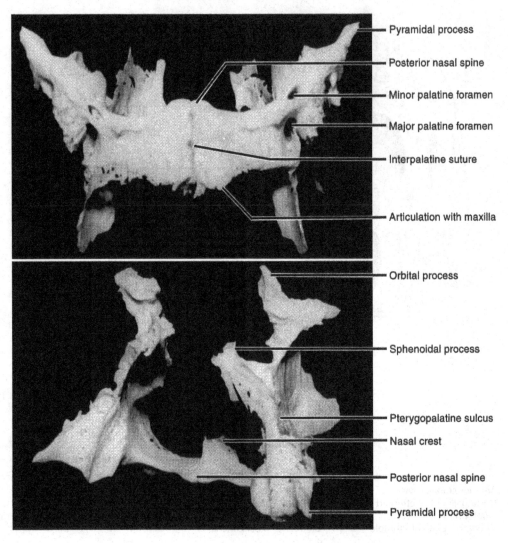

Pyramidal process
Posterior nasal spine
Minor palatine foramen
Major palatine foramen
Interpalatine suture
Articulation with maxilla
Orbital process
Sphenoidal process
Pterygopalatine sulcus
Nasal crest
Posterior nasal spine
Pyramidal process

FIGURE 4-15

Articulated palatine bones as seen from beneath (top) and as seen in perspective from behind (bottom). (From Zemlin and Stolpe, 1967.)

The Zygomatic (Malar) Bones

The zygomatic or malar (L. *mala*, cheek) bone, shown in Figure 4-17, consists of a **body** that is roughly quadrilateral in shape, and four processes: the **frontosphenoidal, orbital, maxillary,** and **temporal.** It is a rather small bone, which, with the zygomatic processes of the maxilla and temporal bone, forms the prominent **zygomatic arch** (or cheekbone).

The zygomatic articulates with the frontal, sphenoid, maxillary, and temporal bones. It contributes to the lateral wall and floor of the orbital cavity. As shown in Figure 4-4, the zygomatic arch is elevated from the side of the skull and, for this reason, presents a *malar (outer) surface* and a *temporal (inner) surface*. Some important muscles of articulation and mastication attach to the zygomatic bone.

The Inferior Nasal Conchae (Inferior Turbinated Bones)

The inferior nasal concha makes up the inferiormost part of the lateral nasal wall. In its general configurations the inferior nasal concha is much like the scroll-like, lateral extensions of the ethmoid bone (to be considered later). The inferior nasal concha articulates anteriorly with the maxilla and posteriorly with the palatine bone, while the inferior border is free. The inferior border forms the lateral and superior boundaries of the inferior nasal meatus. The inferior nasal concha

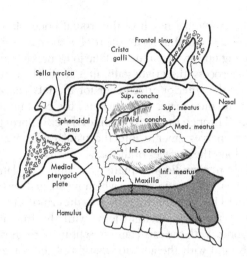

FIGURE 4-16

Lateral wall of nasal cavity, showing relationship of inferior nasal concha to adjacent structures. Also shown are the perpendicular part of the palatine (palat) bone, and the hard palate (shaded).

and its relationship to adjacent structures are shown in Figures 4-13 and 4-16.

The Vomer Bone

The inferior half of the bony septum consists of the vomer (L. plowshare) bone, an unpaired thin quadrilat-eral plate that articulates with the maxillae and palatine bones inferiorly and the perpendicular plate of the ethmoid bone and the rostrum of the sphenoid bone superiorly. The posterior border is free, whereas the anterior border articulates with the cartilaginous septum of the nose. The vomer and adjacent bones are shown in Figures 4-4 and 4-18.

Bones of the Cranium

The Ethmoid Bone

Although the unpaired ethmoid (Gk. *ethmos*, sieve) bone, shown in Figure 4-19, is regarded as a cranial bone, it contributes to the facial skeleton. It is a very delicate and extremely complex bone that is projected down from between the orbital plates of the frontal bone and contributes to the walls of the orbital and nasal cavities as well as to the medial portion of the anterior cranial base. It consists of four parts: the horizontal **cribriform plate,** two lateral masses called the **ethmoidal labyrinths,** and a vertical component consisting of the **perpendicular plate** below and the **crista galli** above. When viewed from above the ethmoid appears roughly cuboidal and when viewed from behind, as in Figure 4-19, it appears to be T-shaped.

The **cribriform** (L. sieve) **plate** serves as a partition, separating the cranial from the nasal cavities. It is received

FIGURE 4-17

The malar or outer surface (top) and temporal or inner surface (bottom) of a zygomatic bone.

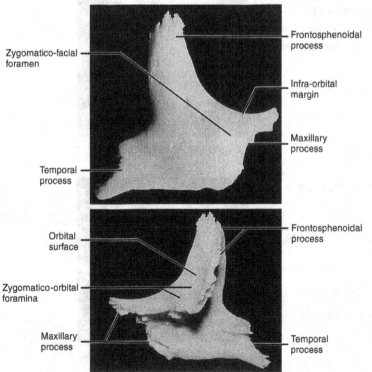

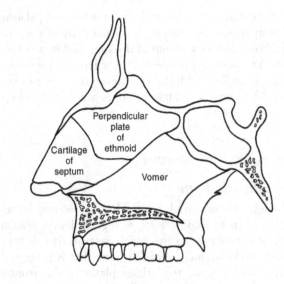

FIGURE 4-18

Schematic of medial wall of nasal cavity showing vomer bone, perpendicular plate of the ethmoid, and the articulation of the nasal bone with the septum.

into the ethmoidal notch of the frontal bone (shown in Figure 4-20), and thus forms the roof of the nasal cavities. Projecting upward from the midline in front is a thick triangular process, the **crista galli,** literally, cock's comb. It serves as the anterior attachment for the **falx cerebri,** a fold of the dura mater that separates the cerebral hemispheres. Through the perforations of the cribriform plate, olfactory nerves emerge into the nasal cavity and pass down along the surfaces of the nasal conchae.

The **perpendicular plate** is a thin, flat lamella, nearly quadrilateral in shape, which is directed vertically downward from the under surface of the cribriform plate. The upper anterior margin joins with the frontal and nasal bones, with the cartilaginous septum of the nose anteriorly, and with the anterior margin of the vomer behind. The posterior margin is thin and articulates with the rostrum of the sphenoid bone (to be discussed later).

Each **ethmoidal labyrinth** consists of thin-walled, highly variable air cells arranged in anterior, middle, and posterior clusters. Unlike other sinuses, the ethmoid air cells are present at birth, but of course the labyrinths are small. A labyrinth is bounded by an orbital plate consist-

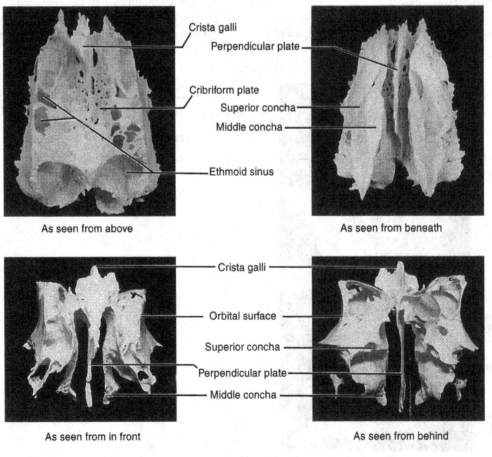

As seen from above　　As seen from beneath

As seen from in front　　As seen from behind

FIGURE 4-19

Various views of the ethmoid bone. (From Zemlin and Stolpe, 1967.)

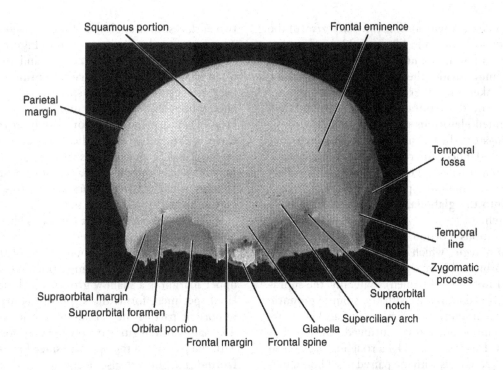

Squamous portion — Frontal eminence — Parietal margin — Temporal fossa — Temporal line — Zygomatic process — Supraorbital margin — Supraorbital foramen — Orbital portion — Frontal margin — Frontal spine — Glabella — Superciliary arch — Supraorbital notch

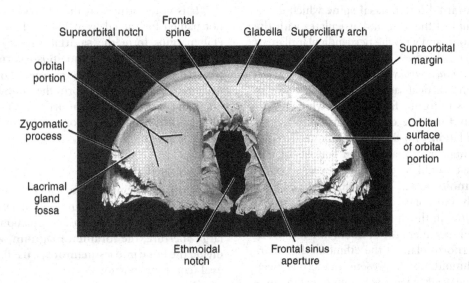

Supraorbital notch — Frontal spine — Glabella — Superciliary arch — Orbital portion — Supraorbital margin — Zygomatic process — Orbital surface of orbital portion — Lacrimal gland fossa — Ethmoidal notch — Frontal sinus aperture

FIGURE 4-20

The frontal bone as seen from the front (top) and from beneath. (From Zemlin and Stolpe, 1967.)

ing of a paper-thin sheet of bone (lamina papyracea) that forms a large area of the medial wall of the orbit. The medial surfaces of the ethmoidal labyrinths comprise the lateral walls of the upper part of the nasal cavity. These are thin bones with scroll-like extensions, the **superior** and **middle nasal conchae,** which have already been discussed as structures of the nasal cavity.

Because of its complexity and numerous articulations, the ethmoid bone demands careful study. It articulates

with fifteen bones: the frontal, sphenoid, nasals, maxillae, lacrimals, palatines, inferior nasal conchae, and vomer.

The Frontal Bone

The unpaired frontal bone, which forms the anterior part of the braincase, consists of a **squamous portion** (the vertical plate or forehead) and an **orbital portion** (the horizontal part that contributes to the roof of the orbital and nasal cavities). The *external surface* of the squamous portion, shown in Figure 4-20, is convex. It may retain a midline **frontal** (or **metopic**) **suture** which, in infancy, divides the frontal bone in two. The midline is flanked on either side, above the supraorbital margins, by the **frontal eminences** (or **tubers**), smooth rounded elevations that are especially prominent in youngsters. Just beneath these eminences are two rather well-defined **superciliary arches,** highly variable in size, but usually larger in the male. The superciliary arches become more prominent medially where they blend into the **glabella,** a prominence just above the nasal notch.

The squamous portion is limited below by the **supraorbital margin,** which delimits the upper boundary of the orbit. This margin is characterized by a **supraorbital notch** (or **foramen**). Laterally, the supraorbital margin is continuous with the stout **zygomatic process.** At the midline, between the supraorbital margins, the squamous portion is continued downward as the nasal part. It is terminated by a rough uneven **nasal notch** which articulates with the paired nasal bones medially and the frontal process of the maxilla and the lacrimal bones laterally. The center of the nasal notch presents a downward directed **nasal spine** which forms part of the septum of the nose and articulates with the nasal bones in front, and with the perpendicular plate of the ethmoid bone behind.

The concave *inner surface* of the squamous portion presents a midline vertical sagittal sulcus, the edges of which meet below to form a **frontal crest** which terminates in a small **foramen cecum,** part of which is formed by articulation with the ethmoid bone.

The horizontal or orbital portion consists of two orbital plates that would be continuous except for the intervening **ethmoid notch.** The orbital surface of the plates is smooth and concave and presents a lacrimal gland fossa, located in the upper lateral orbital margin. In the articulated specimen, the ethmoid notch is occupied by the cribriform plate of the ethmoid. The margins of the ethmoid notch present numerous deep depressions or half-cells which, when united with similar depressions of the ethmoid, complete the **ethmoid air cells** or **sinuses.** On either side of the frontal spine inferiorly may be seen the openings of the **frontal sinuses** which extend backward, lateralward, and upward to an area behind the superciliary arches.

The frontal bone articulates with the unpaired sphenoid and ethmoid bones and the paired parietal, nasal, maxillary, lacrimal, and the zygomatic bones: twelve in all.

The Parietal Bone

The paired parietal bones form, by virtue of their union at the midline, most of the rounded roof of the cranium. Each bone is roughly quadrilateral in shape and presents

two surfaces, four angles, and four margins for inspection. Some landmarks are shown in Figure 4-21.

The *external surface* is convex and smooth and is often characterized by a **parietal eminence** (or **tuber**) near the center. In older specimens, especially, two curved lines arch across the middle of the external surface. They are the **superior** and **inferior temporal lines,** and together they indicate the attachment of the temporal fascia and the muscular origin of the temporalis muscle, a muscle of mastication to be considered later. A small (partietal) foramen is present near the sagittal suture (interparietal margins).

The *inner surface* is concave and is characterized by numerous depressions corresponding to cerebral convolutions and superficial blood vessels of the brain and its connective tissue coverings (meninges). Near the upper margin is a shallow groove which, in the articulated specimen, forms the **superior sagittal sinus,** an important part of the venous system in the braincase. The **sagittal margin** is deeply serrated for articulation with the parietal of the opposite side. The **occipital** and **frontal margins** are also deeply serrated, as contrasted with the sharply beveled **temporal margin** which articulates with the squamous portion of the temporal bone.

It is noteworthy that the *sutures* at the margins are not named for the adjacent bones. Thus, the interparietal margins form the **sagittal suture,** the temporal-parietal margins form the **squamosol suture,** the frontal-parietal margins form the **coronal suture,** and the occipital-parietal margins form the **lambdoid suture.**

In all, each parietal bone articulates with five bones: the occipital, frontal, temporal, sphenoid, and the parietal from the opposite side.

The Occipital Bone

The unpaired occipital bone, which forms the lower and back portions of the cranium, is often described as being trapezoidal in shape. Its most conspicuous landmark is a large aperture, the **foramen magnum,** which serves to divide the bone into a **squamous,** a **basilar,** and two **lateral** (condylar) portions.

The *external surface* of the squama is convex from above downward and from side to side. At the midline, midway between the summit of the bone and the foramen magnum, may be found the **external occipital protuberance** (the most prominent point is denoted in anthropology as the **inion**) from which, directed laterally on either side, are indistinct (especially in young specimens) **superior nuchal lines.** That part of the squama above these superior nuchal lines is for scalp musculature and that part below is for neck muscles (thus the nuchal area). Below and parallel to the superior nuchal lines are the **inferior nuchal lines,** points of attachment primarily for neck muscles.

The *inner surface* is deeply concave, from above downward and from side to side. It is characterized by

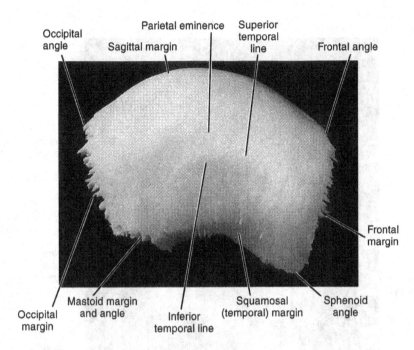

FIGURE 4-21

Right parietal bone, external surface
(top) and inner surface (bottom).

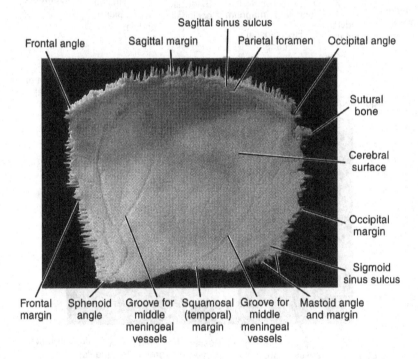

an **internal occipital protuberance** which corresponds
in location to its external counterpart. It is an important
landmark because the inner surface is divided into four
fossae by **transverse** and **longitudinal crests,** all of
which intersect at the internal occipital protuberance.
Collectively, these crests are known as the **cruciform**
(in the shape of a cross) **eminence.**

The parts of the occipital bone lateral to the foramen magnum contain, on their undersurfaces, the **condyles** for articulation with the superior facets of the
first cervical vertebra or atlas. As shown in Figure 4-22,

the condyles are kidney-shaped (reniform) and contain
slightly convex articular surfaces. The base of each condyle presents anteriorly a short **hypoglossal canal,**
while in back is a **condylar fossa,** which carries the
posterior margins of the superior articular processes of
the atlas when the head is tilted sharply back.

The *basilar portion* of the occipital bone is directed
forward and somewhat upward from the foramen magnum. Its lower surface contains a midline **pharyngeal
tubercle** which provides attachment for the fibrous
midline **raphe** of the pharynx, an important part of the

FIGURE 4-22

The occipital bone as seen from behind (top) and from beneath (bottom). (From Zemlin and Stolpe, 1967.)

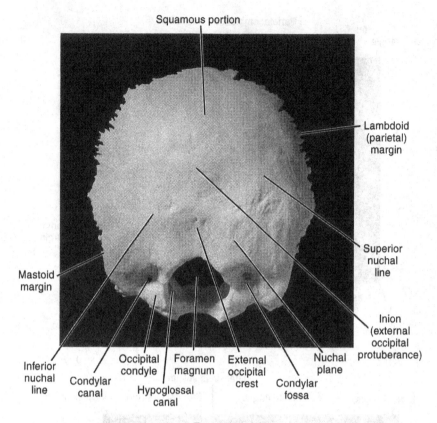

Squamous portion

Lambdoid (parietal) margin

Superior nuchal line

Inion (external occipital protuberance)

Mastoid margin

Inferior nuchal line

Condylar canal

Occipital condyle

Foramen magnum

Hypoglossal canal

External occipital crest

Nuchal plane

Condylar fossa

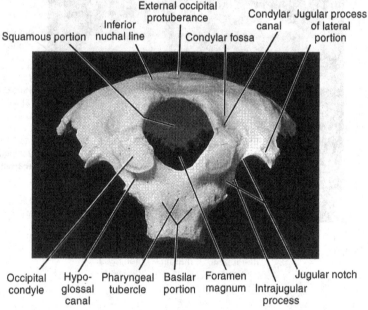

External occipital protuberance

Inferior nuchal line

Condylar canal

Condylar fossa

Jugular process of lateral portion

Squamous portion

Occipital condyle

Hypo-glossal canal

Pharyngeal tubercle

Basilar portion

Foramen magnum

Intrajugular process

Jugular notch

speech mechanism to be described later. In front, the basilar portion articulates (and later fuses) with the body of the sphenoid bone.

The foramen magnum is somewhat oval-shaped, described more accurately as being five-sided. It transmits the vertebral and anterior spinal arteries and marks the junction of the spinal cord and brain.

In all, the occipital bone articulates with six bones: the two parietals, the two temporal bones, the sphenoid, and the atlas.

The Temporal Bones

The paired temporal bones form most of the lateral base and sides of the braincase. Each bone consists of five parts: the **squamous, mastoid, petrous,** and **tympanic** parts and the **styloid process.**

As shown in Figure 4-23, the **squamous** (L. *squamosus,* scalelike) portion forms the lateral, anterior, and upper part of the temporal bone. The outer surface is quite smooth and convex. The outstanding landmark of the outer squamous portion is the long arched **zygomatic process,** which joins with the temporal process of the zygomatic bone to form the zygomatic arch (zygoma). As shown in Figure 4-23, this process is at first directed

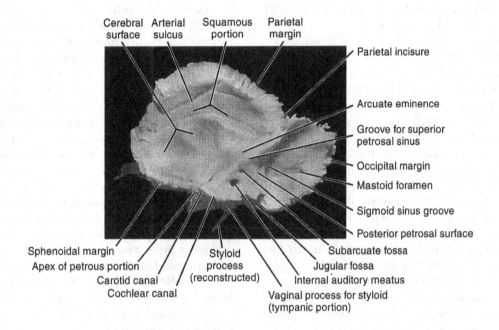

Cerebral surface · Arterial sulcus · Squamous portion · Parietal margin

Parietal incisure
Arcuate eminence
Groove for superior petrosal sinus
Occipital margin
Mastoid foramen
Sigmoid sinus groove
Posterior petrosal surface
Subarcuate fossa
Jugular fossa
Internal auditory meatus

Sphenoidal margin
Apex of petrous portion
Carotid canal
Cochlear canal
Styloid process (reconstructed)
Vaginal process for styloid (tympanic portion)

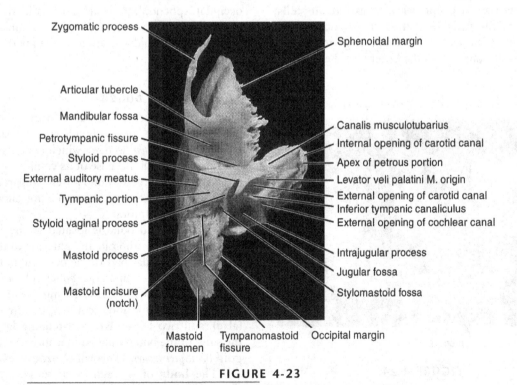

Zygomatic process
Articular tubercle
Mandibular fossa
Petrotympanic fissure
Styloid process
External auditory meatus
Tympanic portion
Styloid vaginal process
Mastoid process
Mastoid incisure (notch)

Sphenoidal margin
Canalis musculotubarius
Internal opening of carotid canal
Apex of petrous portion
Levator veli palatini M. origin
External opening of carotid canal
Inferior tympanic canaliculus
External opening of cochlear canal
Intrajugular process
Jugular fossa
Stylomastoid fossa

Mastoid foramen · Tympanomastoid fissure · Occipital margin

FIGURE 4-23

A right temporal bone as seen from the side (top) and from beneath (bottom).

lateralward and then sharply forward so that the lateral surface is convex and subcutaneous while the medial surface is concave. It provides attachment for the bulk of the masseter muscle, a muscle of mastication. The superior border of the squamous portion is sharply beveled and, for the most part, articulates with the beveled edge of the parietal bone. This type of suture provides good protection against displacement of the two bones, which might be caused by a lateral blow to the head.

The **petrous portion** of the temporal bone is located at the base of the skull between the sphenoid and occipital bones. It is extremely important because it houses the essential parts of the organs of equilibrium and hearing. Because this part of the temporal bone will be described in some detail later, only a few words are necessary here. The petrous (L. *petra*, stone) portion is rough in appearance, having many foramina and canals, and is, as its name suggests, extremely hard.

Below and posteriorly the petrous portion ends as a conical projection called the **mastoid** (Gk. *mastos*, breast) **process,** which provides attachment for the sternocleidomastoid and other neck muscles. The medial limit of the process contains a rather deep **mastoid notch** (incisure) which forms a point of attachment for the digastric muscle. Anteriorly the mastoid process is fused with the squamous portion, below it is fused with the tympanic part, and it also contributes to the formation of the tympanic cavity and the external auditory meatus.

As shown in Figure 4-24, a section through the mastoid process reveals a number of **mastoid air cells,** which are highly variable in their shape and number. The upper part of the process contains large and very irregular air cells, but toward the lower part they become

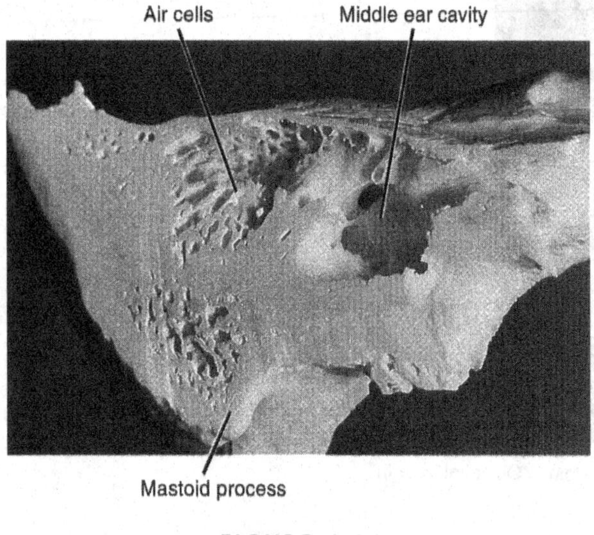

progressively smaller, gradually giving way to marrow. The cells in the upper and front part give way to a rather large **tympanic antrum** (Gk. *tympanon*, drum; L. *antron*, cave), which is bounded above by the **tegmen tympanum,** the roof of the tympanic cavity.

The **tympanic part** is a thick, curved plate of bone, located in front of the mastoid process and just beneath the squamous and petrous portions. Laterally, it presents a rough, free surface which, in life, is continuous with the cartilaginous portion of the external auditory meatus. Its concave posterosuperior surface forms the anterior wall, floor, and part of the posterior wall of the external auditory meatus. Its anteroinferior surface meets the squama at the posterior part of the mandibular fossa in the line of the **petrotympanic** and **tympanosquamosal fissures.** Its posterior border is separated from the mastoid process by the **tympanomastoid fissure.** From the medial part of the inferior surface arises a sheath of bone, the **vaginal process,** which envelops the base of the styloid process.

The prominent **styloid** (Gk. *stylos*, pillar) **process,** a sharp pillar of bone of variable length, and frequently missing in prepared laboratory skulls, serves as the site of origin for three muscles: stylopharyngeus, styloglossus, and stylohyoideus. It also provides attachment to the stylomandibular and stylohyoid ligaments. The **stylohyoid ligament** passes from the extremity of the styloid process, downward and forward, to the lesser horn of the hyoid bone, which is thereby suspended from the skull.

Sutural articulations join each temporal bone to the occipital, sphenoid, parietal, and zygomatic bones, but each temporal bone is joined to the mandible by a freely movable (diarthroidial) joint located in part at the **mandibular fossa.**

The Sphenoid Bone

One of the most complex bones in the skull, and certainly one of the most difficult to understand, is the sphenoid (Gk. *sphen*, wedge), which is shown in Figures 4-25 through 4-28. Because of its complexity, the interested student is urged to find a well-prepared skull, and perhaps a well-prepared instructor, for supplementary information and tuition.

The sphenoid bone is located at the base of the skull, back of the ethmoid and anterior to the foramen magnum and basilar part of the occipital bone. Because of its distinctive shape, the sphenoid bone is often likened to a bat with extended wings, or to a butterfly. It is composed of a **body** (corpus), two **greater wings** (alae), and two **lesser wings** extending laterally from the sides of the body, and two inferiorly directed **pterygoid** (Gk. *pterygodes*, like a wing) **processes.**

The **body** of the sphenoid, roughly cuboidal in shape, contains two **sphenoid sinuses,** separated one from the other by a thin, irregular midline septum. The

Air cells   Middle ear cavity

Mastoid process

FIGURE 4-24

Section through a left temporal bone, showing distribution of air cells in the mastoid region.

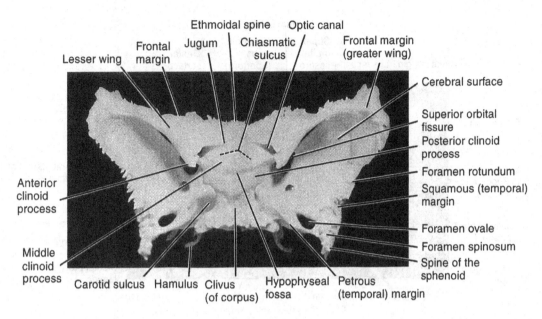

FIGURE 4-25

Sphenoid bone as seen from above.

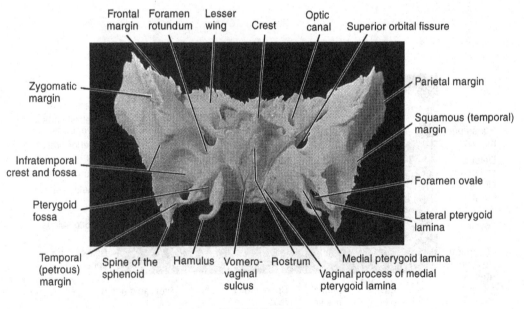

FIGURE 4-26

Sphenoid bone as seen from beneath.

anterior surface of the body forms the posterior wall of the nasal cavity. The wall presents a midline crest for articulation with the perpendicular plate of the ethmoid bone, thus forming part of the bony septum of the nasal cavity. On either side of the sphenoidal crest may be seen the irregular openings into the sphenoidal air sinuses, partially covered by the **sphenoidal conchae.** The conchae are broken in the process of disarticulat-

ing a skull; however, in life they are thin bony membranes fused with the sphenoid, ethmoid, and palatine bones to form the anterior surface of the body, except for the crest. The lateral margin of the anterior surface is rough and articulates with the ethmoid, while the lower anterior margin joins the palatine bones and the upper margin articulates with the frontal bone. The *inferior surface* of the body has a small ridge, the **sphenoidal**

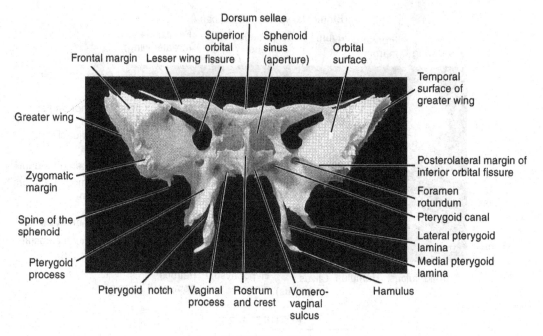

FIGURE 4-27

Sphenoid bone as seen from the front.

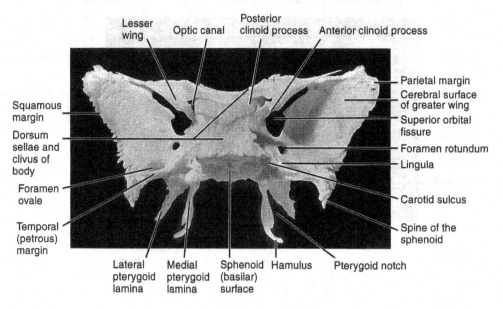

FIGURE 4-28

Sphenoid bone as seen from behind.

rostrum, which articulates with the depression between the alae of the vomer bone.

The *posterior surface* of the sphenoid is not distinctive. Its union with the basilar part of the occipital bone is effected by an interposed layer of cartilage that is ossified by the time young adulthood is reached. The air sinuses of the sphenoid sometimes extend into the basi-

lar part of the occipital bone, as far back as the foramen magnum.

The *superior surface* of the body is a complex arrangement of smooth surfaces, deep grooves, prominent ridges, and processes. Anteriorly, a small projection, the **ethmoid spine,** articulates with the cribriform plate of the ethmoid. Behind this is a smooth surface formed by the union of the lesser wings into a **jugum** (yoke). Its posterior margin is grooved by the **chiasmatic sulcus,** which in life accommodates the optic chiasma (L., Gk. shaped like the letter X). This sulcus connects anteriorly with the **optic canals,** through which the optic nerves and the ophthalmic arteries enter the orbit. Immediately behind the sulcus is the **sella turcica** (literally, Turkish saddle) which, in life, houses the pituitary gland, and within the deepest recess of the sella turcica lies the **hypophyseal fossa.** A small anterior protuberance known as the **tuberculum sellae** forms the posterior wall of the chiasmatic sulcus. A larger protuberance is located behind the hypophyseal fossa. It is known as the **dorsum sellae,** and prominent lateral **posterior clinoid** (Gk. *kline,* bed) **processes** are attached to it. From the dorsum sellae the body becomes continuous with the basilar part of the occipital bone, and together they form the **clivus** (slanted surface) which slants back toward the foramen magnum.

The **lesser wings** are laterally directed plates that arise from the anterior-superior aspect of the body of the sphenoid. They ultimately terminate as sharp points that often can be seen on the posterior margin of the anterior cranial fossa. The *superior surfaces* of the lesser wings form the posterior portion of the anterior cranial fossa, and the region where the two wings join (jugum) has already been discussed. The *inferior surface* of the lesser wings forms the upper boundary for the superior orbital fissure.[3] The anterior margin of the lesser wing is serrated, and it articulates with the orbital plates of the frontal bone. The medial limits of the smooth posterior margin are characterized by the anterior clinoid processes.

The lateral surfaces of the body give rise to the greater wings and to the pterygoid processes. The **greater wings** are directed laterally and at the same time are curved upward and slightly backward. The posterior margin is characterized by a prominent triangle which fits into the angle between the squamous and petrous portions of the temporal bone. The **spine of the sphenoid,** found on the inferior side of the triangle's apex, forms an attachment site for fibers of the tensor veli palatini muscle and the sphenomandibular ligament. On its inferior side along the petrous portion of the temporal bone, the sphenoid is grooved to accommodate the auditory (Eustachian) tube. The cerebral surfaces of the greater wings form part of the middle cranial fossa of the skull. Anteriorly, where the greater wing joins the body, is the prominent **foramen rotundum,** which in life contains the maxillary branch of the trigeminal nerve. Laterally and just behind this foramen is the **foramen ovale.** It transmits the mandibular branch of the trigeminal nerve and meningeal arteries.

The orbital surface of the greater wing is smoothly concave and contributes to the posterior half of the lateral wall of the orbit. Its upper margin is serrated for articulation with the orbital plate of the frontal bone, while its smoothly rounded inferior margin forms the posterolateral margin of the inferior orbital fissure. The medial margin contributes to the lower margin of the superior orbital fissure, and the serrated lateral margin articulates with the zygomatic bone.

The paired **pterygoid processes** descend vertically from the region where the greater wings join the body, just below the foramen rotundum. Posteriorly, each process is divided into a **medial** and a **lateral pterygoid plate** or lamina, and this division results in a V-shaped cleft, the **pterygoid notch,** in addition to a deep **pterygoid fossa.** Anteriorly, the edges of the pterygoid notch articulate with the pyramidal process of the palatine bone. The **lateral plate,** which serves as the origin for the medial and lateral pterygoid muscles (on medial and lateral sides, respectively), has a free posterior edge directed toward the foramen ovale.

The **medial plate** is narrower and forms the posterior boundary of the lateral wall of the nasal cavity. This plate ends inferiorly as a hooklike extension, the **pterygoid hamulus** (L., little hook), to which the tensor palatini muscle attaches. The posterior border provides attachment for the superior constrictor muscle of the pharynx and, at its lower end, the pterygomandibular ligament. The anterior margin of the medial pterygoid plate articulates with the perpendicular plate of the palatine bone, while the anterior border of the lateral pterygoid plate forms the posterior edge of the **pterygomaxillary fissure,** an important landmark for x-ray examination of the skull.

The sphenoid bone articulates with all the bones of the cranium: the occipital, parietal, frontal, ethmoid, and temporal bones. It also articulates with facial bones: vomer, palatine, and zygomatic bones and often with the tuberosities of the maxillary bones. The sphenoid bone forms part of the orbital, nasal, and pharygeal cavities and marks the division between and forms parts of the anterior and middle cranial fossae.

The sphenoid bone has been described in considerable detail; with a grasp of its processes, major landmarks, and its articulations, students are well on their way toward an understanding of this complex structure we call the skull.

The Sinuses

Introduction

From outward appearances the bones of the skull may appear to be solid and massive. As may be seen in Figure 4-13, however, many of the skull bones are but hollow

---

[3]In life, the superior orbital fissure transmits the oculomotor, trochlear, and abducent nerves; the opthalmic branch of the trigeminal nerve; and the meningeal and opthalmic blood vessels.

shells. That is, they contain sinuses (L., hollows), which are air-filled spaces lined by **mucoperiosteum,** a thin membrane formed by the fusion of periosteum and mucous membrane. This membrane, poorly supplied by glandular, nerve, and vascular tissue, is covered by a ciliated (pseudostratified) columnar epithelium characteristic of the respiratory epithelium. Four pairs of accessory sinuses drain into the nasal cavities. Because of their location they are called **paranasal sinuses,** which include the **frontal, maxillary, ethmoid,** and **sphenoid** sinuses, shown in Figures 4-13 and 4-29.

The Frontal Sinuses

The frontal sinuses were shown in Figures 4-13 and 4-16. They are located directly behind the superciliary arches or ridges, shown in Figure 4-20. The frontal sinuses are paired, separated one from the other by a midline bony septum.[4] These sinuses, practically absent at birth, attain their full size only after puberty. The frontal sinus actually develops from one of the anterior ethmoid cells discussed earlier, but it does not start to pneumatize the frontal bone until after the first or second year of life. Developing sinuses can be thought of as outpocketings of nasal mucous membrane. These sinuses drain into the middle meatus of the nasal cavity.

The Maxillary Sinuses

The maxillary sinuses, which were described with the maxillary bones, are the largest of the paranasal sinuses, and they are present at birth. The extent of the sinus cavity may be seen in Figure 4-10. In this photograph, the inferior nasal concha has been removed to expose the opening into the sinus or antrum of Highmore. As might be expected, the maxillary sinuses drain into the middle meatus of the nasal cavity.

The Ethmoid Sinuses

These sinuses, which are present at birth, were discussed in some detail in the earlier description of the ethmoid bone, and they are shown in Figure 4-13. Because of their complexity, the ethmoid sinuses are often referred to as the **ethmoid labyrinth.** You will recall that the cells that comprise these complex sinuses are divided into anterior, middle, and posterior groups. The posterior cells open into the superior meatus of the nasal cavity, while the anterior and middle cells open into the middle meatus.

The Sphenoid Sinuses

We learned earlier that the body of the sphenoid bone contains two sphenoid sinuses, separated one from the other by a highly variable midline septum. These sinuses are not present at birth, and the bone does not begin to pneumatize until about the third year of life. The sphenoid sinuses open into a **sphenoethmoid recess** located above and behind the superior turbinate of the nasal cavity.

Functions of the Sinuses

A number of functions have been attributed to the sinuses, a clear indication that we really don't know what their function is. They have no real significance with respect to speech production, except perhaps for minimal contributions to the resonant characteristics of the skull bones, and there is little support for that contention.

One line of thought is that the sinuses develop because the differential growth of the facial bones away from the cranial bones results in the development of cavity spaces within the bone tissue. The sinuses do reduce the weight of the skull, but the reduction is trivial, because in their absence the space would be occupied by spongy bone and not an equal volume of compact bone.

It is frequently claimed that sinus infections (sinusitis) affect voice quality, and on that basis a resonance function is sometimes assigned to the sinuses. It may be true that voice quality is affected when the sinuses are infected, but it is unlikely that infections of the sinuses affect voice quality. That is to say, there is probably a simultaneous infection of the sinus cavities and the nasal cavities proper, and the combined effects result in changes in voice quality. Since the mucous membrane lining the paranasal sinuses is continuous with that of the nasal cavity, any inflammation of mucous membrane of the nasal cavity is very likely communicated to the mucous membrane of the sinuses. However, the walls of the sinuses are much less sensitive to pain than are their openings or other parts of the nasal mucosa.

The relationship of the maxillary sinus to the upper teeth has important clinical implications because of the frequency with which pain from dental abscess is confused with pain from sinus infection (Deweese and Saunders, 1973). In addition, a remnant of a root tip may enter the maxillary sinus when a tooth is extracted.

The Mastoid Air Cells

The air cells of the mastoid portion of the temporal bone are regarded as diverticula of the tympanic antrum rather than true sinuses. Although the mastoid process is present at birth, it is small and filled with bone. During the first two to six years of life, however, bone is replaced by air cells that bud off from the tympanic antrum. The cells, shown in Figure 4-24, are filled with air and are lined with mucous membrane continuous with that of the tympanic cavity.

---

[4]**Septum** is a Latin term denoting, in general anatomical nomenclature, a dividing wall or partition.

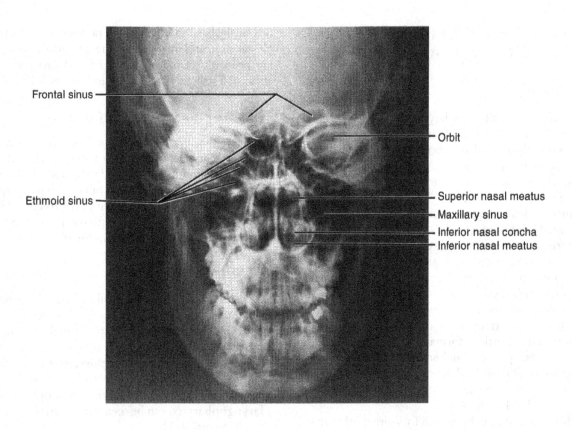

Frontal sinus

Ethmoid sinus

Orbit

Superior nasal meatus

Maxillary sinus

Inferior nasal concha

Inferior nasal meatus

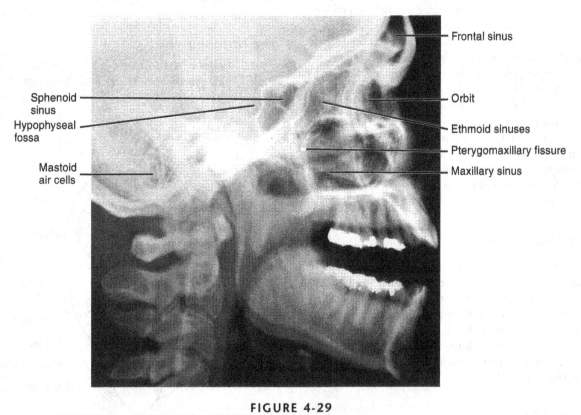

Sphenoid sinus

Hypophyseal fossa

Mastoid air cells

Frontal sinus

Orbit

Ethmoid sinuses

Pterygomaxillary fissure

Maxillary sinus

FIGURE 4-29

Paranasal sinuses as seen by frontal and lateral x-ray.

THE CAVITIES OF THE VOCAL TRACT

Introduction

Earlier we learned that the laryngeal tone is complex, consisting of a fundamental frequency and a rich series of harmonically related overtones. We have also seen that, depending upon the acoustical properties of the vocal tract, certain overtones are reinforced at the expense of others. Resonances in the vocal tract are called **formants,** and we know that information contributing to the intelligibility of speech is conveyed not so much by the frequencies of the energy in the voice or by the amount of power or energy in the voice, but, rather, by the distribution of energy along the frequency domain within the various speech sounds. In other words, changes in the gross configurations (length and cross-sectional area) of the vocal tract result in modifications of the resonant characteristics **(formant frequencies)**; thus, sounds with fairly unique and predictable energy distributions are produced. In these instances the vocal tract filters or modifies the raw material generated by the source at the level of the larynx.

The vocal tract can be excited by sources other than the one at the larynx, to produce those sounds we call consonants. By placing the lower lip against the upper teeth and releasing a puff of air, we are able to produce the [f] sound, and by phonating with the same vocal tract configuration, we generate its voiced counterpart [v]. By placing the tongue to the edge of the upper teeth and releasing a puff of air, we generate a [θ] sound as in "thin." Or, by phonating with the same articulation, we produce the [ð] as in "these." And so on.

The vocal tract may be subdivided, on an anatomical basis, into five cavities: the **buccal, oral, pharnygeal,** and paired **nasal** cavities. For the sake of continuity, we will describe the various cavities at first very briefly. A detailed description will follow in the section titled "The Articulators and Associated Structures."

The Buccal Cavity

The buccal (L. *bucca*, cheek) cavity is highly variable in its shape and dimensions, depending upon the status of the lips and cheeks. It is the small space that is limited by the lips and cheeks externally and by the gums (gingivae) and teeth internally. It communicates with the mouth or oral cavity, with the jaws closed, by the small spaces between the teeth, and by the space on either side behind the last molars or "wisdom teeth."

The Oral Cavity

The oral or mouth cavity proper is bounded anteriorly and laterally by the teeth and alveolar processes, superi-

orly by the hard and soft palates, posteriorly by the palatoglossal arch, and inferiorly by the muscular floor consisting primarily of the tongue. The oral cavity and some associated structures are shown in Figures 4-30 and 4-31.

The Oropharyngeal Isthmus

The port through which the oral cavity communicates with the pharyngeal and nasal cavities is called the oropharyngeal isthmus. It is bounded laterally by the **palatoglossal arch** (anterior faucial pillars), above by the soft palate, and below by the dorsum of the tongue. The palatoglossal arch and the **palatopharyngeal arch** (posterior faucial pillars) can be seen in Figures 4-30 and 4-31.

The Pharyngeal Cavity

The pharynx is a musculomembranous tube extending from the base of the skull to the level of the sixth cervical vertebra behind and the cricoid cartilage in front. It is about 12 cm in length and is oval in cross section, being somewhat wider in its transverse than in the anteroposterior dimension. The cavity of the pharynx, often divided into a **nasopharynx,** an **oropharynx,** and a **laryngopharynx,** can be seen with its associated structures in Figure 4-32.

The pharyngeal tube, which is largely connective tissue and mucoperiosteum superiorly, becomes increasingly muscular as it continues downward toward the esophagus.

The Nasopharynx

Bounded above by the rostrum of the sphenoid bone and the pharyngeal protuberance of the occipital bone, the nasopharynx is limited inferiorly at the level of the

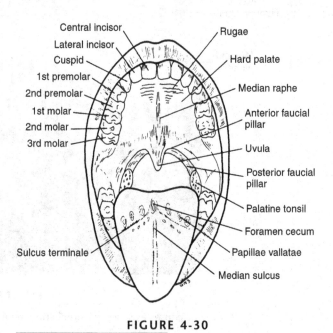

FIGURE 4-30

Schematic of oral cavity and adjacent structures.

FIGURE 4-31

Photograph of oral cavity.

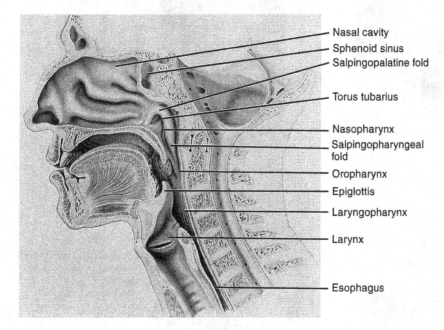

Hard palate

Soft palate

Uvula

Post. faucial pillar
(Palatopharyngeal arch)

Ant. faucial pillar
(Palatoglossal arch)

Tonsil

Pharyngeal wall

Nasal cavity
Sphenoid sinus
Salpingopalatine fold

Torus tubarius

Nasopharynx
Salpingopharyngeal
fold
Oropharynx
Epiglottis
Laryngopharynx
Larynx

Esophagus

FIGURE 4-32

The pharynx and adjacent structures.

soft palate. It communicates anteriorly with the **posterior nares** or the **choanae** of the nasal cavities and laterally with the pharyngeal orifice of the auditory tube.

The Oropharynx

The superior limit to the oropharynx is at the level of the soft palate, while the lower boundary is at the level of the hyoid bone. Anteriorly, it communicates with the oral cavity by way of the palatoglossal and palatopharyngeal arches.

The Laryngopharynx

Bounded above at the level of the hyoid bone, the laryngopharynx is continuous with the esophagus inferiorly.

Anteriorly it communicates with the **aditus laryngis**, the opening of the larynx formed by the epiglottis and aryepiglottic folds.

Thus, in all, the pharynx communicates with the tympanic, oral, laryngeal, and nasal cavities, as well as the esophagus (see Figure 4-32).

The Nose and Nasal Cavities

The nose is defined (Blakiston, 1941) as the prominent organ in the center of the face. The upper part (regio olfactoria) constitutes the organ of smell, and the lower part (regio respiratoria) the beginning of the respiratory tract, in which inspired air is warmed, moistened, and cleaned of impurities. We might add that the nose, highly variable in size and shape, contributes significantly to the general configuration and aesthetics of the facial region (see Figure 4-33).

Terms commonly used to describe the nose include the tip **(apex),** the **base** that includes the nostrils **(nares),** the **root** where the nasal bones join the frontal bone, the **dorsum** (located between the root and the tip), and the **bridge** (the upper part of the dorsum). Only the bridge of the nose has a bony framework. The lower two-thirds has a yielding, cartilaginous framework capable of withstanding certain physical insults.

Cartilages of the Nose

The **septal, lateral,** and **major** and **minor alar** cartilages and their intervening connective tissue have been regarded as a liminal (L. *limen,* threshold) valve, capable of controlling the intake of air.

As can be seen from Figure 4-34, the **major alar** (L. a wing) cartilages form much of the tip of the nose. Smaller **minor alar** cartilages located lateral to the major alae contribute to the general shape of the nose. Cartilaginous extensions of each ala (known as **crura**) form much of the framework of the nostrils and serve to partially separate them. The division of the base into two separate nostrils is completed by part of the **septal** cartilage.

A variable deposit of fibroadipose tissue located in this region accounts for some individual differences in shape. **Lateral nasal** cartilages are located in the middle third of the nose, between the nasal bones above and the major alar cartilages below.

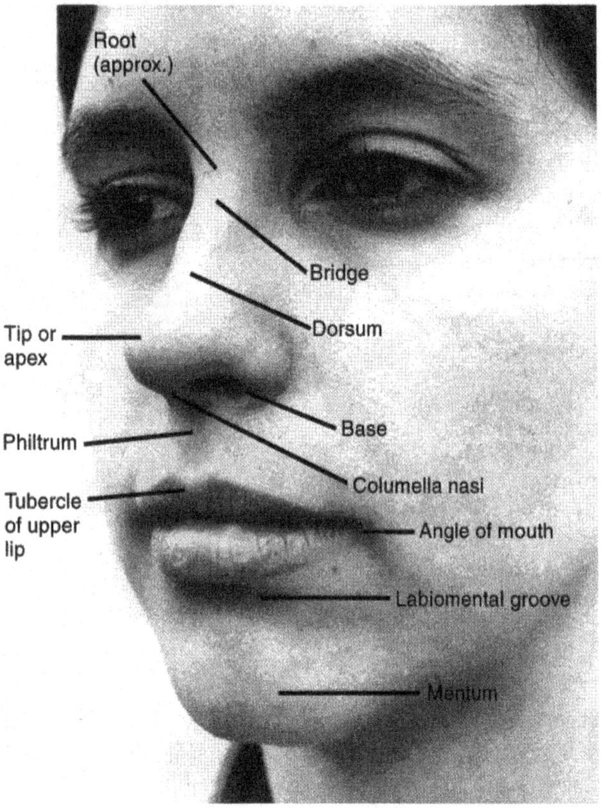

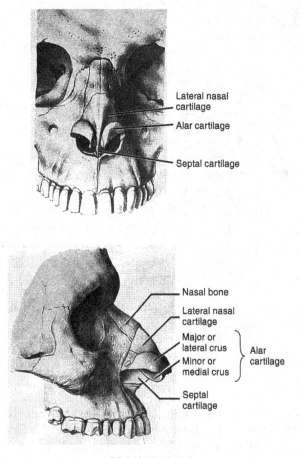

FIGURE 4-34

Framework of the nose. (From Sicher and Tandler, *Anatomie für Zahnartze,* 1928.)

Root (approx.)

Bridge

Dorsum

Tip or apex

Philtrum

Tubercle of upper lip

Base

Columella nasi

Angle of mouth

Labiomental groove

Mentum

FIGURE 4-33

Surface features of the nose.

Muscles of the Nose

The small muscles of the nose are rudimentary (vestigal?) in humans, but they are considered muscles of facial expression. Although their role is usually quite minimal, they may at times be rather significant mediators of secondary cues and facial expression. The five muscles that act directly on the nose are shown schematically in Figure 4-35.

The Procerus Muscle It is a small, triangular unpaired muscle that arises by tendinous slips from the fascia of the lower nasal bones and upper lateral nasal cartilages. The procerus[5] muscle inserts into the skin of the lower forehead between the eyebrows. Some fibers are continuous with those of the scalp muscles (frontalis). When active, the procerus draws down the medial angle of the eyebrow and at the same time wrinkles the skin over the bridge of the nose. These actions may occur when someone is frowning or concentrating, or attempting to reduce the glare of bright light.

The Nasalis Muscle This muscle originates in an area above and lateral to the incisive fossa of the maxilla. The fibers course upward and medially to blend into an aponeurosis that is continuous with the nasalis from the opposite side and with the aponeurosis of the procerus

---

[5]The word **procerus** is from a Latin term denoting long and slender or high, lofty.

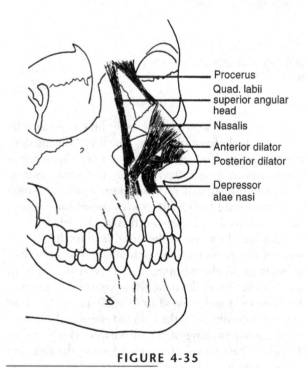

FIGURE 4-35

Muscles of the nose.

muscle. Upon contraction, the nasalis muscle depresses the cartilages of the nose, thereby narrowing the nostrils.

CLINICAL NOTE: This narrowing of the nostrils is a compensatory action sometimes seen in persons with hypernasality, particularly those who also have audible nasal emission.

The Depressor Septi (Depressor Alae Nasi) It arises from the incisive fossa of the maxilla and inserts into the lower border of the cartilaginous nasal septum and adjacent alae of the nose. As the name implies, this muscle depresses the alae of the nose and constricts the nostrils.

The Nasal Dilators Two muscles dilate the nostrils, the **anterior** and **posterior** nasal dilators. The first of these muscles arises from the lower edge of the lateral cartilage of the nose and inserts into the deep surface of the skin covering the alae of the nose. The second arises from the edge of the nasal aperture of the maxilla and adjacent sesamoid cartilages of the nose and inserts into the skin over the posterior and lower part of the alar cartilages.

The angular head of the **quadratus labii superior** (levator labii superioris alaeque nasi), a muscle of facial expression, also dilates the nostrils.

The Nasal Cavities

Consisting of two narrow, approximately symmetrical chambers separated by the nasal septum, the nasal cavities communicate with the exterior by way of the nostrils (**anterior nares**) and with the nasopharynx by way of the choanae (**posterior nares**). The **nasal vestibule** is a slight dilation just inside the aperture of the nostril (Figure 4-36).

The **nasal septum** is a medially placed, vertically directed plate of bone and cartilage. The **anterior cartilaginous portion,** shown in Figure 4-18, is bounded above by the perpendicular plate of the ethmoid bone and below by the vomer bone and the anterior nasal spine. *More often than not, this cartilaginous part of the septum is deviated (buckled) to one side, usually the left.* Severe deviation may cause an ulcerated septum or difficulty in breathing. The **posterior bony portion** is formed by the perpendicular plate of the ethmoid, the rostrum of the sphenoid bone, and the vomer bone. The bony part of the septum seldom deviates from the midline.

The lateral walls of the nasal cavities are composed of the **superior, middle,** and **inferior nasal conchae** (L. *konche,* a shell) and their corresponding nasal passages (or **meatuses,** meati) which are named for the conchae that overlie them (Figure 4-37). The labyrinthine structure of the lateral walls facilitates nasal functions by greatly increasing the surface area of the nasal cavities.

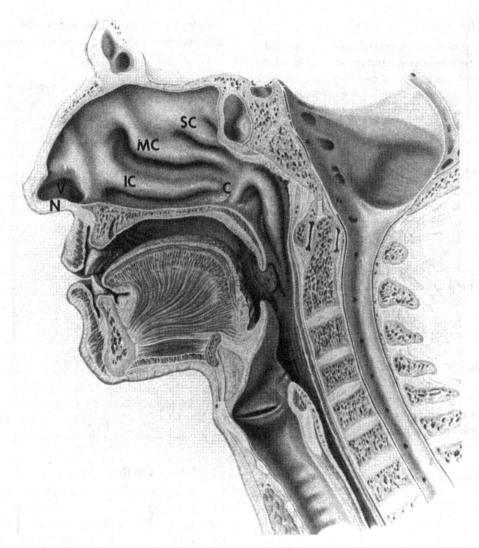

FIGURE 4-36

The lateral wall of the right nasal cavity: nasal vestibule (V), nare (N), choana (C), inferior concha (IC), middle concha (MC), and superior concha (SC).

We have learned that the lateral walls also contain orifices through which the nasal cavities communicate with the paranasal sinuses. A frontal section of the nasal cavities is shown in Figure 4-37, while the lateral and medial walls of the cavities are shown in Figures 4-18 and 4-32, respectively. The floor of the nasal cavities is concave and is formed by the maxillae and palatine bones. The roof is very narrow from side to side and is pierced by the many minute foramina in the cribriform plate of the ethmoid bone. The perforations permit the entrance of the branches of the olfactory nerves, which terminate on the upper septum and adjacent lateral walls.

Functions of the Nose

The nose is constantly exposed to wide ranges in temperature and humidity, and to dusty, dirty atmosphere.

These very conditions give a strong hint regarding its functions. Aside from olfaction, which in humans does little more than augment the sense of taste, the nose has three functions: *temperature, humidity,* and *particle control.*

As mentioned earlier, the nasal turbinates and meatuses constitute a broad surface area covered by mucosa that is overlayed on a specialized ciliated epithelium.

As inhaled air enters the nose, it immediately encounters a tortuous path through the meatuses and over the surfaces of the turbinates. A very rich supply of blood capillaries on the nasal tissue contributes to erectile tissue containing blood or "swell" spaces. Cold air entering the nose causes the blood to engorge the spaces, thus inducing swelling of the turbinates, which in turn encourages heat transfer from the blood to the air being inhaled. A reversed process takes place when very warm air enters the nose. The mechanism is apparently very

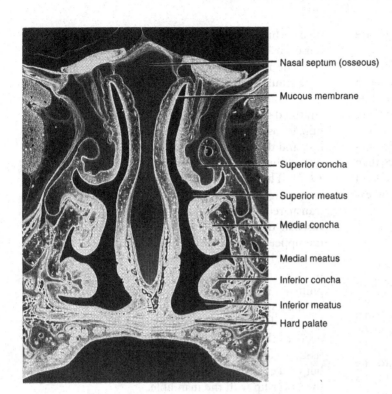

Nasal septum (osseous)

Mucous membrane

Superior concha

Superior meatus

Medial concha

Medial meatus

Inferior concha

Inferior meatus

Hard palate

FIGURE 4-37

Frontal section through the nasal cavities of a fetal head.

efficient, because in the 250 msec or so that it takes inhaled air to pass through the nasal cavities, it can be warmed to very nearly body temperature, whether the outside air is –40°C or +80°C.

Air reaching the nasopharynx has a nearly constant relative humidity of 75 to 80 percent. In the brief interval during which inhaled air passes through the nasal cavities, it receives moisture from the nasal mucous membrane. DeWeese and Saunders (1973) report that as much as 1000 ml of moisture can be evaporated from the nose during a 24-hour interval. Of course, the amount of moisture lost varies with the humidity of the inspired air.

The mucosa of the nose also has a cleansing effect on inhaled air. Bacteria and dust particles are "caught" by the moist mucous blanket lining the cavities. Ciliary action, like that in the remainder of the respiratory tract, constantly propels the mucous blanket, at a rate of about 10 mm per minute, toward the pharynx. Ultimately the mucus and contaminants are swallowed and disposed of in the stomach.

THE ARTICULATORS AND ASSOCIATED STRUCTURES

Functions of the Mouth

The mouth, like other parts of the speech production mechanism, has biological as well as nonbiological functions.

Biological Functions

The mouth establishes communication between the digestive and respiratory tracts and the exterior. It communicates with the pharyngeal cavity by way of the arches (fauces) and with the exterior by way of the buccal orifice or mouth slit. Initiation of the digestive process is also an important biological function. **Ptyalin,** an extremely powerful enzyme contained in the saliva, aids in the breakdown of food by converting starches to maltose or disaccaride (double sugar). Considering the way most people eat, it has but a moment to act before the food departs for the stomach.

Nonbiological Functions

The structures of the mouth may *modify the resonant characteristics of the vocal tract and may also generate speech sounds.* Because of the extremely mobile lips and tongue, the mouth is certainly the most movable and adjustable cavity in the vocal tract. Other mouth structures associated with articulation of speech sounds are the teeth, hard palate, soft palate, cheeks, and lower jaw. In an early experiment dealing with the relative mobility of the articulators, Hudgins and Stetson (1937) found a high degree of consistency between nine subjects. They repeated various syllables, each representing a single articulatory movement, as rapidly as possible. The tip of the tongue was found to be the most mobile articulator, moving 8.2 times per second in the production of "ta ta ta." Values for other articulators were 7.3 per second for the jaw, 7.1 per second for the back of the tongue, 6.7

for the lips, and 6.7 for the soft palate. These values are in essential agreement with subsequent studies.

There are other nonbiological functions of the mouth that perhaps play a less important role in speech and communication. For example, the lips are not only important articulators of speech sounds, but they are also mediators of facial expression. In addition, the movements of the lips and face provide visible secondary cues that facilitate communication far more than most people realize. Face reading is something most of us do quite unconsciously, and it is surprising how expert we are!

The Pyramid of Polyfunction

In a very real sense, separation of the activities of the structures comprising the speech mechanism into biological and nonbiological functions is somewhat artificial, and can be justified only from a strictly operational point of view. This problem has been recognized by Martone (1963), who has outlined an area extending from the sternum to the tip of the nose and onto the outer orifices of the ears. This area has been termed a pyramid of polyfunction, since it contains the organs and structures responsible solely or in part for functions of facial expression, mastication, deglutition, breathing, and speech. This is a truly functional approach, which is worthy of some thought. Such an approach, however, demands some prior knowledge of the descriptive and functional anatomy of the mouth and related structures.

The Lips (Rima Oris)

Anatomy

The lips, which form the orifice of the mouth and part of the external boundary of the buccal cavity, are covered externally by integument (skin) and internally by mucous membrane. Between the skin and mucous membrane are muscular and glandular tissues, and a considerable amount of fat. The lips, shown in Figure 4-38, are often described as being composed of four layers of

tissue, which, in order of increasing depth, are cutaneous, muscular, glandular, and mucous.

The mucous membrane lining the lips and cheeks is continuous with the integument of the lips and the membranous lining of the pharynx. It is covered by stratified squamous epithelium. The skin of the lips terminates as a well-defined line (Cupid's bow on the upper lip), and the **vermilion zone** is the transitional area between the skin and the mucous membrane. (Orban, 1957). The red hue of this zone is due to the epithelium's high content of eleiden, which increases tissue transparency, thus revealing the color of the underlying vascular tissue. In the midline of the vermilion zone of the upper lip is a slight projection called the **tubercle.** A vertical groove connecting this area to the septum of the nose is called the **philtrum** (Gk. love potion). The philtrum is continuous with the **columella** of the nasal septum.

On the lingual or inner surface, the upper lip connects to the alveolar region at the midline by a fold of tissue called the **superior labial frenulum.**[6] A similar but weaker structure, the **inferior labial frenulum,** joins the lower lip with the mandible.

Labial glands, which lie just beneath the mucous membrane, are located on the inner surface of the lip around the orifice of the mouth. Spherical in shape and resembling small peas, they open into the cavity by numerous small orifices. Structurally, they are similar to the salivary glands.

Function

Because the position of the lower lip is somewhat dependent upon mandibular movements, the lower lip is the more mobile of the two. It is also faster. In addition, most of the muscles of facial expression insert into the lips, a feature that contributes to the large repertory of lip movements. Both lips can be compressed to produce **bilabial** consonants such as [p], [b], and [m]. For [p], [b], and [m] production, the lower lip has been found to travel a distance roughly twice that of the upper lip. The lower lip is also less variable in generating a static force level than is the upper lip (Barlow and Netsell, 1986). The upper lip, however, has been found to be more stable than the lower lip (Amerman, 1993). In the production of **labial** consonants, such as [hw] and [w], the lips provide a major constriction, but do not stop the flow of air. **Labiodentals,** such as [f] and [v], are formed by a constriction of the upper incisors and the lower lip. The lips can also be spread (retracted) against the teeth, or they may be rounded or protruded, as in the production

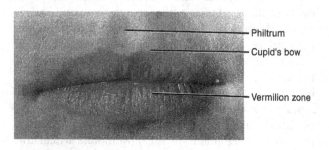

- Philtrum
- Cupid's bow
- Vermilion zone

FIGURE 4-38

Photograph of the lips.

---

[6]A **frenulum** (a small **frenum;** L. bridle) limits the range of movement of a structure.

of [u] or [w]. With the lips spread somewhat, a vowel will have the sound of an [i], but with lip rounding the sound approaches that of a [u].

Lip reflexes can be elicited in response to oral cavity pressure changes. These pressure changes are similar to those that occur during speech production. The results suggest that mechanoreceptors respond to pressure changes as a form of sensorimotor integration for speech production (McClean, 1991).

The Cheeks (Buccae)

The cheeks, like the lips with which they are continuous, are composed externally of skin and internally of mucous membrane, between which may be found facial muscles, the muscles of mastication, glandular tissue, and a rather prominent subcutaneous pad of fat. The mucous membrane of the cheek blends into the gingivae of the mandible and maxillae and is continuous with the mucosa of the soft palate. This membrane is firmly bound to the fascia of the musculature of the cheek and closely follows muscular movements.

Glands

Glands similar to the labial glands, but smaller, are found between the mucous membrane and the musculature of the cheek. Five or six of these glands, larger than the others, open by ducts into the buccal cavity just opposite the last molars. They are called quite appropriately, the **molar glands.** The cheek also contains the duct of the **parotid salivary gland** (Stenson's duct), which opens into the buccal cavity just opposite the second upper molar. The status of the mucous membrane is maintained by the *emollient* (softening) *action* of the mucin content of saliva. This action allows free movement of the membranes without the damaging effects of friction. **Mucin,** a mixture of glycoproteins, is the primary substance of mucus. Saliva also functions as a demulscent, allaying irritation of the mucous membrane within the mouth. A rather constant flow of saliva is essential to normal speech production. We all, at one time or another, have experienced "dry mouth" (possibly from nervousness in a tense speech situation) and the sluggish, ill-controlled movements of the tongue as it contacts the various surfaces of the mouth cavity.

The mouth also receives secretion from the **submaxillary** (submandibular) **salivary glands** by way of **Wharton's ducts,** which open into the underside of the tongue on either side of the **lingual frenulum,** a vertical fold of tissue that extends from the lingual surface of the gum to the inferior surface of the tongue. It also receives secretions from the **sublingual salivary glands** by way of the **ducts of Rivinus,** which open into the cavity medial to Wharton's ducts.

Buccal Fat Pad (Pad of Bichat)

As stated earlier, the deep surface of the cheek musculature is covered by mucous membrane. The superficial surface, however, lies in direct contact with a prominent deposit of fatty tissue called the buccal fat pad. Particularly well developed in infants, it is said to play a role in the suckling activity of nursing babies, and is sometimes called the suckling pad. Supportive evidence of its function is inconclusive.

Muscles of the Face and Mouth

The facial muscles, particularly those of facial expression, are unique in that they are devoid of fascial sheaths characteristic of skeletal muscles. Their size, shape, and extent of development are dependent on, among other things, age, dentition, and sex, as well as intrinsic individual variations. Also, many of their fibers insert directly into the skin. These characteristics make possible the numerous combinations of facial expression we witness in our day-to-day living. The lips are the most mobile part of the face by virtue of the many facial muscles that act upon them. *Because the muscles of the face and lips are so intrinsically related, they exhibit functional unity.*

The Orbicularis Oris Muscle

The principal muscle acting upon the lips is the orbicularis oris, an oval ring of muscle fibers located within the lips and completely encircling the mouth slit. It is a complex muscle that may be thought of as being composed of *intrinsic* as well as *extrinsic muscle fibers*. That is, some fibers are exclusive to the lips, and some fibers from other facial muscles insert into the lips. The muscles of the lips may also be divided into two layers: a *deep layer* of fibers arranged in concentric rings and a *superficial layer* of fibers into which the other muscles of the face converge.

The orbicularis oris is a sphincter muscle (Figures 4-39 and 4-40). When it contracts it closes the mouth and puckers the lips. The extrinsic muscles may be grouped into three sets: **transverse muscles,** which course horizontally from their origin and insert into the orbicularis oris; **angular muscles,** which approach the corners of the mouth obliquely from above and below; and the **labial** or **vertical muscles,** which enter the corners of the mouth directly from above and below. The way these muscles insert into the lips is shown schematically in Figure 4-41.

The transverse muscles pull the lips against the teeth and facilitate compression of the lips for the production of certain consonant sounds, such as the bilabial stops and nasals. The angular muscles are instrumental in producing such expressions as smiling and frowning. The labial or vertical muscles are also important in producing facial

FIGURE 4-39

Superficial facial musculature (muscles of facial expression) as seen from the front.

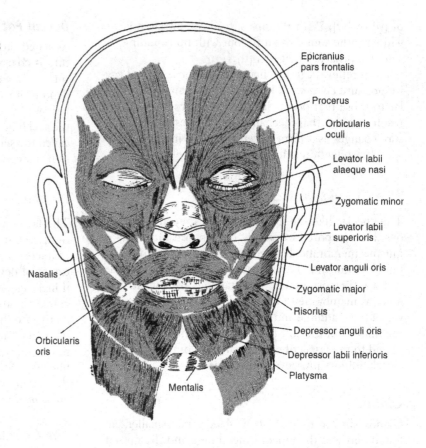

Epicranius pars frontalis

Procerus

Orbicularis oculi

Levator labii alaeque nasi

Zygomatic minor

Levator labii superioris

Levator anguli oris

Zygomatic major

Risorius

Depressor anguli oris

Depressor labii inferioris

Platysma

Nasalis

Orbicularis oris

Mentalis

FIGURE 4-40

Superficial facial musculature (muscles of facial expression) as seen from the side.

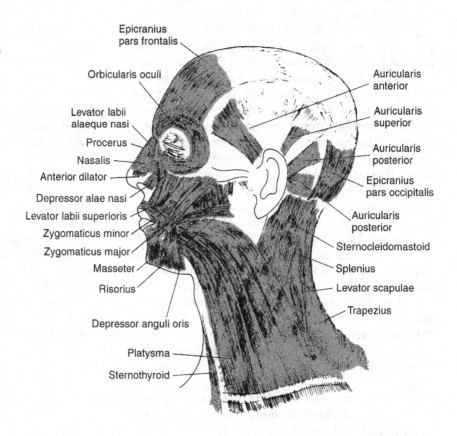

Epicranius pars frontalis

Orbicularis oculi

Levator labii alaeque nasi

Procerus

Nasalis

Anterior dilator

Depressor alae nasi

Levator labii superioris

Zygomaticus minor

Zygomaticus major

Masseter

Risorius

Depressor anguli oris

Platysma

Sternothyroid

Auricularis anterior

Auricularis superior

Auricularis posterior

Epicranius pars occipitalis

Auricularis posterior

Sternocleidomastoid

Splenius

Levator scapulae

Trapezius

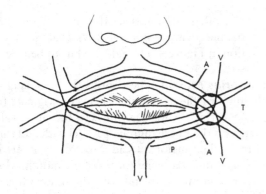

FIGURE 4-41

Schematic of angular (A), vertical (V), transverse (T), and parallel (P) facial muscles that insert into the lips. The modiolus is indicated by the heavy circle, just lateral to the mouth angle.

expression and in addition are important in compressing the corners of the mouth. A fourth group, the **parallel muscles,** is also shown in Figure 4-41. They are not lip muscles in the true sense of the word, but rather are superficial muscles of the integument in the mouth region.

Some eight or nine muscles converge on each of the two angles of the mouth and interlace at a palpable nodular mass, the *modiolus.* It is shown schematically in Figure 4-41. The modiolus is located about 12 mm from the angle of the mouth. Its position is highly variable, between individuals, between world populations, and between various facial expressions and activities.

In electromyographic studies of lip functions it is tempting to attribute certain behavior to specific muscles. Because of the complex interdigitations, isolating single muscle fibers within the lips is hazardous (Blair and Smith, 1986).

The Transverse Facial Muscles

The transverse muscles are the **buccinator** and the **risorius.**

The Buccinator (Bugler's) Muscle The buccinator, shown in Figure 4-42, is the principal muscle of the cheek. The deepest of the facial and of the extrinsic musculature of the lips, it has a complex origin. Its primary origin is from the **pterygomandibular raphe** or

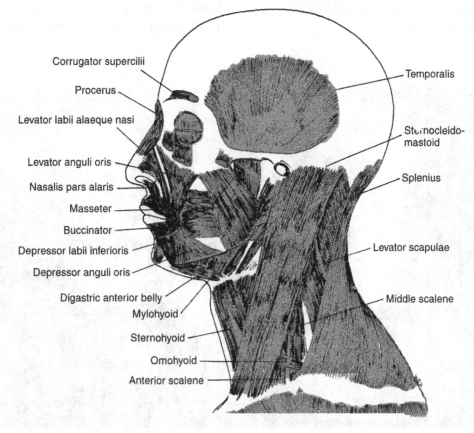

FIGURE 4-42

Deep muscles of the face.

ligament,[7] while the remainder of the fibers arise from the lateral surface of the alveolar process of the maxilla and from the mandible in the region of the last molars. The pterygomandibular raphe is a tendinous structure that runs from the hamulus of the internal pterygoid plate to the posterior limit of the mylohyoid line. It is shown in Figure 4-43. Were it not for the pterygomandibular raphe, the fibers of the superior pharyngeal constrictor and the buccinator would be continuous.

The fibers of the buccinator course horizontally forward and medialward to enter and blend with the muscle fibers of both the upper and lower lips. The fibers of the central portion converge toward the corner of the mouth and decussate before inserting. This means that the lower fibers of the central portion enter the upper lip while the upper fibers enter into the lower lip. The superiormost fibers do not decussate, but rather enter the upper lip; the inferiormost fibers enter the lower lip. Because of this complex arrangement, the buccinator can compress the lips and cheeks against the teeth and draw the corners of the mouth laterally.

Posteriorly, the buccinator is covered by the masseter muscle (to be described later), while anteriorly it is

___

[7]This is an instance where a tendinous inscription between two muscles is referred to as a ligament.

covered by other facial muscles that enter the lips. As a result, the buccinator is not usually as easily seen as the illustration in Figure 4-42 might lead us to believe.

The Risorius Muscle   The risorius (L. *risus*, laughter) is a highly variable muscle that seems to originate from a fascia covering the masseter muscle. Its course is horizontal, with the fibers running parallel with and superficial to the buccinator muscle. Most fibers insert into the skin and mucosa at the corner of the mouth, while a few fibers continue to blend with the muscle fibers of the lower lip. Upon contraction, the risorius helps draw the mouth angle lateralward.

The Angular Facial Muscles

The angular muscles are the **levator labii superior, levator labii superior alaeque nasi, zygomatic minor** and **major**, and **depressor labii inferior.**

The Levator Labii Superior Muscle   The levator of the upper lip has a rather broad origin from the lower margin of the orbit. Some fibers also arise from zygomatic bone and the maxilla. As shown in Figure 4-39, the fibers course downward to insert into the upper lip between the levator anguli oris and the levator labii superior alaeque nasi. The levator labii superior is the

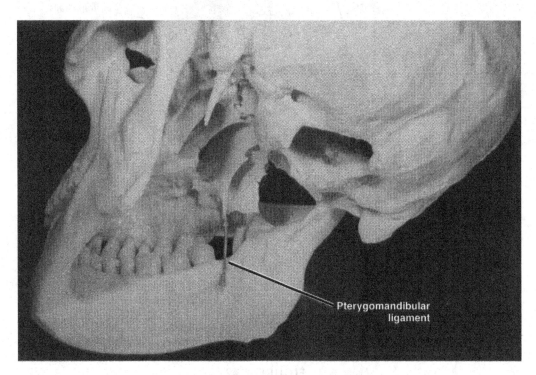

Pterygomandibular
ligament

FIGURE 4-43

A skull as seen in perspective from beneath, showing a reconstruction of the pterygomandibular ligament.

proper elevator of the upper lip, and may evert it somewhat as well.

The Levator Labii Superior Alaeque Nasi Muscle
The levator of the upper lip and dilator of the nostrils takes its origin as a very slender slip of muscle from the frontal process and the infraorbital margin of the maxilla. It courses downward and slightly lateralward, and then divides into two slips, one inserting into the lateral cartilaginous framework of the nose and the other into the orbicularis oris.

The Zygomatic Minor Muscle
The zygomatic minor originates from the facial (malar) surface of the zygomatic bone, in the region of the zygomaticomaxillary suture. The fibers course downward and medially to insert into the orbicularis oris, as seen in Figure 4-39.

The Zygomatic Major Muscle
The zygomatic major is a rather long, slender muscle arising from the malar surface of the zygomatic bone just lateral to the origin of the zygomatic minor. As shown in Figure 4-39, the fibers course downward and medialward to insert into the orbicularis oris and into the integument at the corner of the mouth. Upon contraction, this muscle draws the angle of the mouth upward and lateralward, as in grinning or smiling broadly.

The Depressor Labii Inferior Muscle
The depressor of the lower lip, a small, flat, quadrangular muscle, is located beneath the lower lip just lateral to the midline. It arises from the oblique line of the mandible near the mental foramen. Upon contraction, this muscle draws the lower lip downward and lateralward. It is shown in Figure 4-39.

The Vertical Facial Muscles
There are three pairs of vertical muscles that insert into the orbicularis oris: the **mentalis,** the **depressor anguli oris,** and the **levator anguli oris** muscles. Together they compress the lips and assist in elevating and lowering them.

The Mentalis Muscle
The mentalis (levator menti) is a cone-shaped bundle located at the side of the frenulum of the lower lip. The fibers arise from the incisive fossa (just below the incisors) of the mandible and descend to attach to the skin of the chin. The mentalis raises the lower lip and the mentolabial sulcus (labiomental groove, Figure 4-33), wrinkling the skin of the chin. Because it raises the base of the lower lip, it helps in protruding and everting it in drinking. It is sometimes called the "pouting muscle." Electromyography shows fairly continuous activity in the mentalis, even during sleep, a finding that is unexplained.

The Depressor Anguli Oris Muscle
The depressor of the angle of the mouth is a flat, triangular sheet of muscle superficial and lateral to the fibers of the depressor labii inferior. It arises from the oblique line of the mandible, its fibers interdigitating with those of the platysma (discussed later). The fibers converge as they course vertically upward, and insert for the most part into the orbicularis oris at the angle of the mouth. Some fibers, however, insert into the upper lip (Figure 4-39). Upon contraction, this muscle may either depress the angle of the lip or assist in compressing the lips by drawing the upper lip downward against the lower lip.

The Levator Anguli Oris Muscle
The levator of the angle of the mouth, part of which may be seen in Figure 4-39, seems to be the superior counterpart of the depressor anguli oris. It is a flat, triangular muscle located above the angle of the mouth but deep to the levator labii superior. Its origin, lateral to the ala of the nose, is at the canine fossa on the superficial surface of the maxilla. The fibers converge as they course toward the angle of the mouth, where some fibers insert into the upper lip. Others cross over to insert into the lower lip at the angle. Upon contraction the levator anguli oris draws the corner of the mouth upward and also assists in closing the mouth by drawing the lower lip upward. Upon dissection, the fibers of the levator and depressor anguli oris muscles seem to be common; that is, it appears that the two are actually but one vertically directed muscle originating at the canine fossa of the maxilla and inserting into the mandible.

The Parallel Facial Muscles
The parallel muscles are the **incisivus labii superior** and **inferior** muscles.

The Incisivus Labii Superior Muscle
The incisive muscle of the upper lip is a flat, narrow muscle located deep to the levator labii superior. Its course is parallel to the transverse fibers of the orbicularis oris of the upper lip. The fibers originate on the maxilla at a point just above the canine teeth. They run lateralward to the angle of the mouth where they blend with other fibers of the region. Upon contraction, the incisivis labii superior draws the corner of the mouth medially and upward. In other words, it helps pucker or round the lips.

The Incisivus Labii Inferior Muscle
The incisive muscle of the lower lip is the inferior counterpart of the incisivis labii superior. It is a small narrow muscle located beneath the angle of the mouth and deep to the depressor labii inferior. The muscle arises from the mandible in the region of the lateral incisors. Its fibers course parallel with those of the transverse fibers of the orbicularis oris of the lower lip. They continue to the angle of the mouth

and insert by interdigitating with those of the orbicularis oris. Upon contraction, the muscle draws the corner of the mouth medially and downward.

The Platysma—A Superficial Cervical Muscle

Although the platysma (Gk. *platys*, broad) is a facial muscle, because of its distribution it is usually described as a superficial cervical muscle. It is a thin, flat, and broad muscle that covers most of the lateral and anterior regions of the neck. The platysma arises embryologically from the same primordia that gives rise to all of the facial musculature. Part of the musculature migrates to form a superficial layer that is distributed over the front and sides of the face and neck. This explains why the platysma is supplied by the facial nerve.

The platysma is usually described as originating on the fascia covering the superior parts of the pectoralis major and deltoid muscles, but *this is actually the lower limit of migration of the primordial muscle mass.* Many of the fibers attach to the lower margin of the mandible, back as far as the angle. The anterior fibers interdigitate, in the region of the mental symphysis, with fibers of the muscle of the opposite side, and as can be seen in Figure 4-44, many fibers blend with muscles at the corner of the mouth. The fibers have a broad distribution about the face and can be found contributing to the zygomatic and even the orbicularis oculi muscles.

The functions of this muscle are not fully understood. Gray (1973) states that it draws the lower lip and corner of the mouth laterally and inferiorly, partially opening the mouth. When the entire muscle is contracted voluntarily, the skin of the neck is drawn upward toward the mandible, thus increasing the diameter of the root of the neck and relieving the pressure of a tight collar. This action, known as the **antisphincteric gesture,** probably facilitates the drainage of venous blood from the head and neck.

Electromyography of the platysma has shown it to be active when one is smiling broadly, depressing the jaw against slight resistance, and in speech, especially when the lips are compressed or retracted (Zemlin and Czapar, 1974).

Supplementary Muscles of Expression

The muscles we have been discussing are primarily muscles of facial expression or muscles of the mouth. Other muscles, such as those of the eyelid and scalp,[8] may also be instrumental in facial expression (see Figures 4-39 and 4-40).

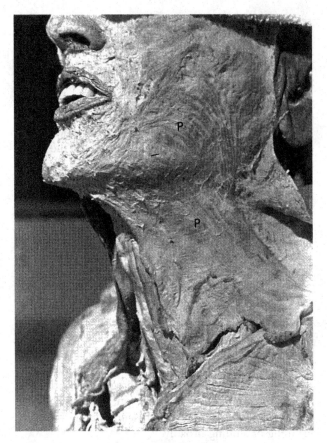

FIGURE 4-44

The platysma muscle (P).

A substantial portion of the cranial vault is covered by a loosely bound subcutaneous fascia which is known as the **galea** (L. helmet) **aponeurotica** or **epicranial aponeuroses.** Its loose attachment to the skull accounts for the mobility of the scalp and also the rapid accumulation of blood (hematoma) under the scalp following a blow to the head.

The **epicranius,** a very extensive but thin muscle attached to the galea, is often described as consisting of an occipital belly (**occipitalis muscle**) and a frontal belly (**frontalis muscle**). The frontalis muscle raises the eyebrows and wrinkles the forehead to convey an expression of surprise.

The **orbicularis oculi** is a sphincterlike muscle surrounding the orbit. It arises from the nasal process of the frontal bone, the frontal process of the maxilla, and a short fibrous band called the palpebral ligament. Because of these attachments the orbicularis oculi is described as consisting of three parts: a **palpebral portion** which gently closes the eyelids as in blinking, an **orbital portion** which firmly closes the eyelids as in winking, and a **lacrimal portion** which is instrumental in drawing tears into the eye.

The **corrugator** (L. to wrinkle) is situated deep to the frontalis and orbicularis oculi. It arises from the medial end of the superciliary ridge and most of its

---

[8]The **scalp** is defined as the hairy integument covering the cranium.

fibers pass upward and lateralward to insert into the skin above the middle of the arch of the eyebrows. A few fibers course downward to insert into the skin, thus drawing the eyebrows downward. Collectively, the muscle fibers of the corrugator wrinkle the forehead by drawing the eyebrows downward and medialward. It is sometimes called the "frowning" muscle, and according to Gray (1973), it may be regarded as the principal muscle in the expression of suffering.

The Teeth

Introduction

We are all aware of the biological as well as some of the nonbiological functions of the teeth. As is the case with so many other structures in the body, specific functions may be ascertained from the name given a tooth. Thus, **incisors** (incisive or cutting teeth) are chisel-shaped with a sharp cutting edge suited for biting or shearing food, while the pointed tusklike **canine** teeth are best suited for ripping or tearing. The **molar** teeth with their flat, broad surfaces are well adapted for crushing and grinding. *Biologically, therefore, the teeth are seen to be the precursors of the digestive process.*

The *nonbiological functions* of the teeth play a vital role in the day-to-day life of a person. The contribution of dental structure to the appearance of the entire face is much discussed, and for good reason. The jaws and teeth, which comprise almost two-thirds of the face, are important determinants of the characteristics of facial structure (Martone, 1963). The teeth and their supporting structures are important for normal speech production. They are directly involved in the production of some consonants, particularly the [f], [v], [θ], and [ð]. Palatography and other recording techniques verify that the tongue makes contact with the teeth during the production of many other sounds, notably those often classified, quite appropriately, linguavelar, linguapalatal, and linguaalveolar. Most essential, however, is our recognition of the important role that teeth play in the production of almost all the sounds we emit, including the vowels.

In those animals that continue to grow throughout life (fish, sharks, etc.), teeth are continually being shed and replaced with new ones whose size is commensurate with general body size. The shed teeth often show little sign of wear. Higher-order mammals, including humans, are provided with two sets of teeth. The first set, which is well developed in utero, makes its appearance in infancy and early childhood. Called **deciduous** (also primary, temporary, milk, baby) teeth, they are smaller and whiter than the permanent teeth and may become extremely worn in the older child.

The **permanent** teeth erupt at an early age and, unless disease intervenes, remain for life. The development of refined carbohydrates (sugar, sweets, etc.) and generally "softer" foods may have contributed to increased tooth decay, gum disease, and loss of teeth, conditions that, in the wild, led to death by starvation. In our society, in spite of their importance, teeth are not vital to sustaining life.

At first appearance a tooth may seem to be nothing more than a small bony tusk protruding from the alveolar ridge. A closer look, however, reveals it to be a dynamic living organ composed of connective tissue, blood vessels, and nerves, as well as inorganic materials. As such, a tooth is subject to disease, infection, and damage, just as is any other part of the body. Before discussing the deciduous and permanent dental arches, it might be of value to look at the general structure of a tooth.

The Structure of a Tooth

A tooth may be divided on an *anatomical basis* into three parts: a crown, root, and neck. That part of a tooth covered by enamel is the **crown.** It comprises about one-third of a tooth. The **root** of a tooth is the part covered by cementum, and it comprises about two-thirds of the tooth. The **neck** is a more or less ill-defined region of transition between the enamel-covered crown and the cementum-covered root. A tooth usually bears a slight constriction at the cementoenamel junction.

The crown of a tooth may also be defined as the visible portion of the tooth, that is, the portion of a tooth projecting above the **gums** or **gingivae** into the oral cavity. The root, then, is that part of a tooth imbedded within the tissue that constitutes the jaw.

In young persons, not all of the enamel-covered crown may be exposed and projected into the oral cavity, while in the case of older persons with worn teeth, the entire crown, neck, and part of the root may be exposed[9] (hence the expression, *getting long in the tooth*, when referring to someone's advanced age).

Sicher and DuBrul (1975) refer to the anatomic crown and anatomic root as the enamel-covered and cementum-covered parts, respectively. That part of the tooth which at any given moment is exposed to the oral cavity is the **functional** (clinical) **crown;** that part which is imbedded in, and in organic connection with, the surrounding tissues is the **functional** (clinical) **root.** In the young, the functional crown is smaller than the anatomical crown, while in older persons, the reverse is true. A schematic section through a tooth is shown in Figure 4-45.

Dentin Dentin (L. *dens*, tooth), which makes up the bulk of the solid portion of a tooth, is sometimes called the ivory of the tooth. It is a yellowish-white avascular

---

[9]Disease of the tissues surrounding the teeth may result in alveolar bone resorption.

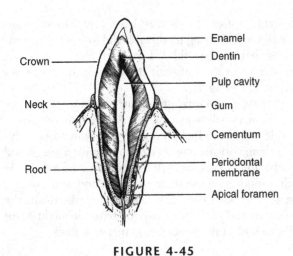

FIGURE 4-45

Schematic section through a tooth.

tissue that does not regenerate but continues to form throughout life, resulting in a gradual diminution of the pulp cavity. Dentin is a mineralized tissue consisting of about one-third animal matter and two-thirds inorganic salts. The animal matter consists of **dental canaliculi,** parallel tubules of protoplasmic substance that course the length of the tooth. These tubules, when disturbed by agents such as bacteria, mechanical pressure, or chemical action, are instrumental in conveying the sensation of pain to the nerves of the dental pulp.

Dental Pulp Dental pulp is tissue rich in nerves and blood vessels. It is contained in the **pulp canal,** which roughly conforms to the general shape of the tooth. The enlarged portion of the canal is called the **pulp cavity.** The pulp canal communicates at its tip or apex with adjacent tissues through the **apical foramen.**

Enamel Enamel, the most dense portion of the tooth and the hardest substance in the body, is about 96 percent mineral by weight. Initially translucent, enamel becomes increasingly yellow with age. Enamel has but one function, to resist abrasion or attrition. It is thickest on the grinding and occlusal surfaces (2.5 mm), becoming progressively thinner toward the neck where it joins the cementum of the tooth. This **cementoenamel junction** is the neck of the tooth.

Cementum A bonelike substance covering the roots of the teeth, cementum is softer than dentin, about 50 percent mineralized. New layers of cementum are deposited throughout life to compensate for tooth movements.

The Periodontal Ligament (or Membrane)

A tooth is suspended in the confining walls of its respective **alveolus** (socket) by connective tissue known as the periodontal ligament. The result is an articulation known as a **gomphosis** (peg-and-socket suture). The arrangement of the white nonelastic fibers in the periodontal ligament facilitates the absorption of mechanical forces on the tooth.

Mechanical pressure on the tooth will lead to a stretching of all or some of the fiber bundles, and thus masticatory pressure is transformed into tension acting on cememtum and bone. Because growth of bone or cementum cannot occur if the growing surface is subjected to pressure, "this transformation of forces is absolutely essential for the normal functional life of a tooth" (Sicher and DuBrul, 1975).

At the neck of the tooth the periodontal ligament is covered by the gingiva (gum). In a healthy mouth the gingivae are pale pink and stippled in appearance, in contrast to the red, smooth, and shiny lining that comprises the oral mucosa.

Dental Morphology

There are four general types of teeth: **incisors, canines, premolars,** and **molars.** They are shown in Figure 4-46.

Incisors The **upper central incisors** (L. *incedere,* to cut into) are chisel-shaped and bear a single root. They are directed somewhat obliquely downward and forward.

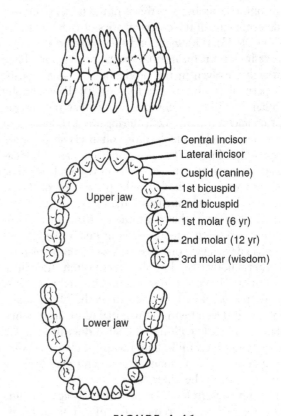

FIGURE 4-46

A permanent dental arch.

The **upper lateral** incisors are smaller than the upper central incisors, have a smaller root, and are far more variable (they are congenitally absent in about 2 percent of the population). The **lower central** incisors are similar in shape to the upper central incisors, but are considerably smaller. In fact, the lower central incisors are even smaller than the lower lateral incisors. Because the anteroposterior diameter of the maxillary dental arch is larger than that of the mandibular arch, the upper one-third of the lower central incisors are overlapped by the upper incisors, a normal relationship known as **overbite.** In addition, the lower incisors are directed more vertically than are the upper incisors. As a consequence, the upper incisors project facially farther than the lower incisors, by about 2 or 3 millimeters, a condition called **overjet.**

As shown in Figure 4-47, the labial (outer) surface of the incisors is convex, while their lingual (inner) surface is concave near the incisal (cutting) edge, becoming abruptly convex toward the base. The convex portion, called the **cingulum** (L. girdle) of the tooth, is prominent only on the upper incisors.

Canines (Cuspids, Eye Teeth) The canines (L. *canis*, a dog) are immediately lateral to the lateral incisors. They are large teeth with a single pointed crown or cusp (L. *cuspis*, point). The upper canines are larger and stronger than the lower canines and have an especially well-developed root.

Premolars (Bicuspids) The premolars are characterized by the development of a true occlusal surface, which in incisors is reduced to an occlusal edge. The occlusal (biting) surface of a premolar usually has two cusps, which accounts for the name bicuspid. They are located posterior to the canines. There are eight premolars in the permanent dental arch and none in the deciduous

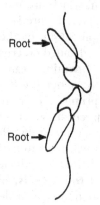

FIGURE 4-47

Lateral view of normal occlusal contact of incisors. The lower incisal edge fits into the concavity of the lingual surface of the upper incisor.

arch. They usually have single flat roots; however, the upper first premolar has a tendency to bear two.

Molars The molars (L. *molaris*, grinding) are the largest teeth. There are 12 in the permanent arch, 6 in each jaw, 8 in the deciduous arch, 4 in each jaw. As shown in Figure 4-46, the molars have large, broad, almost rectangular occlusal surfaces, well adapted to their function. Most often the first molars in the upper jaw are the largest, while the third molars (wisdom teeth) are the smallest. In addition, upper molars have three roots while the lower molars bear but two roots. Interestingly enough, however, the upper molars are usually slightly smaller than the lowers. The grinding surface of the molars is distinctive. The first molar generally has four cusps, the second has three or four, and the third has but three.

Dental Surfaces Because of the curved nature of the dental arches, the application of conventional anatomical descriptive terms is cumbersome. Dental anatomists have, therefore, given special names to the five free surfaces of the teeth.

One surface is the biting or masticatory surface, and since it is in contact with opposing teeth of the opposite jaw, it is called the **occlusal surface.** In the incisors the occlusal surface is reduced to a chisel-like **incisal edge** or **margin.** One surface of each tooth faces the oral cavity, while the other faces either the vestibule of the oral cavity or the buccal cavity. The oral surface is referred to as the **lingual surface** because of its relation to the tongue, while the opposite surface is called the **labial surface** on the incisors and canine teeth and the **buccal surface** on the premolars and molars.[10]

Except for the last molar the other two free surfaces of each tooth are in contact (or nearly so) with adjacent teeth. These are the **approximal surfaces,** and they have been given special names. If we can imagine that curved dental arches have been straightened, as in the pan-oral radiograph shown in Figure 4-48, we see that each tooth has a **mesial surface** (toward the midline) and a **distal surface** (away from the midline).[11]

Directions and regions on the crown are indicated by the terms **occlusally** and **cervically** (toward the neck), and for the root the terms cervically and **apically** are used. These terms are summarized in Figure 4-49.

The Life Cycle of a Tooth

The developmental sequence is essentially the same for deciduous and permanent teeth, and the life cycle of a

---

[10]The terms labial and buccal are sometimes replaced by the term **facial surface,** which applies to all teeth.

[11]For the premolars and molars, the term mesial may sometimes be replaced by **anterior surface,** and the term distal may be replaced by the term **posterior surface.**

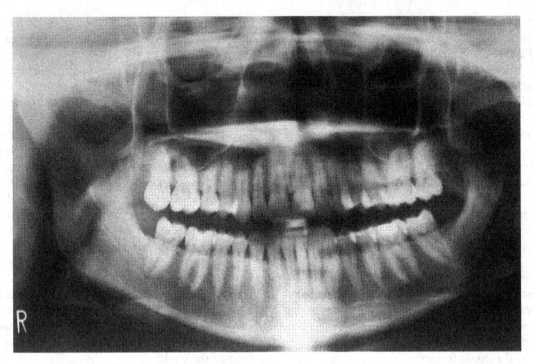

FIGURE 4-48

A pan-oral radiograph of permanent dentition. (Provided by Callahan, Lord, King, and McCabe, orthodontists, Champaign, IL.)

tooth, be it deciduous or permanent, may be considered in four periods: **growth, calcification, eruption,** and **attrition.**

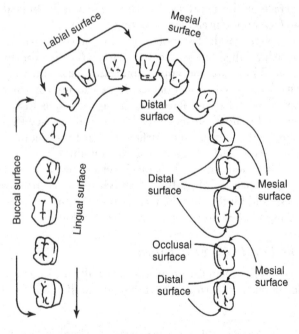

FIGURE 4-49

Summary of dental surfaces.

The growth period includes the beginning formation of the tooth bud, specialization and arrangement of cells to outline the future tooth, and formation of the enamel and dentin matrix. Calcification consists of hardening of the enamel and dentin matrix by deposition of inorganic salts, largely calcium. Eruption consists of the migration of the rather fully developed tooth into the oral cavity, while attrition is the wearing away of the enamel on the contact and occlusal surfaces of the erupted tooth.

Growth The teeth, which are modifications of ectoderm and mesoderm (see Figure 1-9), begin to show the first signs of development during the fifth or sixth week of embryonic life. A detailed description of the embryonic development of dentition can be found in Chapter 7 of this text. At about the 8- or 9-mm stage of development, the primitive oral epithelium begins to bulge into the subjacent mesoderm along a region that will eventually be occupied by the dentition. This horseshoe-shaped thickening in each jaw is called the **dental lamina,** and from it and surrounding cells are produced individual **tooth buds,** which will later develop into teeth. Soon after root development begins, the teeth begin a gradual migration from their crypts to the oral cavity. The origin of the forces which cause the teeth to migrate is not known.

Eruption The usual concept of eruption of teeth is the migration of their crowns into the oral cavity. When the tooth is sufficiently well developed to withstand the stresses to which it will be subjected, it makes its way through the gum, as shown in Figure 4-50. This stage of eruption is called **clinical** (observable) **eruption.** Some time prior to clinical eruption, however, the tooth erupts through the alveolar ridge in a phase known as **intraosseous eruption.** It is interesting to note that calcification of the tooth and development of the root are still in progress during intraosseous eruption. Shortly after this eruption occurs, the bony tissue separating the teeth begins to ossify. This tissue forms the **alveoli,** which are responsible for providing a solid footing for the teeth and the periodontal ligament.

Eruption is sometimes explained on the basis of purely mechanical forces. We have all heard the expression that a child is "cutting teeth." This leads to the impression that a tooth, with brute force cleaves the tissues in its pathway by virtue of the mechanics of tooth growth. It is true, of course, that a growing tooth germ does exert force against the tissues around it and in its pathway. The result, however, is that the affected tissues react to reduce and finally eliminate the unbalanced forces generated by the growing tooth.

Osteoclasts (Gk. *klastos*, broken) are formed in the alveolar bone that is under pressure. They are large, multinucleated cells having the property of bone absorption (resorption), thus clearing the way for the erupting tooth. Intraosseous eruption is shown in Figure 4-51. In the process of the "cutting" of the tooth through the gingivae, pressure leads to the activation of certain enzymes and similar agents which are responsible for the "dedifferentiation" of tissue. The process is a complex one, but it is important to discount pure mechanics.

Like so many phenomena associated with maturation, tooth eruption is a transitory condition that acts as an unbalancing force to which the body reacts. It is the basis for **homeostasis,** or in other words, a tendency toward stability in normal body states.

Attrition Once a tooth has erupted into the oral cavity it is immediately subjected to wear, pressure, and strain. Eventually, even though enamel is the hardest substance in the body, the teeth begin to show signs of wear. This process, called attrition, is shown in Figure 4-50. By definition, attrition is an abrasion or wearing away of the enamel of the teeth by use. The incisive edges of newly erupted permanent incisors bear three small tubercles called **mamelons** which quickly wear away through attrition. Their presence in a young adult suggests malocclusion.

Abnormal or precocious attrition may be seen in the clasping teeth of pipe smokers. The usual sites for normal attrition are the occlusal and approximal (interproximal) surfaces. Continuous eruption of the teeth helps to maintain the spatial relationships while attrition is occurring. It is important to understand that attrition is a normal process. In fact, it is necessary in

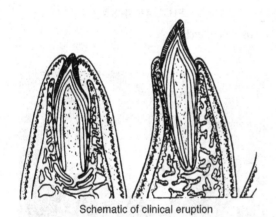

Schematic of clinical eruption

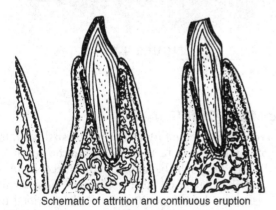

Schematic of attrition and continuous eruption

FIGURE 4-50

Schematic of clinical eruption and attrition of the teeth. (From *Atlas of the Mouth,* courtesy American Dental Association.)

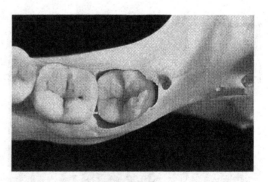

FIGURE 4-51

Photograph of intraosseous eruption of a third molar (wisdom tooth).

maintaining the integrity of the dentition. Attrition and eruption continue throughout the life of an individual, and our teeth wear out about the same time the rest of us wears out. Attrition of occlusal surfaces is readily seen in Figure 4-52.

The Deciduous (Primary) Dental Arch

The deciduous teeth are smaller and fewer in number than are the permanent teeth. In general form, however, they closely resemble their permanent successors. The complete primary deciduous dental arches contain 20 teeth, 10 in the maxillary and 10 in the mandibular arch. The distribution of primary teeth may be expressed by the following formula:

$$I\frac{2}{2}\,C\frac{1}{1}\,M\frac{2}{2} \times 2 = 20$$

$$I = \text{incisor}$$
$$C = \text{canine}$$
$$M = \text{molar}$$

Thus in each dental arch there are two incisors (a central and a lateral), one canine, and two molars. A deciduous dental arch is shown schematically in Figure 4-53, and a photograph of deciduous teeth is shown in Figure 4-54. Because primary teeth are small, gaps may develop between them as the dental arches grow, a condition that should be considered normal.

Eruption of the primary teeth usually begins during the second half of the first year and continues until the end of the second year, as shown in Table 4-1. Normative data are based on relatively large samples of the population and may not necessarily represent the actual sequence of dental eruption for any single child. There may also be deviations ±2 months for eruption of incisors, ±4 months for eruption of molars, and ±6 months for shedding.

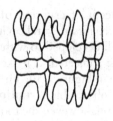

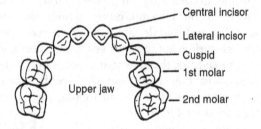

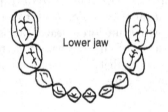

FIGURE 4-53

Deciduous dental arch.

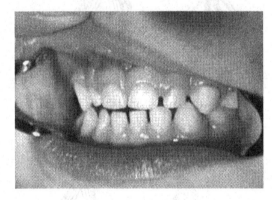

FIGURE 4-54

Deciduous dentition.

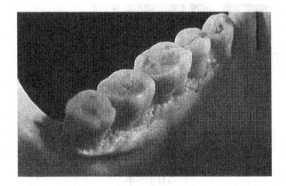

FIGURE 4-52

An example of attrition where the cusps on the molars have worn smooth.

The Mixed Dentition

Toward the end of the fifth or during the sixth year, the first of the permanent teeth may erupt in the deciduous dental arch. This is the beginning of the mixed dentition stage, which will typically span 6 or 7 years. Thus, a child of 6 years may have from 20 to 24 teeth, provided the central incisors have not been shed. The mixed dentition stage ends with the shedding of the second primary molars. Mixed dentition in a prepared skull of a 7-year-old is shown in Figure 4-55. During this period of mixed dentition, the teeth have not moved into their normal

TABLE 4-1

Sequence of eruption and shedding of the deciduous teeth

	Eruption	Shedding
Lower central incisors	6 to 9 mo.	6 to 8 years
Upper central incisors	8 to 10 mo.	7 to 8 years
Upper lateral incisors	8 to 10 mo.	$7\frac{1}{2}$ to $8\frac{1}{2}$ years
Lower lateral incisors	15 to 20 mo.	$6\frac{1}{2}$ to $7\frac{1}{2}$ years
First molars	15 to 21 mo.	$9\frac{1}{2}$ to 11 years
Canines	15 to 20 mo.	9 to 12 years
Second molars	20 to 24 mo.	10 to $11\frac{1}{2}$ years

Eruption of the lower teeth usually precedes eruption of the upper teeth by a short interval.

occlusal relationships. The overbite and overjet seen in normal occlusion may not exist (see Figure 4-47), and the incisors may not even meet when the child bites.

From what has been said thus far regarding the growth of teeth and the development of the alveolar ridge, it ought to be apparent that the dental arch is not simply an inorganic static structure but rather a dynamic, living organ. Proper growth and the health of the entire dental apparatus depends on the balance of forces acting upon the teeth and their supportive structures. The primary teeth are often neglected because they are "only temporary" and are soon to be replaced by permanent teeth. It is important to realize that the health of primary teeth is crucial in maintaining the proper spatial relationships for the permanent teeth. Although the loss of a primary incisor is not particularly serious, premature loss of a cuspid or molar may result in problems such as malocclusion of the permanent dental arch. In *Atlas of the Mouth*, published by the American Dental Association (1956), is the following statement regarding premature loss of permanent teeth:

The first permanent molar is the keystone of the dental arch. The extraction of a lower first molar, without immediate replacement, especially after eruption of the second permanent molar, may result in shifting of the teeth, malocclusion, periodontal injury and caries.

The Permanent Dental Arch

There are two groups of permanent teeth: those that replace the primary teeth and those that have no deciduous predecessors. The first of these are called **successional** permanent teeth; the latter, the permanent molars, are called **superadded** permanent teeth. The development of permanent teeth is essentially the same as that of primary teeth.

Successional Teeth Formation of the successional teeth begins about the tenth week of embryonic life. They first appear as swellings in the same dental lamina that gives rise to the primary teeth, and by the time clinical eruption of the primary teeth has taken place, the successional permanent teeth are well on their way to maturity.

Superadded Teeth The pattern of development of the permanent molars is slightly different from that of the successional teeth. By the fifth month of embryonic life, the dental lamina from which the primary teeth arise has extended posteriorly beyond the growing second primary molars and has become modified into a special dental germ that will become the first permanent molar. This first molar is quite well developed before the first primary teeth erupt. The formation of the special dental germ for the second permanent molar takes place about the same time the first deciduous teeth erupt, and formation of the germ for the third molar coincides with the eruption of the first permanent molars.

Shedding and Eruption During their development, the permanent teeth migrate to the lingual side of the primary teeth and are separated from them by bony partitions. A histological section through an erupted primary tooth and developing permanent tooth is shown in Figure 4-56. As the crown of the permanent tooth reaches maturity, an interesting modification of the corresponding primary tooth and bony partition takes place.

Osteoclasts appear. Gradually, the bony partitions separating the permanent from the primary teeth, as well as the roots of the primary teeth, are resorbed until all that remains of the primary teeth is the crown. The primary teeth are not simply pushed from their corresponding socket by the erupting permanent teeth. The crown is shed when clinical eruption of the permanent teeth is imminent. Many adults (and children) have the impression that the crown of a primary tooth, that part ceremoniously placed under the pillow, constitutes the entire body. They fail to realize that a primary tooth is every bit as complex as its permanent successor. This contributes to the casual attitude toward proper care of primary dentition.

The sequence of eruption for the permanent teeth is shown in Table 4-2. Again, these are normative data and the normal sequence may not be representative of an actual individual sequence of eruption.

Description Each jaw bears a total of 16 permanent teeth: 4 incisors, 2 canines, 4 premolars, and 6 molars. The third molar or wisdom tooth may be congenitally absent (up to 25 percent of some populations), or it may become impacted and fail to erupt. This is especially true of the lower third molar. The upper third molar is rarely impacted.

The size of the molars progressively decreases posteriorly. The permanent incisors are larger than their

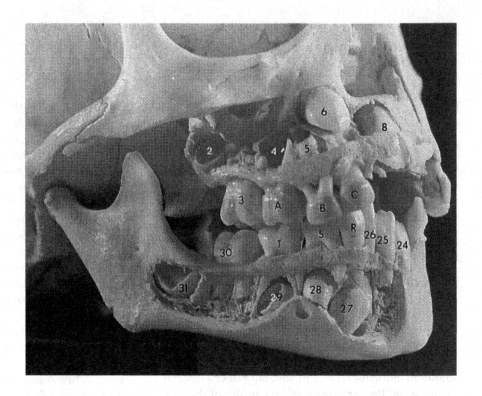

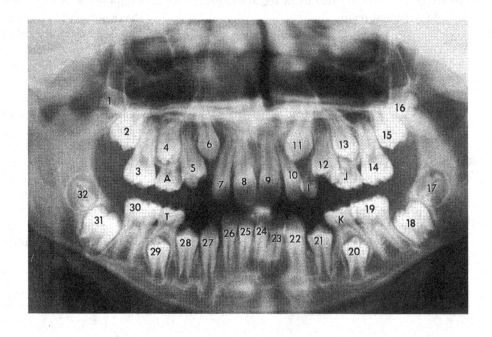

FIGURE 4-55

Mixed dentition as seen in prepared skull of a 7-year-old child (top) and in a living child (bottom). Teeth are identified according to the universal numbering system: third upper-right molar (1), third upper-left molar (16), third left-lower molar (17), third right-lower molar (32). Deciduous teeth are identified in the same manner, only alphabetically.

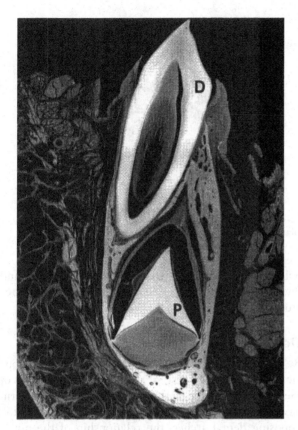

FIGURE 4-56

A histological section through an erupted deciduous tooth (D), and a developing permanent tooth (P).

TABLE 4-2

Sequence of eruption
of the permanent teeth

	Age in Years
Upper central incisors	7–8
Lower central incisors	6–7
Upper lateral incisors	8–9
Lower lateral incisors	7–8
Upper cuspids	11–12
Lower cuspids	9–10
Upper first bicuspids	10–11
Lower first bicuspids	10–12
Upper second bicuspids	10–12
Lower second bicuspids	11–12
Upper first molars	6–7
Lower first molars	6–7
Upper second molars	12–13
Lower second molars	11–13
Upper third molars	17–25
Lower third molars	17–25

The teeth usually erupt earlier in girls than they do in boys.

Occasionally an additional tooth may be found in the region of the upper central incisors. These are called supernumerary teeth.

Anomalies Associated with Tooth Development

Inadequate tooth development or excessive tooth initiation may result in the following anomalies:

Anodontia (absence of teeth) results from a failure of tooth buds to form. A congenital condition called **ectodermal dysplasia** may result in total anodontia, while disturbances of normal sites of development (cleft palate, for example) may result in partial anodontia. The third molars, upper lateral incisors, and mandibular second molars are the teeth that most commonly fail to develop.

Supernumerary teeth result when the dental lamina produces an excessive number of tooth buds. These teeth most often develop in the region of the upper central incisors. **Natal teeth** (present at birth) may be part of the normal primary dentition, or they may be supernumerary, tending to disrupt the position and eruption of adjacent teeth.

Macrodontia, large teeth, and **microdontia**, small teeth, are usually the result of disturbances of embryonic tooth development. Upper lateral incisors may present a slender tapered shape (peg-shaped).

Twinning, a condition in which two teeth are joined together, occurs most often in the mandibular incisors of the primary dentition. Twinning may result from **germination,** the division of a single tooth germ to form a bifid crown on a single root, or from **fusion,** a joining of developing teeth that erupt as a single tooth. **Concrescence** is the fusion of the roots of adjacent teeth resulting from excessive formation of cementum. This type of twinning occurs most often in the maxillary molars.

Amelogenesis imperfecta is a dominant genetic trait that results in a thin layer of abnormal enamel, through which the yellow color of the dentin can be seen. The condition usually affects both primary and secondary dentition.

Dentinogenesis imperfecta (hereditary opalescent dentin) is a condition in which dentin is poorly calcified. The teeth are opaque and pearly and the enamel tends to flake away.

Mottled enamel is found in persons whose drinking water has an excessively high fluoride content (2.0 parts per million). It varies from small white patches to severe brownish discoloration.

Discolored teeth may result from incorporation of certain substances into the developing enamel. All of the tetracyclines (antibiotics) may produce brownish-yellow discoloration. The critical period is from the fourth month of fetal life to the sixteenth year for the permanent teeth (enamel is completely formed on all but the third molars by the eighth year).

Spatial Relationships of the Teeth

In the normal skull, the maxillary arch has a slightly larger diameter and is longer than the mandibular arch. This being the case, the normal relationship between the upper and lower teeth is such that there is a **maxillary overbite.** That is, the upper arch overlaps and confines the lower arch in such a manner that the upper incisors and canines, and to a lesser extent the premolars, bite labial to (outside) the lower teeth. The upper premolars and the upper molars are shifted buccally. The amount by which the upper incisors lie labial (anterior) to the lower incisors is the **overjet,** as illustrated in Figure 4-47. Normal overjet is 2–3 mm.

The normal relationship between the teeth of the upper and lower arches is such that (excepting the upper third molars and lower central incisors) each tooth is opposed by two teeth of the opposite arch. The lower-arch molars are positioned one cusp (one-half tooth) ahead of the upper-arch molars, and it is this relationship that forms the basis for classification of occlusion. This was illustrated schematically in Figure 4-46, and a photograph of healthy, mature permanent dentition is shown in Figure 4-57.

During the process of eruption of the permanent teeth, spaces may develop between them. This condition, called **diastema,** is considered normal and is usually self-correcting. It is illustrated in Figure 4-58.

In the habitual relaxed jaw position, the teeth do not meet as they do in centric occlusion,[12] but are

_____

[12]**Centric occlusion** refers to the mandible being central to the maxilla (i.e., there is full occlusal contact of the upper and lower teeth).

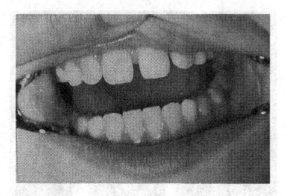

FIGURE 4-58

Diastema in a 9-year-old child.

held slightly apart. The space between the upper and lower teeth is called the **freeway space,** or **interocclusal clearance.**

Occlusion

By definition, occlusion means the full meeting or contact, in a position of rest, of the masticating surfaces of the upper and lower teeth. In actual practice, the term has come to include the alignment of the teeth in the opposing dental arches, the relationship of the upper and lower arches to each other, as well as the positioning of individual teeth. When the opposing occlusal surfaces meet in centric occlusion, the forces generated by the muscles of mastication are distributed over a large area of alveolar bone. In malocclusion, only a few teeth may touch, and the force is distributed over a much smaller area. In adulthood, malocclusions are a leading cause of loss of teeth.

Angle's Classification In 1899, Angle proposed a system of classification of three main types of occlusion (see Figure 4-59). The relationship of the upper and lower jaw is determined by observing the teeth in centric occlusion.

In **Class I (normal) occlusion,** the cusps of the first mandibular molar interdigitate ahead and inside of the corresponding cusps of the opposing maxillary teeth. This occlusion provides a normal facial profile. In a **Class I malocclusion** the _molar relationship is normal,_ and the variation lies in the anterior (mesial) portion of the dental arch.

A **Class II malocclusion** occurs when the cusps of the first mandibular molars are behind and inside the opposing molars of the maxillary arch. This is the most common of the occlusal discrepancies and is found in about 45 percent of the population. A Class II malocclusion also results in an _increased overjet,_ the appearance of a _receding chin,_ and a _decrease in lower facial height._

In a **Class III malocclusion** the cusps of the first mandibular molar interdigitate a tooth (or more) ahead

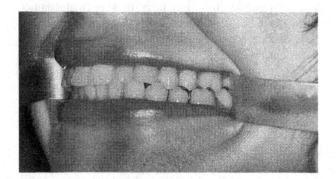

FIGURE 4-57

Photograph of healthy, permanent dentition.

FIGURE 4-59

Examples of types of occlusions.

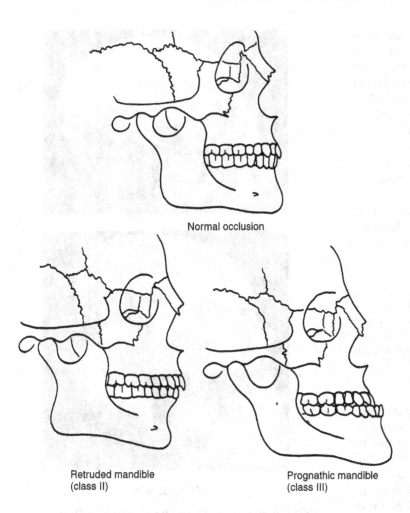

Normal occlusion

Retruded mandible
(class II)

Prognathic mandible
(class III)

of the opposing maxillary incisors, giving the appearance of a *prognathic jaw* and an *increase in facial height*.

The terms neutrocclusion (Class I), distocclusion (Class II), and mesiocclusion (Class III) are falling into disuse.

Crossbite Normally the mandibular teeth are overlapped by the maxillary teeth. A reversal of this relationship is called a crossbite, and it may involve a single tooth or an entire arch.

Malpositioned Teeth Certain terms have come into general use in describing the positions of individual teeth.

1. **Axiversion**—improper axial inclination. The following terms specify which way the teeth are "tipped":

     Distoversion (tilting distally)

     Labioversion (tilting toward the tongue, or out of the arch lingually)

     Mesioversion (tilting mesially).

2. **Infraversion**—a tooth that has not erupted sufficiently to reach the line of occlusion.

3. **Supraversion**—a tooth that has grown past the normal line of occlusion. It extends too far into the oral cavity. A snag tooth.

4. **Torsiversion**—a tooth that is rotated on its long axis. *Twisted* is an acceptable substitute.

Open and Closed Bites Occasionally, in the course of dental development, the anterior teeth fail to erupt sufficiently to reach the line of occlusion (infraversion), or the posterior teeth have erupted past the normal line of occlusion (supraversion). In either case a condition known as **open bite** results; that is, the anterior teeth are unable to approximate, and a persistent space exists between them. Conversely, either due to infraversion of the posterior teeth or supraversion of the anterior teeth, the posterior teeth fail to meet, a condition known as **closed bite.** These conditions of open and closed bite need not necessarily occur bilaterally but may occur only on one side of the dental arch. In that case, a condition known as a **lateral open bite** exists. An open bite may be detrimental to the general health of an individual and may contribute to the production of defective speech.

Effects of Evolution As might be expected, the masticatory apparatus in modern humans is less well developed than that of our anthropoid predecessors. A fairly well-established difference is the loss of the third molar and general reduction of the dentition. Note, in the photograph of the dentition of an ape (Figure 4-60), the large canine teeth and three premolars. Another feature associated with the evolution of Homo sapiens is a reduction of the facial skeleton, which is manifested in decreased facial protrusion. This can be seen by comparing the lateral view of the facial skeleton of an ape with that of a modern human, as shown in Figure 4-61. Sicher and DuBrul (1975) point out, however, that the reduction in the length of the jaws and the reduction of the dentition are not taking place at an equal pace.

> It seems the shortening of the jaws is, in modern man, already further advanced and more firmly fixed than the shortening of the dentition. The reduction of space for the third molars is enhanced in many individuals by the fact that the third molars erupt at a time when the general growth of the individual and that of the jaws is already nearing its end.

Orthodontics We have probably all heard a statement to the effect that an individual's teeth are too large for the mouth, a statement that could also imply that the mouth is too small for the teeth. Or a child has her dad's teeth and her mother's mouth, and this explains the crowded teeth. Whatever the reason, the imbalance between the length of the jaws in an anteroposterior direction and the length of the dental arch can lead to problems that require the attention and therapeutic management of specialists in dentistry.

The disharmony in dentition may begin to manifest itself at an early age and will be recognized by a dentist

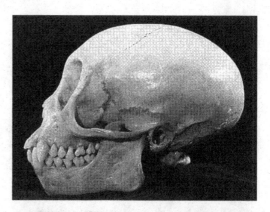

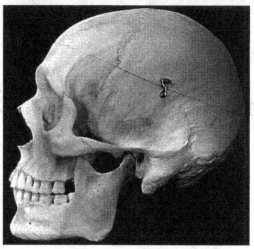

FIGURE 4-61

Lateral view of the facial skeleton of an ape (top) and of a modern adult male (bottom).

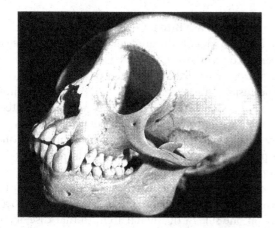

FIGURE 4-60

The dentition of an ape. Note the large canine teeth, the three premolars, and the comparatively large jaws relative to the remainder of the facial skeleton.

or a pedodontist. **Pedodontics** is a specialty within dentistry concerned with the diagnosis and treatment of the teeth and mouth in children. Children who are developing crowded teeth or malocclusion may then be referred to an orthodontist (Gk. *orthos*, straight). **Orthodontics** is a branch of dentistry that deals with the prevention and correction of irregularities of the teeth and malocclusion, and with associated facial problems. One phase of orthodontics deals with the reduction or elimination of an existing malocclusion and its secondary characteristics. It is called **corrective orthodontia**. **Interceptive orthodontia** is concerned with the elimination of a condition that might lead to the development of a malocclusion, whereas **preventive orthodontia** is a phase of orthodontics concerned with the preservation of what appears to be normal occlusion. Orthodontic treatment is instrumental in reducing the number of dental caries (L. rottenness), prevention of premature loss of teeth, and it can be effective in maintaining a normal, healthy balance between dentition and the facial skeleton.

Stated very simply, the role of an orthodontist is to design an appliance that will shift the position of a tooth in the jaw.

When prolonged force of a surprisingly small magnitude is applied to a tooth, the body reacts to correct the state of imbalance. Elevated force on one side of a tooth results in the formation of **osteoclasts** that resorb alveolar bone, with a simultaneous formation of **osteoblasts** on the relieved side of the tooth. As a consequence the tooth literally shifts position in the mouth. Teeth can be moved individually or in groups within the jaw, caused to rotate on their axes; the growth of the jaws can even be controlled by proper applications of force.

Almost all orthodontic appliances have but one function, and that is to apply a steady, controlled force to move teeth into their proper position. The basic tool available to the orthodontist is called an **appliance,** although we may casually refer to braces on the teeth.

We have seen how crowding can be the consequence of teeth that are simply too large for the jaw. We may also encounter instances where the jaw is too small for the teeth. This can be one of the serious consequences of mouth breathing (Massler and Schour, 1958), and unless treated at an early age, serious crowding of the teeth can result. In addition, the palate may become so high that it actually imposes constraints on the amount of air that can pass through the nasal meati, making unrestricted nose breathing extremely difficult. It is interesting that this condition, which may be a consequence of mouth breathing, in turn, encourages it. This is a runaway situation.

The Tongue

Introduction

The primary biological function of the tongue is in taste, mastication, and deglutition. It moves food into position to be crushed by the teeth, helps mix the food with saliva, and later sweeps the place clean before forming the food into a bolus. It finishes the job by shoving the bolus into the pharynx.

The tongue is without doubt the most important and the most active of the articulators. It functions to modify the shape of the oral cavity and thus the resonance characteristics of the oral and associated cavities. The tongue also acts as a valve to either inhibit or stop the flow of air and, in conjunction with the teeth, alveolar processes, and palate, may act as a noise generator. At times, it functions both as a noise generator and a modifier of the laryngeal tone, as in the production of voiced consonants. Indeed, the tongue is a very remarkable structure, able to assume many different configurations and positions in amazingly rapid sequences.

It is primarily due to high innervation and to the complex arrangements of the muscle fibers making up the bulk of the tongue that such rapid and subtle sequences of movement are possible.

Description

On an anatomical basis the tongue may be divided into a **blade** and a **root.** It may also be divided into four regions based on the relationship of the tongue to the roof of the mouth. As seen in Figure 4-62, the portion of the tongue

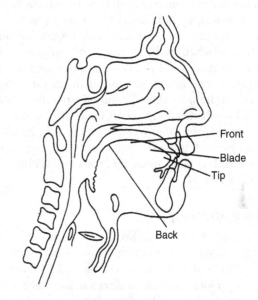

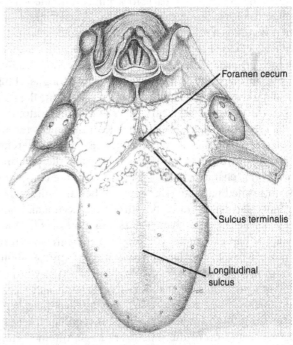

FIGURE 4-62

Divisions of the dorsum of the tongue (top) and major surface landmarks of the dorsum (bottom).

nearest the front teeth is called the **tip,** the part below the upper alveolar ridge is the **blade,** the part just below the hard palate is called the **front** and the part beneath the soft palate is the **back** of the tongue.

The configuration of the tongue at rest is such that the front and back parts of the dorsum bear nearly a right-angle relationship to one another, a consequence of our being upright animals. This change in orientation adds versatility to tongue movements and is one reason we are able to speak. The tongue is "slung" by muscles from the roof of the mouth and the base of the skull. It can be raised, retruded, or both, but the tongue is also fastened, by muscles, to the inner surface of the mandibular symphysis, to the hyoid bone, and the pharynx. It is attached by ligaments to the epiglottis. The tongue can move, and the jaw can move, and the two can move in opposite directions, or in the same direction, and at the same time. Because the tongue is free in a horseshoe-shaped region on its undersurface, the sides and tip are capable of movement that is independent of its main mass. This means the tip and sides can curl up or down and, in some of us, fold back on itself (like the tongue of a toad).

Surface Anatomy

The tongue's development from two embryonic primordia is reflected in the adult form by differences in surface characteristics and sensory innervation. The dorsum is divided by a **longitudinal median sulcus,** which is continued from the front back to a pit of variable extent called the **foramen cecum** (L. *caecum,* blind). The foramen cecum is a remnant of the embryonic origin of the thyroid gland. From the foramen cecum, a shallow V-shaped groove called the **sulcus terminalis** courses anteriorly and laterally to the margins of the tongue. This landmark separates the anterior two-thirds of the dorsum from the posterior one-third (see Figure 4-62 bottom).

The surface areas on either side of the sulcus terminalis are anatomically and functionally quite different. The area in front of the sulcus terminalis, the **palatine surface,** is characterized by projections of the corium or dermis called **papillae** (L., nipple). They are thickly distributed over the entire two-thirds of the dorsum and give the surface its characteristic roughness. The four types of papillae that have been identified are shown in Figure 4-63. The **vallate** (circumvallate) **papillae,** about ten in number, form a V- or chevron-shaped row on the dorsum just anterior to the foramen cecum and sulcus terminalis. They contain taste buds at their periphery. The **fungiform** (mushroom-shaped) **papillae** found at the sides and tip of the tongue are large, rounded eminences, red in color and covered with secondary papillae. Taste buds are liberally distributed over them. **Filiform** (threadlike) **papillae** are the most common. They are

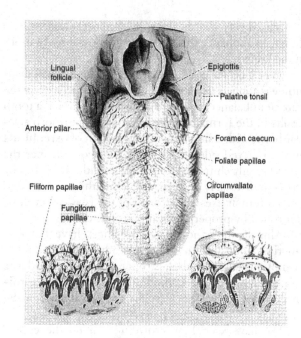

FIGURE 4-63

The tongue as seen from above. (From *Atlas of the Mouth,* courtesy American Dental Association.)

arranged in lines or rows that parallel the vallate papillae, except at the tip where their direction is transverse. The **simple papillae,** similar to the papillae of the skin, cover the entire mucous membrane as well as the surface of the larger papillae.

The posterior third of the tongue, the **pharyngeal surface,** is smoother in appearance than the palatine surface. It is somewhat nodular because it contains numerous mucous glands and an aggregate of lymph glands that collectively comprise the **lingual tonsil.** Sometimes remnants of the thyroid gland can be found in this region.

At rest, the undersurface of the tongue is in contact with the floor of the mouth. The **lingual frenulum (frenum),** shown in Figure 4-64, extends from the floor of the mouth at the midline to the underside of the tongue, and from the lingual frenulum, we get the expression "tongue-tied" as an explanation for certain speech problems. In fact, sometimes the frenulum extends to near the tip of the tongue and may interfere with tongue protrusion. The frenulum stretches with age, however, and rarely presents a problem.

Superficial Anatomy

The mucous membrane covering the inferior surface of the tongue is thin, squamous, and identical to the membrane lining the rest of the oral cavity. The mucous membrane on the pharyngeal surface is quite thick, but freely movable, while the membrane covering the ante-

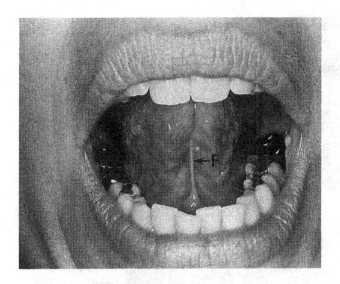

FIGURE 4-64

Intraoral view of the lingual frenulum (F).

rior portion of the dorsum is quite thin and closely attached to the musculature of the tongue. The membrane consists of a layer of connective tissue called the **corium** (L. hide) or **dermis,** which in the skin is subjacent to the epidermis. The corium is a dense feltlike network of fibrous connective tissue liberally supplied with elastic fibers that can be traced through the lingual musculature to the fibrous midline septum of the tongue. The corium plays an important role, because it forms part of the "skeleton" of the tongue.

Deep Structures

If muscle contraction is to decrease the distance between two points, the muscle must have attachments on the structures to be moved. The muscle cannot simply arise within the mass of an organ, follow a particular course, and then terminate without attachments. The corium, the fibrous midline septum, and the deep connective tissue of the lingual mucosa (lamina propria) form the **skeleton of the tongue** and to a large extent account for its protean nature.[13]

There are eight (or nine) muscles of the tongue, which may be divided into intrinsic and extrinsic muscle groups. Because the two groups are interwoven to such a large extent, it is difficult to trace the path of a particular extrinsic muscle once it has entered the tongue. It is even difficult to determine whether fibers are from the intrinsic or extrinsic muscles.

Because the tongue is divided into two lateral halves by its median fibrous septum, all the lingual musculature is regarded as paired, and the two halves seem to be individually supplied by motor and sensory nerves and blood vessels. This becomes apparent in hemiplegia and some other forms of brain disease, where the tongue, when protruded, may deviate to one side.

The Intrinsic Muscles of the Tongue

There are four intrinsic lingual muscles: the **superior longitudinal,** the **inferior longitudinal,** the **transverse,** and the **vertical** muscles. They are shown in Figures 4-65 and 4-66.

The Superior Longitudinal Muscle (Superior Lingualis) The superior longitudinal muscle is often described as a thin layer of oblique and longitudinal muscle fibers lying just deep to the mucous membrane of the dorsum of the tongue. The muscle actually occupies a substantial portion of the tongue. Fibers arise from the submucous fibrous tissue (described earlier) close to the root and from the median fibrous septum.[14] Confined to the middle portion of the tongue, the superior longitudinal muscle never quite reaches the apex or dorsum, but it can usually be traced to the hyoid bone. The fibers course anteriorly to the edges of the tongue and terminate in the fibrous membrane.

Upon contraction, the muscle tends to shorten the tongue and thereby turn the tip upward. The oblique fibers may assist in turning the lateral margins upward, giving the dorsum a concave or troughlike appearance.

The Inferior Longitudinal Muscle (Inferior Lingualis) The inferior longitudinal consists of a bundle of muscle fibers located on the undersurface of the tongue, somewhat laterally. It courses between the genioglossus and hyoglossus muscles, and longitudinal muscle fibers interdigitate with them. Muscle fibers of the inferior longitudinal muscle extend from the root to the apex of the tongue. Some muscle fibers arise from the hyoid bone, while anteriorly a few fibers may blend with those of the styloglossus. Upon contraction this muscle either shortens the tongue or pulls the tip downward.

The Transverse Muscle (Transverse Lingualis) The transverse muscle fibers arise from the median fibrous septum and course directly in a lateral direction to terminate in the submucous fibrous tissue at the lateral margins of the tongue. The course of the lateralmost fibers is somewhat radiate, as can be seen in Figure 4-67. As a consequence of this fanlike distribution, some fibers

---

[13]Proteus, a sea god and son of Oceanus and Tethys, was noted for his ability to assume many different forms. Thus, **protean** means anything that readily changes appearance, character, or principles.

[14]The septum may be seen in the frontal section of Figure 4-66.

FIGURE 4-65

Frontal sections through the tongue of a five-month fetus.

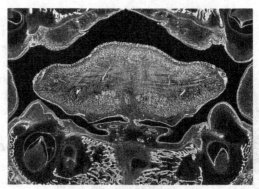

Through the tip

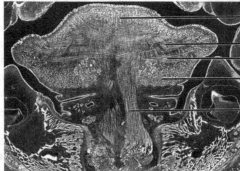

Superior longitudinal muscle

Vertical muscle

Transverse muscle

Inferior longitudinal muscle

Genioglossus muscle

Through the blade

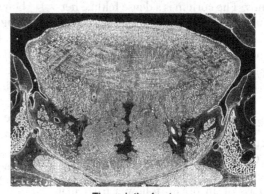

Through the front

of the transverse muscle seem to ultimately take the same course as the vertical fibers. Contraction of the transverse muscle causes the tongue to narrow and to become elongated.

The Vertical Muscle (Vertical Lingualis) The vertical muscle fibers originate from the mucous membrane of the dorsum of the tongue. They course vertically downward, and somewhat laterally, to terminate at the sides and inferior surface of the tongue. As can be seen in Figures 4-65 and 4-66, the fibers are confined to the lateral portion of the tongue. They are also more highly developed anteriorly. The vertical muscle flattens the tongue.

The Extrinsic Muscles of the Tongue

Four muscles originate from adjacent structures and insert into the tongue. They are the **genioglossus,** the **styloglossus,** the **palatoglossus,** and the **hyoglossus.** The extrinsic tongue muscles and associated structures are shown schematically in Figure 4-68.

The Genioglossus Muscle (Geniohyoglossus) The genioglossus (Gk. *genein,* chin), which forms the bulk of the tongue tissue, is the strongest and largest of the extrinsic muscles. It is a flat, triangular muscle located close to the median plane. Part of the genioglossus may be seen in Figure 4-65, and it is shown schematically in Figure 4-68. It originates from the superior mental spine

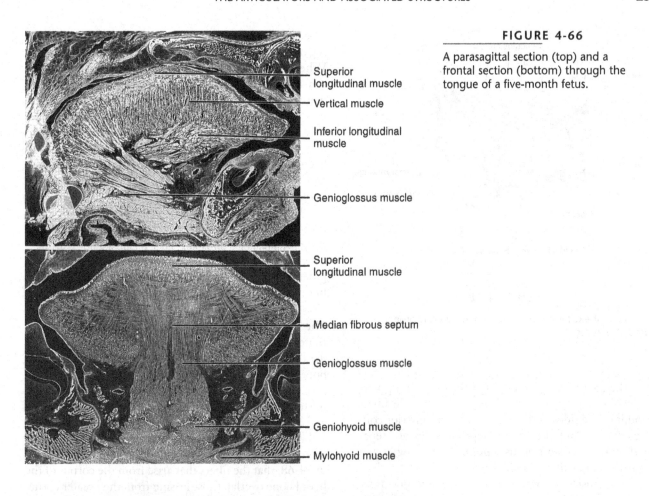

FIGURE 4-66

A parasagittal section (top) and a frontal section (bottom) through the tongue of a five-month fetus.

Superior longitudinal muscle

Vertical muscle

Inferior longitudinal muscle

Genioglossus muscle

Superior longitudinal muscle

Median fibrous septum

Genioglossus muscle

Geniohyoid muscle

Mylohyoid muscle

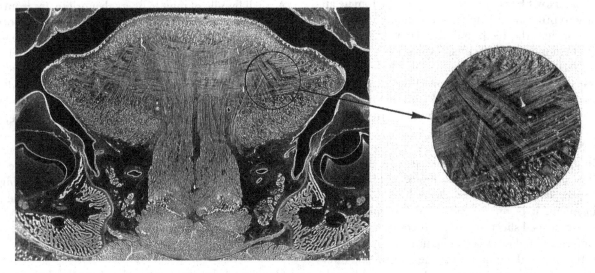

FIGURE 4-67

A greatly enlarged section through a fetal tongue, showing the radiating nature of the vertical and transverse intrinsic muscles of the tongue.

(on the posterior surface of the mandibular symphysis). The lowermost fibers course to the hyoid bone and attach by a thin aponeurosis to the upper part of the body.

The remainder of the fibers radiate fanlike to the dorsum of the tongue and insert into the submucous fibrous tissue on either side of the midline in an area extending

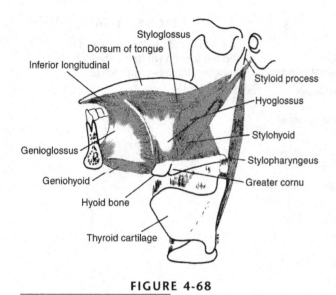

FIGURE 4-68

Schematic of extrinsic tongue musculature and some associated structures.

from the root to the tip, although the extreme tip may be devoid of genioglossus fibers. A few muscle fibers blend into the sides of the upper pharynx (superior constrictor). The muscles of the opposite sides are separated by the median fibrous septum of the tongue, but toward the apex they blend.

This muscle accounts for many tongue positions. The **posterior fibers** draw the whole of the tongue anteriorly to protrude the tip from the mouth or to press the tip against the teeth and alveolar ridges. Certain states of emotion are sometimes expressed by the use of the posterior muscle fibers. Contraction of the **anterior fibers** is responsible for retraction of the tongue, while contraction of the entire muscle draws the tongue downward, thus making the dorsum like a trough.

The Styloglossus Muscle The styloglossus is the smallest of the three muscles that arise at the styloid processes. Beginning from the anterior and lateral surface of the styloid process and from the stylomandibular ligament, it begins to radiate almost immediately into a fan-shaped sheet of muscle. It courses downward and anteriorly, and as shown in Figure 4-68, some fibers enter the side of the tongue near the dorsum and interdigitate with those of the inferior longitudinal muscle. The remainder of the fibers overlap and blend with fibers of the hyoglossus muscle.

Upon contraction, the styloglossus draws the tongue upward and backward and thus may be considered to be a true *antagonist of the genioglossus muscle.* It may also draw the sides of the tongue upward, thus assisting the intrinsic muscles in making the dorsum concave or troughlike.

The Palatoglossus Muscle The palatoglossus may be regarded as a muscle of the tongue or of the palate. When considered a muscle of the tongue, it is sometimes referred to as the **glossopalatine** muscle. It originates from the anterior surface of the soft palate, where it is continuous with its fellow from the opposite side. The fibers course downward and somewhat laterally to insert into the sides of the tongue, where they blend and become continuous with those of the transverse lingual, and with the superficial fibers of the styloglossus and hyoglossus muscles.

Upon contraction, the palatoglossus may either lower the soft palate or raise the back of the tongue to groove the dorsum. This muscle, with its mucous membrane covering, forms the palatoglossal arch (anterior faucial pillars); it will be referred to again in the section dealing with the arches and soft palate.

The Hyoglossus Muscle The hyoglossus, a thin quadrilateral sheet of muscle, originates from the upper border of the greater cornu and from the corpus of the hyoid bone. The fibers course vertically, diverging slightly before inserting into the lateral submucous tissue of the posterior half of the tongue. These fibers interdigitate and become continuous with those of the palatoglossus. Other fibers of the hyoglossus change their course and interlace with fibers of the styloglossus. Note, in Figure 4-68, that the fibers that arise from the corpus of the hyoid bone overlap those arising from the greater cornu. A small bundle of muscle fibers that originates from the lesser cornu and the region of the union of the corpus and greater cornu follows a parallel course with the hyoglossus muscle and inserts into the intrinsic muscles at the sides of the tongue for the most part, while some fibers continue to the tip of the tongue. This bundle of muscle fibers is sometimes considered a part of the hyoglossus, or it may be known as a separate muscle, the **chondroglossus.**

Besides functioning to retract and depress the tongue, the hyoglossus and chondroglossus may elevate the hyoid bone. Thus, it may be seen that there is an implicit relationship between the muscles of the tongue and those of phonation.

Anomalies of the Tongue

Congenital abnormalities of the tongue include **macroglossia** (very large) and **microglossia** (very small). Both are extremely rare. Macroglossia may occur in cretinism, Down syndrome, and acromegaly (due to pituitary disease). Only rarely is a **bifid** tongue encountered. A condition called **pseudomacroglossia** may exist in abnormalities associated with a very small jaw (micrognathia) such as Pierre Robin and Treacher Collins syndromes. In the case of Pierre Robin syndrome, especially, mandibular growth takes place within a few months, and the condition is relieved.

Black hairy tongue (lingua nigra) is a condition in which the filiform papillae become elongated, usually in the region just in front of the sulcus limitans. It may be due to chronic intraoral bleeding or to prolonged antibiotic therapy. Because of the presence of blood in the mouth, there is a characteristic **fetor ex ore** (a nice way to say very bad breath). Other conditions include rashes, discoloration, and dry furry tongue, usually associated with fever and dehydration.

The Tongue as an Articulator

The various tongue positions and configurations are mediated by lingual musculature and to a lesser extent by lower jaw movement. The movements of the tongue due to contractions of the extrinsic and some of the intrinsic muscles are shown schematically in Figure 4-69. We must realize that any given tongue position or configuration (that departs from a position of rest) is almost always the result of contraction of a complement of muscles. If we were to speculate on the consequences of all the various combinations of muscle contraction, the repertory of tongue postures becomes staggering.

Motor Control MacNeilage and Sholes (1964), using small surface electrodes, made electromyographic recordings of muscle activity from 13 locations on the tongue of a single subject during the phonation of 17 different types of [p]-vowel-[p] monosyllables. In addition, x-ray data and anatomical information were uti-

lized to describe the action of specific tongue muscles during vowel production. They found, for example, that the posterior portion of the genioglossus contracts to move the tongue anteriorly, thus increasing the depth of the oropharynx, particularly for those vowels that exhibit a high tongue position. The authors were able to assign specific functions to many of the extrinsic tongue muscles, but discrete activity of intrinsic muscles was not possible. As a result of this study, the overall picture of the motor control of the tongue that emerges is one that might be expected from knowledge of the complexity of the tongue musculature and the speed and accuracy with which it functions.

The impression is not one of the **ballistic movements** seen in simple musculature. Ballistic movements result from sudden contractions of single muscles that cease abruptly before the movement ceases. Tongue movement, on the other hand, seems to be a complex pattern of finely graded changes in activity in which one or two of the muscles produce most of the movement, and others cooperate in movement, stabilize adjacent structures, or actively oppose the movement.

Highly skilled subjects (supranormal) such as trumpet players and public speakers do not differ from "normal" subjects in terms of their tongue strength, but they do have greater endurance (Robin, et al., 1992).

Articulatory Paramenters Hardcastle (1976) lists just seven articulatory parameters which can account for the wide range of tongue positions and configurations during speech. The parameters, shown schematically in Figures 4-70 and 4-71, are as follows:

1. **Horizontal forward-backward movement of the tongue body,** mediated primarily by the posterior part of the genioglossus. Movement that takes place during production of low-back vowels. In the production of an [ɑ] sound, for example, it doesn't matter much what is done with the tip of the tongue, the sound changes very little from the [ɑ].

2. **Vertical upward-downward movement of the tongue body,** mediated by the styloglossus and palatoglossus, with inferior longitudinal muscle acting in synergism. Probably used in central vowels and for palatal consonants.

3. **Horizontal forward-backward movement of the tip-blade,** mediated by the transversus and posterior geniohyoid. Important in retroflex articulations.

4. **Vertical upward-downward movement of the tip-blade,** mediated by superior longitudinal, often accompanied by parameters 1 and 2. Used in production of [i], [t], and [n], and in [s].

5. **Transverse cross-sectional configuration of tongue body, convex-concave in relation to**

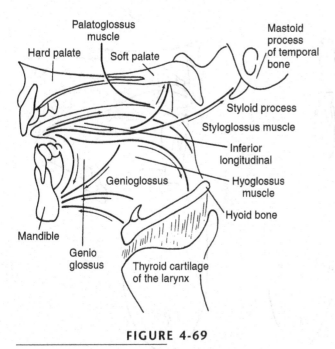

FIGURE 4-69

Functional diagram of tongue musculature.

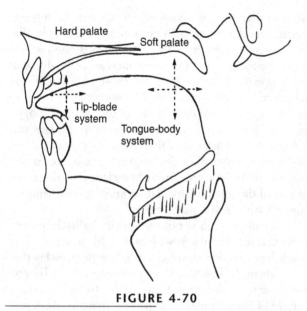

FIGURE 4-70

Sagittal view of tongue illustrating lingual articulatory parameters 1–2. (Modified after Hardcastle, 1976, with permission.)

palate. Hardcastle lists the styloglossus, palatoglossus, and transversus as the protagonists for these configurations, which occur for [t].

6. **Transverse cross-sectional configuration extending throughout the whole length of the tongue, particularly the tip and blade—degree of central grooving,** such as occurs in [s]. Muscles responsible for grooving are the transversus and verticalis. The styloglossus and palatoglossus may act synergistically.

7. **Surface plane of the tongue dorsum—spread or tapered,** for articulation of [t], [s], [l], and [i], [e], mediated by transversus and hyoglossus.

In terms of the number of parameters used in sound production, the vowels are the least complex, utilizing primarily parameters 1 and 2, while alveolar stop consonants utilize parameters 1, 2, 3, 4, and 7. Grooved fricatives such as [s] require maximum participation of all articulatory parameters.

FIGURE 4-71

(Top) Lingual articulatory parameter 5; on the right the vertical broken line shows the point at which the coronal plane section was taken. (Center) Lingual articulatory parameter 6; on the right the vertical broken line shows the point at which the coronal plane was taken. (Bottom), Lingual articulatory parameter 7. (Modified after Hardcastle, 1976, with permission.)

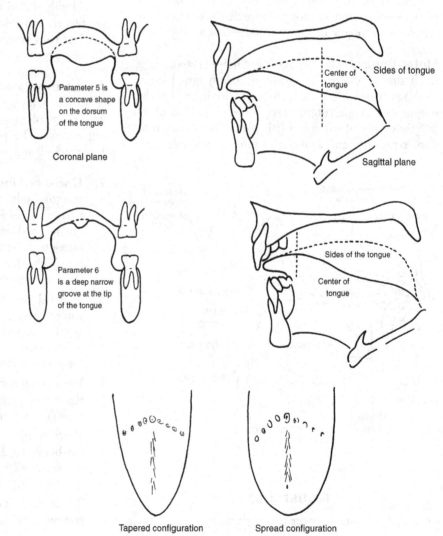

The Mandible

Introduction

The principal function of the mandible is mastication, and it contributes to speech production by modifying the resonant characteristics of the vocal tract. It also houses the lower teeth, which are important articulatory structures. The mandible and teeth comprise the lower facial skeleton. Lower lip and tongue postures are dependent, somewhat, upon jaw movement. Although the maximum jaw opening may exceed 50 mm, for speech the vertical movement amounts to 7–18 mm, with a slight (2–3 mm) anterior-posterior component.

Although jaw movement is very slight during normal speech production, inadequate, inappropriate, or sluggish movements may contribute to articulatory defects. The rapidity of jaw movements is surprising, for although it is a massive structure, it is exceeded in mobility only by the tip of the tongue. The maximum rate of movement of the jaw is about 7.5 per second (producing "pa pa pa"), while the maximum rate of movement for the tip of the tongue is about 8.2 per second (producing "ta ta ta"). We should also note that the jaws never completely close during speech production, and so we should be very cautious about attributing articulation disorders to malocclusion or misaligned teeth. On the other hand, an open-mouth position increases vocal intensity 4–5 dB, something orators and singers should be aware of.

The primary movements of the jaw are elevation and depression. It may also be protruded and retracted, as well as moved laterally in a grinding motion, or movements may be combined. Normal mobility of the lower jaw is dependent upon the integrity of the temporomandibular joint. The anatomy of this joint is noteworthy because improper temporomandibular articulation may result in malocclusion, and conversely, such disturbances as overclosure may be due to improper dentition and to malocclusion.

The Temporomandibular Joint

The mandible, which is the only truly movable bone in the face, articulates with the temporal bone by means of a joint that permits both hingelike movement and gliding action, or in other words, a **ginglymoarthrodial joint.** This articulation between the condyle of the mandible and the anterior part of the mandibular fossa of the temporal bone is called the temporomandibular joint. It can be palpated (L. *palpare*, to touch) by placing a finger just in front of and a little below the opening of the external auditory meatus, while the jaw is alternately depressed and elevated.

Description As shown schematically in Figure 4-72, the condyle of the mandible rests in the **glenoid** or **mandibular fossa.** The fossa is divided into two parts by a

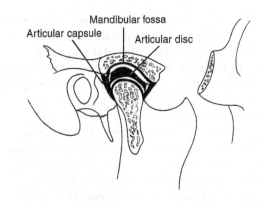

FIGURE 4-72

Schematic of temporomandibular joint.

narrow cleft, the **petrotympanic fissure.** The anterior part of the fossa, formed by the squamous portion of the temporal bone, is smooth, covered with fibrocartilage, and articulates indirectly with the condyle of the mandible. That is to say, the condyle is separated from the fossa by an **articular disc** or **meniscus** (Gk. *meniskos,* crescent). The posterior portion of the mandibular fossa is formed by the tympanic plate and is nonarticular. The **articular capsule,** a thin envelope completely surrounding the joint, is attached to the articulatory surfaces of the mandibular fossa and to the neck of the condyle of the mandible.

Sicher and DuBrul (1975) point out that the articulatory surfaces of the bones in the temporomandibular joint are not covered by the usual hyaline cartilage, but rather by a fibrocartilage devoid of vascular tissue. Another unique characteristic of this joint is that the two articulating complexes of bones carry the teeth, and their shape and position influence certain movements of the joint. And, finally, we must realize that the right and left temporomandibular joints constitute a *single bilateral articulation.*

The roof of the articulatory (mandibular) fossa is thin and translucent. This suggests that the fossa, which houses part of the articular disc and part of the condyle of the mandible, is normally not a stress-bearing functional component of the temporomandibular joint. Stress is absorbed between the condyle and articular disc, and between the disc and the thickened anterior part of the fossa known as the **articular eminence.** The entire articulatory fossa is lined by fibrous tissue which is thickened in the region of the articular eminence, but in the roof it is hardly thicker than periosteum. This is added evidence that the fossa does not function as a stress-bearing part of the temporomandibular articulation (Sicher and DuBrul, 1975).

Ligaments The **temporomandibular** or **lateral ligament** is composed of two short bundles (fasciculi) which extend from the malar surface of the articular tubercle at the root of the zygomatic arch. As shown in Figure 4-73, the fibers converge as they course down and backward to insert along the back of the neck of the mandible. A deep layer of ligamentous fasciculi terminates on the lateral aspect of the condyle. The temporomandibular ligament is part of a system of ligaments that restricts movement at the joint. It prevents down and backward displacement of the condyle, away from the articular eminence.

The remaining ligaments are located on the medial apsect of the temporomandibular joint. The **spheno-mandibular ligament,** shown in Figure 4-73, is regarded as an accessory ligament to the temporomandibular ligament because it has no influence on mandibular movements. It arises on the small spine of the sphenoid angle, then courses down and obliquely laterally, to insert on the **lingula** of the mandibular foramen.

The **stylomandibular ligament** is another accessory ligament. As shown in Figure 4-73, it extends from the styloid process of the temporal bone to the region of the angle of the mandible.

The Mandibular Depressors (Inframandibular Muscles)

Three of the four muscles responsible for depressing the mandible have previously been described as elevator

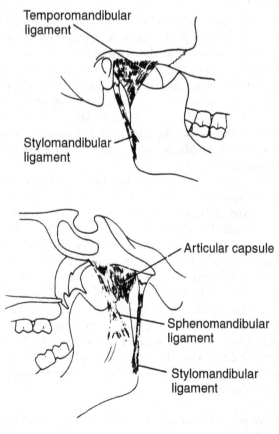

Temporomandibular ligament

Stylomandibular ligament

Articular capsule

Sphenomandibular ligament

Stylomandibular ligament

FIGURE 4-73

Schematic of temporomandibular ligaments.

muscles of the larynx. Those muscles, the **digastricus,** the **mylohyoid,** and the **geniohyoid,** will be quickly reviewed. The fourth muscle, the **lateral (external) pterygoid,** is sometimes classified as a mandibular protractor (protrusor), but it also functions as a depressor of mandible.

Digastricus The digastricus consists of an anterior and a posterior belly, united by a central or intermediate tendon. The posterior belly arises from the mastoid process (mastoid notch) of the temporal bone and then courses anteriorly and inferiorly to the corpus of the hyoid bone. The anterior belly arises from the inner surface of the lower border of the mandibular symphysis and courses posteriorly and inferiorly to the intermediate tendon that is held in position at the side of the corpus and greater horn of the hyoid bone by a tendinous loop.

Contraction of this muscle will raise the hyoid bone, or with the hyoid bone fixed, it will assist in depressing the jaw. The anterior belly draws the hyoid bone upward and forward, while the posterior belly draws the hyoid bone back and upward.

Mylohyoid The mylohyoid forms the muscular floor of the mouth. It originates from the mylohyoid line of the mandible, which extends from the last molars to the mental symphysis. The fibers course inferiorly and medially to join with their fellows from the opposite side at the midline raphe. The posteriormost fibers, however, insert into the corpus of the hyoid bone.

The effect of this muscle is probably minimal, but it cannot be discounted. We must realize that even minor adjustments of the mandible will affect the total balance of the skull on its occipital condyles. That in turn will require adjustments of the pre- and postvertebral cervical musculature.

Geniohyoid The geniohyoid is located just superior to the medial border of the mylohyoid muscle. It arises from the inferior mental spine on the posterior surface of the mental symphysis. The fibers course posteriorly and inferiorly to be inserted into the anterior surface of the hyoid bone and upon contraction may assist in elevating the larynx or depressing the mandible.

Because the jaw depressor muscles attach to the hyoid bone, any resistance to depression will result in elevation of the hyoid bone unless it is fixed in place. This is one of the functions of the sternohyoid muscles. We can begin to appreciate that the simple act of opening the mouth is in fact extraordinarily complex, and mandibular movement is but a small part of the total process of speech production.

The Lateral Pterygoid Muscle The lateral pterygoid muscle originates from two heads, one from the lateral portion of the greater wing of the sphenoid bone and the other from the lateral surface of the lateral pterygoid plate. The fibers converge as they course horizontally backward to insert into the **pterygoid fossa,** a depression on the anterior neck of the condyle of the mandible, and into the anterior margin of the articular disc of the temporomandibular articulation.

Its action is complex, but in brief it protrudes the mandible, causing the condyle to slide down and forward on the articular eminence. Contraction of the muscle on just one side moves the jaw in a grinding fashion. The lateral pterygoid muscle is shown in Figure 4-74.

The Mandibular Elevators

The jaws are approximated by those muscles that draw the mandible upward. There are three mandibular elevators: the **masseter,** the **temporalis,** and the **medial pterygoid** muscles.

The Masseter Muscle The masseter (Gk. *maseter,* chewer), shown in Figure 4-75A, is the most powerful of the muscles of mastication. A thick, flat, quadrilateral muscle that covers the lateral surface of the mandibular ramus, it is composed of an external and an internal layer. The *external fibers,* which form the bulk of the muscle, arise from the zygomatic arch by means of an extensive, thick aponeurosis. The fibers course inferiorly and somewhat posteriorly to be inserted into the angle and lateral surface of the ramus of the mandible. The *internal* or *deep fibers* are much less extensive. They arise from the posterior surface of the lower border and from the full length of the medial surface of the zygomatic arch. The fibers course downward and forward to be inserted into the upper half of the ramus and the lateral surface of the coronoid process of the mandible.

Upon contraction, this muscle closes the jaws. The superficial portion exerts a force that is at right angles to the occlusal plane of the molars, so pressure is brought to bear on the teeth in the molar region. The deep portion, in addition to elevating the mandible, has a retract-

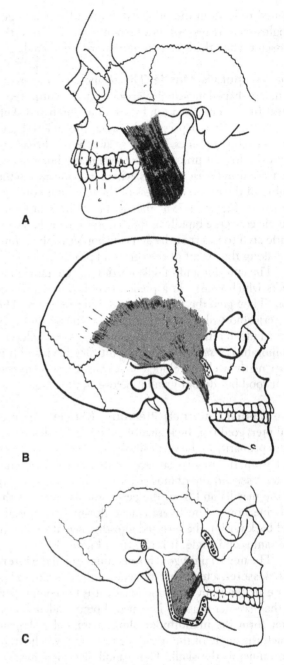

B

C

FIGURE 4-75

(A) Schematic of masseter muscle (external layer).
(B) Schematic of temporalis muscle. (C) Schematic of the medial pterygoid muscle (internal pterygoid).

ing function that is important in closing movements. *The masseter is a muscle adapted for power.* It is composed of a considerable amount of tendinous tissue, arranged in layers with interposed short muscle fibers. This means that, as a whole, the muscle contracts slowly, but powerfully. The masseter is especially well developed in the herbivores, which grind their food before swallowing.

Weber and Smith (1987) found reflex responses to direct mechanical stimulation in the masseter. They also

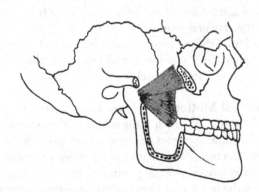

FIGURE 4-74

Schematic of lateral pterygoid muscle (external pterygoid).

elicited reflexes in the orbicularis oris inferior and genioglossus muscles. A reflex response was found in the masseter when the lip and tongue were stimulated.

The Temporalis Muscle The temporalis is a broad, thin, fan-shaped muscle that arises from the entire **temporal fossa.** The fossa can be seen on a prepared skull as a very shallow depression between the superior and inferior temporal lines. The fossa sweeps in a broad arc from the frontal process of the zygomatic bone across the frontal and parietal bones, where it terminates in the region of the mastoid process of the temporal bone. As shown in Figure 4-75B, the fibers of the temporalis muscle converge rapidly as they course under the zygomatic arch to insert at the anterior border of the ramus and along the extent of the coronoid process.

The anterior and middle portion of the muscle has fibers which course in a predominantly vertical direction. They give the muscle an elevating function. The posteriormost fibers have a horizontal course, and they contribute in retraction of the mandible. As a whole, the temporalis is a *snapping muscle*, built for speed, and it is particularly well developed in carnivores which tear their food but do not grind it before swallowing.

The Medial (Internal) Pterygoid Muscle The medial pterygoid is a thick quadrilateral muscle that originates primarily in the vertically directed pterygoid fossa, and from the medial surface of the lateral pterygoid plate. A second slip of muscle arises from the tuberosity of the maxilla and from the perpendicular plate of the palatine bone. The fibers course downward, laterally, and backward, to be inserted into the medial surface of the ramus and angle. It is shown in Figure 4-75C.

The medial pterygoid is sometimes called the **internal masseter,** a term that is operationally descriptive because anatomically and functionally it is the counterpart of the masseter muscle. The medial pterygoid and masseter form the **mandibular sling,** a muscular sling in which the angle of the mandible rests and which straps the ramus to the skull. The mandibular sling forms a functional articulation between the mandible and maxilla, with the temporomandibular joint acting as a guide.

Mandibular Movement

Because of the interposed articular disc, the temporomandibular joint, in a real sense, constitutes a true double joint, one between the disc and the articular eminence (the **upper joint**) and another between the condyle of the mandible and the disc (the **lower joint**). Due to the nature of the joint and the geometric arrangement of the muscles that act across the joint, mandibular movement is complex. The direction of muscle action forces on the

mandible are shown schematically in Figure 4-76A, and the principal movements due to muscle action are summarized as follows:

1.	**Raising:**	**a.** internal pterygoid
		b. masseter
		c. temporalis
2.	**Lowering:**	**a.** external pterygoid
		b. geniohyoid
		c. digastricus (anterior belly)
		d. mylohyoid
		e. genioglossus
3.	**Protrusion:**	**a.** external pterygoid
		b. internal pterygoid
4.	**Retraction:**	**a.** temporalis (posterior part)
		b. mylohyoid
		c. geniohyoid
		d. digastricus (anterior belly)
		e. geniohyoid
5.	**Lateral:**	**a.** external pterygoid
		b. temporalis (posterior part)

Mandibular movements influence lip posture, tongue position, and oral cavity configuration, in addition to changes in pharyngeal cavity dimensions. Jaw position may also influence laryngeal height. This complex mandibular movement can be "decomposed" into translational and rotational movements, however.

Translational Movement The upper joint performs a translatory movement. This means that all points on the jaw move in the same straight or curved direction. In the jaw, the disc and condyle as a unit slide down (or up) along the posterior slope of the articular eminence. This type of motion can be executed bilaterally, when the mandible is simply protruded or retracted, or it can take place unilaterally, which produces a lateral swing of the jaw to one side.

In both protrusion and retraction, the articular discs and the mandible slide forward and downward, or upward and backward, with the condyles in firm contact with the articular eminences. This is illustrated in Figure 4-76B. Gliding action occurs between the articular disc and articular eminence, and as a result, the condyle is carried forward and backward.

Rotational Motion The lower joints perform a rotational motion, in which some points of the jaw move in one direction, about an axis, and others move in the opposite direction. A familiar example of simple rotational motion is a door swinging about an ordinary hinge. In the jaw the hinge movement occurs around a horizontal

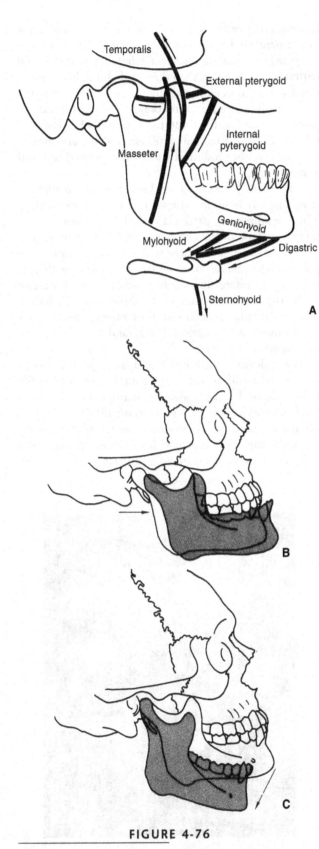

FIGURE 4-76

Summary of muscle actions (A), illustration of translatory motion of the mandible (B), and rotational motion (C).

axis that runs through the centers of the two condyles, as illustrated in Figure 4-76C.

Combined Movements Under normal circumstances both translational and rotational movements take place. That is, sliding in the upper joints and rotation in the lower joints are usually combined, but the predominance of one type of motion over the other is highly variable, depending upon circumstances.

In the opening movement the condyles rotate against the articular discs around a transverse axis, and at the same time they slide down and forward along the slope of the articular eminence of the mandibular fossa. During maximum opening of the jaw, anterior gliding action may bring the articular capsule out of the mandibular fossa so that the condyle moves under the articular tubercle of the zygomatic process of the temporal bone. When this **(subluxation)** occurs, a very definite sharp snap may be felt, and heard! Mandibular movements for speech have been modeled after a pattern generated for chewing activities. Electromyography has revealed muscle action patterns that are quite distinctive from those of chewing (Moore, et al., 1988).

Anomalies of the Temporomandibular Joint

Although the symptom complex known as **temporomandibular joint–pain dysfunction syndrome (TMJ syndrome)** described by Schwartz (1956) is not common, it is about three to four times more common in women. The symptom complex consists of

1. Facial pain and muscle spasm.

2. Reduced mandibular movement, precipitated by a sudden or continuous stretching of the masticatory musculature.

3. Joint noises, clicking, popping, and grating sounds that accompany jaw movements.

Rest, heat, sedatives, muscle relaxants, and occlusal adjustment have all been successful in the treatment of most acute and traumatic disorders of the temporomandibular joint. These treatments are also applicable to **myofacial–pain dysfunction (MPD) syndrome,** in which the patient is usually female and under 40 years of age. MPD is often idiopathic (of unknown causation).

In 1934 Costen described a symptom complex that included ear and balance problems, headaches, burning sensations in the mouth and throat, and varying degrees of **trismus** (spasm of muscles of mastication). Costen attributed this symptom complex to a disturbed temporomandibular joint due to overclosure of the jaws resulting from loss of the posterior teeth. Subsequent research has failed to support the enthusiastic ascribing of these symptoms to dental malocclusion.

Thickening and displacement of the articular meniscus is often found to be responsible for the pain and noises associated with temporomandibular joint disorders. Other causes include direct trauma (repeated dislocations) and arthroses. Chronic dislocation and subluxation (partial dislocation) are generally the result of muscular imbalance and are more common in women. The mandible can be dislocated only forward. Reduction of a dislocation is accomplished by depressing the jaw with the thumbs placed on the molar teeth and at the same time elevating the chin. The downward pressure overcomes the spasms of the masticatory musculature, while elevating the chin rotates the condyle backward.

Ankylosis[15] of the mandible often follows infections and traumatic and developmental disorders. If bilateral ankylosis occurs in childhood, the result may be a micrognathic recession of the chin. If unilateral ankylosis occurs, the ramus on the unaffected side becomes elongated, resulting in asymmetry of the lower face.

The temporomandibular joint permits movements in three planes: **vertical plane** (opening and closing), **anterior-posterior plane** (protrusion and retrusion), and **horizontal plane** (laterally). This three degree-of-freedom movement is dependent not only upon the integrity of the temporomandibular joint, but on the muscles of mastication.

The Palate

The contribution of the palate to speech production may be stated quite simply. *It modifies the degree of coupling between the nasopharynx and the remainder of the vocal tract.* It consists of a fixed bony plate in front and a muscular valve behind, although it is often described as consisting of three parts: the **alveolar arch,** the bony **hard palate,** and the muscular **soft palate.** A side-view schematic of the palate was shown in Figure 4-18, while the hard palate as seen from beneath was shown in Figure 4-12, and in frontal section in Figure 4-13. The alveolar arch, you will recall, consists of the bony, tooth-bearing processes of the maxillae and its mucous membrane covering.

The Hard Palate

The hard palate is formed by the medial projections of the **palatine processes** of the maxillae, which articulate at the midline and contribute to about the anterior

three-fourths of the bony roof of the mouth and floor of the nasal cavity. As may be seen in Figure 4-10, the palatine processes are thicker in front, where they blend with the alveolar arch, than they are behind. Posteriorly, the palatine processes articulate with the horizontal plates of the paired palatine bones. They comprise the posterior one-fourth of the hard palate. The posterior borders of the horizontal plates are free and are continued back at the midline to form the **posterior nasal spine.**

The hard palate is covered by a mucous membrane that is tightly bound to the subjacent mucoperiosteum. This membrane is particularly well developed on the posterior slope of the alveolar arch, where it presents a series of transverse ridges or wrinkles called **rugae.** The palatal rugae, which become less prominent with age, probably facilitate linguapalatal articulation. Posterior to the rugae and continued back throughout the length of the palate may be seen a **midline raphe,** which is subject to individual variation. Rugae and a midline raphe may be seen in Figure 4-77.

Occasionally a clinical examination of the mouth may reveal a midline ridge that courses more or less the full extent of the hard palate. This ridge may consist of thickened periosteum and mucous membrane, but more often it is the result of an **exostosis** (bony outgrowth) along the site of the intermaxillary suture. In anatomy a bulging or swelling is known as a **torus,** and so in this

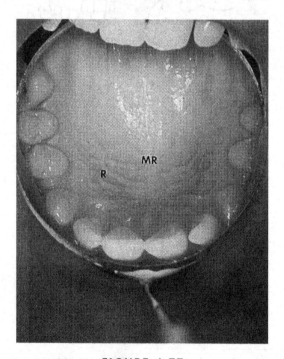

FIGURE 4-77

Photograph of the roof of the mouth showing the rugae (R) and a midline raphe (MR).

---

[15]**Ankylosis** (*ankylo-,* crooked + *-osis,* a process, often pathological) is the fusion of joints due to disease, trauma, or abnormal development.

instance we have a **torus palatinus.** The mucoperiosteum around the periphery of a torus can be expected to have a bluish tint. The presence of a torus is of little or no consequence, except for a person being fitted with a dental appliance. An example of a torus palatinus, which occurs in roughly twenty percent of the population, is shown in Figure 4-78.

The Palatal Vault (Arch)

As shown in Figures 4-10 and 4-13, the hard palate is thick at its anterior and lateral margins, becoming progressively thinner toward the midline. As a result, the inferior surface is arched transversely as well as anteroposteriorly. The extent of the palatal vault varies considerably from individual to individual and is dependent to a large extent upon the status of dentition. Edentulous jaws have a tendency to atrophy, with a resultant *flattened appearance* of the palate. The height of the palatal vault has direct bearing on the acoustic properties of the oral cavity and may well contribute to individual voice characteristics.

Topographical descriptions of the palatal vault are possible by means of a **palatopograph,** a measuring instrument that provides contour lines of an individual palatal vault. Early descriptions of palatal vaults were provided by Bloomer (1943); they included the *height of the*

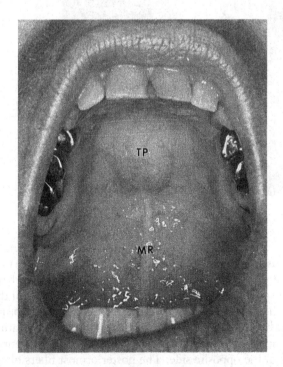

FIGURE 4-78

An example of a torus palatinus (TP) and midline raphe (MR).

vault, the *angle of the slope*, and the *palatal area at various planes*. Palatal vaults also have been classified in terms of their *geometric configurations*. Crane and Ramstrum (1943) have described three basic palatal shapes: *trapezoid, triangular*, and *ovoid*. The significance of palatal configurations has yet to be determined quantitatively.

The Soft Palate (Velum)

The soft palate is attached anteriorly to the posterior free border of the palatine bones. Attachment is by means of a **palatal aponeurosis,** which is particularly well developed anteriorly and less so posteriorly. Laterally, muscle fibers of the soft palate are continuous with those of the superior pharyngeal constrictor muscle. The soft palate is directed posteriorly and when relaxed hangs curtainlike into the oropharynx.

The arrangement of muscle fibers in the soft palate is such that it may be *elevated, lowered*, or *tensed*. Five muscles are responsible for the mobility of the soft palate. Two are **depressor relaxers** (palatoglossus and palatopharyngeus), two are **soft palate elevators** (levator palati and uvular), and one is a **depressor-tensor** (tensor palati). About a third of the palate is composed of connective tissues, fairly evenly distributed, while muscle tissues (3–23%) seem to be confined to the midpoint of the palate (Ettema and Kuehn, 1994).

As the soft palate is raised or lowered, it modifies the general configuration and consequently the resonant characteristics of the vocal tract. In the production of various nasal sounds, the palate is lowered, thus adding length and complexity to the vocal tract and, as we might expect, a concomitant modification of the quality of the emitted tone. Normally, the soft palate is elevated, as in Figure 4-79A, for the production of vowel sounds and is lowered for those sounds we identify as nasals. The palate is also lowered, as in Figure 4-79B, during normal breathing. A closer look at the anatomy of the soft palate ought to put us in a better position to appreciate its capabilities and contributions to the production of speech.

The musculature of the soft palate, and of the pharynx with which it is so intimately related, is difficult to visualize. One reason for the difficulty lies in the approach used in dissection of the palate and pharynx. The pre- and postvertebral musculature, the cervical vertebrae, and the base of the skull are removed to expose the posterior wall of the pharynx (see Figure 4-80). The posterior wall of the pharynx is then opened longitudinally, revealing the membranous lining of the pharynx, the nasal and oral cavities, and the aditus of the larynx, as shown in Figure 4-81. Only after the membranous lining is removed can the intricate system of palatal and pharyngeal musculature be seen. Sagittal sections of the head are also dissected, but the normal spatial relationships are lost.

FIGURE 4-79

Lateral head x-rays showing the position of the soft palate during vowel production (A) and during breathing (B).

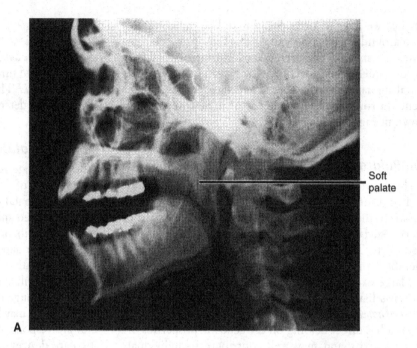

A

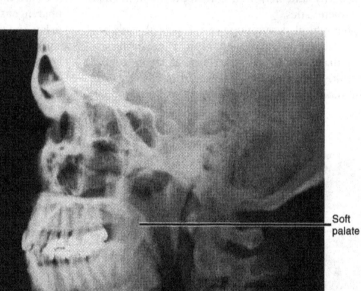

B

The Tensor Palati (Tensor Veli Palatini) The base of the skull with the lateral and medial pterygoid plates, the foramen ovale, carotid canal, and the sphenopetrosal fissure is shown in Figure 4-82. The tensor palati arises as a ribbonlike muscle, from a thin plate immediately in front of the sphenopetrosal fissure at the base of the medial pterygoid plate. It also receives fibers from the spine and angle of the sphenoid bone, and from the anterolateral wall of the cartilaginious portion of the auditory (Eustachian) tube. The muscle descends vertically between the medial pterygoid plate and the medial

pterygoid muscle, becoming quite narrow and tendinous. The **tendon** winds around the hamulus of the medial pterygoid plate and then passes medialward, where it expands to a **palatal aponeurosis.** Some fibers of the fanlike aponeurosis are attached to the posterior border of the hard palate (the horizontal plate of the palatine bone) while medially the fibers fuse with the aponeurosis of the opposite side. The posteriormost fibers blend into the connective tissue and musculature of the soft palate. In a sense, the palatine aponeurosis forms a fibrous "skeleton" of the soft palate.

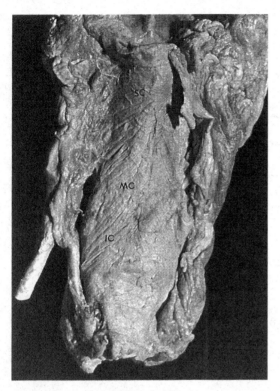

FIGURE 4-80

The pharynx and associated structures as seen from behind: superior constrictor (SC), middle constrictor (MC), inferior constrictor (IC).

The tensor palati has two important functions, and the significance of its action is easily overlooked. Note in Figure 4-83 that the hamulus of the medial pterygoid

plate is somewhat below the level of the hard palate. This means that when the tensor palati muscles contract, force is exerted in a downward and lateral direction, causing the palatal aponeurosis to become tensed and lowered somewhat. At the same time, the tensor palati pulls the membranous anterolateral wall of the auditory tube away from its stationary cartilaginous medial wall, causing the cartilage to "unwind" and open the normally collapsed tube. *This permits air pressure within the middle ear cavity to equalize with atmospheric pressure.*

The Levator Palati (Levator Veli Palatini) The bulk of the soft palate is formed by the levator palati muscle. It is a deceptively complex muscle, arising from the apex of the petrous portion of the temporal bone and from the posteromedial plate of the cartilaginous framework of the auditory tube. It is a cylindrical muscle that courses downward, medially, and forward to insert into the soft palate, as shown in Figure 4-84. In sagittal views of the palatal complex, the palatal elevator forms a ridge or **torus** (L., a round swelling) as seen in Figure 4-85. The fibers of the levator palati are distributed along the upper surface of the soft palate, interdigitating with their fellows from the opposite side.

In a sense the two palatine elevators form a muscular sling for the soft palate. Note, in Figure 4-85, the posterior portion of the soft palate is almost at right angles to the plane of the hard palate. The action of the palatine elevators is to raise the vertical position of the soft palate into a horizontal position and to stretch the palate slightly backward. This action is complemented by the simultaneous tensing action of the tensor palati.

FIGURE 4-81

The pharynx as seen after a longitudinal incision through its posterior wall, revealing the nasal and oral cavities and the aditus of the larynx.

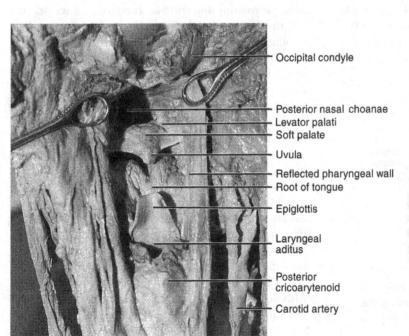

Occipital condyle

Posterior nasal choanae
Levator palati
Soft palate

Uvula

Reflected pharyngeal wall
Root of tongue

Epiglottis

Laryngeal aditus

Posterior cricoarytenoid

Carotid artery

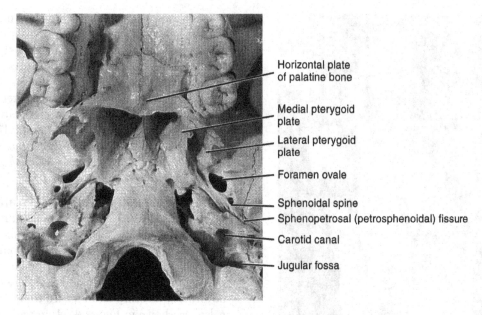

Horizontal plate
of palatine bone

Medial pterygoid
plate

Lateral pterygoid
plate

Foramen ovale

Sphenoidal spine

Sphenopetrosal (petrosphenoidal) fissure

Carotid canal

Jugular fossa

FIGURE 4-82

Detail of the base of the skull, showing the lateral and medial pterygoid plates, the foramen ovale, carotid canal, and the sphenopetrosal fissure.

The result of this complex action is that the soft palate is brought into contact with the posterior pharyngeal wall to close off the nasal cavities from the oral cavity, as shown in Figure 4-79A.

Research has shown that levator muscle activity (force) tends to occur in the lower region of its operating range in relation to its activity in a blowing task. It seems, in fact, that speech production demands are quite modest ones in comparison with the muscles' operating ranges (Kuehn and Moon, 1994). For example, young adults are capable of generating pulmonary pressures in the 140–240 cm H_2O range, while the requirements for speech are in the modest range of from 6–10

cm H_2O. Levels of lip force used for speech are only 10–20 percent of the maximum forces possible (Barlow and Abbs, 1983).

The Musculus Uvulae (Azygos Uvulae) The uvular (azygos) muscle is often regarded as a paired muscle, although anatomy texts may describe it as unpaired, hence the word **azygos,** which means unpaired. It arises from the nasal spines of the palatine bones and from the adjacent palatine aponeurosis. It courses posteriorly the length of the soft palate and inserts into the **uvula,** a midline pendulous structure of the soft palate.

Upon contraction this muscle shortens and lifts the soft palate, but its function is not entirely free from debate. For example, it may function as an important articulator in some languages, although it seems to play no particular role in the English language. Although the uvula, shown in Figure 4-80, is often regarded as a degenerate or vestigial remnant, it is present only in the higher mammals (Kaplan, 1960; Palmer and LaRusso, 1965).

There is a considerable variation in the length and thickness of the uvula, and very long uvulas were at one time amputated to "prevent the patient from gagging on it." A long uvula probably causes no symptoms whatever, regardless of its length (DeWeese and Saunders, 1973).

A **bifid uvula** occurs in about 1 out of 75 people. Although it is comparatively rare, it does have important clinical significance because it signals that a person may have a submucous cleft of the soft palate. The soft

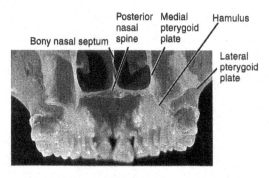

Bony nasal septum

Posterior
nasal
spine

Medial
pterygoid
plate

Hamulus

Lateral
pterygoid
plate

FIGURE 4-83

The base of the skull as seen from behind, showing the hamulus of the medial pterygoid plate, in relation to the hard palate.

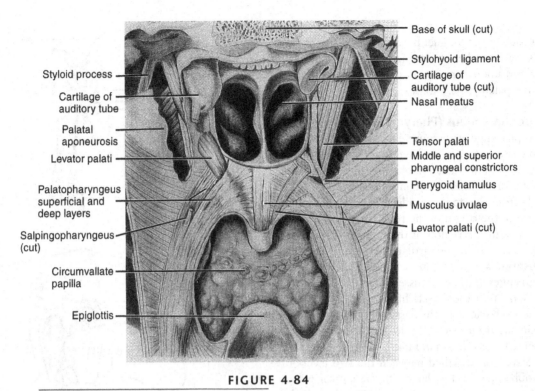

FIGURE 4-84

The levator palati muscle, as viewed from behind (drawing by Therese Zemlin).

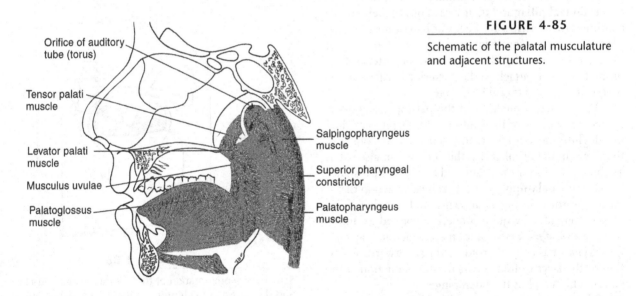

FIGURE 4-85

Schematic of the palatal musculature and adjacent structures.

palate may at first glance appear to be normal because of the intact mucous membrane, when actually a deficiency of muscular tissue may exist. A bifid uvula and a soft palate with a bluish tint (especially in the midline) suggest that the palate is short and lacks appropriate musculature. Hypernasality often results from a submucous cleft of the soft palate.

The Palatoglossus (Glossopalatinus) Muscle The palatoglossus is described by various authors as a pha-

ryngeal muscle; others see it as a muscle of the palate, or as a muscle of the tongue. We described it earlier as an *extrinsic muscle of the tongue*. It arises from the lower surface of the palatine aponeurosis, where it is continuous with the muscle from the opposite side. The fibers pass down, forward, and laterally and insert into the sides of the tongue, where they blend with the longitudinal fibers in the dorsum. This muscle, with its mucous membrane covering, comprises the **palatoglossal arch** (anterior faucial pillar). Upon contraction, it may depress the soft palate or, with the soft palate fixed, it may raise the sides and back of the tongue. Because the course of this muscle is semicircular, it also acts as somewhat of a sphincter and upon contraction decreases the distance between the palatoglossal arches.

The Palatopharyngeus (Pharyngopalatine) Muscle

The palatopharyngeus is a muscle of the soft palate, and at the same time a *longitudinal muscle of the pharynx*. It is a long fleshy bundle that arises from the soft palate, where many of its fibers are continuous with those of the muscle from the opposite side. Part of its complexity stems from the origin of the remaining fibers, some of which arise in the region of the pterygoid hamulus, while others arise from the cartilage of the auditory tube (they constitute a slender slip of muscle called the **sal-pingopharyngeus,** to be discussed later).

Very soon after the muscle fibers arise, they are divided into two fasciculi by the descending levator palati. One fasciculus passes over the levator palati and one passes beneath it, as shown in Figure 4-84. In effect, the levator palati is sandwiched between the two layers of the palatopharyngeus. Just lateral to the levator palati, the two fasciculi blend into a single ribbonlike muscle. Although the muscle has an extensive origin, the fibers quickly converge in the **palatopharyngeal fold** or **posterior faucial pillar** and then spread out as their course continues the muscle into the lower half of the pharynx. Most of the fibers insert into the mucous membrane of the lateral wall of the pharynx, while the anteriormost of the fibers may attach to the posterior border and superior horn of the thyroid cartilage.

The principal function of the palatopharyngeus is to guide the bolus of food into the lower pharynx during deglutition. Because of the semicircular course of the fibers in the oropharynx, this muscle can also act as a sphincter to lower the palate and decrease the distance between the **palatopharyngeal arches,** an action that is quite vigorous during swallowing and gagging. This muscle may also be quite properly regarded as an *extrinsic muscle of the larynx*, since its contraction may raise the larynx or tilt the thyroid cartilage forward. Elevation of the larynx often occurs during phonation at the extreme high end of the pitch range.

The schematic representation of the palatal musculature and its assumed functions during speech, as shown in Figure 4-86, is taken from Fritzell (1969). It is especially useful because in its elegant simplicity, it summarizes the assumed functions of all the musculature.

The Tonsils

A small triangular space, wider below than above, exists between the palatoglossal and palatopharyngeal arches. This space, called the **tonsillar fossa,** is partially filled

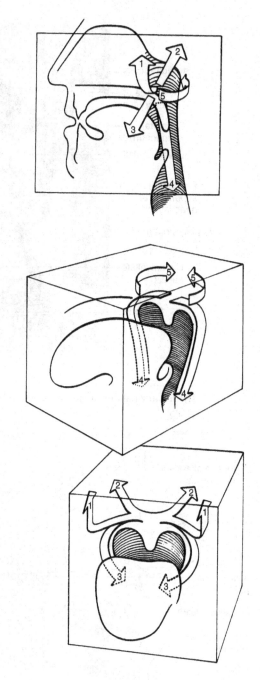

FIGURE 4-86

Schematic representation of the velopharyngeal muscles and their actions: (1) tensor, (2) levator, (3) palatoglossus, (4) palatopharyngeus, (5) superior constrictor. (From Fritzell, 1969).

by masses of lymphoid tissue referred to as the palatine tonsils. They are part of a complete ring of tonsillar tissue surrounding the entrance to the oropharynx. This ring, called **Waldeyer's ring** consists of the **palatine tonsils** laterally, the **adenoids** superiorly, and the **lingual tonsil** inferiorly. Tonsils may also be found at the entrance to the *auditory* (Eustachian) tube and are known appropriately as *tubal tonsils*.

Lingual Tonsil

The lingual tonsil is a collection of lymph follicles that covers much of the root of the tongue.

Adenoids (Pharyngeal Tonsil)

The adenoids consist of an aggregate of lymphoid tissue located in the posterior wall of the nasopharynx. In childhood and even into the teens, the adenoids are usually *hypertrophied* (greatly enlarged). In a longitudinal study employing serial cephalometric laminagraphy, Subtelny and Koepp-Baker (1956) examined the growth of adenoid tissue in fifteen subjects, some of whom were followed from shortly after birth to adolescence and/or adulthood. They found adenoid tissue to follow a predictable growth cycle. Shortly after birth the soft tissue which forms the roof of the nasopharynx slopes obliquely downward and backward to blend into the posterior pharyngeal wall. Adenoid tissue is not readily

identifiable until at least six months of age, and by two years it is usually developed to the extent that it may occupy as much as one-half the nasopharyngeal cavity. Thereafter the adenoid tissue continues to grow at a slower pace until the peak of growth is reached at about nine to ten years. After this growth peak is reached, the growth pattern seems to reverse itself; that is, the tissue begins to atrophy, and its mass decreases substantially. By adulthood the adenoid tissue has usually completely atrophied. The growth pattern of adenoid tissue is shown schematically in Figure 4-87. Note the concave roof of the nasopharynx in the infant, which with the downward and forward growth of adenoid tissue becomes convex, as in the adolescent. In the adult, the nasopharynx once more resumes a concave appearance. The authors stress, however, that although the growth of adenoid tissue is in an anterior and downward direction, the growth of the facial skeleton is also in an anterior and downward direction. The result is that the dimensions of the nasopharynx are held in a fine state of balance. Facial growth will be discussed at greater length later in the chapter.

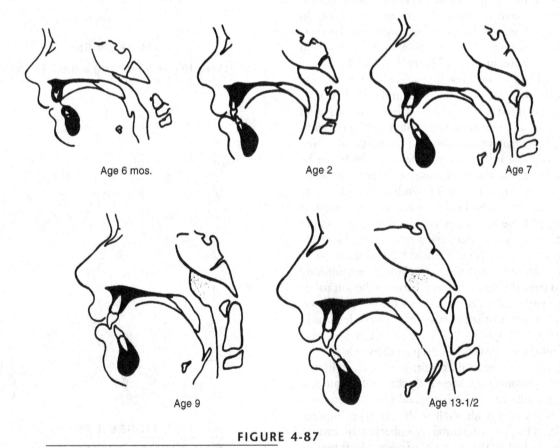

Age 6 mos.   Age 2   Age 7

Age 9   Age 13-1/2

FIGURE 4-87

Tracings of lateral cephalometric x-rays of the same individual depicting the growth of adenoid tissue from infancy to the peak of adenoidal growth. (From *Plastic and Reconstructive Surgery,* 18, no. 3, 1956. Courtesy J. D. Subtelny and H. Koepp Baker.)

Palatine Tonsils

While the lingual tonsils and adenoids are not readily visible, the palatine tonsils are easily seen in an oral examination. They are relatively large in young children, sometimes to the extent that they almost obstruct the opening into the oropharynx. They shrink or atrophy, however, shortly after puberty. Although the medial or pharyngeal surface of the palatine tonsil is free and visible, the lateral surface is imbedded in the pharyngeal wall. It is retained in position by a fibrous capsule. The rough appearance of the visible portion of the tonsil is accounted for by the presence of from twelve to fifteen orifices that lead into crypts or recesses called **tonsillar fossulae.** The fossulae branch out and extend deeply into the tonsil structure. A small space superior to the tonsil is called the **supratonsillar fossa** and, in cases of abscessed tonsil tissue, is frequently the site of pus collection.

Relevance to Speech

The tonsilar ring is probably a defense mechanism against bacterial invasion of the body, and for this reason it is often the locus of infection. Organisms fill the tonsillar crypts and appear as small whitish masses at the openings of the fossulae. In small children such whitish masses are almost continuously present, especially in the palatine tonsils. Relatively large tonsils in a 10-year-old child are shown in Figure 4-88A, and the tonsils in a 15-year old are shown in Figure 4-88B. Chronic or repeated infections may result in a spread of the disease to the adenoids, the auditory tube, and middle ear. In addition, enlarged adenoids may affect production of nasal sounds and contribute to certain voice problems. Chronic hypertrophy may also lead to mouth breathing and a syndrome called **adenoid facies,** which can be particularly serious during the age when the facial skeleton is approaching maturity. The arch of the palate may become very high, the bridge of the nose widened. A shortening of the upper lip, labioversion of the upper incisors, an elongated face, and a dull staring facial expression are all seen in the adenoid facies (Figure 4-89).

The adenoids may also contribute to establishing **velopharyngeal closure** (closure between the soft palate and the pharyngeal walls). Sometimes the soft palate may be slightly short, or the pharynx particularly deep, as in the subject of Figure 4-90. This child has a normal palate, but the pharynx is too deep to allow velopharyngeal closure. The acoustic result, of course, is hypernasality. Occasionally, a congenitally short soft palate may accomplish adequate velopharyngeal closure because a normal pharynx is made shallow due to hypertrophied adenoids. Thus, a congenital velopharyngeal insufficiency is masked by the presence of adenoids. It may be unmasked, however, by surgical removal of the ade-

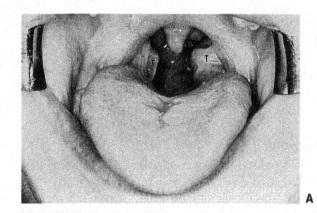

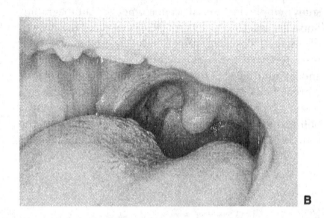

FIGURE 4-88

Tonsils (T) in a 10-year-old child (A) and in a 15-year-old (B).

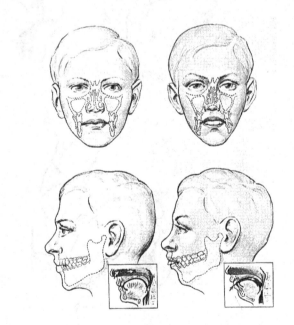

FIGURE 4-89

Adenoid facies. (From *Atlas of the Mouth,* courtesy American Dental Association.)

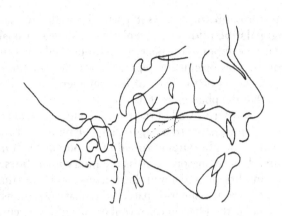

FIGURE 4-90

Tracings of a lateral head x-ray of a child with a normal palate and a deep pharynx. (X-ray from which tracing was made provided by Center for Craniofacial Anomalies, University of Illinois. Courtesy Dr. Samuel Pruzansky.)

noids, and temporary (as is usually the case) or permanent hypernasality may result. Brodnitz (1959) asserts that permanent or irreversible hypernasality rarely results from adenoidectomy. However, the matter is not at all free from debate. On the basis of radiographic and longitudinal study of a large number of children and young adults, Subtelny and Koepp-Baker (1956) con-

cluded that in some instances an irreversible nasal quality may appear in speech subsequent to adenoidectomy. The relationship between hypernasality and adenoidectomy has been recognized by Mason (1973) who suggests that speech disorders following adenoidectomy can be prevented by proper preoperative evaluation.

The Pharynx

From our description of the speech mechanism thus far, it seems that many of the contributing structures have biological as well as nonbiological functions. The pharynx, called the "gateway to the gut" by Sicher and DuBrul (1975), forms the upper part of both the respiratory system and the digestive tract. From Figure 4-91, we see that the upper part of the pharynx, which forms a substantial portion of the supralaryngeal speech mechanism, has a dual function, while below the larynx, its function is again quite specific. In the adult male, the distance between the level of the vocal folds and the lips is about 17 cm.

The pharynx, a cone-shaped musculotendinous tube extending from the base of the skull to the level of the sixth cervical vertebra, is about 12 cm long. It is about 4 cm wide at its extreme width superiorly and about 2 cm from front to back. It narrows considerably until, at the level of the larynx in front and the sixth vertebra behind,

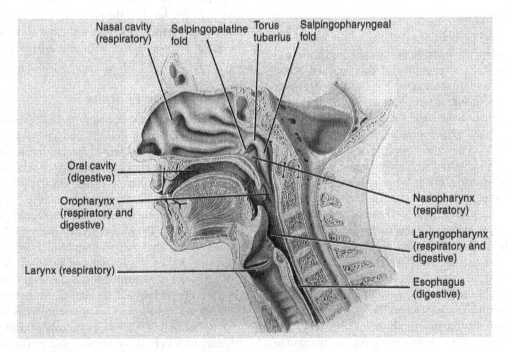

FIGURE 4-91

A biofunctional representation of the pharynx and adjacent structures.

it is about 2.5 cm in width. At its lowest extreme the pharynx is continuous with the esophagus, and at this level the front and back pharyngeal walls are in direct contact with one another and separate only to permit the passage of food into the esophagus. In a sense the muscular arrangement of the entire pharynx is much like that of the gut. It is circular and sphincterlike, although toward the base of the skull, the pharynx can actually dilate a little.

The contributions of the pharynx to speech production are not fully understood. It is known for certain that its function is one of resonance and that it contributes significantly to the acoustic properties of the vocal tract and to modifications of the energy distribution in the source material generated at the level of the larynx. The pharynx is not a particularly dynamic structure in speech production. That is, variations in the size and configuration of the vocal tract are mediated not so much by changes in the muscular walls of the pharynx, but rather by modifications resulting from movements of the tongue and of the soft palate with which the pharynx is so closely associated and to elevations and depressions of the larynx. Recently, however, cinefluorography and electromyography have shown that changes in the configurations of the pharynx do take place during speech production, but these changes are not particularly well understood.

As stated earlier, the cavity of the pharynx can be divided into nasal, oral, and laryngeal portions.

The Nasopharynx

The superior and posterior boundaries of the nasopharynx are formed by the rostrum of the sphenoid bone and by the pharyngeal protuberance of the occipital bone. The inferior boundary is set at the level of the soft palate. Anteriorly, the nasopharynx communicates with the posterior choanae of the nasal cavities; laterally it communicates with the pharyngeal orifice of the auditory (Eustachian) tube. Thus, the nasopharynx has a posterior-superior wall and lateral walls. The anterior wall is deficient since the pharynx opens into the nasal cavities.

A prominent landmark of the lateral wall of the nasopharynx is the **pharyngeal ostium of the auditory tube.** This tube courses laterally, backward, and slightly upward to the middle ear cavity. The pharyngeal (medial) end of the cartilaginous skeleton of the auditory tube causes a distinct elevation of the mucous membrane. As a result, the posterior portion of the somewhat triangular ostium is characterized by a prominence called the **torus tubarius** (cushion of the tube). As shown in Figure 4-91, a fold of mucous membrane courses vertically downward from the posterior margin of the torus tubarius. This fold, called the **salpingopharyngeal fold,** contains the salpingopharyngeal muscle. A similar but smaller fold courses from the upper margin

of the torus tubarius to the soft palate. It is called the **salpingopalatine fold.** The nasopharynx widens in a small area just posterior to the pharyngeal ostium and the torus tubarius. This prominent depression is called the **pharyngeal recess** or the fossa of Rosenmuller. It is at this point that the pharynx is at its widest.

The posterior wall of the nasopharynx, you will recall, is characterized by an aggregate of lymphatic tissue known as the **pharyngeal tonsil (adenoids).** A second landmark in the nasopharynx is the **pharyngeal bursa.** It is a midline depression in the mucous membrane that extends from the superior part of the pharyngeal tonsil as far up as the pharyngeal protuberance of the occipital bone.

The Oropharynx

The oropharynx extends from the soft palate, above, to the level of the hyoid bone, below. Anteriorly, it communicates by way of the arches (fauces) with the oral cavity. Structures in the oropharynx are located on the lateral walls. They are the palatine tonsils and the palatopharyngeal arches (posterior faucial pillars).

Whereas the nasopharynx is relatively static in nature, and always patent, *the oropharynx is comparatively dynamic.* This is due to the mobile soft palate and base of the tongue which extends into its lumen.

The Laryngopharynx

The laryngopharynx extends from the hyoid bone, above, to the level of the sixth cervical vertebra, below. It is funnel-shaped, being much wider above than below, where it communicates with the **aditus laryngis** (the entrance to the larynx).

Muscles of the Pharynx

The pharyngeal tube is composed of three layers of tissue: a fibrous coat called the pharyngeal aponeurosis, a mucous coat, and a relatively strong muscular layer.

The **pharyngeal aponeurosis** is attached above to the pharyngeal tubercle of the occipital bone, the petrous portion of the temporal bone, the cartilage of the auditory tube, and the medial pterygoid plate of the sphenoid bone. From the medial pterygoid plate it descends along the pterygomandibular ligament to the posterior end of the mylohyoid ridge of the mandible, from where it is continued to the lateral margins of the tongue, the stylohyoid ligament, the hyoid bone, and the thyroid cartilage. The aponeurosis is well defined above, but below it loses its density and gradually disappears as a definite structure, and at the same time it gives way to musculature. The attachments of the pharyngeal aponeurosis to the base of the skull are schematized in Figure 4-92. *In a sense the muscular portion of the pharynx is suspended from this aponeurosis.*

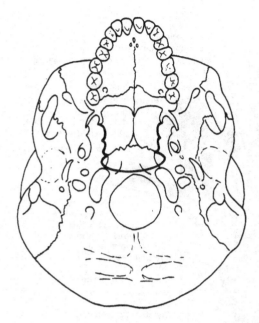

FIGURE 4-92

Schematic illustrating attachments (heavy line) of pharyngeal aponeuroses to the base of the skull.

The mucous membrane of the pharynx is continuous with that of all the cavities with which it communicates.

The muscles of the pharynx consist of three pairs of constrictors: the superior, middle, and inferior (Figures 4-93 and 4-94). From an anatomical standpoint the pharynx is composed of eight muscular parts, as illustrated in Figure 4-94, and as shown in Table 4-3. The superior constrictor consists of the first four of these parts, the middle constrictor of parts five and six, while parts seven and eight comprise the inferior constrictor.

The Superior Constrictor Muscle   The superior constrictor is the weakest and yet the most complex of the pharyngeal muscles. It consists of four rather distinct muscle bundles.

The first, the **pterygopharyngeal muscle**, arises from the lower third of the medial pterygoid plate and from its hamular process. The fact that its fibers have been consistently found to blend with those of the palatopharyngeus muscle has important implications for velopharyngeal mechanics.

Fibers of the superior pharyngeal constrictor also arise from the **pterygomandibular raphe.** This raphe, you will vividly recall, is a tendinous inscription that divides the buccinator muscle from the pharyngeal constrictor musculature. The fibers that arise from the raphe are sometimes called the **buccopharyngeus muscle.**

The third part of the superior constrictor, the **mylopharyngeus muscle**, is composed of fibers arising from the posterior part of the mylohyoid line and the adjacent alveolar process of the mandible.

The fourth part, the **glossopharyngeus muscle**, is composed of a few fasciculi from the sides of the tongue.

The fibers of the superior pharyngeal constrictor curve back, then medialward and obliquely upward, to be inserted into the midline pharyngeal raphe. The superiormost fibers fail to reach the base of the skull in an area lateral to the midline on either side. Consequently, a nonmuscular space exists in a region between the levator palati muscle and the base of the skull. This space, filled in by glandular and connective tissue (pharyngeal aponeurosis), is referred to as the **sinus of Morgagni.**

The Middle Constrictor Muscle   The middle constrictor is somewhat fan-shaped. It is composed of muscle fibers from two relatively distinct regions. Much of the middle constrictor is derived from fibers arising from the superior border of the greater horn of the hyoid bone. These fibers constitute the **ceratopharyngeus muscle.** The remainder of the fibers make up the **chondropharyngeus muscle** which arises from the lesser horn of the hyoid bone and from the stylohyoid ligament.

The fibers of the middle constrictor radiate as they course backward and medialward to be inserted into the

TABLE 4-3

Muscles of the pharyngeal constrictors

Constrictor	Component	Origin
Superior	1. pterygopharyngeus	medial pterygoid plate
	2. buccopharyngeus	pterygomandibular raphe
	3. mylopharyngeus	mylohyoid line
	4. glossopharyngeus	sides of tongue
Middle	5. ceratopharyngeus	greater horn of hyoid bone
	6. chondropharyngeus	lesser horn of hyoid bone
Inferior	7. thyropharyngeus	thyroid cartilage
	8. cricopharyngeus	inferior horn of thyroid cartilage and from cricoid cartilage

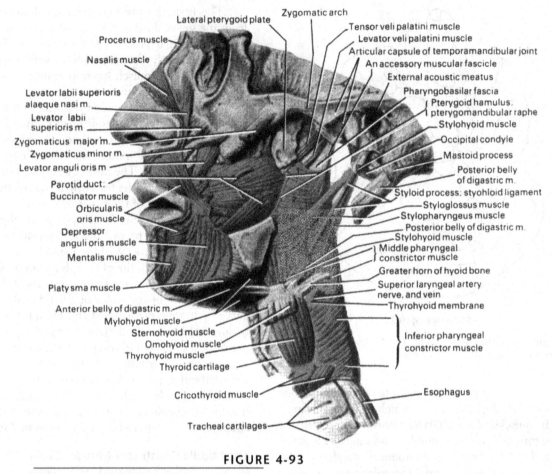

Zygomatic arch
Lateral pterygoid plate
Procerus muscle
Nasalis muscle
Tensor veli palatini muscle
Levator veli palatini muscle
Articular capsule of temporamandibular joint
An accessory muscular fascicle
External acoustic meatus
Levator labii superioris alaeque nasi m.
Pharyngobasilar fascia
Pterygoid hamulus; pterygomandibular raphe
Levator labii superioris m
Stylohyoid muscle
Zygomaticus major m.
Occipital condyle
Zygomaticus minor m.
Mastoid process
Levator anguli oris m
Posterior belly of digastric m.
Parotid duct;
Styloid process; styohloid ligament
Buccinator muscle
Styloglossus muscle
Orbicularis oris muscle
Stylopharyngeus muscle
Posterior belly of digastric m.
Depressor anguli oris muscle
Stylohyoid muscle
Mentalis muscle
Middle pharyngeal constrictor muscle
Greater horn of hyoid bone
Platysma muscle
Superior laryngeal artery nerve, and vein
Anterior belly of digastric m.
Thyrohyoid membrane
Mylohyoid muscle
Sternohyoid muscle
Omohyoid muscle
Inferior pharyngeal constrictor muscle
Thyrohyoid muscle
Thyroid cartilage
Cricothyroid muscle
Esophagus
Tracheal cartilages

FIGURE 4-93

Pharyngeal and facial musculature as seen from the side. (From Clemente, 1975.)

medial pharyngeal raphe. The inferiormost fibers course somewhat downward beneath the superior fibers of the inferior constrictor. The middle fibers course transversely, while the superior fibers course obliquely upward to overlap the inferior fibers of the superior constrictor.

The Inferior Constrictor Muscle The inferior constrictor, the thickest and the strongest of the pharyngeal muscles, is widely distributed. Most of the fibers arise from the lamina and superior horn of the thyroid cartilage. In addition, however, *a substantial part of the inferior constrictor is a continuation of the sternothyroid musculature.* If the sternothyroid is freed from its sternal attachments and reflected forward, as in Figure 4-95, a large number of muscle fasciculi on its deep surface will be seen to continue into and contribute to the inferior pharyngeal constrictor. The fibers that arise from the thyroid cartilage (and from the sternothyroid) are called the **thyropharyngeus muscle.** We learned in the preceding chapter that the thyropharyngeus may influence the angular relationships between the thyroid laminae. An additional group of muscle fibers arises from the cricoid cartilage and the inferior horn of the thyroid cartilage. These

fibers, which constitute the **cricopharyngeus muscle,** are often complemented by additional fibers which are continuations of the cricothyroid muscle.

From their origins, the muscle fibers of the inferior constrictor abruptly diverge fanlike as they course backward and medialward, where they interdigitate with their fellows from the opposite side, thus forming the midline pharyngeal raphe. The inferiormost fibers course in an obliquely downward direction to encircle and blend with muscle fibers of the esophagus. These fibers probably contribute to the sphincteric action of the esophagus.

CLINICAL NOTE: These inferior fibers may play an important role in the development of esophageal speech by a person who has had a laryngectomy. It is the cricopharyngeus muscle that often functions as the **pseudoglottis.**

The remainder of the fibers of the inferior constrictor course in an increasingly vertical direction, with the superiormost fibers coursing almost vertically.

ynx is carried upward with it. Simultaneously, the ary-epiglottic folds are approximated, and the arytenoid cartilages are drawn upward and forward, all of which serves to prevent the bolus from entering the larynx. In response to successive contractions of the superior and middle constrictors, the bolus slides over the posterior surface of the epiglottis, past the sealed entrance to the larynx, and into the lower pharynx.

An electromyographic investigation of the muscles of the superior pharyngeal constrictor showed greatest activity during reflexive behavior (swallowing and gag). Less activity was found during production of the word /hawk/ and a modified Valsalva maneuver. Vowel production produced activity levels that were just above the inactive or baseline level (Perlman, et al., 1989). In addition, Perlman and Liang (1991) used the Fourcin Electroglottogram to measure laryngeal displacement during swallowing. They suggested that the instrument has clinical utility.

The fact that the epiglottis folds down to cover the entrance to the larynx (laryngeal aditus) during swallowing has been verified repeatedly by radiography (Ardran and Kemp, 1951, 1952, 1967). The epiglottis is reported to make two distinct movements in covering the laryngeal aditus. The first movement occurs where the epiglottis attaches to the thyroid cartilage. The first movement is from the vertical rest position to a horizontal position followed by a second movement that takes place as the bolus passes through the pharynx. This movement brings the upper one-third of the epiglottis below the horizontal. These movements seem to be the result of anterior displacement of the hyoid bone and of thyroid cartilage-hyoid bone approximation. Perlman et al. (1995) propose that, as the larynx elevates during swallowing and the hyoid bone moves anteriorly, the paired lateral hyoepiglottic ligaments exert traction on the upper third of the epiglottis to bring it to a position below the horizontal.

The Last Stage

The last stage consists of contraction of the inferior pharyngeal constrictor, which compresses the bolus into the esophagus and at the same time initiates **peristalsis,** which is the wormlike contraction of the alimentary canal. These stages are not discrete maneuvers but follow in rapid succession, as often as 300 times per hour when we are eating.

Growth of the Head[16]

The skull is not simply a static organic hitching post for the speech musculature; rather, it is a dynamic, living structure, capable of differential growth, capable of adjusting to environmental influences, and capable of disease.

Methods of Study

Aside from measurements of the various structures of the skull, two principal methods of study of skull growth have been employed. The first is known as **vital staining.** It involves injection of bone-penetrating dyes such as alizarin red into growing animals, usually monkeys. Preparations reveal layers of stained bone and provide an index of growth. The second technique involves **serial x-ray studies** of animal and human skulls during the growth period. X-ray studies have the advantage of being applicable to living humans, and they also reveal the growth of soft tissue, such as the soft palate and pharynx. The value of any x-ray film is largely dependent upon the methods used to analyze it. Still cephalic x-rays have been used successfully in studies of the growth of the skull structures (Broadbent, 1930, 1937; Brodie, 1940, 1941; Subtelny, 1957) as well as of soft tissues (King, 1952; Subtelny and Koepp-Baker, 1956; Subtelny, 1957; and Willis, 1952).

X-rays have also been useful in specifying articulatory gestures during production of speech sounds (Chiba and Kajiyama, 1958; Fant, 1970, 1973; and Hardcastle, 1976).

Cineradiographic films taken during speech production have proven extremely valuable. Examples are the in-depth study by Perkell (1969) and studies reported by Fritzell (1969); Amerman et al. (1970); and Moll and Daniloff (1971).

Researchers have generally employed **cephalometric roentgenography,** or the measurement of the head by x-ray, to assess the structural and functional integrity of the speech mechanism. Cephalometry and craniometry (measurements of the skull) have applicability in anthropology, dentistry, and orthodontia, but it is essential that a standardized methodology be employed.

Cephalometry

The head should be oriented in the **Frankfort horizontal plane,** which passes through the orbitale and porion, as shown in Figure 4-96B. The **orbitale** is the lowest point of the infraorbital rim, while the **porion** is the most lateral point on the uppermost margin of the external auditory meatus. It is cartilaginous and does not appear on an x-ray, however, so the **tragion** is often used instead. It is the most forward point on the supratragal notch. The **tragus,** shown in Figure 4-96A, is a tab on the ear that projects back and slightly outward on the anterior rim of the entrance to the ear canal. The following landmarks, measure points, lines, and planes are useful for describing the skull. A lateral head x-ray is shown in Figure 4-97, and a partial tracing of the same x-ray, containing a number of abbreviated reference

---

[16]Prenatal growth of the head is presented in Chapter 7, Embryology.

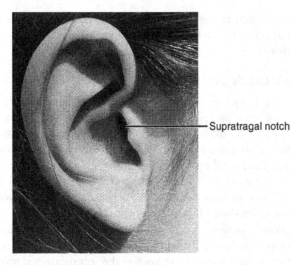

A

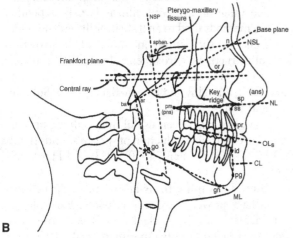

B

FIGURE 4-96

(A) Photograph of an ear, illustrating the supratragal notch.
(B) A partial tracing of the x-ray shown in Figure 4-97, illustrating some reference lines and planes that are used in cephalometry.

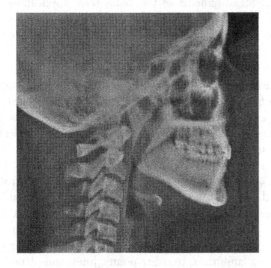

FIGURE 4-97

Lateral head x-ray of a normal female adolescent. (Courtesy Center for Craniofacial Anomalies, University of Illinois.)

points used in cephalometric studies, is shown in Figure 4-96B. Some reference lines or planes are also shown. Inferior, lateral, and frontal views of a prepared skull are shown in Figures 4-98 and 4-99, along with some anthropologic landmarks that are in fairly common use.

Landmarks and Measure Points

1. **A point (A),** an arbitrary measure point taken at the innermost curvature from the maxillary anterior nasal spine to the crest of the maxillary alveolar process, signifying the approximate juncture of the basal or supporting maxillary bone and the alveolar bone (apical base). Also called the **subspinale (ss).** In the cleft palate population this surface is often convex due to anomalous dentition and/or displacement of the anterior portion of the larger cleft segment.

2. **Anterior nasal spine (ans),** the median, sharp bony process of the alveolar process at the midline between the maxillary central incisors.

3. **Articulare (ar),** the intersection between the contour of the external cranial base and the dorsal contour of the condylar head.

4. **Auricular point (au p),** the center of the external auditory meatus.

5. **Basion (ba),** the most forward and lowest point on the anterior margin of the foramen magnum. This point is not well defined on lateral head x-rays, so the Bolton point is often used instead.

6. **Bolton point (bp),** the most superior point on the concavity behind the occipital condyle.

7. **Bregma (br),** the point at which the sagittal and coronal sutures meet.

8. **Glabella (gl),** the most anterior point on the midsagittal plane, between the superciliary arches.

9. **Gnathion (gn),** the lowest point of the median plane in the lower symphysis of the mandible. It is easily palpated in the living.

10. **Gonion (go),** the lowest, posterior, and most outward point on the angle of the mandible. In a lateral head x-ray the gonion can be located by bisecting the angle between tangents to the lower and posterior borders of the mandible, as shown in Figure 4-96.

11. **Infradentale (id),** the highest interdental point on the alveolar mucosa between the mandibular central incisors.

12. **Inion (in),** the most prominent point, at the midline, of the external occipital protuberance.

13. **Key ridge (kr),** the lowest point on the zygomaticomaxillary ridge, also known as the **zygomaxillare.**

14. **Lambda (la),** intersection of the sagittal and lambdoidal sutures on the cranial vault.

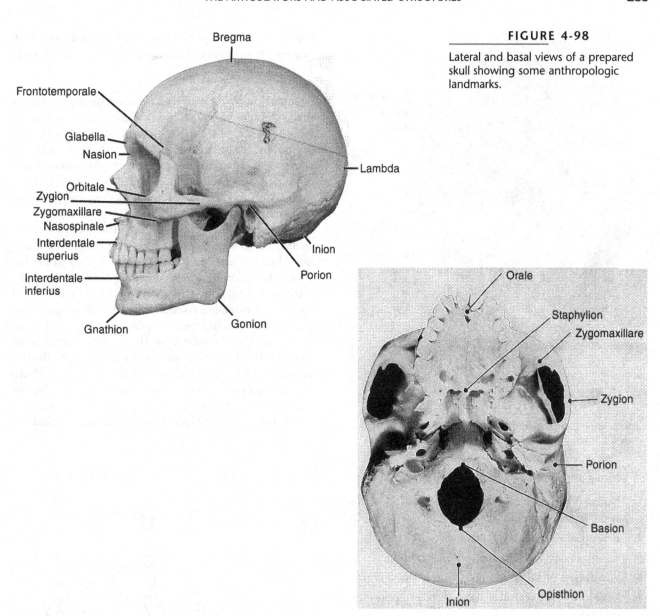

FIGURE 4-98

Lateral and basal views of a prepared skull showing some anthropologic landmarks.

15. **Menton (m),** the lowest point from which the face can be measured.

16. **Nasion (n),** the middle point located on the frontonasal suture intersected by the midsagittal plane.

17. **Orbitale (or),** the lowest point on the margin of the orbit.

18. **Pogonion (pg),** the most anterior prominent point on the chin.

19. **Porion (p),** the midpoint on the upper edge of the external auditory meatus. In cephalometrics, it is located in the middle of the ear rods.

20. **Posterior nasal spine (pns),** process formed by the uniting ends of the posterior borders of the horizontal plates of the palatine bones.

21. **Prosthion (pr),** the lowest interdental point on the alveolar mucosa in the medial plane between max-

illary central incisors. Also defined as the lowest and most prominent point on the upper alveolar arch. It is used to measure *facial length* not facial height.

22. **Pterygomaxillare (ptm),** the point where the pterygoid processes of the sphenoid and maxillary bones begin to form the pterygomaxillary fissure. The lowest point is used in cephalometrics.

23. **Sella (s),** the center of the Sella turcica.

24. **Sella turcica (s),** the pituitary (hypophyseal) fossa of the sphenoid bone.

25. **Tragion (t),** the notch just above the tragus of the ear.

26. **Tuberculum sellae (ts),** anterior boundary of sella turcica.

27. **Vertex (v),** the highest point of the head (in midsagittal plane).

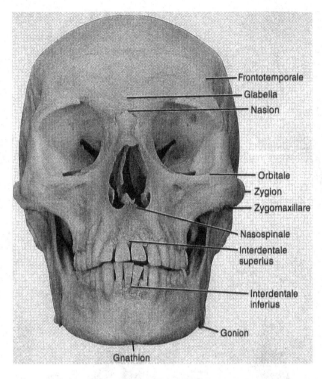

FIGURE 4-99

Frontal view of a prepared skull showing some anthropologic landmarks.

Lines and Planes

1. **Bolton's plane,** nasion to Bolton point (also called Broadbent-Bolton line).

2. **Broadbent's line,** nasion to sella.

3. **Cranial base line,** nasion to Bolton's point.

4. **Facial line** or **facial plane,** nasion to pogonion.

5. **Frankfort horizontal plane,** orbitale to porion, or tragion.

6. **Hard palate** or **palatal plane,** anterior to posterior nasal spines.

7. **Huxley's line,** nasion to basion.

8. **Nasion-sella line (n-s),** sella to nasion.

9. **Occlusal plane (Ols),** a line drawn between points representing one-half of the incisor overbite and one-half of the cusp height of the last occluding molars.

Most of these references are in general use, and the reader is likely to encounter many of them in literature that deals with orthodontic and cleft palate problems, as well as normal and abnormal speech functions. References used to analyze still x-rays of the head are also applicable to frame-by-frame analysis of cineradiographics films. Specific measurements are made in the study of velopharyngeal closure and in studies of the growth of

the facial region. A partial tracing of a lateral x-ray of an oropharyngeal region, including soft tissues, is shown in Figure 4-100.

Measurement Procedures Measurements frequently made include the length and thickness of the soft palate and the vertical height and horizontal depth of the nasopharynx. These measures are usually made with the subject at rest and during sustained phonation of the vowel [ɑ]. In addition, the ratio between the length of velar tissue and horizontal depth of the pharynx is also evaluated (Subtelny, 1957).

These measures are made as follows: the base of the skull is delineated from the face and pharynx by drawing a line (cranial base line) from the nasion to the basion or Bolton's point. A second line, drawn through the reference points for the anterior and posterior nasal spines and extended to the soft tissue of the posterior pharyngeal wall, indicates *the plane of the hard palate*; by measuring the distance from the posterior nasal spine (pns) to the posterior pharyngeal wall (ph), an effective measure of *the horizontal depth of the nasopharynx* is obtained. In order to study *the vertical height of the nasopharynx*, the distance from the posterior nasal spine to the cranial base line is measured. According to Subtelny,

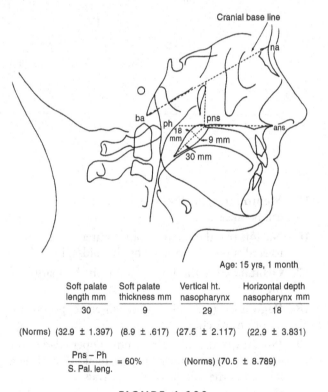

Soft palate length mm	Soft palate thickness mm	Vertical ht. nasopharynx	Horizontal depth nasopharynx mm
30	9	29	18
(Norms) (32.9 ± 1.397)	(8.9 ± .617)	(27.5 ± 2.117)	(22.9 ± 3.831)

$$\frac{Pns - Ph}{S.\ Pal.\ leng.} = 60\%$$ (Norms) (70.5 ± 8.789)

FIGURE 4-100

Tracing of lateral head x-ray showing measures to assess adequacy of velopharyngeal tissues. (Norms taken from Subtelny, 1957.)

this distance is measured along a line perpendicular to the cant of the hard palate and projected to intersect the cranial base line, as in Figure 4-100. The *length of the soft palate* at rest may be obtained by measuring the distance from the posterior nasal spine to the tip of the uvula; when the oral surface of the soft palate can be delineated from the dorsum of the tongue, the *greatest thickness of the soft palate* may also be measured.

Subtelny's Study An example of the uses to which such measures may be put is seen in a longitudinal cephalometric radiographic study by Subtelny (1957), who in an attempt to facilitate long-range rehabilitation planning for young children with a cleft of the palate, studied the progressive growth and development of the velum, nasopharynx, and associated structures. Serial cephalometric x-rays of thirty normal subjects, with x-ray records from infancy to early adulthood, were evaluated. The sample included an equal number of males and females. The x-rays were taken using a technique developed by Broadbent (1930, 1931), in which the subjects' heads were stabilized by means of a specially constructed head holder. Thus, the subjects could be repositioned to obtain comparable successive x-rays over intervals of time. The x-ray films studies were taken every three months during the first year of life, every six months from one to three years, and at yearly intervals through the eighteenth year.

Some of Subtelny's findings are summarized as follows:

Growth in length of the soft palate was most rapid during the early years of life, with a marked and consistent increase in length until about 1½ to 2 years, at which time there was a leveling off of growth until approximately 4 to 5 years of age. Thereafter, the average growth was consistent but not as rapid as during the first years of life.

Changes in thickness of the soft palate were the most rapid during the first year of life, and in succeeding years the average growth was slight until maximum thickness was reached at 14 to 16 years.

Subtelny found that in the infant, the soft palate, as it rests against the dorsum of the tongue, gives the appearance of being almost in line with the hard palate as it slopes downward toward the oropharynx, as shown in Figure 4-101. With growth, however, the soft palate was found to approach more of a parallel relationship with the posterior pharyngeal wall, as in Figure 4-102. Subtelny noted that this change in angularity of the soft palate is closely correlated with the downward and forward growth of the facial skeleton described by Broadbent (1937) and Brodie (1941) and the increased vertical height of the pharynx found by King (1952).

As shown in Figure 4-103, with growth of the facial skeleton, the hard palate moves in a parallel manner

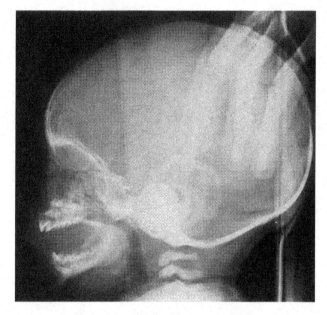

FIGURE 4-101

Lateral headplate of a normal infant. The soft palate is almost in line with the hard palate and perpendicular to the posterior wall of the pharynx. (Courtesy Center for Craniofacial Anomalies, University of Illinois.)

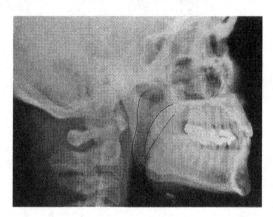

FIGURE 4-102

Lateral head x-ray of an adult showing the slope of the soft palate and its relationship to the posterior pharyngeal wall.

away from the base of the skull. Subtelny was interested in determining the concomitant changes of the vertical height of the nasopharynx. He found that the average vertical height doubled from early infancy to early adulthood, with the most profound changes occurring during the first year and a half of life. These findings support those of King (1952).

Along with the downward and forward growth of the facial skeleton and the increase in height of the nasopharynx, there is an increase in the horizontal depth of the nasopharynx. The growth rate remains rather

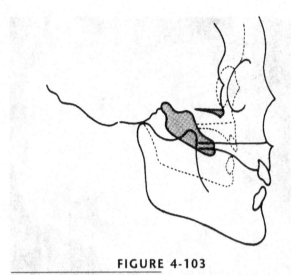

FIGURE 4-103

Schematic of superimposed lateral head x-rays illustrating downward and forward growth of the facial skeleton.

gradual from infancy through early adulthood. The data revealed fluctuations in depth, however, that probably reflect the growth of adenoid tissue on the posterior pharyngeal wall.

Subtelny also determined the proportional amount of velar tissue available for establishment of velopharyngeal closure. That is, the horizontal depth of the pharynx was stated in proportion to or as a percentage of the length of the soft palate. He found that the depth of the nasopharynx approximated a 2:3 ratio, relative to the length of the soft palate. Individual differences, which varied considerably, are reflected by the large standard deviations in Table 4-4. The results, however, suggest that a figure of 60 to 70 percent would indicate adequate tissue for velopharyngeal closure. Higher percentages would suggest less likelihood of proper closure. The subject in Figure 4-104, for example, has a much higher percentage, in spite of considerable adenoid tissue. Such a value suggests that

TABLE 4-4

Means and standard deviations based on ratios computed from horizontal measurements of the nasopharynx over the length of the soft palate

Age in Years	Number of Ratios	Percentage Means $\dfrac{(Pns\text{-}Ph)}{Soft\ Palate\ Length} = \%$	Standard Deviations
.25	10	73.8	12.7516
.50	14	66.3	8.6944
.75	14	65.2	8.9528
1	17	68.6	14.6142
1.50	16	62.5	11.5912
2	18	67.1	14.1381
2.50	19	60.0	8.6470
3	27	65.1	11.3986
4	27	65.1	14.1092
5	26	68.7	9.6563
6	23	66.3	15.0549
7	27	69.6	14.1922
8	23	68.7	13.6498
9	24	66.0	13.1667
10	26	68.3	9.8647
11	25	66.3	10.1304
12	23	68.3	9.5014
13	22	66.2	8.3813
14	17	70.0	9.1434
15	17	70.5	8.7881
16	17	71.4	6.9858
17	10	72.6	11.4739
18	6	70.2	6.9927

From J. D. Subtelny, "A Cephalometric Study of the Growth of the Soft Palate," *Plastic and Reconstructive Surgery,* 19, 1957.

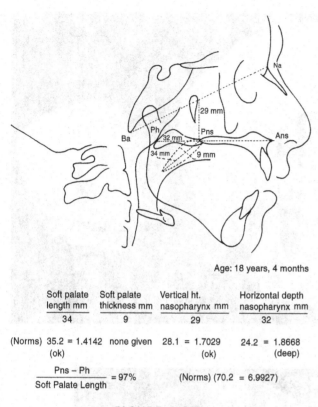

Age: 18 years, 4 months

Soft palate length mm	Soft palate thickness mm	Vertical ht. nasopharynx mm	Horizontal depth nasopharynx mm
34	9	29	32

(Norms) 35.2 = 1.4142   none given   28.1 = 1.7029   24.2 = 1.8668
      (ok)   (ok)   (deep)

$$\frac{Pns - Ph}{Soft\ Palate\ Length} = 97\%$$ (Norms) (70.2 = 6.9927)

FIGURE 4-104

Tracing of a lateral head x-ray of a subject with questionable velopharyngeal competence.

with atrophy or surgical removal of adenoid tissue, the result might well be irreversible hypernasality.

Influences on Growth of the Skull

Study of the growth of the skull is necessarily complicated by the fact that its two parts, the brain capsule and the masticatory facial skeleton, are integrated into one anatomic and biological unit. The complications arise because the growth of the brain capsule is entirely dependent upon the growth of the brain itself, whereas growth of the facial skeleton is dependent upon muscular influences and growth of the teeth and tongue. The two parts of the skull not only follow different paths of development, but their chronological sequence is different. For example, the brain has reached about 90 percent of its physical development by the age of ten years, whereas the dentition and jaws are but beginning their final growth period, which goes on until about the twentieth year.

Growth of Bone and Cartilage

It is important in the study of the growth of the skull to appreciate the mechanisms of bone and cartilage growth. Because of the rigidity of the calcified bone, **interstitial** (expansive) **growth** is impossible. Bone tissue, therefore,

can grow only by **apposition** or **addition.** Other connective tissue, such as cartilage, grows interstitially. This requires cell division to produce **fibroblasts** (connective tissue cells) plus new collagenous (elastic) fibers and cementing substances.

Hyaline cartilage is capable of both interstitial and appositional growth. Interstitial growth is initiated by division of the cartilage cells (chondrocytes), which then grow to produce new hyaline substance. Appositional growth can take place only where the cartilage is covered by a layer of perichondrium. Cells in the perichondrium (which is connective tissue) differentiate into **chondroblasts,** which in turn produce the ground substance of hyaline cartilage. **Hyaline cartilage** is found at three primary locations at birth: parts of the nasal skeleton, the spheno-occipital synchondrosis (plus parts of the occipital bone that are joined by a synchondrosis), and the mandibular condyle. *Growth at sutures is initiated by proliferation of connective tissue at the suture, and not by apposition of new bone.*

The Infant Skull

At birth the skull, relative to the body, is quite large. The facial portion is small, however, as can be seen in Figure 4-105, by comparing the skull of a newborn infant to that of an adult. The facial portion of the infant skull is equal to about one-eighth of the bulk of the cranium, compared to about one-half in the adult. With the skulls in the Frankfort horizontal plane, the adult skull measures 20.5 cm in height, while the facial height (nasion to gnathion) measures 11.1 cm. Facial height, therefore, comprises about 54 percent of the total height of the skull. The infant skull, 11.1 cm in height, has a facial height of 3.5 cm, which is about 35 percent of the total height.

Some additional differences become obvious from inspection of the photographs. The adult mandibular height is 9.0 cm, which is equal to 43 percent of the total skull height and 81 percent of the facial height, while the infant mandible is 2.0 cm in height, which amounts to 20 percent of the total skull height and 57 percent of the total facial height. These differences can be attributed in large part to the lack of development of alveolar bone on the maxillae and mandible.

The difference in the height of the middle ear cavity relative to the palatal plane is significant, but more about that later. In the adult the floor of the middle ear cavity is much higher than in the infant. This is especially evident in the lateral headplate shown in Figure 4-106. Notice in the frontal x-ray of the infant skull that the nasal cavities are located almost entirely between the orbits, and that the lower border of the anterior nasal aperture is just below the level of the orbital floor. In the adult the difference in these two levels is about 2.0 cm.

FIGURE 4-105

The skull of a newborn infant compared with the skull of an adult.

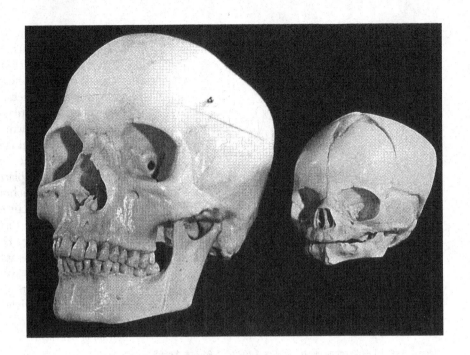

FIGURE 4-106

X-ray plates of an infant skull showing relationship of middle ear to plane of hard palate.

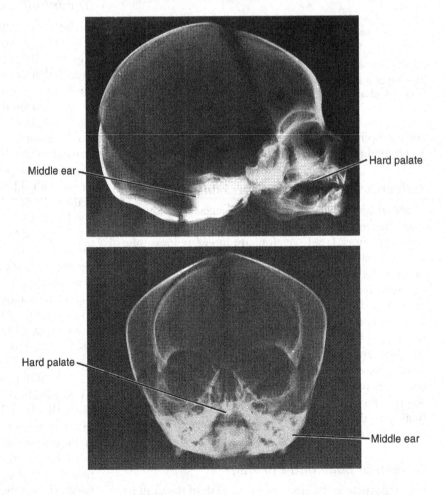

In the infant the frontal and parietal eminences are prominent, and the skull is widest at the parietal eminences, while the adult skull is usually widest at the level just above the mastoid processes of the temporal bones.

The glabella, superciliary arches, and mastoid processes are not as well developed in the infant skull.

Unossified membranous regions can be seen at the various angles of the parietal bones. They are called fontanelles—from a French word denoting a spring or filter. An anterior and posterior midline fontanelle can be seen in Figure 4-107, and an anterolateral (sphenoid) and posterolateral (mastoid) fontanelle can be found on either side. The anterior fontanelle marks the region where the vault of the cranium is highest in the adult, so it is often called the **bregmatic fontanelle.**

Growth of the Cranium

The posterior and lateral fontanelles are usually obliterated shortly after birth, while the bregmatic fontanelle does not close until after the middle of the second year. This is an important point, because *during the first two years of life the brain capsule and brain just about triple in volume.* The rate of growth then begins to slow down until about the seventh year, after which the annual growth is very slight. The brain capsule reaches about 90 percent of growth and volume by the tenth year.

Growth of the Facial Skeleton

After the first year, the facial skeleton grows considerably faster than the cranium. During this growth period, in which the skull grows in all three dimensions—height, width, and depth—the original relationship between the facial skeleton and the neurocranium is maintained. That is, the plane of the palate, the occlusal plane, and the plane of the lower border of the mandible maintain a constant angular relation to the base of the skull. During periods of growth the parallel relationships of these three planes vary only slightly.

Maxillary Growth There are three primary sites of growth of the maxillary complex, which includes the maxillae and the palatine bones. These three sites are the frontomaxillary, the zygomaticomaxillary, and the zygomaticotemporal sutures. As shown in Figure 4-108, they lie in planes in such a way that *growth has the effect of shifting the entire maxillary complex downward and forward.* During this growth period, the anteroposterior depth of the bony palate almost doubles, whereas the transverse growth is much less. This is illustrated schematically in Figure 4-109.

Growth of the palate is due to apposition. The increase in transverse diameter of the maxillae is brought about by appositional growth at the medial palatine suture and also by the influence, at the junction of the palatine processes and the maxillary complex, of the downward and lateral growth of the pterygoid plates of the sphenoid bone. By the end of the fifth year, the palate has attained about five-sixths the width of a mature palate, and it has reached maximum transverse development by ten years.

Growth in *facial height* is most pronounced during the first six months of life while the deciduous incisor

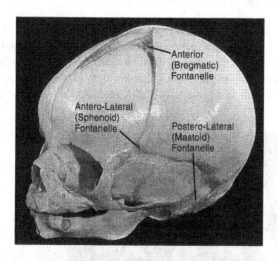

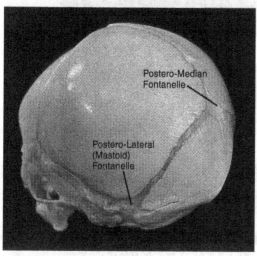

FIGURE 4-107

Photographs of an infant skull illustrating the location of the fontanelles.

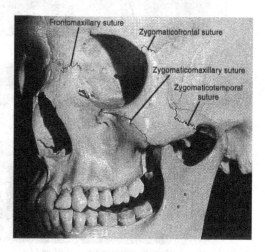

FIGURE 4-108

Illustration of the primary sites of growth of the maxillary complex, which have the effect of shifting the face downward and forward.

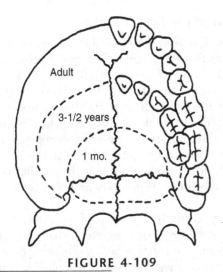

FIGURE 4-109

Schematic of anterior and transverse growth of the palate and dental arch.

teeth are developing, and between the ages of seven and eleven when the permanent incisors and cuspid teeth are erupting. Studies of the *anteroposterior growth* of the maxillae show three periods of rapid growth: at ages five to six, when the first molars are developing and erupting; at age eleven; and at age sixteen, when the second and third molars are descending and erupting.

Mandibular Growth The height of the body of the mandible is gained by apposition of bone on its external (labial) surfaces. Growth is much the same as that on the alveolar process of the maxilla. That is, growth in the lingual direction is accomplished by a heavy deposition of bone on the posterior edge of the ramus. Continual proliferation of hyaline cartilage below the articulating surface of the mandibular condyle and replacement of cartilage by deposition of bone account for the development that lowers the mandible and its occlusal plane.

As evidence of the extent of the growth of the mandible, the height and length of the posterior border of the ramus, as measured from the angle to the temporomandibular joint, more than doubles during the period of development. Compared with the growth mechanism of the maxilla, the growth of the mandible is unique. Whereas maxillary growth is primarily sutural and appositional, growth of the mandible is due to interstitial growth in the hyaline cartilage of the condyle.

Infancy and Childhood. At birth, the body of the mandible is but a mere shell, containing the alveoli (tooth sockets) for the deciduous dentition. There are two incisors, one cuspid, and two molar teeth in each quadrant. As shown in Figure 4-110, the angle of the ramus with

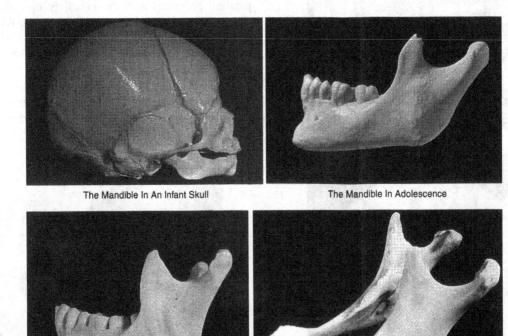

The Mandible In An Infant Skull

The Mandible In Adolescence

The Mandible In Young Adulthood

The Mandible In Old Age Following The Loss Of The Teeth

FIGURE 4-110

Changes in the mandible with age.

the mandibular plane is obtuse, about 170 degrees. Shortly after birth the two halves of the mandible become joined at the symphysis, beginning from below, a process that is usually completed by the end of the first year. As stated previously, the body of the mandible elongates in an anteroposterior direction to provide room for the three additional permanent teeth that will be developing in the region behind the mental foramen.

Because of the increasing dental development and consequent growth of the alveolar process, the depth of the body of the mandible increases. The mandibular angle becomes less and less obtuse, and at four years is about 140 degrees. In the adult mandible the alveolar and subdental portions occupy about equal space. The ramus is almost vertical with the mandibular angle, being about 110 degrees to 120 degrees.

Effects of Aging. In old age the body of the jaw becomes reduced in its vertical dimension. This is due to absorption of the alveolar process subsequent to the loss of teeth. The ramus again becomes increasingly oblique, with the mandibular angle measuring about 140 degrees.

Although totally edentulous jaws are not encountered as frequently as they once were, the specimen shown in Figure 4-111 illustrates the importance of maintaining the normal biomechanical processes in the jaws. The canine teeth are natural, while the four incisors are a pontic (L. *pontis*, bridge). In other words, the incisors are the part of a bridge which substitutes for absent teeth, both aesthetically and functionally. Note that the alveolar bone is relatively healthy where the bridge is located, especially when compared to the remainder of the jaw. The loss of alveolar bone in the edentulous portion can be attributed to disuse atrophy. The rest position of the mandible is dependent upon the musculature that comprises the mandibular sling and the temporalis muscle. This means that the angle of the mandible in the rest position remains fairly stable and decreases

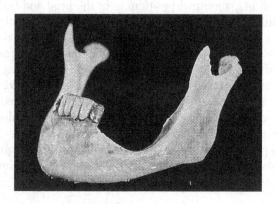

FIGURE 4-111

Partially edentulous mandible showing the consequences of alveolar bone resorption. The alveolar bone is relatively healthy where the bridge is located, when compared to the remainder of the jaw.

gradually only after all the teeth are lost. All this points to the importance of proper dental care.

Sex Differences in the Skull

Until the onset of puberty there is very little difference between the male and female skull. However, the adult female skull is as a general rule smaller than the adult male skull. That is, the size of the female cranium is about 10 percent smaller, and the overall structure is characterized by a less well-defined development of bony crests, ridges, and processes. The walls of the bones of the female skull are also thinner than are those of the male, and the glabella, superciliary arches, and mastoid processes are less prominent. In addition, the air sinuses are smaller in the female skull.

According to Gray (1973), the upper margin of the orbit is sharp, the forehead vertical, the frontal and parietal eminences are prominent, and the cranial vault is generally somewhat flattened. The contour of the face is more rounded, the facial bones are less rough, and the jaws and teeth are smaller than the male structures. Sicher and Dubrul (1975) state that the general outline of the female skull is more similar to the outline of the skull of a child than the outline of the adult male skull. They also point out that these differences are superficial and probably are correlated to muscular activity.

The differences in musculature development of the skulls of adult males and females have been greatly reduced in modern humans, to the extent that determination of sex on the basis of morphology of the skull may at times be very difficult, or impossible. In addition, the difference in overall cranial volume is well correlated with purely somatic qualities. That is, adult females are generally smaller and less muscular than adult males.

CONTRIBUTIONS OF THE ARTICULATORS

Research Techniques

Challenges

Much of what is known about the complex and highly integrated process of speech production has been learned by introspection, and much has also been learned by attempts to quantify various parameters of articulation and its relationship to laryngeal and respiratory behavior. An impressive battery of instrumentation has emerged for research purposes. But, in spite of a high degree of sophistication in the use of instrumentation, the rapid changes that occur during speech production are very difficult to specify. Very precise measurements are valuable to researchers interested in speech synthesis and to linguists.

As Fujimura (1961) has pointed out, when an experimenter tries to produce a syllable by means of an electrical analog, he may find he is unable to give in advance a detailed specification of the rates at which the component parts of the speech mechanism must move. Although information regarding the behavior of the articulators may be derived from detailed acoustic analysis of speech, the analysis often turns out to be postdictive rather than predictive. The specific changes in the states of the articulators necessary to produce a given modification of the acoustic event are not known until after the analysis, and even then certain assumptions often must be made. Simultaneous acoustic and physiological measures are vital to an understanding of the dynamics of the speech processes, but they are difficult to obtain.

Aerodynamic Measurements

One of the earliest instruments to find its way into the laboratory was the **spirometer,** which is used mainly to assess pulmonary functions. It has also been used to assess the structural and functional integrity of the speech mechanism, but its utility is limited due to a lack of resolution. Very small, yet probably significant, differences in air expenditure during speech will not be detected by a spirometer.

Instruments are available, however, that provide precise measures of air flow through the vocal tract and of air pressure within the oral cavity. **Air-pressure sensors** are coupled to a subject either through a catheter (through a nostril, or the corner of the mouth) or by means of a mouthpiece. Pressure variations in the oral cavity cause the sensor to generate a pressure-dependent electrical voltage, which is recorded (usually by a graphic ink recorder). These devices have been used to measure intraoral air pressure during consonant production (Arkebauer, et al., 1967). Air flow through the vocal tract is generally measured at the mouth by means of a **pneumotachograph.** (See Figure 3-66 and a description in Chapter 3.)

Electromyography

A number of studies of speech physiology have been conducted using electromyography, a muscle activity recording technique. Electromyography and its shortcomings were discussed briefly in Chapter 1. With proper control techniques, the relative activity of a muscle or muscle group and its possible contribution to the speech process can be determined (Fritzell, 1969).

Photography

Single-frame and motion-picture photography (of lip and jaw movements, for example) are techniques that have shed light on speech production (Fujimura, 1961).

Radiography

Single-frame lateral **x-rays** and **cineradiography** (motion picture radiography) have been used extensively in the study of tongue placement in vowel production, in consonant articulation, and in the dynamics of articulation.

Russell (1928) made early use of lateral head x-rays in an effort to study articulation during vowel production. He concluded that vowels had no constant characteristics with respect to resonant cavities or tongue positions and that the traditional vowel triangle was fallacious. Trevino and Parmenter (1932) questioned the conclusions of Russell, basing their criticism on inadequate control of head position during the x-ray exposures, thus rendering serial x-rays unsuitable for comparison, one with the other. In 1934 Kelly and Higley, using a specially designed head holder to eliminate the posture artifact, analyzed x-rays of 10 subjects producing the vowels [u], [o], [ɑ] and [e]. They concluded that the traditional vowel triangle was valid, except for [o]. In 1937 Holbrook and Carmody analyzed over 500 lateral head x-rays of subjects producing vowels and consonants in English and other languages. They found that the standard vowels tended to be produced with the tongue in a rather definite posture, which supported the general notion of a vowel triangle or vowel quadrilateral.

The development of motion-picture radiography (combined with image intensification) has provided researchers with a valuable technique for observing tongue, jaw, and palatal movements during the production of continuous speech and during such otherwise unobservable events such as swallowing. The value of the information is largely dependent upon control measures used during filming.

Certain factors, which have been discussed by Moll (1965), should be taken into account. For example, the methods used should place as few restrictions as possible on the normal activity of the speech mechanism. Head stabilizers, abnormal positioning of the head and neck, sedation, or topical anesthesia should not be used unless their effects are taken into consideration. A great deal of what we know about speech dynamics has been learned from radiography. *The single most important shortcoming of the technique is* **radiation hazard,** *and today very few institutions permit radiographic research to take place.* New techniques are being developed, however, that reduce filming time and radiation exposure. One of them, a computer-controlled **x-ray microbeam technique,** holds much promise (Fujimura, et al., 1973; Sawashima, 1976; Kiritani, 1977).

Palatography

An early technique for study of tongue placement is called palatography, and at one time it was probably the most thoroughly exploited method of investigating tongue placement during speech. It is still used by descriptive phoneticians and speech scientists to record areas of linguadental and linguapalatal contact during the production of various sounds (Hardcastle, 1974). In **direct palatography,** the hard palate, lingual surfaces of the teeth, and the soft palate are all dusted, by means of an anatomizer, with a dark powder prior to the production of the sound in question. A mixture of charcoal and powdered sweetened chocolate is very satisfactory. It adheres to the palate very well, tastes good, and is easily rinsed away when the experiment has been completed. Once the sound has been produced, a small oval mirror is inserted into the oral cavity, and the entire roof of the mouth can be either examined directly or photographed as in Figure 4-112. The technique is limited by the fact that only isolated sounds can be sampled and studied.

In 1964 Palmer reported a technique of **indirect palatography** that permitted continuous recording of linguapalatal contacts. A series of transducers, imbedded in a thin artificial palate, operated upon contact with the tongue. These contacts were monitored visually by means of a series of miniature lamps mounted on a pictorial display of the roof of the mouth. The technique permitted prolonged continuous recordings of tongue-palatal contact during the production of conversational speech. More recent applications of palatography incorporate computer techniques that provide computer generated displays and analyses of the dynamics of linguapalatal contact during speech (Fletcher, et al., 1975).

Articulation Tracking Devices

Tracking devices, especially those employing **strain gauge** systems, have proven useful (Abbs and Gilbert, 1973; Müller and Abbs, 1979, Barlow and Abbs, 1983). As the name implies these devices respond electrically to distortion, the more distortion the more electrical response. Strain gauges have been employed in measures of extent and rapidity of lip, jaw, and velar movements. This is an inexpensive and comparatively noninvasive technique (no needles or catheters). Moller et al (1971) used strain gauges to measure velar movement, and Proffit et al (1965) measured lingual force during speech using strain gauges.

Another articulation tracking system, known as **ultrasound,** is produced by placing an ultra-high-frequency sound transmitter against the skin. The sound is transmitted through the tissues until a discontinuity of tissue property is encountered, and the sound is then reflected to be received again at the surface of the skin. Very much like an echo, the distance from the source to the reflecting wall can be determined by the time it takes for the sound to return. Ultrasound has been used for measurements of the lateral pharyngeal wall (Minifie, et al., 1970; Skolnick, et al., 1975; Hawkins and Swisher, 1978) and tongue movements (Minifie, et al., 1970). One shortcoming with ultrasound is that it is not always possible to specify just what it was that produced the discontinuity that resulted in the reflection. Did the sound reflect from the lateral wall of the pharynx, or did it reflect from a bony structure?

Speech Production: A Review

We have seen that a steady-state, unmodulated, subglottal air supply can be placed under pressure by introducing resistance to the outward flow of air while the forces of exhalation are brought to bear. Resistance to air flow can occur at a number of points along the vocal

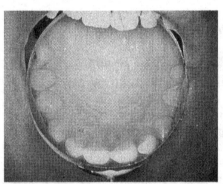

A

Undusted palate

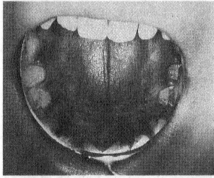

B

Dusted palate

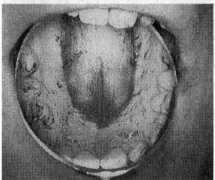

C

Palatogram illustrating linguapalatal contact (d)

FIGURE 4-112

An example of a direct palatogram, in which the palate is dusted with dark powder. The powder is "wiped" away during linguapalatal contact to reveal tongue placement during articulation of various speech sounds.

tract. We have already seen how resistance to air flow at the laryngeal level generates a glottal tone. We must realize, however, that the vibrating movements of the vocal folds themselves are not the source of vibrations we ultimately hear as speech sounds. *The vibratory movements are the instigators of speech sounds.*

This may seem puzzling at first, until we recognize that whenever the vocal folds are blown apart by the elevated subglottal pressure, a short-duration burst of air is released into the vocal tract. With the vocal folds vibrating at a rate of 150 times per second, a burst of air is released into the vocal tract each 1/150 seconds. The effect of each of these transient bursts of energy is to excite the relatively dormant supraglottal air column, which then vibrates for a short duration. The amplitude of the vibrations dies away quickly, but the rapid succession of energy bursts serves to maintain the air column in vibration.

Vibrations that die away quickly do so because the vibratory energy is being dissipated. We call these vibrations **damped.** So the acoustic result of vocal fold vibration is that a rapid series of **damped vibrations** is generated in the supraglottal vocal tract. It is a tone generated within the vocal tract as a consequence of vocal fold vibration. A series of damped vibrations is shown in Figure 4-113.

When the value of subglottal pressure and volume velocity (air flow) through the glottis is known, subglottal power can be computed and compared to the acoustic power of the voice at some distance from the lips. The efficiency of conversion of subglottal power to acoustic power turns out to be extremely low. If the conversion were efficient, however, we would deafen ourselves with the intensity of our own voices.

Vibrations generated by the vocal folds have just three parameters—**frequency, intensity,** and **duration**—and by themselves carry very little meaning. In order to produce speech as we know it, the character of the vocal tract vibrations must be modified by the structures that lie between the vocal folds and the mouth opening. To a large extent, these modifications can be accounted for by the principle of **resonance** and its antithesis, **damping.**

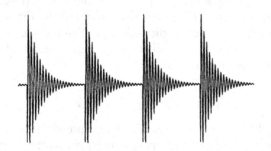

FIGURE 4-113

A series of damped vibrations.

Resonance

Natural Frequency

Almost all matter, under appropriate conditions, will, when energized by an outside force, vibrate at its own natural frequency. We have seen how the frequency of the vibrating vocal folds, energized by an air stream, is a direct function of tension and an inverse function of mass. A swing in the backyard or the limbs on a tree, when driven by gusts of wind, will tend to swing at a rate that is most appropriate. It is a common experience to anyone who has had the pleasure of sitting on a swing that no matter how hard the effort, no matter how hard one "pumps," the rate of frequency of each successive round trip remains the same. The extent of the excursion of the swing may vary with effort, but not the rate!

Forced Vibration

The swing has a "natural period or frequency," and it takes an unreasonable amount of effort to cause it to travel at an "unnatural period"; that is, we would have to force it into vibration. The term for such vibration is forced vibration. If the outside force is removed from a system vibrating at its natural frequency, it will continue to vibrate for some considerable length of time. The damping forces are slight. The vibrations of something vibrating at an unnatural frequency, or executing forced vibration, will, when the outside driving force is removed, cease quite abruptly. Such a system is said to be *highly damped.*

Radiation of Energy

The tines of a tuning fork vibrate with maximum force and for a maximum length of time at their natural frequency, and at no other. Thus, if the natural period of a tuning fork is 200 Hz and if it is driven by a vibratory force that contains 100, 200, 300, 400, and 500 Hz components (a complex tone, that is), the fork will vibrate at the 200 Hz rate, even if the 200 Hz component is not the most intense in the series. The tuning fork absorbs the energy of the 200 Hz component, and we say it resonates to 200 Hz. By the same token, *anything that absorbs energy at a specific frequency radiates energy best at that same frequency.* Vibrating systems always resonate at their natural frequencies when they can! They do not absorb energy well at frequencies other than their natural frequencies.

Resonant Frequencies of Vibrating Air Columns

Air columns also have their own natural frequencies, just like swings and trees. This is exemplified in the pipes of an organ or, better yet, in the vocal tract of a speech mechanism. A simple experiment will demonstrate how an air column may be set into vibration.

Almost everyone has blown across the top of a narrow-necked bottle to produce a deep, mellow tone, called an **edge tone.** No matter how intense the air stream (within certain limits), the bottle resonates at just one frequency. The air particles in the bottle may vibrate with greater excursions due to increased breath force, but they vibrate no faster. In other words, the sound may become louder, but never higher in pitch. The vibrating air column has a natural frequency, or to put it another way, the bottle will resonate at a specific frequency. If water is added, the air column is shortened and the resonant frequency increases. Thus, the resonant frequencies of vibrating air columns may be manipulated by modifying the size and configuration of the cavities.

An edge tone is one way to set an air column into vibration, but there are other ways. If the bottle is held an inch or so from the lips and a puff of air is released into it (call them bilabial puffs, for want of a better term), a short-duration note is emitted from the mouth of the bottle. The pitch of the note, although it is of short duration, is the same as when the air column is set into vibration by means of an edge tone. Adding water to the bottle raises the pitch, just as in the previous experiment. If we could now place our bottle over the isolated vibrating vocal folds mentioned earlier, we should not be surprised to find that the air column in the bottle is set into vibration at the same rate as before, and not at the vibratory rate of the vocal folds. The implication, of course, is that although the vocal folds may vibrate and release puffs of air at some particular frequency, the rate of vibration of the air column in the bottle is determined solely by its length and configuration. The resonating cavity in the bottle absorbs energy, contained in the puffs of air, only at the natural frequency of the bottle.

The air column is driven into vibration for a short duration with each discrete puff of air that is emitted by the vocal folds. *The rate at which the air column is driven into vibration determines the pitch, while the frequency or frequencies at which the air column resonates determines the quality of the tone.* This is the reason, for example, that the speech mechanism is capable of producing a certain vowel sound over a large part of the pitch range while a static vocal tract configuration is maintained.

The Source-Filter Theory of Speech Production

The following expression is a symbolic equation of the functions involved in the production of any particular speech sound:

$$|P(f)| = |U(f)| \cdot |H(f)| \cdot |R(f)|$$

It states that the **sound pressure spectrum** $P(f)$ at some distance from the lips is the product of the **volume velocity spectrum** generated by the source, or in other words the amplitude versus frequency characteristics of the source $U(f)$, the frequency–selective gain function of vocal transmission $H(f)$, and the radiation characteristics at the lips $R(f)$, where volume velocity through the lips is converted to sound pressure. The vertical bars tell us that we are concerned with only the magnitude of these functions, while the notation (f) denotes function of frequency.

The expression, which in a sense says that the speech wave as it is emitted is the response of the vocal tract to one or more sound sources, forms much of the basis for the source-filter theory of speech production described in detail by Fant (1970).

Characteristics of the Source

In 1958 Flanagan computed some of the properties of the glottal sound source by using the familiar glottal-area-as-a-function-of-time graphs of vocal fold vibration that can be extracted from ultra-high-speed motion pictures of the internal larynx during phonation. We saw a number of such graphs in the previous chapter. Using normative data for subglottic pressure, Flanagan was able to calculate from glottal area functions, **glottal resistance,** which in turn provided an indication of air flow through the glottis, or in other words, **volume velocity** or $|U(f)|$ in our equation. Glottal area and derived volume velocity curves for a single vibratory cycle of the vocal folds are shown in Figure 4-114. The vibratory rate of the vocal folds is given as F_0, while the subglottic pressure is given as P_s.

The **amplitude spectrum** (amplitude as a function of frequency) for the glottal area curve of Figure 4-114 is shown in Figure 4-115, and from it we learn that the

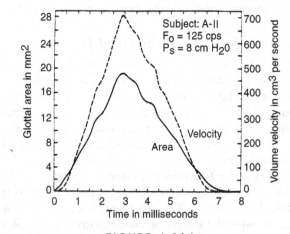

FIGURE 4-114

Glottal area and derived volume velocity. (From Flanagan, 1958.)

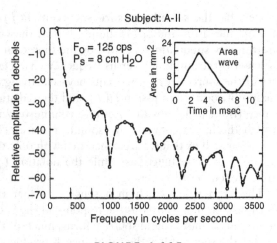

FIGURE 4-115

Amplitude spectrum for glottal area curve. (From Flanagan, 1958.)

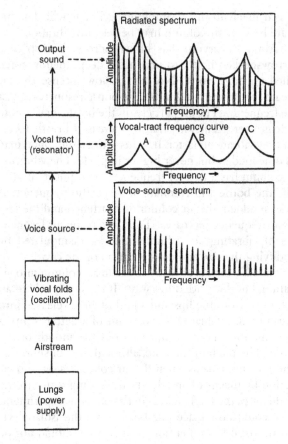

FIGURE 4-116

Schematic voice-source spectrum. (From "The Acoustics of the Singing Voice" by Johan Sundberg. Copyright 1977 by Scientific American, Inc. All rights reserved.)

laryngeal tone is complex, composed of a **fundamental frequency** which is determined by the vibratory rate of the vocal folds, and a number of **partials** with frequencies that are integral multiples of the fundamental frequency. That is, the partials are harmonics of the fundamental frequency. Thus, with the vocal folds vibrating at a rate of 100 times per second, the composition of the laryngeal buzz would include a 100 Hz component and components that were integral multiples of 100. That is, 100, 200, 300, 400 . . . Hz components would be found in the tone. In addition, the amplitude of the partials or harmonics can be seen to decrease at a rate of about 12 decibels per octave. This is the **source spectrum** generated by the larynx. This is the raw material of which speech is mostly made. The schematic voice-source spectrum shown in Figure 4-116 is in a sense a pictorial representation of the source-filter theory. *The amplitude of its many harmonics decreases uniformly as frequency increases. This represents the source spectrum for our voiced sounds.*

Transfer Function of the Vocal Tract

Of the three factors in the source-filter equation, the acoustical properties of the vocal tract are the most directly related to the perceived differences among speech sounds. We have identified this as the *frequency–selective gain function of vocal tract transmission*, or $|H(f)|$ in our equation, which is also known as the transfer function of the vocal tract.

A **transfer function** is illustrated in Figure 4-117. It shows a quantity X entering, and a quantity Y leaving a box. Y is related to X in accordance with the function placed inside the box. A **resonance curve** is a graphic representation of the transfer function of a resonator. A mass-spring vibrator is shown in Figure 4-118. The upper end of the spring is fastened to a variable speed crank.

If the **mass** M is displaced and then released, it will bob up and down at its natural or **resonant frequency** f. Now let the crank revolve at a frequency f, and if f is varied slowly, the amplitude of **vibration** A of the mass will change and will reach its maximum A_{max} when $f = f_0$. The mass is forced to vibrate at frequency f of the crank, and when $f = f_0$ maximum energy transfer occurs and

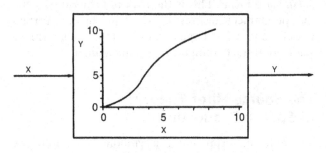

FIGURE 4-117

A graphic representation of a transfer function where Y is related to X according to the transfer function placed inside the box.

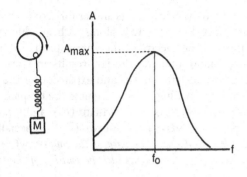

FIGURE 4-118

A mass-spring vibrator that vibrates with maximum amplitude at f_0. When $f = f_0$, maximum energy transfer occurs. The resonant frequency of the mass-spring vibrator is f_0, and the graph on the right represents the transfer function of the mass-spring vibrator.

amplitude reaches its maximum. This is **resonance,** and the graph in Figure 4-118 represents the **transfer function** of the mass-spring vibrator. *Resonance curves of the vocal tract represent its transfer function.*

The Vocal Tract as a Uniform Tube

Measurements of the vocal tract from the glottis to the lips reveal that the configuration approximates that of a uniform tube. That is, the **cross-sectional area** is fairly uniform throughout the length of the vocal tract, which is on the average about 17.5 cm in adult males, 14.7 cm in adult females, and 8.75 cm in very small children.

The fact that our uniform tube has about a 90 degree bend is of no consequence from an acoustical standpoint. This means that we can represent the vocal tract as a uniform tube 17.5 cm in length, closed at one end, as in Figure 4-119. *We must represent the tube as closed at one end because of the high resistance at the glottis compared to virtually no resistance at the lip opening.*

A tube closed at one end will resonate or absorb energy best at a frequency which has a wavelength (λ) four times the length of the tube. For a tube 17.5 cm in length, closed at one end, the wavelength of the first resonant frequency is 70 cm. If we take the velocity of sound to be 340 meters per second (the value near room temperature), the resonant frequency, which is given by the **fundamental wave equation,** is

$$f = \frac{V}{\lambda} = \frac{340 \text{ meters/second}}{70 \text{ centimeters}} = 485.7 \text{ Hz}$$

The first resonant frequency of our model of the vocal tract is 485.7 Hz. *Tubes closed at one end and open at the other resonate at frequencies that are odd-numbered multiples of the lowest resonant frequency.* If we round the first resonant frequency off to 500 Hz, the second resonance

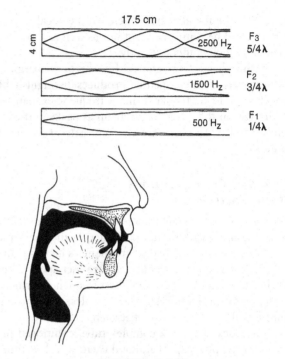

FIGURE 4-119

The vocal tract represented as a tube of uniform cross-sectional area, 17.5 cm in length, and closed at one end. Its first resonant frequency has a wavelength four times the length of the tube, and successive resonant frequencies are odd-numbered multiples of the first.

will have a frequency of 500 × 3, or 1500 Hz, and the third resonance will have a frequency of 500 × 5, or 2500 Hz. Only the first three resonant frequencies need to be specified for any given vowel, although the vocal tract actually has four of five of these resonances, which are called **formants.** Formants correspond to standing waves of air pressure oscillations in the vocal tract.

Formant Frequencies (Resonances)

The closer a particular partial in the source spectrum is in frequency to a formant frequency, the more its amplitude at the lips is increased. If the frequency of a partial in the source is the same as that of a formant frequency, the amplitude radiated at the lips will be maximum.

Suppose, for example, that the glottal tone has a fundamental frequency of 100 Hz. The harmonics in the glottal spectrum will be multiples of 100, and so the fifth harmonic will have a frequency of 500 Hz, the fifteenth will have a frequency of 1500 Hz, and so on. The harmonics in this glottal tone coincide exactly with the formant frequencies of the vocal tract model. If the fundamental frequency were 120 Hz, the fifth harmonic would have a frequency of 600 Hz, the thirteenth a frequency of 1560, and the twenty-first harmonic will have a frequency of 2520 Hz. These frequencies are close enough to the formant frequencies of the vocal tract so they too will be reinforced, but not as well as those frequencies which coincide exactly.

As Sundberg (1977) states, "It is this perturbation of the voice source envelope that produces distinguishable speech sounds: particular formant frequencies manifest themselves in the radiated spectrum as peaks in the envelope, and these peaks are characteristic of particular sounds."

Effects of Configurations of the Vocal Tract

Resonances or formant frequencies are determined by the shape and length of the vocal tract. As the vocal tract is lengthened, all the formant frequencies decrease, and as it is shortened, the frequencies are increased. Thus, we should expect to find the highest frequency formants in children and the lowest in adult males, with those of adult females somewhere in between.

The vocal tract is a complex tube, comprised primarily of the pharyngeal and oral cavities and, at times, the nasal cavities. We know that the vocal tract is capable of resonating to, or reinforcing, some of the partials in the glottal spectrum. *The glottal tone is shaped by the configurations of the vocal tract.* A tracing of a lateral x-ray of a person producing a neutral vowel is shown in Figure 4-120. Also shown are an idealized glottal spectrum, and the spectrum of the glottal tone after it has been shaped by the resonant characteristics of the vocal tract.

Changes in the cross-sectional area of the vocal tract will also shift individual formant frequencies.

Some schematic vocal tracts in various configurations are shown in Figure 4-121, along with graphic representations of the spectra of the vowels produced. Generally speaking, opening the jaw results in vocal tract constriction near the glottis and expansion of the tract at the mouth opening. This influences the frequency location of the lowest or first formant (F_1), and it *tends to rise as the jaw is opened.* Formant two (F_2) is especially *influenced by the shape of the back of the tongue*, while formant three (F_3) is *influenced by the position of the tongue tip.*

The modifications of the vocal tract that are necessary to produce the speech sounds in our repertory are reasonably well documented. For example, phoneticians learned long ago that rather specific tongue positions are associated with production of certain vowel sounds. Because the tongue is so highly variable and makes contact with so many structures in the mouth, adequate descriptions of tongue positions are very difficult. In practice, the configuration of the tongue is described by specifying its gross position during the production of vowels, together with the degree of lip rounding.

Radiation Resistance

To complete our equation for the source-filter theory of speech production, the radiation characteristics at the lips $|R(f)|$, where volume velocity through the lips is converted to a sound pressure pattern (speech), must be considered. Air molecule displacement is greater for high intensity than it is for low intensity sounds, which means that air molecule displacement is greater for the

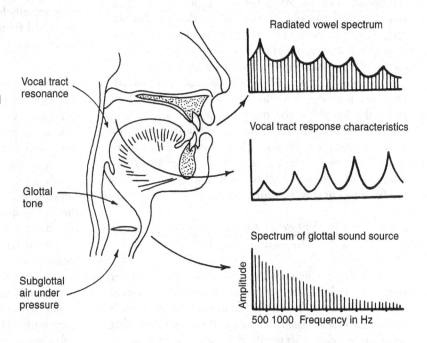

FIGURE 4-120

Schematic tracing of an x-ray of a person producing a neutral vowel; spectrum of glottal sound source and of the vocal tract acoustical response characteristics (transfer function). The radiated vowel spectrum is shown at the top of the figure.

Vocal tract resonance

Glottal tone

Subglottal air under pressure

Radiated vowel spectrum

Vocal tract response characteristics

Spectrum of glottal sound source

Amplitude

500 1000 Frequency in Hz

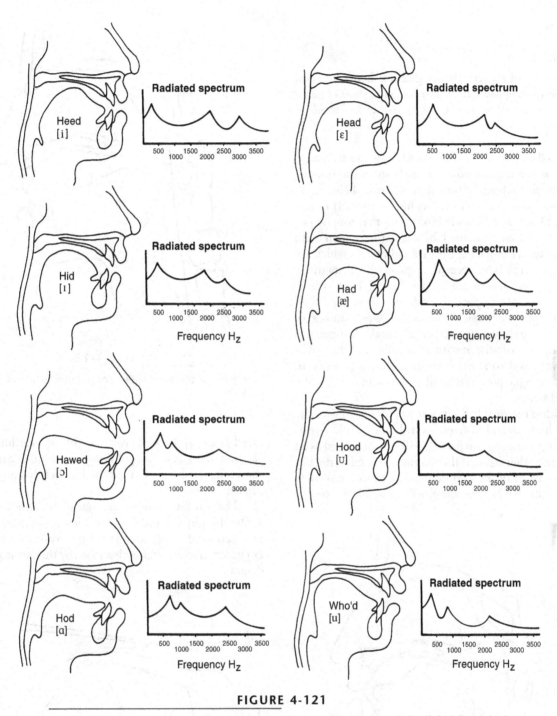

FIGURE 4-121

Partial tracing of x-rays of a subject producing the vowels in the words *heed, hid, head, had, hod, hawed, hood,* and *who'd.* The radiated vowel spectrum is also shown schematically.

low frequency sounds in the glottal spectrum than it is for the high frequency sounds. When the air pressure wave at the lips is radiated, the low frequency–large displacement air molecule movement encounters greater resistance by the air which the pressure wave is exciting than does the high frequency–small displacement air molecule movement. Radiation resistance "favors" high frequencies as opposed to low frequencies at a rate of about 6 decibels per octave. The upshot of radiation resistance is that the original 12 decibel slope of the glottal sound source is reduced to a slope of 6 decibels per octave.

Vowels

Classification

Four aspects of an articulatory gesture shape the vocal tract for vowel production. They are the *point of major constriction, degree of constriction, degree of lip rounding,* and *degree of muscle tension.*

The Cardinal Vowels The position of the tongue is defined as the highest point of the body of the tongue. It is difficult to describe tongue positions as being high, low, front, back, and so forth, without some sort of reference. Denes and Pinson (1963) state that tongue positions are often described by comparing them with positions used for making the cardinal vowels, which are a set of vowels whose perceptual quality is substantially the same regardless of the language used. They constitute *a set of standard reference sounds whose quality is defined independently of any specific language.* X-ray studies of speakers have shown that rather predictable tongue positions can be associated with the qualities of the cardinal vowels, and so it has become common practice to compare tongue positions of all vowels with those of the cardinal vowels.

Within reasonable limits a vowel produced with the tongue high up and in front, as in Figure 4-122 (without the tip touching the palate), will be recognized as an [i]. On the other hand, if the tongue is moved to the opposite extreme of the oral cavity, that is, low and back, as in Figure 4-123, the vowel will probably be recog-

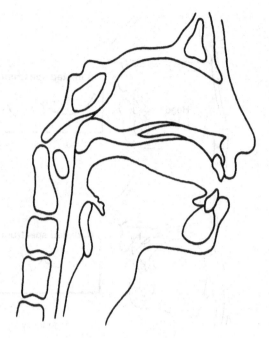

FIGURE 4-123

Schematic of tongue position for the production of the [ɑ] vowel.

nized as an [ɑ]. In all there are eight such cardinal vowels, and their relative physiologic positions are often shown in the form of a cardinal vowel diagram, as in Figure 4-124.

The cardinal vowels are useful because they describe the physiologic limits of tongue position for the production of vowel sounds; all the vowels we produce fall within the boundaries described by the cardinal vowel diagram.

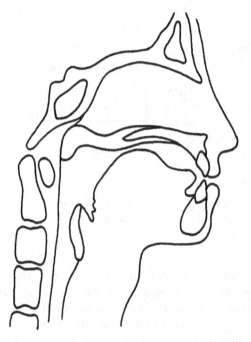

FIGURE 4-122

Schematic of tongue position for the production of the [i] vowel.

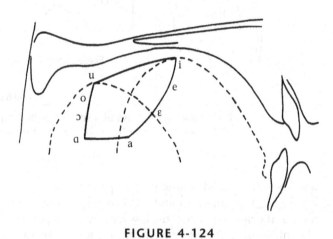

FIGURE 4-124

Relative physiological positions for articulation of the cardinal vowels. Range of vowel articulation is shown in solid line. Close, back, and front tongue shapes are shown in dashed lines.

The Vowel Quadrilateral The traditional vowel triangle—or perhaps better, the vowel quadrilateral—is shown in Figure 4-125. It indicates the articulatory positions of the commonly recognized vowels, in English, relative to the cardinal vowels.

Vowels are also classified according to their positions relative to the palate. In normal production, when the tongue is high and near the palate, the vowel produced is called a **close vowel,** and when the tongue is low, pulled toward the bottom of the oral cavity, the vowel is called **open.** Those sounds produced with the tongue near the center of the vowel quadrilateral are called the **central** or **neutral vowels.**

We can also describe the articulatory position of the tongue as being either toward the front of the oral cavity or toward the back. The [i], for example, is a **close front vowel,** while the [u] is a **close back vowel.** On the other hand, [æ] is an **open front vowel,** while [ɑ] and [ɔ] are **open back vowels.** Lip rounding and degree of muscle tension are also used to classify vowels.

Lip Rounding Certain vowels are produced with the lips in a comparatively spread position. The vowels [i] as in team, [ɪ] as in miss, [ɛ] as in said, and [æ] as in bad are some examples. They can be contrasted with rounded vowels such as [ɔ] as in hawk, [o] as in coat, [ʊ] as in wood, and [u] as in soup.

Muscle Tension In addition, certain vowels seem to require more heightened muscular activity for their production than others, although the mechanisms have yet to be documented. This has given rise to **tense-lax** distinctions, which may serve to differentiate vowels which share almost precisely the same place of constriction, degree of constriction, and lip rounding. The [i] vowel, for example, is classified as a tense vowel, while its physiological or phonetic neighbor [ɪ] is a lax vowel. Pretty much the same holds for the [e] (tense) and [ɛ] (lax), as well as [u] and [ʊ].

Other properties can be associated with the tense-lax feature. One of them is duration. *Tense vowels are longer in duration, and at the same time they are more powerful acoustically than are their lax partners.*

Diphthongs A group of speech sounds very similar to vowels is called the diphthongs. They are sometimes described as blends of two consecutive vowels, spoken within the same syllable. That is, a syllable is initiated with the articulators in the position for one vowel; they then shift with a smooth transition movement toward the position for another vowel. The transition movement may bridge two, three, or even more vowels.

Vowel Articulation

In Figure 4-120, an outline of the configuration of the vocal tract during production of a neutral vowel is shown, and as shown earlier, it can be represented by an equivalent simple resonator model. A graphic representation of the amplitude of the harmonics in the glottal source, as a function of frequency (**glottal spectrum**), is shown to the right of the vocal tract. An **acoustic response curve** illustrating the transfer function of the vocal tract is also shown, and finally, at the top of the illustration is a diagrammatic representation of the **sound spectrum** of the radiated neutral vowel. The **harmonics** in the glottal tone are shown every 125 Hz (which implies a vibratory rate of the vocal folds of 125 Hz). *The radiated vowel spectrum in general has the same shape as the source spectrum, with five notable exceptions:* the **spectral peaks** at 500, 1500, 2500, 3500, and 4500 Hz. They represent the formants of the vocal tract, but in talking about the spectral peaks, we have a tendency to identify them as "formants," which is not entirely correct. *Formants are the property of the vocal tract.* The first formant for any vowel is identified as F_1, the second formant F_2, the third formant F_3, and so on.

The vocal tract does not affect the frequency of the harmonics in the glottal source, but rather it reinforces the amplitudes of those harmonics that coincide or nearly coincide with the natural frequencies of the vocal tract. As a person phonates at different fundamental frequencies while maintaining a constant vocal tract configuration, the distribution of the harmonics in the glottal tone will be altered, but the frequencies of the spectral peaks in the vowel being produced remain the same. *Changes in the source characteristics do not cause changes in the transfer function of the vocal tract.*

Each vowel in our language system is characterized by its own unique energy distribution or spectrum, which is the consequence of the cross-sectional area properties and length of the vocal tract. Changes in the

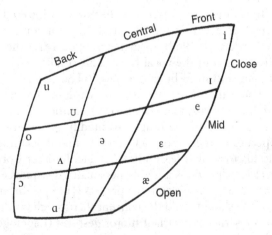

FIGURE 4-125

Tongue positions for English vowels as represented by the vowel quadrilateral.

acoustic properties are mediated by the articulators, and we can, to some extent, predict what will happen to the formant distribution as movements of the articulators take place. The principal articulators for vowel production are the tongue, jaw, and lips, and the length of the vocal tract can be modified by movements of the larynx.

Our simple resonator model will have to become complex if we are to have a repertory of more than one vowel. To change the frequency locations of the formants in our model, different sections of the tube can be given various diameters and lengths. These modifications can represent lip rounding or protrusion, various degrees of vocal tract constriction due to tongue height or position, or changes in mandibular height as shown schematically in Figure 4-126.

There are just three physical parameters that can be manipulated by our articulators: the overall *length of the vocal tract*, the *location of a constriction* along the length of the vocal tract, and the *degree of constriction*.

Length of the Vocal Tract We saw earlier that the first formant frequency will have a wavelength that is four times the length of the tube. This explains why the formant frequencies of an adult female vocal tract are higher than the formant frequencies of an adult male vocal tract. *The frequencies of the formants are inversely proportional to the length of the vocal tract.*

Constrictions of the Vocal Tract Constrictions also affect the frequency of the formants. It is interesting to note that any constriction in the vocal tract will cause F_1 to lower, and the greater the constriction, the more F_1 is lowered. On the other hand, the frequency of F_2 is lowered by a back tongue constriction, and the greater the constriction the more F_2 is lowered.

We begin to see that no single formant can be assigned to any particular region of the vocal tract. That is, we can't say that F_1 "belongs" to the pharynx, F_2 belongs to the oral cavity behind the tongue, and so forth. For example, we have just seen that F_1 will be lowered by any constriction in the vocal tract and that F_2 will be lowered by a back tongue constriction. However, front tongue constrictions will raise the frequency of F_2 while at the same time F_1 will be lowered.

Increasing Length of Vocal Tract The same can be said for the consequences of lip rounding, or depression of the larynx, either of which increases the effective length of the vocal tract, and so all formants are lowered (Lindblom and Sundberg, 1971). Lip protrusion can increase the effective length of the vocal tract by about 1 cm (Fant, 1970; Perkell, 1969), which will cause a decrease in the frequency of F_1 of about 26 Hz. This small shift in frequency can be perceptually significant (Flanagan, 1955).

In addition, the larynx may be raised or lowered by as much as 2 cm during the production of contextual speech (Perkell, 1969), to increase or decrease the effective length of the vocal tract. This results in a concomitant shift in F_1 by as much as 50 Hz.

These motor gestures (lip protrusion, changes in level of the larynx) may accompany "traditional" articulatory gestures of the tongue to modify the acoustical properties of the vocal tract in a way that is seemingly contradictory, or at least unpredictable. In other words, speech production is a highly personalized sequence of events, and to some extent the process is unique for each of us. We should avoid the concept that speech production is a series of invariant motor gestures (Ladefoged, et al., 1972).

Spectrographic Analyses Figure 4-121 shows partial tracings of x-rays of a subject producing the vowels in

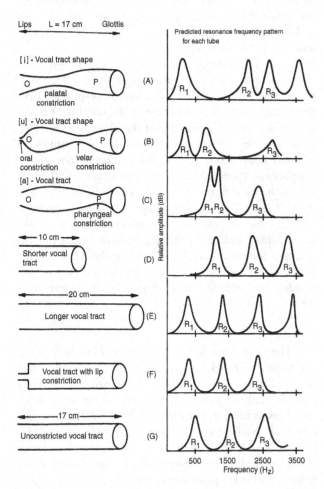

FIGURE 4-126

Formant distribution patterns for vocal tracts that differ in length and constrictions at various places along the vocal tract. (G) shows the formant distribution for a neutral vowel. (From Daniloff, Schuckers, and Feth, *The Physiology of Speech and Hearing: An Introduction,* Prentice Hall, Englewood Cliffs, N.J., 1980.)

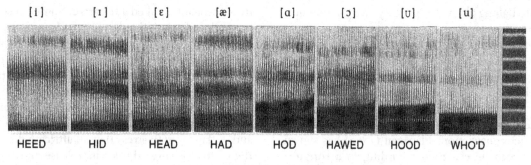

[i]   [ɪ]   [ɛ]   [æ]   [ɑ]   [ɔ]   [ʊ]   [u]

HEED   HID   HEAD   HAD   HOD   HAWED   HOOD   WHO'D

FIGURE 4-127

Excerpts of spectrographic analyses of the vowels in the same word series as in Figure 4-121. The centers of each gray bar on the right are separated by 500 Hz.

the words *heed, hid, head, had, hod, hawed, hood,* and *who'd,* in addition to the spectrum for each of the vowels. Figure 4-127 contains excerpts of spectrographic analyses of the vowels in the same word series. Notice that for the words *heed, hid, head,* and *had,* the frequency of F_1 is rising, while F_2 is lowering. Inspections of the tracings of x-rays in Figure 4-121 reveal the changes in cross-sectional area in the region of the tongue constriction that account for these shifts in formant distribution.

Graphic representations of the relationships between the frequency of the first formant and that of the second formant have been employed to represent certain physiological dimensions in vowel production. In 1948, Joos, as well as Potter and Peterson, demonstrated that when the frequency of the first formant is plotted against the frequency of the second formant, the graph assumes the shape of the conventional vowel diagram but rotated to the right by 45°, as shown in Figure 4-128. Note that the frequency scale is linear below 1000 Hz and logarithmic above 1000 Hz. It approximates the relationship between the frequency of a sound and judgments of pitch (Koenig, 1949). The frequency of the formants is higher for the female than for the male, while the formant frequencies for the child are substantially higher than those of either of the adults. The differences in frequencies do not follow a simple proportionality in overall size of the vocal tract, however. Fant (1973) attributes the disparity to the *ratio of pharyngeal cavity length to oral cavity length,* which tends to be greater in males than in females.

Vowels in General American English Before leaving the topic of vowel production, we should add that the vowels in general American English are normally produced exclusively by vocal fold excitation of the vocal tract. During normal speech the vocal tract is held in a relatively constant configuration while a vowel is being produced. During contextual speech the vowels may lead into consonants or to other vowels, as in diphthongs, so it is not surprising to see short duration transitions or

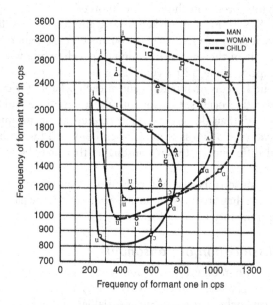

FIGURE 4-128

Loops which resemble the vowel diagram constructed with the frequency of the second formant plotted against the frequency of the first formant for vowels by a man, a woman, and a child. (After Peterson and Barney, 1952.)

formant shifts leading into or out of relatively steady state vocal tract configurations.

Another characteristic of vowels is that they are usually sounded with virtually no coupling between the oral and nasal cavities. Excessive coupling between the vocal tract and nasal cavity will result in nasalized speech sounds, but more about that later.

Consonants

Comparison of Vowels and Consonants

We have been dealing with the consequences of air flow resistance at the level of the larynx and with vowel production. We should also examine some of the consequences of constrictions and airway resistance that can be generated along the vocal tract by the tongue, lips, and jaw movements.

The consonants, which are characterized physiologically by an obstruction of the vocal tract, are often described by place and manner of articulation, and whether they are voiced or unvoiced. Consonants are often said to be the constrictive gestures of speech, but most vowels are also characterized by a certain degree of vocal tract constriction. Flanagan (1965) has shown how vowels can be classified according to a **tongue-hump-position/degree-of-constriction scheme**. In Table 4-5, each vowel is shown with a key word containing the vowel. This is not unlike the **close-open/front-back scheme** described earlier, but the notion that *constriction in the vocal tract is a relative term* requiring interpretation should be reinforced.

Since consonants often initiate and terminate syllables, it is no surprise that consonants comprise about 62 percent of the sounds in running speech, while vowels comprise about 38 percent. This means we can expect about 1.5 consonants to occur in each syllable for each vowel that occurs. Consonants also carry more "information" than do vowels. That is, contrast in meaning between two words is more often conveyed by a minimal difference between consonants than it is between vowels.

Consonants are not only more constrictive than vowels; they are more rapid and account in large part for the transitory nature of speech.

Classification of Consonants

As shown in Figure 4-129, and as can be seen in the consonant classification chart (Table 4-6), **place of articulation** includes use of the lips (labial or bilabial), the gums (alveolar), hard palate (palatal), the soft palate (velar), or the glottis (glottal). **Manner of articulation** describes the degree of constriction as the consonants initiate or terminate a syllable. For example, if closure is complete, the consonant is called a **stop**; if incomplete,

the consonant is called a **fricative.** Some consonants can be produced as sustained sounds and are termed **continuants.** When the complete blockage of air is followed by an audible release of the impounded air, such consonants are sometimes called **plosives.** In other instances complete closure is followed by a rather slow release of the impounded air; a stop is released as a fricative. These consonants, [tʃ] and [dʒ], are called **affricates.** Carrell and Tiffany (1960) stress that an affricate depends upon the shift or change during its release and is not to be thought of as a simple stop-plus-fricative combination.

Other sounds, called **glides,** are produced by rapid movements of an articulator, and the noise element is not as prominent as in stops and fricatives. Examples are [j], [w], and [r]. The **liquids,** [r] and [l], are distinctive consonants because of the unique manner in which the tongue is elevated. The liquid [l] is also called a **lateral** because the breath stream flows more or less freely around the sides of the tongue.

The glides and liquids, because they may be used as either vowels or consonants, are sometimes called **semivowels.** In certain phonetic contexts they may be syllabic and consequently serve as vowels, while in other contexts these sounds either initiate or terminate syllables and therefore function as consonants.

Voiced/Unvoiced Consonants produced with the vocal folds vibrating are called, appropriately, voiced sounds.

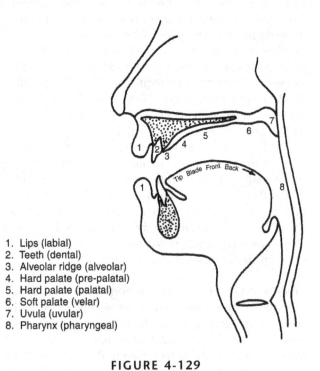

1. Lips (labial)
2. Teeth (dental)
3. Alveolar ridge (alveolar)
4. Hard palate (pre-palatal)
5. Hard palate (palatal)
6. Soft palate (velar)
7. Uvula (uvular)
8. Pharynx (pharyngeal)

FIGURE 4-129

A schematic sagittal section of the head showing articulators and places of articulation.

TABLE 4-5

Vowels

Degree of Constriction	Tongue Hump Position		
	Front	Central	Back
High	[i] eve	[ɝ] bird	[u] boot
	[ɪ] it	[ɚ] over	[ʊ] foot
Medium	[e] hate	[ʌ] up	[o] obey
	[ɛ] met	[ə] alarm	[ɔ] raw*
Low	[æ] at		[ɑ] father

*This vowel could be classified as low-back, as shown in Figure 4-125.

TABLE 4-6

Classification of English consonants by place and manner of articulation

Place of Articulation	Stops		Fricatives		Nasals		Glides and Liquids	
	Voiceless	Voiced	Voiceless	Voiced	Voiceless	Voiced	Voiceless	Voiced
Labial	[p]	[b]				[m]	[hw]	[w]
Labiodental			[f]	[v]				
Dental			[θ]	[ð]				
Alveolar	[t]	[d]	[s]	[z]		[n]		[l]
Palatal	[tʃ]	[dʒ]	[ʃ]	[ʒ]				[j][r]
Velar	[k]	[g]				[ŋ]		
Glottal			[h]					

Their primary excitation source is the larynx, with a secondary constriction somewhere along the vocal tract resulting in noise being generated. Radiation of the sound is from the mouth. If sufficient intraoral pressure is generated so as to result in turbulent air flow, the source is said to be a noise source, and the consonant is unvoiced or voiceless. Often a given articulatory gesture is associated with a pair of consonants that differ only in the voiced-unvoiced feature. Pairs of "related" consonants are called **cognates.** The voiced [b] and unvoiced [p] constitute a cognate pair and the [s] and [z], [f] and [v] are other examples.

Stops Stop consonants are dependent upon complete closure at some point along the vocal tract. With the release of the forces of exhalation, pressure is built up behind the occlusion until the pressure is released very suddenly by an impulsive sort of movement of the articulators. As shown in Table 4-6, articulation for stops normally occurs at the lips in the production of [b] and its voiceless cognate [p], with the tongue against the alveolar ridge for the [d] and [t] pair, and with the tongue against the palate for the cognates [g] and [k].

Production of the stop consonants is very dependent upon the integrity of the speech mechanism. The articulators must be brought into full contact, firmly, to resist the air pressure being generated. The elevation of intraoral pressure requires an adequate velopharyngeal seal, but the air pressures generated during speech production are surprisingly low. In 1967, Arkebauer, Hixon, and Hardy measured intraoral pressures during the production of selected consonants, by means of a polyethylene tube positioned in the oral-pharyngeal cavity. Children as well as adults served as subjects. Intraoral pressure associated with most consonants fell within the 3- to 8-cm H_2O range. In addition, *air pressures for the voiceless consonants were found to be significantly higher than for the voiced consonants.* This, of course, reflects the pressure

drop across the vocal folds, or in other words, the **transglottal pressure differential.**

Voice-Onset-Time (VOT). Contrasting stop consonants as voiced or voiceless is not without its difficulties. Both voiced and voiceless stops are produced with a short interval of complete silence. When stop consonants occur in the middle of a vowel-consonant-vowel (VCV) sequence, a true distinction between the voiced and voiceless categories may be difficult to perceive.

Definition. A phenomenon called voice-onset-time (VOT) may be an important cue for the voiced-voiceless distinction in either a consonant-vowel (CV) or a vowel-consonant-vowel (VCV) environment. *Voice-onset-time is the time interval between the articulatory burst release of the stop consonant and the instant vocal fold vibration begins.* The time interval is measured using the **instant of burst release** as the reference (**t = O**). This means laryngeal pulsing prior to the burst release results in **negative VOT,** while pulsing after the release gives us a **positive VOT** value, as illustrated in Figure 4-130. Generally speaking, if VOT is 25 msec or more, the phoneme will be perceived as **voiceless.** If VOT is less than about 20 msec, it is perceived as **voiced** (Stevens and Klatt, 1974). Some voiced stops are produced with **prevoicing** or negative VOT values (Figure 4-130). The critical VOT value lies between 20 and 25 msec for the distinction between voiced and voiceless consonants, which suggests that VOT is not the only cue for distinction. Research has shown that VOT increases as place of articulation moves from alveolar to velar.

Hoit et al. (1993) found VOT to be dependent on lung volume. VOT was longer at high lung volume and shorter at low lung volume in most cases. Their findings point out the need to take lung volume into account when using VOT as an index of laryngeal behavior.

Universality. Voice-onset-time, as a perceptual cue, seems to be a nearly universal linguistic phenomenon.

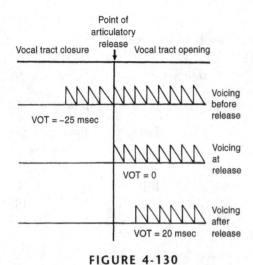

FIGURE 4-130

Schematic illustration of voice-onset-time. At the top, voicing begins 25 msec before burst release of the consonant and so it has a negative VOT of 25 msec. In the middle, voicing begins at the moment of consonant release, and it has a VOT of 0. At the bottom, voicing begins 20 msec after the consonant release, and it has a VOT of +20 msec.

Lisker and Abramson (1964) found that voice-onset-time was an adequate cue for a voiced-voiceless distinction in eleven different languages. The authors also found that voice-onset-time was sensitive to place of articulation. Velars, for example, had consistently longer VOT values that did labials and apicals.

Other Aspects of Voicing Distinction. Even the early investigators of voice-onset-time, however, realized that voicing distinction may not be made solely on the basis of the time interval between burst release and voice onset (Klatt, 1975). The implication is that other acoustical aspects of the complex feature of voicing onset should be considered.

When the glottis remains open after the release of a burst there is an aperiodic excitation of supraglottal cavities so that noise is generated. In other words, voiceless consonants are **aspirated.** In English, at least, when voicing is present, aspiration is not, and when aspiration is present, voicing is normally absent. This may be an important cue (Winitz, et al., 1975).

Another acoustic feature thought to be a perceptual cue is the presence (or absence) of formant transitions. For a voiced stop there is a well-defined rapid transition of the formants, after the onset of voicing (Stevens and Klatt, 1974). For a voiceless stop, however, the formant transitions have been completed before voice onset takes place.

Pitch change in a vowel may also influence the perception of the preceding consonant as voiced or voiceless (Haggard, et al., 1970).

Interestingly, though, newborn infants seem to be able to distinguish between voiced and voiceless con-

sonants, obviously without having acquired language (Eimas, 1976), and this has led to the hypothesis that humans are born with linguistic feature detectors (Eimas and Corbit, 1973).

Fricatives Fricatives are generated by a *noise excitation* of the vocal tract. The noise is generated at some constriction along the vocal tract. Five common points or regions of constriction for the production of fricative consonants are used in the English language, and except for the [h] consonant, which is generated at the glottis, all voiced fricatives have **voiceless cognates.** Place and manner of articulation of the fricative consonants, along with key words, are shown in Table 4-7.

Glides and Liquids Glides and liquids are characterized by voicing, radiation from the mouth, and a lack of nasal coupling. These sounds almost always precede vowels, and they are very vowel-like, except that they are generated with more vocal tract constriction than are the vowels. Place of articulation for glides and liquids is shown in Table 4-8.

Nasals The three nasal consonants, [m], [n], and [ŋ], are produced by excitation from the vibrating vocal folds. They are voiced, but at the same time complete constriction of the vocal tract by the lips, by the tongue at the alveolar ridge, or by the dorsum of the tongue against the hard and/or soft palate takes place. The nasopharyngeal port is opened wide so the transmission

TABLE 4-7

Fricative consonants

Place of Articulation	Voiced	Unvoiced
Labiodental	[v] vote	[f] far
Dental	[ð] then	[θ] thin
Alveolar	[z] zoo	[s] see
Palatal	[ʒ] beige	[ʃ] she
Glottal		[h] how

TABLE 4-8

Glides and liquids

Place of Articulation	Voiced
Palatal	[j] you
Labial	[w] we
Palatal	[r] red
Alveolar	[l] let

pathway is the nasal cavity complex. This means that *most of the sound radiation is from the nostrils.*

This complex articulatory gesture results in an increase in the overall length of the vocal tract, which will lower the frequencies of all the formants. On the other hand, because of the tortuous acoustic pathway through the nasal cavities, and the fact that now two acoustic resonance systems are acted upon by the glottal impulse, rather than just one, the amplitudes of the resonances are reduced somewhat. In addition, because of the interaction between the nasal cavities and the vocal tract, the resonances are not so well defined as they are for nonnasal vowel production. A schematic diagram of the vocal apparatus is shown in Figure 4-131. For the production of the nasal consonants, the soft palate is fully lowered so the oral and nasal cavities become resonant systems that are operating in parallel. In the case of the [m], a bilabial nasal consonant, and [n], an alveolar nasal consonant, the size of the oral cavity behind the constriction is acoustically significant. The effect is to increase the length of the acoustic tube, and a lowering of F_1 (mostly) takes place. In fact, for the nasals, the frequency of F_1 is usually below 250 Hz.

When the oral cavity constriction is near the velum as in the [ŋ], the effect of the oral cavity "shunt" is minimal, so the resonator consists of just the pharyngeal and nasal cavities. The formant distribution for the [ŋ] is not very different from that of vowels. The formants

have less amplitude and, as stated earlier, are less well defined than those of vowels, but because of the increased effective length of the resonating system, F_1 is found at about 250 Hz, F_2 at 1000, and F_3 at 2000 Hz.

As shown in Figure 4-131, the lowered velum results in two resonant systems that are placed side by side. In other words, two parallel resonant systems, each with substantially different configurations, are excited by the same glottal sound source. One of the consequences of the interaction of the two parallel systems is that the formants usually associated with vowel production are substantially modified in frequency and amplitude, and formants normally found in one or the other system simply don't appear in the radiated spectrum. It is tempting to think that formants fail to materialize because the acoustic energy is absorbed by the complex acoustical pathway of the nasal cavities, but this is simply not the case. These changes are sometimes attributed to a phenomenon called **antiresonance,** which is a consequence of the interaction between the two parallel acoustical systems. A discussion of antiresonances is beyond the intended scope of this textbook; the interested reader will have to turn to Chiba and Kajiyama (1958), Flanagan (1965), and Fant (1970).

Antiresonances often occur when a single excitatory source is coupled to two parallel acoustical systems as in Figure 4-131, or when a single resonant system is excited at some place other than at either end. Vowels are normally produced with glottal excitation, and they can be specified by just their formants. Consonants, including the nasal consonants, on the other hand, are produced with excitation somewhere along the length of the vocal tract, and acoustically, the result is two parallel resonant systems, similar to those shown schematically in Figure 4-131. Consonants are therefore specified by both formants (resonances) and by antiresonances.

Specification For many years the place and manner of articulation of speech sounds have been studied by means of repeated careful introspection and critical observation of the speech mechanism. The classifications that evolved usually represented idealized articulations during the production of idealized sounds, often produced in isolation. Variations were known to occur, due to individual speech habits and to the influences of immediately adjacent sounds during continuous speech, but the variations were difficult to quantify or specify. One reason for the difficulty is the rate of production of speech sounds. Most of the syllables we utter are fairly simple combinations of consonants and vowels. About 75 percent of all the syllables used in speech are either CVC, CV, or VC combinations, and we utter about 5 syllables per second in conversational speech. This means we generate about 12.5 phonemes per second. It is difficult to track physiological events that rapid.

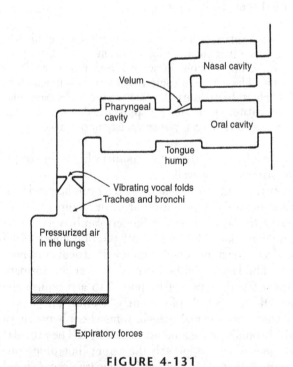

FIGURE 4-131

Schematic diagram of the functional components of the vocal tract. The soft palate is lowered to couple the nasal cavity, the pharyngeal, and oral cavities. (Modified after Flanagan, 1965.)

Some Aspects of Contextual Speech

Speech is the most elegant of serially ordered and complex neuromotor behavior humans are capable of producing. Acquired very early in life, speech largely determines our ability to later read and write.

It is tempting, at first, to explain contextual speech as a sequential production of speech sounds, where each sound follows another as independent entities. True, this is largely the type of serially ordered neuromotor behavior that takes place when we write, but it cannot be applied to contextual speech because individual speech sounds, produced in isolation, would have no contextual identity with adjacent speech sounds. Try, for example, to say the phrase, *his speech*, by producing the isolated [h] followed by the vowel [ɪ] and finally [z], and then attempt to put these sounds together like beads on a string. What happens to the [s] in the word *speech*? This is a task that is physically impossible. How do we do it? How do we arrange our motor gestures so that one sound *blends* into the next, and so that the production of one sound is the logical consequence of its predecessor?

If "beads on a string" will not work, we might seek an explanation through the use of a **stimulus-response** model, in which serially generated gestures are temporally ordered by means of a chain of reflexes. The production of one speech element elicits a reflexive response which leads to the production of the next element, as illustrated in Figure 4-132. The response is in the form of **kinesthetic feedback** (awareness of movement), and it leads to the successive sound. A stimulus-response model doesn't differ very much from "beads on a string." For example, the articulatory gesture for the final [p] is not exactly the same as it is for the initial [p]. In addition, a motor gesture that produces one particular sound is not inevitably followed by a single specific sound. Thus, [p] can be followed by [r], [l], and the entire vowel repertory. While stimulus-response behavior undoubtedly plays a

role in contextual speech production, there must be some other factor or factors that are responsible for the serially ordered and temporally appropriate sequence of sounds we call speech. One factor is that we have a very complex and elaborate cerebral cortex covering our otherwise primitive brain.

When we listen to contextual speech, it becomes apparent that what we hear is not a series of discrete phonemes, but rather, a *stream of speech sounds*.

Targets

The purpose of speaking is to generate a stream of speech sounds that produce purposeful consequences. The target is the production of the correct sounds. Achievement of this target requires that the respiratory target is adequate for the laryngeal and articulatory requirements, that the laryngeal target is adequate for the articulatory target, and that the articulatory target meets the criteria for a correct sound. Traditionally, we have regarded the articulatory gestures that produce speech sounds in isolation as the gestures that set the standard for articulation during contextual speech. It would be difficult to generate a substantial argument in defense of these articulatory targets. What we hear as properly produced sounds, either in isolation or contextual speech is really the criterion. It is possible for more than one combination of articulatory gestures to produce vocal tract configurations that have the same auditory effect. As Lindau et al. (1972) state,

> What a speaker aims at in vowel production, his target, is a particular configuration in an acoustic space where the relations between formants play a crucial role. The nature of some vowel targets is much more likely to be auditory than articulatory. The particular articulatory mechanism a speaker makes use of to attain a vowel target is of secondary importance only.

And we might add, the same argument holds for consonant articulation as well.

At times the same auditory effect can be produced by articulatory compensation or be due simply to individual articulatory behavior. Singers can be very expert at compensation. The open mouth position singers often use places constraints on "traditional" articulatory postures. The larynx can be lowered to decrease formant frequencies, the lips can be pursed to accomplish the same effect, or a little of each may be effective.

During contextual speech, somewhere between 10 and 15 sounds per second are articulated. The articulatory gesture may approach the target, but time constraints do not allow the ideal target (the same sound produced in isolation) to be attained. The articulators may undershoot or overshoot the ideal target. If the auditory target is reached, however, the criteria have been

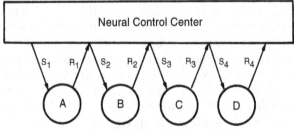

S = command to produce sound (stimulus)
R = kinesthetic feedback (response)
A, B, C, D = successive speech sounds

FIGURE 4-132

A stimulus-response model of speech production in which the articulatory gesture of one sound elicits a response that produces the next sound. (Based on Daniloff, et al., 1980.)

met. *A near miss is good enough if it works.* Targets, then, are both auditory and articulatory.

Phonetics and Phonemics

Phonetics is essentially taxonomy (classification according to natural relationships), in which speech sounds are described and classified relative to the cardinal vowels, or place and manner of articulation. **Phonemes,** on the other hand, are abstract sound units that convey or impart **semantic differences.** The words "bill," "pill," "till," "dill," "kill," "gill" all mean something different because of the initial phonemes. The meanings of all these words can also be changed by adding an [s] to their endings. Not all differences in sounds result in changes in the meaning of a word, however. A vowel can be short or long, or nasalized, and "bill" is still "bill." Speech sounds produced in approximately the same way and which do not have phonemic significance are called **allophones** of the phoneme.

Segmental Features

We have explored the articulation of vowels and consonants, and in grade school we learned that a syllable is one or more speech sounds constituting an uninterrupted unit of utterance. A syllable can form a whole word (boy) or part of a word (A-mer-i-ca). Speech sounds are also called **segments.** Thus, vowels, consonants, and syllables are composed of the following segmental features:

List of Segment-Type Features (Fant, 1973)

Feature Number	Feature
	Source Features
1	voice
2	noise
3	transient
	Resonator Features
4	occlusive
5	fricative
6	lateral
7	nasal
8	vowellike
9	transitional

In one and the same sound segment, it is possible to find almost any combination of these segmental-type features. Features are a useful means of viewing the contrast between speech as beads on a string and speech as a continuous succession of gradually varying and overlapping patterns. Figure 4-133 illustrates various concepts. From the top,

A) A sequence of ideal nonoverlapping phonemes (beads on a string).

B) A sequence of minimal sound segments, the boundaries of which are defined by relatively distinct changes in the speech wave structure.

FIGURE 4-133

Schematic representation of sequential elements of speech. (A) The ideal phoneme sequence (beads on a string). (B) and (C) Acoustic aspects. (D) The degree of phoneme-sound correlation. (From Fant, 1973.)

A

B

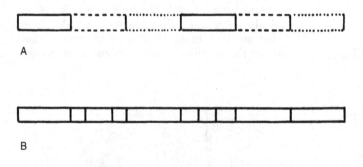

C

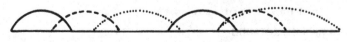

D

C) One or more of the sound features characterizing a sound segment may extend over several segments.

D) A continuously varying importance function for each phoneme describing the extent of its dependency on particular events within the speech wave. Overlapping curves without sharp boundaries. (From Fant, 1973.)

From Figure 4-133 we see that the number of successive sound segments within an utterance is greater than the number of phonemes. Fant says,

> Sound segments may be decomposed into a number of simultaneously present sound features. Boundaries between sound segments are due to the beginning or end of at least one of the sound features but one and the same sound feature may extend over several successive sound segments. A common example would be the continuity of vocal cord vibrations over a series of voiced sounds.

Suprasegmental Elements

Extending across speech segments are the suprasegmental elements which consist of the prosodic features of pitch, loudness, and duration. They impart stress, intonation, and inflection to speech. Prosodic features are important in conveying emotion, and even meaning to speech. For example, you can change the emotional content and the meaning of the sentence, "I don't want it," by stressing different words and varying inflectional patterns. These features are called suprasegmental because they often extend past segmental boundaries.

Transitions

When we examine sequences of sounds as they occur in contextual speech, the role of the consonants seems to be to interrupt the vowels in an utterance. That is, the consonants seem to permit vowels to be "turned on and off," and the very nature of consonant articulation will influence the vowel-shaping gestures that immediately precede and follow consonants. One of the consequences of this consonant articulation is that what we tend to think of as relatively steady-state vowel articulation is in reality characterized by **formant transitions,** which reflect articulation into and out of consonants. Formant transitions are also characteristic of diphthongs, as can be seen in Figure 4-134. The first and second formants, especially, reflect the movement of the articulators in the production of "Roy was a riot in leotards." *The shifts of the first formant reflect the manner of articulation* (where the tongue produces the vocal tract constriction) and *the shifts of the second formant reflect the place of articulation,* which is important in recognition of plosive consonants.

The spectrograms in Figure 4-135 illustrate this latter point. Here, a vowel-consonant (VC) is shown. As the vowel approaches the plosive consonant the second formant "bends" toward the **burst frequency** that is characteristic of the consonant. For the production of [b] or [p], the second formant of the vowel [ɑ] bends toward the burst frequency of those consonants, approximately 1000 Hz. Whereas for [t] or [d], the second formant bends toward a burst frequency of about 2000 Hz.

Formant transitions of the vowel provide a cue for the perception of the consonant. The significance of these transitions has been recognized by Fant (1973) and others. Fant states,

> The time-variation of the F-pattern across one or several adjacent sounds, which may be referred to as the F-formant transitions, are often important auditory cues for the identification of a consonant supplement-

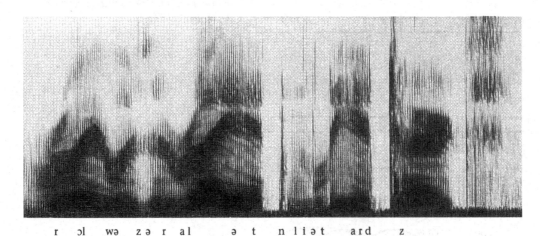

r   ɔɪ   wə   zə   r   aɪ   ə   t   n   liə   t   ard   z

ROY WAS A RIOT IN LEOTARDS

FIGURE 4-134

Spectrogram of the phrase *Roy was a riot in leotards* illustrating the diphthongs that occur.

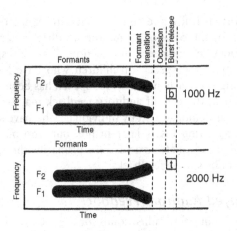

FIGURE 4-135

Schematic spectrograms of a VC in which a vowel is followed by the [b] or [p], where the second formant "bends" toward the burst frequency of the consonant that is located at about 1000 Hz (top) and in which the vowel is followed by the consonants [t] or [d]. Here, the second formant bends toward the burst frequency of the consonant that is located at about 2000 Hz (bottom).

ing the cues inherent in the composition of the sound segments traditionally assigned to the consonant.

Coarticulation

Coarticulation or **assimilation** occurs when two or more speech sounds overlap in such a way that their articulatory gestures occur simultaneously. In the word *class*, the [l] of the cluster [kl] is usually completely articulated before the release of the plosive. We overlap our articulatory gestures, and while one sound is being produced, the articulators are getting "set" to produce the next sound. This, of course, results in a large number of allophonic variations that listeners may not even perceive.

CLINICAL NOTE: When producing consonant clusters, particularly those beginning with stops, very young children may articulate both consonants correctly but the consonants may not be fully coarticulated, for example, the word *blue* may resemble the word *balloon* minus the [n]. Such a variance, though not unusual for a young child, should be noted because future evidence of improved coarticulation may indicate that speech is still maturing. Also, an articulation test or phonological exam should provide an exact record of what the examiner heard, whether or not it was considered significant at the time of testing.

During production of the word *heed*, the lips are somewhat retracted, while in production of the word *who'd*, the lips are pursed, even before the [h] is sounded. Coarticulation is one reason why our "beads on a string"

speech production model is so unsatisfactory. Our idealized articulation and their targets are corrupted by the production of the preceding and successive sounds. This means articulatory overlap can be **anticipatory** (right to left, RL) or **carryover** (left to right, LR), as shown in Figure 4-136. In either instance, RL or LR, the articulatory targets must he compromised in order to facilitate smooth transitions from one sound to the next, and this is the nature of human speech.

Coarticulation is, by the very nature of the rapidity of speech sound production, a necessary component of speech physiology and is one reason that human-machine communication systems have been so difficult to develop.

CLINICAL NOTE: The complexity of coarticulation also explains why integration (or carryover) of newly acquired sounds into conversational speech outside of the therapy session is often such a stumbling block in articulation therapy. It may be that we expect too much too soon. Unless these sounds can be produced rapidly, with absolutely smooth RL and LR transitions in all phonetic environments, attempts to use them will interrupt the natural flow of contextual speech.

Coarticulation is sometimes described as the spreading of features. This means that features such as voicing,

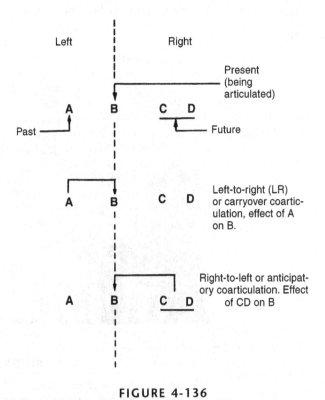

FIGURE 4-136

Illustration of right-left and left-right coarticulation.

nasalization, place and manner of articulation, can all be coarticulated, although *manner of articulation is the least resilient of the features.* Modifications in manner of articulation usually produce a phonemic distinction rather than an allophonic variation.

Coarticulation often occurs with *nasality.* When a vowel precedes a nasal consonant, the soft palate has been seen to lower during the vowel production, and it too is nasalized. This feature (nasality) may spread over two, three, or more vowels preceding the nasal consonant.

Coarticulation also occurs in *voicing.* In the word *Baja* [bɑhɑ], for example, the [h], which is traditionally classified as a voiceless consonant, is almost completely voiced in most contextual speech. Said slowly, however, the [h] is indeed voiceless. This is illustrated in the spectrograms of Figure 4-137.

The Role of Feedback in Speech Production

Auditory Feedback

It is very difficult to say something in the way it is intended to be said, without hearing what is being said, while it is being said. As was shown in Figure 1-34, auditory feedback is a principal avenue by which we monitor our speech production. Control of speech is often likened to a **servo-system,** in which sensors sample the output of a system, and compare it with the input. The difference (error signal) is used to correct the input so that the output is what it is supposed to be. This is shown

as **mutual influence** and **feedback** in Figure 1-34. Almost any interruption of auditory feedback will result in degradation of speech production. This is especially evident in the speech of children who have lost their hearing very early in life. Once speech has been well established, the role of auditory feedback may be diminished, as demonstrated by individuals who have suffered severe hearing losses later in life, but who manage to maintain adequate articulation, primarily through the use of kinesthetic feedback.

Delayed Auditory Feedback

It takes but a few milliseconds for the speech sounds we generate to reach our ears. A number of experiments conducted in the early 1950s used a modified tape recorder in addition to headphones through which the subject listened while speaking. The tape recorder delayed the input to the ears of the subject by about 200 msec. The system, called delayed auditory feedback, produces profound speech degradation for most people. Speech becomes hesitant, slurred, and repetitive (much like stuttering), and the prosodic features suffer dramatically. Timing and inflections are inappropriate, and extremely difficult to accommodate to delayed auditory feedback. The effects can be heard even after a subject has had hours of practice trying to "beat the system."

Motor Feedback

There is also interaction between the motor and other sensory modalities, which although mostly unconscious,

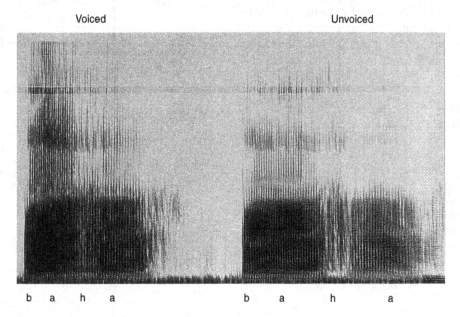

Voiced   Unvoiced

b   a   h   a   b   a   h   a

FIGURE 4-137

An example of coarticulation of voicing during the production of the word Baja [baha], which is almost completely voiced. When said slowly, the [h] in Baja is unvoiced as shown in the right spectrogram.

control our entire speech production mechanism. Muscles, tendons, and mucous membrane have elaborate and sensitive stretch, pressure, tactile, and other receptors that deliver information about the extent of movements, degree of muscle tension, speed of movement, and much more. This information is returned to the brain and spinal cord where it is integrated into serially ordered neural commands for the muscles of speech (and locomotor) mechanisms. These receptors are for the most part very quick to adapt. That is, they send information only while movement is taking place. Once a structure has gotten to where it is supposed to go, we needn't be reminded where it is. In Figure 4-138, a lower motor (efferent) neuron transmits an impulse (Nl) to a muscle, which then contracts. This muscle movement stimulates a receptor (R), and it transmits information to the **comparator** by way of an afferent (sensory) neuron. At the same time, information about the initial neural impulse has also been transmitted to the comparator, which weighs the difference between the afferent and efferent neural impulses. Comparator output then transmits "compensatory information" back to the lower motor neuron.

Facilitation of Compensatory Movement

One important role of the feedback mechanism is to facilitate compensation in the event of disease or disorder. If an anesthetic is applied to the oral cavity (in the case of a bilateral mandibular block in the dentist's office, for example), there is a loss of tactile and stretch receptor feedback, along with a loss of pain. Although speech remains intelligible, articulatory exactness and timing suffer, not unlike the speech of someone who has overindulged in alcohol.

In 1976 Abbs et al. reported that when muscle spindle feedback from the mandibular muscles was disrupted, jaw movements were delayed and were often undershot. Again, in 1975, Folkins and Abbs demonstrated that when the jaw was suddenly restrained during articulation of [p], the lips were able to compensate, and bilabial closure occurred in 20 to 30 msec.

To more fully appreciate the neural control of speech production we should become acquainted with the nervous system, the subject of Chapter 5.

BIBLIOGRAPHY AND READING LIST

Abbs, J., and B. Gilbert, "A Strain Gauge Transduction System for Lip and Jaw Motion in Two Dimensions: Design Criteria and Calibration Data," *J. Sp. Hrng. Res.*, 16, 1973, 248–256.

————, J. Folkins, and M. Sivarjan, "Motor Impairment Following Blockade of the Infraorbital Nerve: Implications for the Use of Anesthetization Techniques in Speech Research," *J. Sp. Hrng. Res.*, 19, 1976, 19–35.

Abramson, A. S., and L. Lisker, "Voice Onset Time in Stop Consonants," in Haskins Laboratories, *Status Report on Speech Research*, SR-3. New York: Haskins Laboratories, 3, 1965, 1–17.

Amerman, J., "A Maximum-Force-Dependent Protocol for Assessing Labial Force Control," *J. Sp. Hrng. Res.*, 36, 1993, 460–465.

Amerman, J., R. Daniloff, and K. Moll, "Lip and Jaw Coarticulation for the Phoneme /æ/," *J. Sp. Hrng. Res.*, 13, 1970, 147–161.

Angle, E. H., "Classification of Malocclusion," *Dental Cosmos*, 41, 1899, 248–264, 350–357.

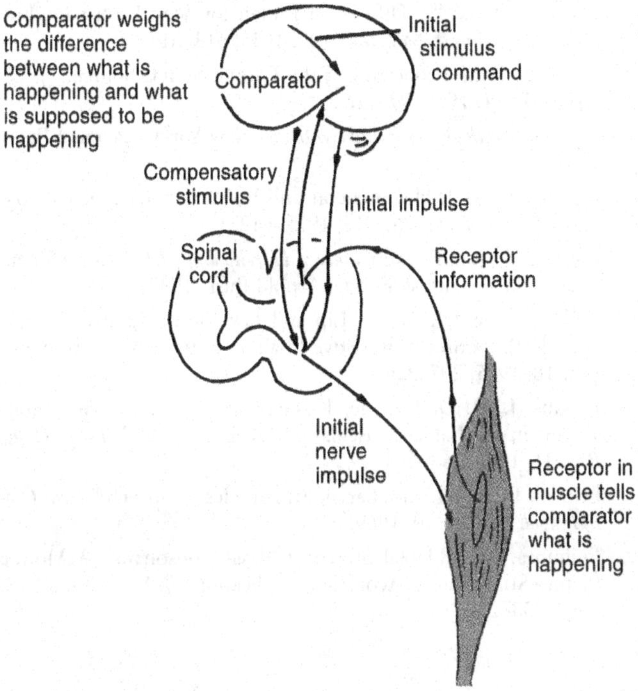

FIGURE 4-138

Schematic of a feedback system in which a comparator (the brain), weighs the difference between the input signal to a muscle and output signal generated by the contraction of the muscle.

Ardran, G., and F. Kemp, "The Mechanism of the Larynx, Part II: The Epiglottis and Closure of the Larynx," *Brit. Jour. Rad.*, 40, 1967, 372–389.

Ardran, G., and F. Kemp, "The Protection of the Laryngeal Airway During Swallowing," *Brit. Jour. Rad.*, 25, 1952, 406–416.

Ardran, G., and F. Kemp, "The Mechanism of Swallowing," *Proc. of the Royal Soc. of Med.*, 44, 1951, 1038–1040.

Arey, L., *Developmental Anatomy: A Textbook and Laboratory Manual of Embryology.* Philadelphia: W. B. Saunders, 1966.

Arkebauer, H., T. Hixon, and J. Hardy, "Peak Intraoral Air Pressures During Speech," *J. Sp. Hrng. Res.*, 10, 1967, 196–208.

Barclay, J. R., "Noncategorical Perception of a Voiced Stop: A Replication," *Perception and Psychophysics*, 11, 1972, 269–273.

Barlow, S., and J. Abbs, "Force Transducers for the Evaluation of Labial, Lingual, and Mandibular Motor Impairments," *J. Sp. Hrng. Res.*, 26, 1983, 616–621.

Barlow, S., and R. Netsell, "Differential Fine Force Control of the Upper and Lower Lips," *J. Sp. Hrng. Dis.*, 29, 1986, 163–169.

Bell-Berti, F., "An Electromyographic Study of Velopharyngeal Function in Speech," *J. Sp. Hrng. Res.*, 19, 1976, 225–240.

Blair, C., "Interdigitating Muscle Fibers Throughout Orbicularis Oris Inferior: Preliminary Observations," *J. Sp. Hrng. Res.*, 29, 1986, 266–269.

Blair, C., and A. Smith, "EMG Recording in Human Lip Muscles: Can Single Muscles Be Isolated?" *J. Sp. Hrng. Res.*, 29, 1986, 256–266.

Blakiston's New Gould Medical Dictionary, 5th ed. New York: McGraw-Hill, 1941.

Bloomer, H. H., "A Palatopograph for Contour Mapping of the Palate," *J. Amer. Dent. Assn.*, 30, 1943, 1053–1057.

———, "Observations of Palatopharyngeal Movements in Speech and Deglutition," *J. Sp. Hrng. Dis.*, 18, 1953, 230–246.

Broadbent, B. H., "Roentgenographic Method of Measuring Biometric Relations of the Face and Cranium," White House Conference on Child Health and Protection, 1930, Report of Committee A, Growth and Development, Sect. 1, p. 23.

———, "New X-ray Technique and Its Application to Orthodontia," *Angle Orthod.*, 1, 1931, 45.

———, "The Face of the Normal Child," *Angle Orthod.*, 7, 1937, 209.

Brodie, A. G., "Some Recent Observations on the Growth of the Face and Their Implications to the Orthodontist," *Amer. J. Orthod. and Oral Surg.*, 26, 1940, 741.

———, "On the Growth Pattern of the Human Head from the Third Month to the Eighth Year of Life," *Amer. J. Anat.*, 89, 1941, 209.

Brodnitz, F. S., *Vocal Rehabilitation.* Rochester, Minn.: Whiting Press, 1959.

Calnan, J., "The Error of Gustaf Passavant," *Plastic and Reconstruct. Surg.*, 13, 1954, 275–289.

Carrell, J., and W. Tiffany, *Phonetics: Theory and Application to Speech Improvement.* New York: McGraw-Hill, 1960.

Cates, H., and J. V. Basmajian, *Primary Anatomy.* Baltimore: Williams & Wilkins, 1955.

Chiba, T., and M. Kajiyama, *The Vowel—Its Nature and Structure.* Tokyo: Phonetic Soc. of Japan, 1958.

Clemente, C., *Anatomy—A Regional Atlas of the Human Body.* Philadelphia: Lea & Febiger, 1975.

Cooper, F. S., "Research Techniques and Instrumentation: EMG," *Proceedings of the Conference: Communicative Problems in Cleft Palate*, ASHA Report No. 1, 1965, 153–168.

Cooper, W. E., "Selective Adaptation for Acoustic Cues of Voicing in Initial Stops," *J. Phonetics*, 2, 1974, 303–313.

Costen, J., "A Syndrome of Ear and Sinus Symptoms Dependent upon Disturbed Function of the Temporomandibular Joint," *Ann. Otol., Rhin., Laryng.*, 43, 1934, 1–15.

Crane, E., and G. Ramstrum, "A Classification of Palates," unpublished Master's thesis, University of Michigan, Ann Arbor, 1943.

Daniloff, R., G. Schuckers, and L. Feth, *The Physiology of Speech and Hearing: An Introduction.* Englewood Cliffs, N.J.: Prentice-Hall, 1980.

Denes, P., and E. Pinson, *The Speech Chain.* Baltimore: Waverly Press, 1963.

DeWeese, D., and W. Saunders, *Textbook of Otolaryngology*, 4th ed. St. Louis: C. V. Mosby, 1973.

Dickson, D., and W. Dickson, "Velopharyngeal Anatomy," *J. Sp. Hrng. Res.*, 15, 1972, 372–382.

———, and W. Maue, *Human Vocal Anatomy.* Springfield, Ill.: Charles C Thomas, 1970.

Eimas, P. D., "Speech Perception in Early Infancy," in L. B. Cohen and P. Salapatek, eds., *Infant Perception.* New York: Academic Press, 1976.

———, and J. D. Corbit, "Selective Adaptation of Linguistic Feature Detectors," *Cognitive Psychology*, 4, 1973, 99–109.

———, W. E. Cooper, and J. D. Corbit, "Some Properties of Linguistic Feature Detectors," *Perception and Psychophysics*, 13, 1973, 247–252.

Ettema, S., and D. Kuehn, "A Quantitative Histological Study of the Normal Human Soft Palate," *J. Sp. Hrng. Res.*, 37, 1994, 303–313.

Fant, G., *Acoustic Theory of Speech Production*, The Hague: Mouton, 1970.

———, *Speech Sounds and Features*, Cambridge, Mass.: M.I.T. Press, 1973.

Flanagan, J. L., "A Difference Limen for Vowel Formant Frequency," *J. Acoust. Soc. Amer.*, 27, 1955, 613–617.

———, "Some Properties of the Glottal Sound Source," *J. Sp. Hrng. Dis.*, 1, 1958, 99–116.

———, *Speech Analysis and Synthesis.* New York: Academic Press, 1965.

Fletcher, S., M. J. McCutcheon, and M. Wolf, "Dynamic Palatography," *J. Sp. Hrng. Res.*, 18, 1975, 812.

Fogh-Anderson, P., *Inheritance of Harelip and Cleft Palate.* Copenhagen: NYT Norkisk Forlag, Arnold Busk, 1942.

Folkins, J., and J. Abbs, "Lip and Jaw Motor Control During Speech: Responses to Resistive Loading of the Jaw," *J. Sp. Hrng. Res.*, 18, 1975, 207–220.

Folkins, J., R. D. Linville, K. Garrett, and C. Brown, "Interactions in the Labial Musculature During Speech," *J. Sp. Hrng. Res.*, 31, 1988, 253–264.

Fritzell, B., "The Velopharyngeal Muscles in Speech," *Acta Oto-Laryngol.* Suppl, 250, 1969, 5–81.

Fujimura, O., "Bilabial Stop and Nasal Consonants: A Motion Picture Study and Its Acoustical Implication," *J. Sp. Hrng. Res.*, 4, 1961, 233–247.

————, S. Kiritani, and H. Ishida, "Computer-Controlled Radiography for Observation of Movements of Articulatory and Other Human Organs," *Comput. Biol. Med.*, 3, 1973, 371–384.

Gay, T., "Effect of Speaking Rate on Diphthong Formant Movements," *J. Acoust. Soc. Amer.*, 44, 1968, 1570–1573.

Goffman, L., and A. Smith, "Motor Unit Territories in the Human Perioral Muscles," *J. Sp. Hrng. Res.*, 37, 1994, 975–984.

Gray, H., *The Anatomy of the Human Body*, 29th ed., C. M. Goss, ed. Philadelphia: Lea & Febiger, 1973.

Hagerty, R. F., and M. J. Hill, "Pharyngeal Wall and Palatal Movement in Post-Operative Cleft Palates and Normal Palates," *J. Sp. Hrng. Res.*, 3, 1960, 59–66.

————, H. S. Pettit, and J. J. Kane, "Posterior Pharyngeal Wall Movement in Adults," *J. Sp. Hrng. Res.*, 1, 1958, 203–210.

Haggard, M., S. Ambler, and M. Callow, "Pitch as a Voicing Cue," *J. Acoust. Soc. Amer.*, 47, 1970, 613–617.

Hardcastle, W., "The Use of Electropalatography in Phonetic Research," *Phonetica*, 25, 1972, 197–215.

————, "Instrumental Investigations of Lingual Activity During Speech: A Survey," *Phonetica*, 29, 1974, 129–157.

————, *Physiology of Speech Production*. London: Academic Press, 1976.

Hardy, J. C., "Air Flow and Air Pressure Studies," *Proceedings of the Conference: Communicative Problems in Cleft Palate*, ASHA Report No. 1, 1965, 14–152.

Harrington, R., "A Study of the Mechanism of Velopharyngeal Closure," *J. Sp. Dis.*, 9, 1944, 325–344.

Hawkins, C., and W. Swisher, "Evaluation of a Real Time Ultrasound Scanner in Assessing Lateral Pharyngeal Wall Motion During Speech," *Cleft Palate J.*, 15, 1978, 161–166.

Hoit, J., N. Solomon, and T. Hixon, Effect of Lung Volume on Voice Onset Time (VOT)," *J. Sp. Hrng. Res.*, 36, 1993, 516–521.

Hoit, J., P. Watson, T. Hixon, P. McMahon, and C. Johnson, "Age and Velopharyngeal Function During Speech Production," *J. Sp. Hrng. Res.*, 37, 1994, 295–302.

Holbrook, R. T., and F. J. Carmody, "X-ray Studies of Speech Articulations," *University of California Publications in Modern Philology*, 20, 1937, 187–238.

Hudgins, C. V., and R. H. Stetson, "Relative Speed of Articulatory Movements," *Arch. Neerl. Phon. Exper.*, 13, 1937, 85–94.

Hutchinson, J., K. Robinson, and M. Herbonne, "Patterns of Nasalance in a Sample of Normal Geronotologic Speakers," *J. Comm. Dis.*, 11, 1978, 469–481.

Joos, M., "Acoustic Phonetics," *Language*, 24, Suppl., 1948, 1–136.

Kaplan, H. M., *Anatomy and Physiology of Speech*. New York: McGraw-Hill, 1960.

Keaster, J., "Studies in the Anatomy and Physiology of the Tongue," *Laryngoscope*, 1940, 222–257.

Keefe, M., and R. Dalton, "An Analysis of Velopharyngeal Timing in Normal Adult Speakers Using a Microcomputer Based Photodetector System," *J. Sp. Hrng. Res.*, 32, 1989, 39–48.

Kelly, J., and L. B. Higley, "A Contribution to the X-ray Study of Tongue Position in Certain Vowels," *Archives of Speech*, 1, 1934, 84–95.

King, E. W., "A Roentgenographic Study of Pharyngeal Growth," *Angle Orthod.*, 22, 1952, 23.

Kiritani, S., "Articulatory Studies by the X-ray Microbeam System," in M. Sawashima and F. S. Cooper, eds., *Dynamic Aspects of Speech Production*. Tokyo: University of Tokyo Press, 1977.

Klatt, D., "Voice Onset Time, Frication, and Aspiration in Word-Initial Consonant Clusters," *J. Sp. Hrng. Res.*, 18, 1975, 686–706.

Koenig, W., "A New Frequency Scale for Acoustic Measurements," *Bell Laboratories Record*, 27, 1949, 299–301.

Kuehn, D., "A Cineradiographic Investigation of Velar Movement Variables in Two Normals," *Cleft Pal. Jour.*, 13, 1976, 88–103.

Kuehn, D., and J. Moon, "Levator Veli Palatini Muscle Activity in Relation to Intraoral Air Pressure Variation," *J. Sp. Hrng. Res.*, 37, 1994, 1260–1270.

Kuehn, D., and N. Azzam, "Anatomical Characteristics of Palatoglossus and the Anterior Faucial Pillar," *Cleft Palate Jour.*, 15, 1978, 349.

Ladefoged, P., J. DeClerk, M. Lindau, and G. Papcun, "An Auditory Motor Theory of Speech Production," UCLA Phonetics Laboratory, *Working Papers in Phonetics*, 22, 1972, 48–76.

Liberman, A. M., K. S. Harris, P. D. Eimas, L. Lisker, and J. Bastian, "An Effect of Learning on Speech Perception: The Discrimination of Durations of Silence with and Without Phonetic Significance," *Language and Speech*, 4, 1961, 175–195.

————, K. S. Harris, J. A. Kinney, and H. Lane, "The Discrimination of Relative Onset Time of the Components of Certain Speech and Nonspeech Patterns," *J. Exp. Psych.*, 61, 1961, 379–388.

Lieberman, P., *Intonation, Perception, and Language*. Research Monograph No. 38. Cambridge, Mass.: M.I.T. Press, 1967.

Lindau, M., L. Jacobson, and P. Ladefoged, "The Feature Advanced Tongue Root," UCLA Phonetics Laboratory, *Working Papers in Phonetics*, 22, 1972, 48–76.

Lindblom, B., and J. Sundberg, "Acoustical Consequences of Lip, Tongue, Jaw, and Larynx Movement," *J. Acoust. Soc. Amer.*, 50, 1971, 1166–1179.

Lisker, L., "Closure Duration and the Intervocalic Voiced-Voiceless Distinction in English," *Language*, 33, 1957, 42–49.

————, and A. S. Abramson, "A Cross-Language Study of Voicing in Initial Stops: Acoustical Measurements," *Word*, 20, 1964, 384–422.

————, and A. S. Abramson, "Some Effects of Context on Voice Onset Time in English Stops," *Language and Speech*, 10, 1970, 1–28.

Lubker, J., and K. May, "Palatoglossus Function in Normal Speech Production," *Papers from the Institute of Linguistics*, University of Stockholm, 17, 1973, 17–26.

————, B. Fritzell, and J. Lindquist, "Velopharyngeal Function: An Electromyographic Study," Speech Transmission Lab., Royal Institute of Technology (KTH) QPR, 4, 1970, 9–20.

Lundstrom, A., *Introduction to Orthodontics*. New York: McGraw-Hill, 1960.

MacNeilage, P. F., and G. N. Sholes, "In Electromyographic Study of the Tongue During Speech Production," *J. Sp. Hrng. Res.*, 7, 1964, 209–232.

Martone, A. L., "The Phenomenon of Function in Complete Denture Prosthodontics," a collection of reprints from *J. Prosthet. Dent.* St. Louis: C. V. Mosby, 1963.

Mason, R., "Preventing Speech Disorders Following Adenoidectomy by Preoperative Evaluation," *Clinical Pediatrics*, 12, 1973, 405–414.

Massler, M., and E. Schour, *Atlas of the Mouth*. Chicago: American Dental Assn., 1958.

Mattingly, I. G., A. M. Liberman, A. K. Syrdal, and T. Halwes, "Discrimination in Speech and Nonspeech Modes," *Cognitive Psychology*, 1971, 131–157.

McClean, M., "Lip Muscle EMG Responses to Oral Pressure Stimulation," *J. Sp. Hrng. Res.*, 34, 1991, 248–251.

Minifie, F., T. Hixon, C. Kelsey, and R. Woodhouse, "Lateral Pharyngeal Wall Movement During Speech Production," *J. Sp. Hrng. Res.*, 13, 1970, 584–594.

Moll, K. L., "Velopharyngeal Closure on Vowels," *J. Sp. Hrng. Res.*, 5, 1962, 30–37.

———, "Photographic and Radiographic Procedures in Speech Research," *Proceedings of Conference: Communicative Problems in Cleft Palate*, ASHA Report No. 1, 1965, 129–139.

———, and R. Daniloff, "An Investigation of the Timing of Velar Movements During Speech," *J. Acoust. Soc. Amer.*, 50, 1971, 678–684.

Moller, K., R. Martin, and R. Christiansen, "A Technique for Recording Velar Movement," *Cleft Palate J.*, 8, 1971, 263–276.

Moore, C., "Symmetry of Mandibular Muscle Activity as an Index of Coordinative Strategy," *J. Sp. Hrng. Res.*, 36, 1993, 1145–1157.

Moore, C., A. Smith, and R. Ringel, "Task-Specific Organization of Activity in Human Jaw Muscles," *J. Sp. Hrng. Res.*, 31, 1988, 670–680.

Müller, E., and J. Abbs, "Strain Gauge Transduction of Lip and Jaw Motion in the Midsagittal Plane: Refinement of a Prototype System," *J. Acoust. Soc. Amer.*, 65, 1979, 481–486.

Nishimura, H., R. Semba, T. Tanimura, and O. Tanaka, *Prenatal Development of the Human with Special Reference to Craniofacial Structures: An Atlas*. Bethesda, Md.: U.S. Department of Health, Education, and Welfare, National Institutes of Health, 1977.

Orban, B. J., *Oral Histology and Embryology*, 4th ed. St. Louis: C. V. Mosby, 1957.

Osborne, G., S. Pruzansky, and H. Koepp-Baker, "Upper Cervical Spine Anomalies and Osseous Nasopharyngeal Depth," *J. Sp. Hrng. Res.*, 14, 1971, 14–22.

Palmer, J. M., "A Continuous Recording Technique for the Palatograph," Paper presented at Chicago, Ill., 1964 ASHA Convention.

———, and D. A. LaRusso, *Anatomy for Speech and Hearing*. New York: Harper & Row, 1965.

Passavant, G., *Ueber die Verschliessung des Schlundes beim Sprechen*. Frankfort a. M.: J. D. Sauerländer, 1863.

———, "Ueber die Verschliessung des Schlundes beim Sprechen," *Archiv. fur. Pathol. Anat. u. Physiol.*, 46, 1869, 1.

Patten, B., *Human Embryology*. Philadelphia: Blakiston, 1946.

———, "The Normal Development of the Facial Region," in S. Pruzansky, ed. *Congenital Anomalies of the Face and Associated Structures*, Springfield, Ill.: Charles C Thomas, 1961.

Perkell, J., *Physiology of Speech Production: Results and Implications of a Quantitative Cineradiographic Study*. Cambridge, Mass.: M.I.T. Press, 1969.

Perlman, A., and H. Liang, "Frequency Response of the Fourcin Electroglottograph and Measurement of Temporal Aspects of Laryngeal Movement during Swallowing," *J. Sp. Hrng. Res.*, 34, 1991, 791–795.

Perlman, A., E. Luschei, and C. Dumond, "Electrical Activity from the Superior Pharyngeal Constrictor During Reflexive and Nonreflexive Tasks," *J. Sp. Hrng. Res.*, 32, 1989, 749–754.

Perlman, A., D. Van Daele, and M. Otterbacher, "Quantitative Assessment of Hyoig Bone Displacement from Video Images During Swallowing," *J. Sp. Hrng. Res.*, 38, 1995, 579–585.

Perrier, P., L. J. Roe, and R. Sock, "Vocal Tract Area Function Estimation from Midsagittal Dimensions with CT Scans and a Vocal Tract Cast: Modeling the Transition with Two Sets of Coefficients," *J. Sp. Hrng. Res.*, 35, 1992, 53–67.

Peterson, G., and H. Barney, "Control Methods Used in a Study of the Vowels," *J. Acoust. Soc. Amer.*, 24, 1952, 175–184.

Pisoni, D. B., and J. H. Lazarus, "Categorical and Noncategorical Modes of Speech Perception Along the Voicing Continuum," *J. Acoust. Soc. Amer.*, 55, 1974, 328–333.

Potter, R., and G. Peterson, "The Representation of Vowels and Their Movements," *J. Acoust. Soc. Amer.*, 20, 1948, 528–535.

Proffit, W., J. Palmer, and W. Kydd, "Evaluation of Tongue Pressure During Speech," *Folia Phoniat.*, 17, 1965, 115–128.

Pruzansky, S., ed., *Congenital Anomalies of the Face and Associated Structures*. Springfield, Ill.: Charles C Thomas, 1961.

Raphael, L. J., "Preceding Vowel Duration as a Cue to the Perception of the Voicing Characteristics of Word-Final Consonants in American English," *J. Acoust. Soc. Amer.*, 51, 1972, 1269–1303.

———, M. F. Dorman, and F. Freeman, "Vowel and Nasal Duration as Cues to Voicing in Word-Final Stop Consonants: Spectrographic and Perceptual Studies," *J. Sp. Hrng. Res.*, 18, 1975, 389–400.

Robin, D., A. Goel, L. Somodi, and E. Luschei, "Tongue Strength and Endurance: Relation to Highly Skilled Movements," *J. Sp. Hrng. Res.*, 35, 1992, 1239–1245.

Russell, G. O., *The Vowel*. Columbus: Ohio State University Press, 1928.

Sawashima, M., "Current Instrumentation and Techniques for Observing Speech Organs," *Technocrat*, 9, 1976, 19–26.

Schwartz, L., "A Temporomandibular Joint Pain–Dysfunction Syndrome," *J. Chronic Dis.*, 3, 1956, 284–293.

Sicher, H., "The Growth of the Mandible," *J. of Periodontia*, 16, 1945, 87–93.

———, *Oral Anatomy*. St. Louis: C. V. Mosby, 1949.

———, and E. L. DuBrul, *Oral Anatomy*, 6th ed. St. Louis: C. V. Mosby, 1975.

———, and J. Tandler, *Anatomie für Zahnartze*. Vienna and Berlin: Springer, 1928.

Skolnick, M., J. Zagzebski, and K. Watkin, "Two-Dimensional Ultrasonic Demonstration of Lateral Pharyngeal Wall Movement in Real Time—A Preliminary Report," *Cleft Palate J.*, 12, 1975, 299–303.

Stevens, K. N., and D. H. Klatt, "Role of Formant Transitions in the Voiced-Voiceless Distinction for Stops," *J. Acoust. Soc. Amer.*, 55, 1974, 653–659.

Subtelny, J. D., "A Cephalometric Study of the Growth of the Soft Palate," *Plastic and Reconstructive Surg.*, 19, No. 1. 1957, 49–62.

———, and H. Koepp-Baker, "The Significance of Adenoid Tissue in Velopharyngeal Function," *Plastic and Reconstructive Surg.*, 12, 1956, 235–250.

Summerfield, A. Q., and M. P. Haggard, "Perceptual Processing of Multiple Cues and Contexts: Effects of Following Vowel upon Stop Consonant Voicing," *J. Phonetics*, 2, 1974, 279–295.

Sundberg, J., "Acoustics of the Singing Voice," *Scientific American*, 236, March 1977.

Swanson, C. P., *The Cell*, 2nd ed. Englewood Cliffs, N.J.: Prentice-Hall, 1964.

Trevino, S. N., and C. E. Parmenter, "Vowel Positions as Shown by X-ray," *QJS*, 17, 1932, 351–369.

Weber, C., and A. Smith, "Reflex Responses in Human Jaw, Lip and Tongue Muscles Elicited by Mechanical Stimulation," *J. Sp. Hrng. Res.*, 30, 1987, 70–79.

Willis, R. H., *A Cephalometric Study of Size Relationships of the Normal Male Soft Palate*, Master's thesis in dentistry, Department of Orthodontia, University of Washington, Seattle 1952.

Winitz, H., C. LaRiviere, and E. Herriman, "Variations in VOT for English Initial Stops," *J. of Phonetics*, 3, 1975, 41–52.

Zemlin, W., and C. Czapar, "The Platysma Muscle," Paper presented at 1974 ASHA Convention, Detroit.

———, and S. Stolpe, *The Structure of the Human Skull*. Champaign, Ill.: Stipes, 1967.

Zlatin, M. A., and R. A. Koenigsknecht, "Development of the Voicing Contrast: Perception of Stop Consonants," *J. Sp. Hrng. Res.*, 18, 1975, 541–553.

The Nervous System

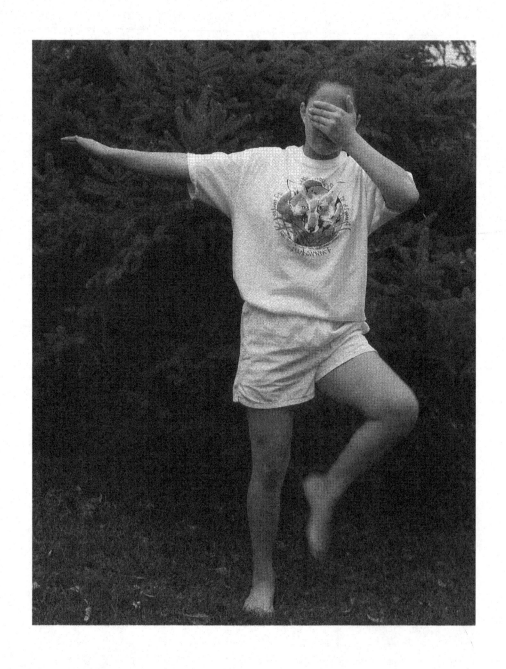

INTRODUCTION

Virtually all of our behavior, the observable as well as the unobservable, is, in the final analysis, mediated by the nervous system. The nervous system is incomprehensively complex, being composed of billions of highly specialized cells called **neurons** (Gk. nerves). Estimates of the number of neurons in the nervous system vary from 10 billion to over a 100 billion, each of which may "connect" with as many as 1,000 to 100,000 other neurons. A neuron is unique because its response to a stimulus results in a short-duration change of state, which in turn can act as a stimulus for adjacent nerve and muscle cells.

Some of our behavior, however, is not so directly under the control of the nervous system; changes in body and blood chemistry may also result in modifications of our behavior. These changes often are the result of the secretions of the glandular system, in particular the **endocrine system** (Gk. *endon*, within + *krinein*, to separate) or, in other words, secreting internally.

The nervous and endocrine systems are usually regarded as two separate systems. Functionally, however, they have far more in common than we might realize. Certain endocrine glands, for example, stem from the same embryonic tissue that gives rise to the nervous system. Together the endocrine and nervous systems constitute a highly integrated behavior-controlling mechanism that is responsible for almost all that we do.

Very grossly, the internal activities such as the life processes are regulated to a large degree by the endocrine system, while the observable behavior is mediated by the nervous system. We may also say that the nervous system is responsible for quick actions, while the endocrine system functions in producing much slower reactions that may extend over some period of time.

Simple animals living in their uncomplicated environments do not require a complex nervous system, as is evident from the simple nerve net of the hydra. Larger animals, composed of a larger number of cells, make more frequent and complex adaptations to their environments, so they require increasingly complex nervous systems. Even in the lowly planaria, for example, there is a well-defined anterior brain, with large lateral nerves coursing caudally. Size of an animal, however, should not be equated directly with the complexity or size of its nervous system. An adult human with a weight of about 180 pounds will have a brain that weighs about 3 pounds (1360 grams), while a full-sized bull moose, weighing about 1600 pounds, has a brain that weighs less than a pound and will fit snugly into the palm of your hand.

Among some of the higher invertebrates and all of the vertebrates, the network of nerve fibers, in spite of its complexity, has proven inadequate in some respects, and a supplementary endocrine system has evolved. In this system, specific chemical agents, released either directly or indirectly into the blood, circulate to various parts of the body where they produce a specific effect of comparatively long duration. Because the endocrine system is so closely linked with the nervous system, this chapter will conclude with a brief description of the endocrine glands and some of their effects.

But, even before we embark on our study of the nervous system, a host of questions surface, awaiting answers. Neuroscientists have the same questions, and others, which are unanswered. How or why did the brain evolve? What changes take place in the brain when we learn, or forget something? Is my brain *me*? Why do we have a "right" and a "left" brain, and to what extent do they have exclusive functions? Can the brain ever understand itself? Why does the brain "destroy" itself in some people? How does the brain produce its own pain killers for the body? What is consciousness?

TOOLS OF THE TRADE

A number of investigative techniques and tools are at the disposal of the neuroscientist. One of the most frequently used is the **microscope** and an associated camera. Microscopy dates back to 1647, when Leewenheck observed neural tissue with a simple lens. The introductions of alcohol (Reil, 1809) and chromic acid (Hannover, 1844) as tissue hardeners were important advances in improving the morphological integrity of sectioned tissue. In 1842, Stilling and Wallack devised a primitive **microtome** for cutting sections of tissue. Subsequent introductions of imbedding media such as paraffin wax, collodion, and celloidin marked the beginning of histology as we know it today. Diverse staining techniques proved invaluable for observing various aspects of the same tissue. Some stains revealed the nucleus of a neuron, others the soma or cell body, and still others revealed just the protoplasmic extensions of the nerve cell body.

Initially the light microscope was the standard optical device. Improvements include fluorescent microscopy, electron microscopy, dark field, polarized light, and interference microscopy combined with photography, including time lapse.

Clinical neurologists have been able to relate selective lesions to subsequent behavior. Noninvasive radiographic imaging such as x-ray, magnetic resonance imaging, nuclear magnetic resonance, positron emission tomography, single photon emission, and computed tomography all have enabled the contemporary neuroscientist to visualize certain aspects of the astronomical complexity of the nervous system. Neural transplant techniques and tissue culture are valuable research techniques, as are embryology and comparative physiology. The very early research on the axon, for example, was conducted on the squid.

Early researchers have left their names as monuments to their contributions. They include Reil (1807), Remak (1836), Purkinje (1837), Kuhn (1862), Deiters (1865), Ranvier (1871), Golgi (1871), Ramón y Cajal (1908), and Nissl (1892), all of whom are historically recorded as pioneers in neurology.

GENERAL ORGANIZATION OF THE NERVOUS SYSTEM

The fibers and cells that make up the nervous system are distributed unevenly throughout the body. The brain contains billions of neurons and nerve fibers, while the ear lobe has but a few sensory fibers. It is difficult to discuss the nervous system as it really is—a single, highly integrated behavior-regulating system. With the realization that no single element of the nervous system can be justifiably treated in isolation from the remainder of the nervous system, we can divide it into individual subsystems, at least for descriptive purposes. Here again, however, we may encounter difficulties. Some of our divisions may be made on an anatomical basis, while others may be made on a functional basis. With these potential hazards in mind, let us proceed.

Divisions of the Nervous System

On a functional basis almost all of the neurons in the nervous system can be categorized as either **somatic** or **autonomic.**

Somatic neurons are those involved either with the production of observable events or with the reception of environmental events and changes. **Autonomic neurons,** on the other hand, are involved chiefly with life processes, such as those that occur in the viscera, blood vessels, and glands, and they are often referred to as the unconscious activities of the body. Broadly speaking, *somatic fibers are involved in voluntary activities,* while *autonomic fibers are involved with involuntary activities.* Even at birth the autonomic nervous system is sufficiently developed to maintain a healthy internal environment. Heart and respiratory rates are carefully regulated, digestion proceeds on schedule, and all of the other internal affairs of the body go on, with absolutely no thought on the part of the host.

The autonomic (self-controlling) nervous system is aptly named. Also from a *functional standpoint,* neurons or their processes can be classified either as **efferent** (conducting away from the neuron cell body or from the central nervous system) or **afferent** (conducting toward the neuron cell body or toward the central nervous system).

On an *anatomical basis* we can divide the entire nervous system into the central and peripheral nervous systems. The **central nervous system** is that part which is surrounded and protected by the cranial bones and the vertebral column and consists of the brain and spinal cord. The **peripheral nervous system** can be divided into the cranial and spinal nerves, plus their peripheral combinations, and the autonomic nervous system. The **autonomic system,** in turn, can be subdivided into the **sympathetic** (thoracolumbar) and **parasympathetic** (craniosacral) systems. The divisions of the nervous system are shown in Figure 5-1.

Neurons, Nerves, and Nerve Tracts

The basic functional unit of the nervous system is a highly specialized cell known as a neuron. It includes a **cell body** and all of its extensions or **nerve processes,** of which there are essentially two types: (1) **dendrites** (Gk. tree), being *afferent,* conduct nerve impulses toward the cell body, and (2) **axons** (Gk. axis), being *efferent,* conduct nerve impulses away from the cell body.

We rarely discuss individual neurons or their components in functional neuroanatomy or neurophysiology. Rather, we discuss **nerves** which are typically composed of *bundles of axons and/or dendrites from numerous neurons.* **Sensory nerves** are exclusively afferent, **motor nerves** are exclusively efferent, and **mixed nerves,** as you might

---

FIGURE 5-1

The divisions of the nervous system.

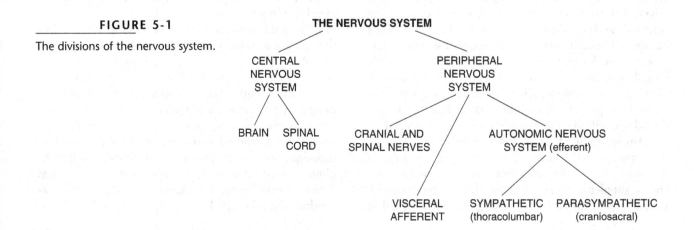

expect, are comprised of both afferent and efferent nerve processes.

Bundles of axons or dendrites in the peripheral nervous system are called nerves, but, in the central nervous system, these bundles are called nerve tracts. A **nerve** typically is composed of axons and dendrites that have a variety of functions, such as reporting pain, temperature, muscle tension, limb movement, limb position, or delivering motor impulses to muscles. **Nerve tracts** are composed of groups of axons or dendrites that have but one, very specific function.

The Synapse

One of the most important aspects of the functioning nervous system is the way in which neural impulses get from one part of the body to another. The initial neural impulse is an electrical-chemical wave that is propagated much like a burning train of gunpowder, as illustrated in Figure 5-2. Note the discontinuity in the gunpowder train between "neurons." It represents an actual space (microscopic), called the **synaptic cleft,** between two neurons in a chain. As the gunpowder reaches its termination, the small mound at the very end burns vigorously, generating heat that ignites the mound of gunpowder in the subsequent or adjacent **(postsynaptic)** "neuron." There has been a *transmission* of the "burning impulse," but *without an actual physical continuity of tissues* at the neural synapse (Gk. *synapsis,* contact).

Neural synapses permit the impulse to travel in just one direction, and here is where the gunpowder model begins

to break down. It would be a simple matter to add something to the "presynaptic" mound of gunpowder to cause it to burn a little more vigorously and in the process facilitate the transmission of the burning impulse. We could also place a shield or barrier between the two mounds to inhibit the transmission of the impulse. One of the remarkable features of *neural tissue* is that it *is capable of manufacturing its own chemical agents to inhibit or facilitate neural transmission*. About 30 types of **neurotransmitters** have been discovered, many of them in just recent years. Some are excitatory, some inhibitory, which means that neural transmission can be influenced by drugs that have properties similar to neurotransmitters, and much of what is known about the nervous system has been learned in just this way.

The Central Nervous System

The Brain

In even the most primitive forms of vertebrate animals the central nervous system consists of a hollow spinal cord which is expanded in the head region into that structure we call the brain. The term brain is from an old Anglo-Saxon word *braegen*, which means the center of the nervous system. In Greek, however, the word *enkephalos* pertains to the mass of nerve tissue housed within the bony confines of the head.

The brain, in a sense, is *an enlargement of the spinal cord*. It is not segmented functionally the way the spinal cord is, however, and it is a highly specialized part of the nervous system, responsible for those higher-level functions that make us human—the ability to reason and to use a complex language system. As shown in Figure 5-3,

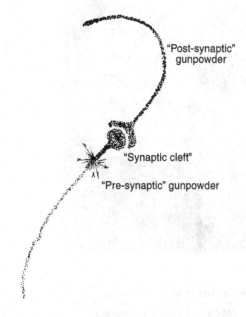

"Post-synaptic" gunpowder

"Synaptic cleft"

"Pre-synaptic" gunpowder

FIGURE 5-2

Gunpowder analogy illustrating propagation of neural impulse and transmission of the impulse across the synaptic cleft.

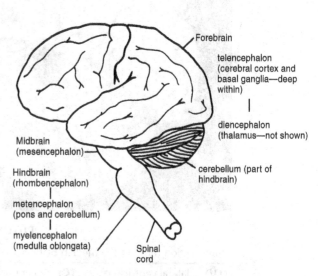

Forebrain

telencephalon (cerebral cortex and basal ganglia—deep within)

diencephalon (thalamus—not shown)

Midbrain (mesencephalon)

Hindbrain (rhombencephalon)

metencephalon (pons and cerebellum)

myelencephalon (medulla oblongata)

cerebellum (part of hindbrain)

Spinal cord

FIGURE 5-3

The major divisions of the brain: the hindbrain (rhombencephalon), the midbrain (mesencephalon), and the forebrain (telencephalon and diencephalon).

the brain can be divided into a **hindbrain, midbrain,** and **forebrain.**

Hindbrain The hindbrain is also known as the **rhombencephalon,** a term that describes its shape (Gk. *rhombos,* a spinning top). The rhombencephalon in turn is divided into a **metencephalon** (Gk. *meta,* after + *enkephalos,* brain) and a **myelencephalon** (Gk. *myelos,* marrow). In the adult the myelencephalon, an enlarged region where the spinal cord merges into the brain, is called the **medulla oblongata,**[1] (Figure 5-3). The fluid-filled central canal of the spinal cord also enlarges in the hindbrain, where it is known as the **fourth ventricle.**

The upper or rostral portion of the hindbrain is called the **metencephalon.** The prominent dorsal region of the metencephalon is formed by the **cerebellum** (little brain), while ventrally the metencephalon is an upward continuation of the medulla oblongata called the **pons.** It is aptly named because it functions as a bridge to join the two hemispheres of the cerebellum

and to connect the cerebellum with the cerebrum and with the spinal cord. The cerebellum, a heavily convoluted structure, is an important integrating center for coordinated regulation of limb movement, balance, and posture. Like the cerebrum or forebrain, the cerebellum is composed of a **cortex** (L. bark, shell) of *gray matter* and an **interior** of *white matter* and *gray nuclei.*

Midbrain The midbrain, also called the **mesencephalon** (Gk. *mesos,* middle), is essentially a connecting link between the forebrain and hindbrain. It also contains some important nuclei instrumental in regulating and coordinating movements. The fluid-filled cavity of the mesencephalon is called the **cerebral aqueduct.** It connects the fourth ventricle of the hindbrain with the ventricles of the forebrain.

Forebrain The forebrain can be divided into the **diencephalon** and the **telencephalon.** The structures that constitute the diencephalon are located lateral to the third ventricle (shown in Figure 5-4). The thickened lateral walls of the diencephalon are formed by the thalamus (Gk. *thalamos,* inner chamber) and by the hypothalamus. The **thalamus** is a principal relay and integration center

---

[1]**Medulla** is a general anatomical term used to designate the middle or innermost portion of an organ or structure.

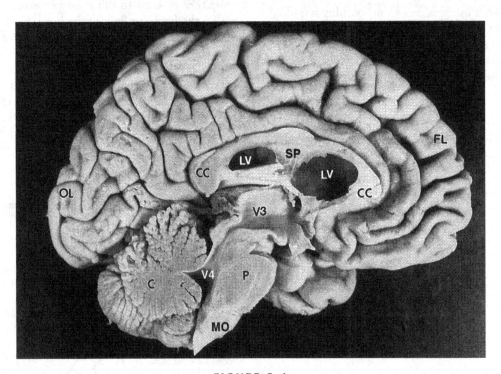

FIGURE 5-4

Brain section through the median plane showing ventricles and associated structures.

(LV)	lateral ventricle	**(C)**	cerebellum	**(MO)**	medulla oblongata
(V3)	third ventricle	**(CC)**	corpus callosum	**(OL)**	occipital lobe
(V4)	fourth ventricle	**(FL)**	frontal lobe	**(P)**	pons
(SP)	septum pellucidum				

The major structures of the diencephalon are located lateral (deep) to the third ventricle.

for sensory information delivered to the telencephalon. The **hypothalamus** consists of a number of nuclei that influence and control visceral activities, water balance, temperature, sleep, and metabolic functions, among other things.

The **telencephalon** (Gk. *telos*, far off, at a distance) is the largest part of the human brain. It consists of the **cerebrum**, two highly convoluted **cerebral hemispheres** separated by a deeply penetrating **longitudinal fissure.** The convolutions of the surfaces of the hemispheres are known as **gyri** (L. circle), and they are separated by depressions called **sulci** (L. *sulcus*, a furrow). Some of the more prominent gyri and sulci have had names assigned to them. The **lateral** and **central sulci** are used as references to divide each cerebral hemisphere into separate parts or **lobes,** but the names assigned to the lobes are based on the cranial bones with which they are most closely associated. As shown in Figure 5-5, the **frontal lobe** is located in front of the central sulcus while the **parietal lobe** is located behind the central sulcus and above the lateral sulcus. The **temporal lobe** is located below the lateral sulcus. The **occipital lobe** is difficult to outline because there is no well-defined sulcus separating it from the temporal and parietal lobes.

Frontal sections through the cerebral hemispheres reveal a cortical layer of gray matter and an internal aggregate of multilayered gray and white matter that collectively are known as the **basal ganglia** (or nuclei). They are shown in Figures 5-6 and 5-7.

The Brain Stem Referring to structures as parts of the fore-, mid-, or hindbrain can be cumbersome, so the term brain stem is often used to designate structures of the diencephalon, the mesencephalon, the pons, and the medulla oblongata. The cerebellum is connected to the brain stem, but is not considered a part of it.

The brain stem contains a number of ascending and descending nerve tracts and numerous nuclei that comprise major integrating centers for both sensory and motor functions. It contains the nuclei for most of the **cranial nerves** (nerves that supply the head) as well as centers associated with regulation of visceral, endocrine, behavioral, and metabolic functions. The brain stem is also associated with most of the special senses (vision and hearing in particular), and it controls muscular activity in the head and part of the neck.

The Spinal Cord

The lower (caudal) end of the medulla oblongata is prolonged into, and is continuous with, the spinal cord. It extends from the level of the upper border of the first cervical vertebra to about the lower border of the first lumbar vertebra.

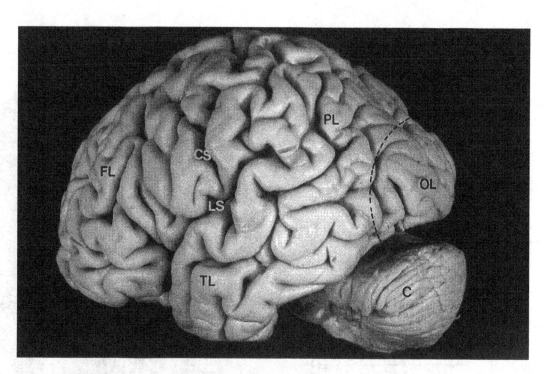

FIGURE 5-5

Lateral surface of cerebrum and cerebullum

(C)	cerebellum	**(LS)**	lateral sulcus	**(PL)**	parietal lobe
(CS)	central sulcus	**(OL)**	occipital lobe	**(TL)**	temporal lobe
(FL)	frontal lobe				

FIGURE 5-6

Frontal section of cerebrum showing relationship of basal ganglia and internal capsule **(IC)** to other structures. Basal ganglia consists of the caudate nucleus **(CN)** and lenticular nucleus, which is composed of the putamen **(P)** and globus pallidus **(GP).** The above region is known as the *striate bodies.*

CC	corpus callosum
CR	corona radiata
LF	longitudinal fissure
LV	lateral ventricle
SP	septum pellucida
T	thalamus

Note the asymmetry—due in part to imperfect sectioning.

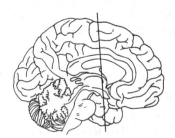

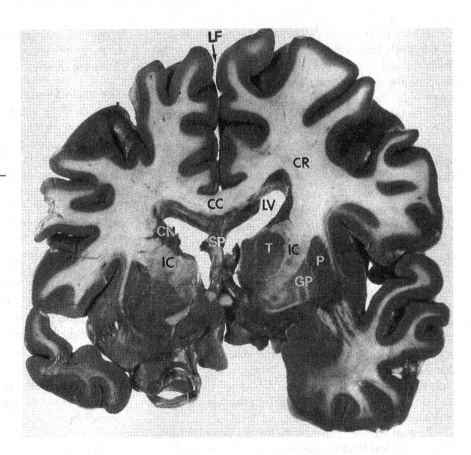

FIGURE 5-7

Transverse section of cerebrum showing relationships of

CN	caudate nucleus
CR	corona radiata
IC	internal capsule
LVAH	lateral ventricle (anterior horn)
T	thalamus

CCs	corpus callosum (splenium of)
CCt	corpus callosum (trunk of)
CV	cerebellum (vermis of)
I	insula
LF	longitudinal fissure
LS	lateral sulcus
LVIH	lateral ventricle (inferior horn)

FL frontal **OL** occipital **TL** temporal lobes

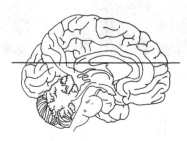

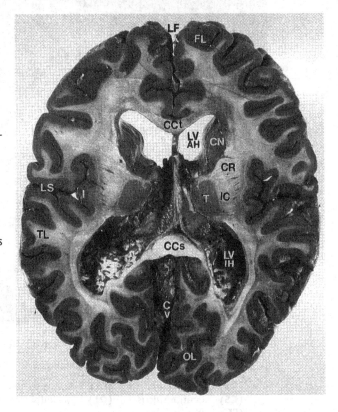

A transverse section of the spinal cord reveals a central core of gray matter surrounded by white matter. The **gray matter,** consisting of two crescent-shaped bodies joined across the midline by a **transverse commissure** of gray matter, has the appearance of the letter **H** or the shape of a butterfly. A frontal plane through the transverse commissure divides each crescent into a **ventral** (or anterior) **horn** and a **dorsal** (or posterior) **horn,** each of which extends the full length of the spinal cord.

Generally speaking, the nerve cells and processes in the ventral horns are associated with motor functions, while those of the dorsal horns are associated with receptor (sensory) and coordinating functions. The ventral horns contain **lower motoneurons** (motor neurons), the axons of which leave the spinal cord as the motor roots of the spinal nerves. The dorsal horns contain a large number of **internuncial neurons** (connecting neurons) and axons from neurons in the dorsal root ganglia (Figure 5-8). They enter the spinal cord as sensory roots of the spinal nerves.

The spinal cord has pronounced enlargements in the cervical and thoracic regions. This is due to the increased number of neurons in the gray matter supplying the muscles of the upper and lower extremities. The white matter is divided into **ventral, lateral,** and **dorsal columns** (funiculi), each of which contains both ascending and descending tracts.

The Meninges

The brain and spinal cord are completely surrounded by three layers of protective connective tissue known as the meninges (Gk. *meninx,* membrane). The outermost is called the **dura mater** (L. hard + *mater,* mother). The **arachnoid mater,** as its name suggests, is a weblike membrane, and it loosely invests the brain. The innermost **pia mater** (gentle mother), a highly vascular membrane that invests the brain very closely, gives fresh brains their bright pink color. A space between the arachnoid and pia mater is filled with **cerebrospinal fluid,** which enters the space from the fourth ventricle and circulates around the brain and spinal cord.

The Peripheral Nervous System

The peripheral nervous system is by definition that part of the nervous system which is *located outside the bony confines of the skull and vertebral column.* It includes the 12 pairs of cranial nerves and their ganglia, dorsal and ventral roots of the spinal nerves, the 31 pairs of spinal nerves and their dorsal root ganglia, peripheral nerves, and the ganglia and nerve processes of the autonomic nervous system, as illustrated in Figure 5-9.

Spinal and Cranial Nerves

Individual spinal nerves are formed by the merging of their dorsal and ventral spinal **nerve roots.** Immediately after merging, a **dorsal** and **ventral ramus** is given off, each of which carries fibers from both the dorsal and ventral roots. *Since dorsal roots are sensory and ventral roots are motor in function, all rami are mixed (carrying both motor and sensory fibers).* The **motor fibers** of the spinal nerves arise

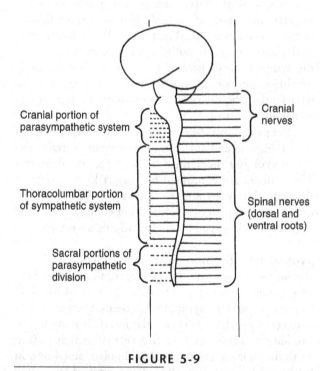

FIGURE 5-9

A schematic of the peripheral nervous system. It includes the 12 pairs of cranial nerves, the dorsal and ventral roots of the 31 pairs of spinal nerves, and the autonomic nervous system.

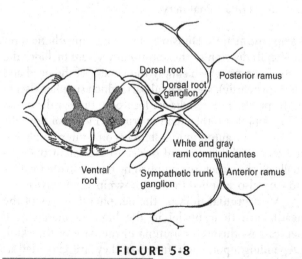

FIGURE 5-8

Schematic of a transverse section through the spinal cord, showing the butterfly-shaped gray matter and the arrangement of a typical spinal nerve.

from cell bodies in the ventral column of the gray matter in the spinal cord, while **sensory fibers** arise from cell bodies located in ganglia outside the cord (Figure 5-8).

By the same token **motor cranial nerves** arise from cell bodies (their **nuclei of origin**) within the brain stem, while **sensory cranial nerves** arise from groups of cells outside the brain. These cells may form ganglia on the trunks of nerves, or they may be located in the peripheral sense organs such as the eyes and nose. The central processes of the sensory nerves course to the brain stem (mostly) and end by arborizing around nerve cells that form their **nuclei of termination.** The nuclei of termination of the sensory nerves are connected with the cerebral cortex.

Autonomic Nervous System

The autonomic nervous system controls the internal environment of the body, while the remainder of the peripheral nervous system reacts to and adjusts to the external environment. As its name implies, the autonomic nervous system is *self-regulating*. This means we don't have to think about the adjustments almost constantly taking place within us.

The autonomic nervous system, which is sometimes referred to as the **visceral efferent system,** is divisible into a **sympathetic** (or thoracolumbar) division and a **parasympathetic** (or craniosacral) division. Both are composed of efferent nerves that supply the heart, the glandular tissue of the body, and the smooth muscle of the viscera, eyes, etc. The principal control center is in the nuclei of the hypothalamus. The primary role of the sympathetic division is to accommodate the body for threatening or stressful conditions, while that of the parasympathetic division is to reinstate the normal internal environment.

Preganglionic fibers of autonomic nerve cells in the brain stem and spinal cord accompany certain cranial nerves and the ventral roots of the spinal nerves. These fibers are continued to ganglia located outside the central nervous system. The axons of the ganglion cells are called **postganglionic fibers.** They supply the viscera, the glands, and smooth and cardiac muscle.

Sympathetic Division In the sympathetic division of the autonomic system, a long nerve trunk flanks the vertebral column on either side, from the base of the skull to the coccyx. This **sympathetic trunk** presents interconnected ganglia at fairly regular intervals along its entire length. There are usually 3 cervical ganglia, 10 to 12 in the thoracic region, 4 in the lumbar, and 4 or 5 in the sacral regions. Branches of the sympathetic trunk form a number of **plexuses** (L. braids), which also contain ganglia. As shown in Figure 5-10, nerve fibers to and from the sympathetic trunk connect it with the ventral rami of the spinal nerves. These connecting nerve fibers,

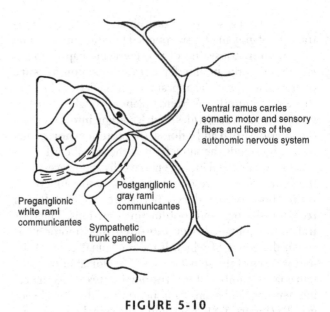

FIGURE 5-10

A schematic of the relationship of the pre- and postganglionic fibers and the ganglia of the sympathetic trunk of the autonomic nervous system. The preganglionic fiber (white ramus) leaves the spinal cord to synapse with ganglia in the trunk. The postganglionic fiber (gray ramus) returns to the spinal cord and emerges along with other fibers in the ventral ramus of a spinal nerve.

known as **rami communicantes,** are composed of pre- and postganglion fibers.

Typically, a myelinated preganglionic fiber (white ramus) leaves the spinal cord by way of a ventral root and courses to a sympathetic trunk ganglion where a synapse occurs with an unmyelinated (gray ramus) postganglionic cell. The axon of this postganglionic cell (sometimes quite long) leaves the sympathetic trunk and courses to its destination, at least part way, with the ventral ramus of a spinal nerve.

Parasympathetic Division The parasympathetic (craniosacral) division of the autonomic system includes the cranial nerves, which supply the viscera of the head and neck (primarily), and a sacral part, which supplies viscera in the pelvis. The ganglia are located at or near the organ being supplied rather than in trunks. Fibers of both divisions of the autonomic system become intermingled in the thorax, abdomen, and pelvis, to the extent that virtually all the structures supplied by the sympathetic division are also supplied by the parasympathetic division.

Most **cranial nerves** (the peripheral nerves of the head) have their nuclei in the brain stem, and the nerves pass through foramina in the base of the skull. Depending upon their function they are classified as motor, sensory, or mixed. Although cranial and spinal nerves have similar origins, they differ because cranial nerves are not all mixed nerves, they do not have dorsal and ventral roots or rami, and not every nerve has a ganglion. Cranial nerves transmit information from the special senses and from receptors,[2] while their output is to muscles of the eyes, face, jaw, tongue, pharynx, and larynx. They also provide the parasympathetic supply to the viscera of the head and neck.

Cranial nerves are designated by Roman numerals (I through XII) in accordance with the order in which they leave the brain or brain stem. Their names reflect either their *structure* (e.g., trigeminal), *function* (e.g., olfactory), or *distribution* (e.g., facial). Since most of the **motor nuclei** for the cranial nerves (located in the brain stem) receive bilateral cortical representation, lesions "above" nuclei (supranuclear) usually have a transitory effect. The facial nerve, to be discussed later, is an interesting exception.

There we have it—*the nervous system once over lightly.* This remarkable part of us is due, in large part, to the fascinating process called *natural selection.* We are dependent upon our brains, and they have become increasingly complex. We have become less and less dependent upon our dentition, and so it regresses.

FUNCTIONAL ANATOMY OF THE CENTRAL NERVOUS SYSTEM

The primitive neural tube differentiates into five secondary brain vesicles and the spinal cord, all of which constitute the central nervous system. The secondary brain vesicles are the telencephalon, diencephalon, mesencephalon, metencephalon, and myelencephalon.

The Meninges

In addition to the protection provided the central nervous system by the bones of the skull and vertebral column, the brain and spinal cord are surrounded by three layers of nonnervous connective tissue collectively known as the meninges. Spaces between the meningeal layers contain **cerebrospinal fluid** that moistens, lubricates, and protects the brain and the spinal cord. The brain virtually floats in the fluid.

Dura Mater

The outermost of the meninges is the dura mater, a tough two-layered membrane that functions as a pro-

tective sheath for the brain and spinal cord and as a lining for the cranial vault (Figure 5-11). It also extends out with cranial and spinal nerves to form **epineurium,** a connective tissue covering for the peripheral nerves.

The outer layer of the dura is periosteal and the inner layer meningeal. These two layers are closely bound together in the cranium, except where they are separated to form **venous sinuses,** and where the meningeal layer forms **fibrous septa** between the major parts of the brain. The outer layer is closely attached to the inner surface of the cranium by means of fine fibrous projections into the bone tissue. The attachment is closest along the sutures and at the margin of the foramen magnum. As we will see in detail later, the sinuses of the dura form a complex system of channels which drain venous blood from the brain into the internal jugular vein, and from there to the heart. Cerebrospinal fluid also drains into the dural sinuses by way of projections of the arachnoid mater into the sinuses (the arachnoid granulation).

The meningeal layer of dura forms four major folds that separate the large parts of the brain, and which divide the cranial vault incompletely into compartments. One is the **falx** (L. sickle) **cerebri,** which extends into the longitudinal fissure between the two cerebral hemispheres. It courses from the crista galli of the ethmoid bone in front, to the occipital protuberance behind, where it becomes continuous with a transverse shelf of dura, the **tentorium** (L. a tent) **cerebelli.** It separates the cerebellum from the occipital lobes of the cerebral hemispheres.

A small triangular fold of dura that separates the two cerebellar hemispheres is called the **falx cerebelli,**

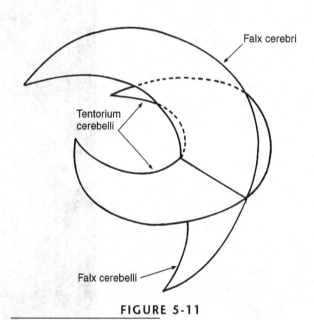

FIGURE 5-11

Schematic of the folds that are formed by the meningeal layer of the dura mater. The diaphragma sella is not shown.

---

[2]**Receptors** are terminals of sensory nerves that respond to various types of stimulation. **Proprioceptors** provide information about body position, balance, and equilibrium, especially during locomotion. **Exteroceptors,** such as those in the skin and mucous membrane, respond to pressure, temperature changes, and pain. **Interoceptors** transmit impulses from the viscera.

while the fourth fold is called the **diaphragma sella.** It forms a covering over the sella turcica and the hypophysis (pituitary gland). The anterior projections of the tentorium cerebelli are continuous with the diaphragma sella. The dura of the spinal cord, which forms a loose sheath around it, is continuous with just the meningeal layer. The periosteal layer attaches to the foramen magnum and does not continue into the vertebral canal. **Epidural spaces** exist between the dura and the vertebral canal and between the dura and spinal cord. The epidural space is occupied by loose areolar tissue (trabeculae) and a number of blood vessels.

Arachnoid Mater

The arachnoid (Gk. *arachno*, spider) mater is so called because of its resemblance to a spider's web. Notice, in Figure 5-12A the gossamer appearance of the cerebral hemisphere with its arachnoid mater. Although the middle cerebral artery (MCA) can be seen in Figures 5-12A and 5-12B, the arachnoid itself is devoid of vascular

---

FIGURE 5-12

Views of the brain with and without the arachnoid mater. In A, a lateral view, the middle cerebral artery is indicated by an arrow. In B, the middle cerebral artery is indicated by an arrow, as are the arachnoid granulations. In C, the brain as it appears with the arachnoid removed.

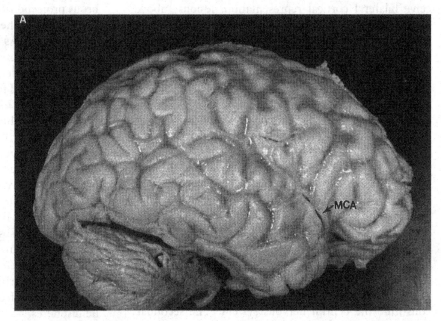

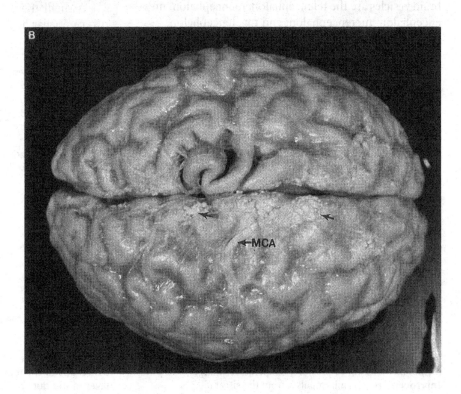

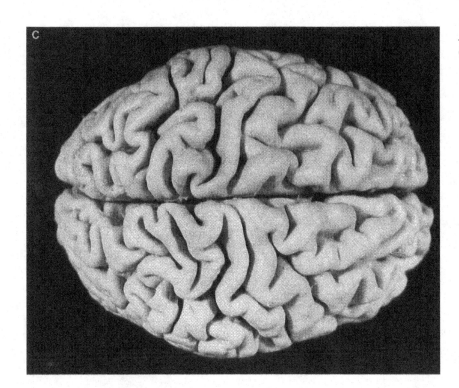

FIGURE 5-12

Continued

tissue. It is a delicate membrane of reticular fibers, the outer and inner aspects of which are lined by mesothelium. The arachnoid mater loosely invests the brain and spinal cord, but does follow the convolutions, except at the longitudinal fissure (falx cerebri) and the tentorium cerebelli. The arachnoid is separated from the inner surface of the dura only by a thin layer of fluid in the **subdural space.**

A **subarachnoid space** also exists, but is almost wanting over the surface of the hemispheres of the brain. At the height of the convolutions, the arachnoid and subjacent pia mater come into close contact, where they are called the **leptomeninges** (Gk. *leptos,* slender, delicate). The arachnoid bridges the sulci, leaving an increased subarachnoid space, and where **subarachnoid cisterns** are formed the space between the brain and arachnoid is extensive (Figure 5-13).

In regions adjacent to the superior sagittal sinus small tufts of arachnoid project into the sinus channel. These tufts, called **arachnoid granulations** (or villi), provide a means of resorption of cerebrospinal fluid into the venous bloodstream. The arachnoid granulations are indicated by arrows in Figure 5-12B. Note that a small parasagittal region of arachnoid mater has been torn away from the surface of the brain. This happens due to adhesions between the arachnoid and the dura maters. The hydrostatic pressure[3] of cerebrospinal fluid

---

[3]**Hydrostatic** pertains to a liquid in a state of equilibrium.

exceeds that of the venous pressure, and the granulations act as one-way valves that permit cerebrospinal fluid flow from the subarachnoid space into the superior sagittal sinus (Figure 5-13).

Pia Mater

The deepest layer of the meninges, called the pia mater, is an extremely vascular membrane held together by a loose network of areolar tissue, trabeculae from which connect the arachnoid to it. The highly vascular nature of the pia is responsible for the pink color of a fresh brain specimen. The pia very closely follows the convolutions and irregularities of the surface of the brain and spinal cord. The pia even extends into the ventricles, where it, together with the ependyma, forms the **choroid plexus** of the lateral, third, and fourth ventricles. The choroid plexuses are the major sites of formation of cerebrospinal fluid. In Figure 5-14, notice that granular appearance of the lateral ventricles (LV), which is due to the tufts of the choroid plexus.

The Brain

The Telencephalon (Forebrain)

The cerebral hemispheres are very nearly mirrored images of one another when seen in a sagittal section, as in Figure 5-15. When seen in detail, however, there are some very obvious differences between the right and left hemispheres, not only in neuron distribution, but in

FIGURE 5-13

Subarachnoid cisterns shown schematically.

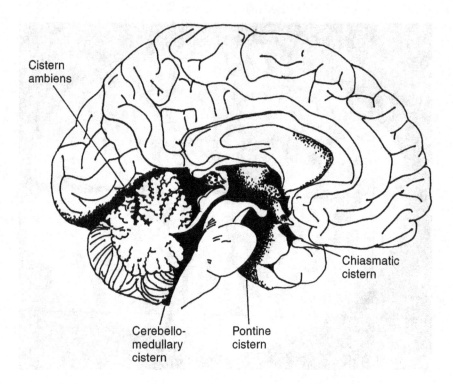

Cistern ambiens

Chiasmatic cistern

Cerebello-medullary cistern

Pontine cistern

function as well. This is particularly true in regions devoted to speech production and to language. A brain specimen as seen from above is shown in Figure 5-16. Obvious differences between the right hemisphere (RH) and the left hemisphere (LH) can be seen, to the extent

that identification of the central sulcus in the left hemisphere can be risky. Each hemisphere has three surfaces—a convex lateral, a plane medial, and an irregular inferior surface—all characterized by a maze of folds and depressions. Each fold is known as a **gyrus,** while a de-

FIGURE 5-14

The granular appearance of the lining of the lateral ventricle **(LV)** is due to the secretory choroid plexus, which is found in the lateral, third, and fourth ventricles.

CC	corpus callosum
CS	cingulate sulcus
FL	frontal lobe
LF	longtitudinal fissure
OP	occipital pole

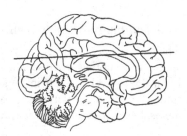

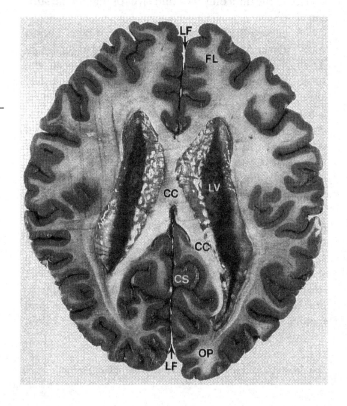

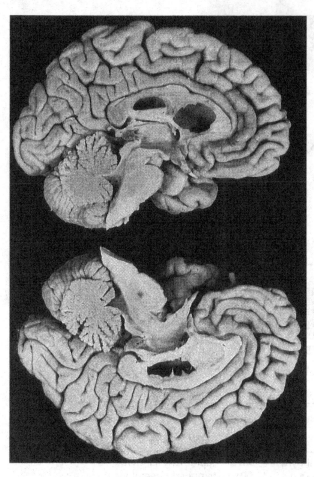

FIGURE 5-15

When seen in a sagittal preparation such as this one, the two cerebral hemispheres appear to be mirror images of one another. Grossly this seems to be true, however many significant differences exist between the right and left hemispheres. This is particularly true in those regions of the brain devoted to speech production and to language.

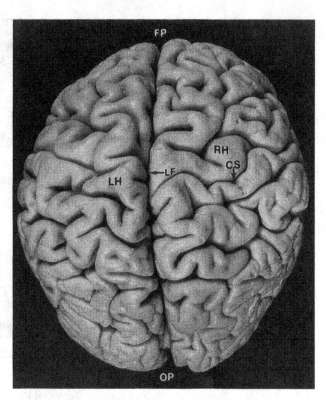

FIGURE 5-16

A brain specimen as seen from above. Note the differences between the convolutions in the right **(RH)** and left **(LH)** hemispheres. The central sulcus **(CS)** is easily identified in the right hemisphere, but is less obvious in the left.

pression is called a **sulcus** or, if particularly deep, a **fissure.** The terms sulcus and fissure are sometimes used interchangeably. The prominent lateral sulcus, for example, is often called the lateral fissure.

Cerebral Fissures There are a number of important fissures in the brain that serve as reference landmarks. The **longitudinal cerebral fissure** has already been mentioned. It separates the two cerebral hemispheres. The separation is only partial in front and behind, but in the middle, it penetrates to the **corpus callosum,** a prominent band of commissural fibers that unites the two hemispheres. The meningeal fold that extends into the fissure is the **falx cerebri.**

The cerebrum and cerebellum are separated from one another by a deeply penetrating **transverse fissure,** and the meningeal fold that extends into it is called the **tentorium cerebelli,** as shown in Figure 5-11.

The Lateral Surface The **central fissure** (or sulcus, of Rolando) begins about midway between the inferior and superior borders of the lateral surface of each hemisphere (Figure 5-17A). It courses obliquely upward to terminate near the midpoint of the superior border. The central fissure can be difficult to locate on a brain specimen because of the inconsistent shape of the surrounding gyri.

The **lateral fissure** (or sulcus, of Sylvius) begins at the inferior border of the lateral surface of each hemisphere and courses obliquely upward to terminate, slightly more than halfway back. The junction of the central fissure with the lateral fissure in the frontal lobe is the **motor area for speech.**

Lobes The central and lateral fissures help to divide the cerebral hemispheres into four lobes—**frontal, temporal, parietal,** and **occipital**—but they are named after the cranial bones to which they are immediately adjacent. An **insular lobe** (island of Riel) is also identified in each hemisphere. It lies deeply buried at the bottom of the lateral fissure and can only be seen when the lips of the fissure, the **opercula** (L. a cover or lid), are separated. The insula has visceral functions that are not well understood.

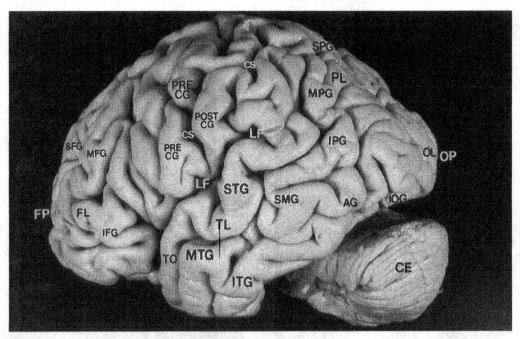

FIGURE 5-17A

Lateral surface of cerebral hemisphere and cerebellum **(CE).**

Gyri	Frontal lobe	Temporal lobe	Parietal lobe	Occipital lobe
Superior	**SFG**	**STG**	**SPG**	
Middle	**MFG**	**MTG**	**MPG**	
Inferior	**IFG**	**ITG**	**IPG**	**IOG**

AG	angular gyrus	**POST CG**	postcentral gyrus	**SMG** supramarginal gyrus
CS	central sulcus	**PRE CG**	precentral gyrus	**TO** temporal operculum
LF	lateral fissure			

Frontal Lobe. The lateral surface of the frontal lobe presents the precentral, superior, and inferior frontal sulci for examination, and they divide the surface into the superior frontal, middle frontal, inferior frontal, and precentral gyri. The **precentral gyrus** is particularly noteworthy because it is the area associated with the common motor pathway to the skeletal muscles. The *left inferior frontal gyrus* is more heavily convoluted than is the right one and is referred to as **Broca's speech area.**

Parietal Lobe. The parietal lobe contains the postcentral and the intraparietal sulci. As shown in Figure 5-17A, the **postcentral sulcus** courses parallel to the central fissure. The area between the two, the **postcentral gyrus,** is the principal somatic sensory area. In addition, the parietal lobe presents the **superior** and **inferior parietal gyri** (or lobules). The inferior parietal lobule is further divided into the angular and supramarginal gyri. The **angular gyrus** is especially important for comprehension of the written word. If the *left angular gyrus* is damaged, the ability to read and write may be lost (**alexia** and **agraphia**) even though the person may retain the ability to speak and to comprehend speech.

Occipital Lobe. The occipital lobe, which is relatively small and pyramidal in shape, bears a **lateral occipital sulcus** that divides the lateral surface into a **superior** and **inferior gyrus,** both of which are continuous in front with the parietal and temporal lobes.

Temporal Lobe. The temporal lobe is divided into **superior, middle,** and **inferior temporal gyri** by two sulci that course parallel with the lateral sulcus. The temporal lobe also presents a superior surface that extends deeply into the cerebrum, forming the inferior border of the lateral fissure. Parts of the gyri partially covering the insula are called the **temporal operculum.** Much of the **cortical center for hearing** is located on this superior surface.

The Medial Surface A brain must be severed through the midline in order to view the medial surface of a hemisphere. The most prominent structure seen is the **corpus callosum.** It forms the floor of the longitudinal sulcus and part of the roof of the lateral ventricle. Composed of myelinated fibers, it reciprocally interconnects virtually all the cortical regions of the two hemispheres. The parts of the corpus callosum are the rostrum, genu, body (trunk), and splenium (Figure 5-17B). Once the

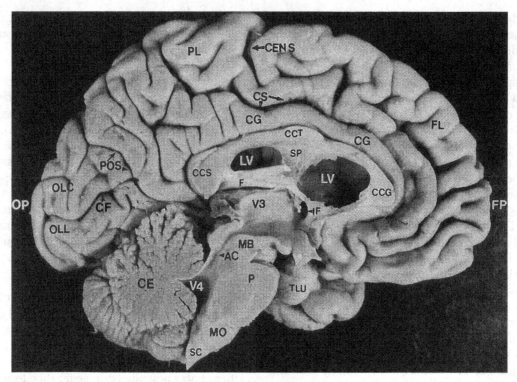

FIGURE 5-17B

Sagittal section through the brain illustrating some prominent landmarks.

AC	aqueduct cerebri	**F**	fornix	**OP**	occipital pole
Corpus callosum		**FL**	frontal lobe	**P**	pons
CCG	(genu)	**FP**	frontal pole	**PL**	parietal lobe
CCS	(splenium)	**IF**	interventricular foramen	**POS**	parietal-occipital sulcus
CCT	(trunk)	**LS**	lateral sulcus	**SC**	spinal cord
CE	cerebellum	**LV**	lateral ventricle	**SP**	septum pellucidum
CEN S	central sulcus	**MB**	midbrain	**TLU**	temporal lobe (uncus)
CG	cingulate gyrus	**MO**	medulla oblongata	**V3**	third ventricle
CS	cingulate sulcus	**OLC**	occipital lobe (cuneus)	**V4**	fourth ventricle
CF	calcarine fissure	**OLL**	occipital lobe (lingula)		

fibers have crossed the midline, they radiate fanlike to nearly all parts of the cerebral cortex.

The corpus callosum plays an important role in **cross hemispheric transfer** of learned discriminations, sensory experiences, and memory. It is interesting to note that complete surgical section of the corpus callosum does not result in any obvious neurological deficits, but these patients show a functional independence of the two hemispheres with respect to memory, perceptual, cognitive, and certain volitional activities. The hemispheres do not communicate with one another, and information experienced in the nondominant (right) hemisphere cannot be communicated by means of speech or writing. There is, however, no impairment of linguistic expression by the dominant hemisphere. This type of behavior tells us that linguistic expression and complex thought processes are organized almost exclusively in the dominant (left) hemisphere.

A medial view of a cerebral hemisphere reveals the **parietooccipital sulcus,** which courses down and for-

ward as a rather deep cleft and joins the calcarine (L. spur-shaped) fissure just below and behind the corpus callosum. The **calcarine fissure** extends from the occipital pole to the region of the posterior limit of the parietal lobe. This fissure divides the occipital lobe into a wedge-shaped **cuneus** and a **lingual gyrus** (Figure 5-17B). The **cingulate** (L. girdle) **sulcus,** which begins near the anterior limits of the corpus callosum, runs nearly parallel to its upper surface, but near the splenium it turns dorsally and terminates on the superomedial border of the hemisphere where it is known as the **marginal sulcus.** The superior frontal gyrus and paracentral gyrus both course parallel to the cingulate gyrus, while the portion of the parietal lobe caudal to the paracentral lobule is known as the **precuneus.**

The medial aspect of the temporal lobe presents the **parahippocampal** (or hippocampal) **gyrus,** the **uncus** (L. hook), and the **fornix** (L. arch) structures, which are associated with the olfactory sense and the limbic system.

The Limbic Lobe and Limbic System Not a true lobe in the usual sense, the **limbic lobe** consists of the most medial margins (i.e., the limbus) of the frontal, parietal, and temporal lobes. Together, these margins encircle the upper part of the brain stem. The **limbic system,** which is dominant in reptiles, is a very primitive part of our nervous system. Phylogenetically, it is thought to be between 200 and 300 million years old. *It is associated with temperature regulation, feeding, anger, and sexual functions.* Its major components include the **hippocampus, fornix, cingulate gyrus, mammillary bodies, amygdala, uncus,** and **olfactory bulbs** (Figure 5-18).

The limbic system receives sensory information from, and returns its output to, the reticular formation in the brain stem, and it connects to the frontal lobes and hypothalamus. These projections mediate our "animal behavior" such as smell, taste, thirst, hunger, anger, fear, and sexual arousal. Much of this behavior can be "overridden" by the higher functions of the cerebral cortex. The limbic system has also been implicated in *short-term memory.* Bilateral lesions of the hippocampus and amygdala result in short-term memory loss, but long-term memory is retained.

The Inferior Surface The inferior surface of the cerebrum can be described as two parts: (1) the large part consisting of the inferior surfaces of the temporal and occipital lobes and (2) the orbital surface of the frontal lobes. Prominent gyri on the posterior part include the **lingual, occipitotemporal,** and **parahippocampal gyri** and the **uncus.** The orbital surface of the frontal lobe contains the **olfactory bulbs** medially, dorsal to which can be seen some structures of the **hypothalamus.** They include the mammillary bodies, tuber cinereum, infundibulum, hypophysis, and the optic chiasma (Figures 5-19 and 5-20).

White Matter of the Cerebrum The extensive subcortical white matter of the cerebrum contains three types of fibers: (1) **projection fibers,** which convey impulses from remote regions to and from the cerebral cortex; (2) **association fibers,** which interconnect various cortical regions in the same hemisphere; and (3) **commissural fibers,** which interconnect corresponding cortical regions of the two hemispheres.

The common central mass of white matter, which contains projection, association, and commissural fibers, has an oval-shaped appearance in horizontal sections and is termed the **semioval center,** as shown in Figure 5-21.

Projection Fibers. Afferent and efferent fibers transmitting impulses to and from the cerebral cortex enter the white matter in fan-shaped bundles that converge toward the brain stem. These radiating projection fibers form the **corona radiata** (Figures 5-22A, 5-22B). As these fibers near the brain stem, they form a compact band of white matter called the **internal capsule,** which is flanked medially and laterally by nuclear (gray) masses called the **basal ganglia.** When seen in horizontal sections, the internal capsule presents an anterior and posterior limb, and the junction of the two is called the **genu** (see Figure 5-23).

Association Fibers. Fibers that interconnect various regions of the cortex may be either long or short. **Short fibers** connect cells in adjacent convolutions. **Long fibers,** which interconnect cortical regions within the same

---

FIGURE 5-18

Structures comprising the limbic system. (From "Opiate Receptors and Internal Opiates," by Solomon H. Snyder. Copyright 1977 by Scientific American, Inc. All rights reserved.)

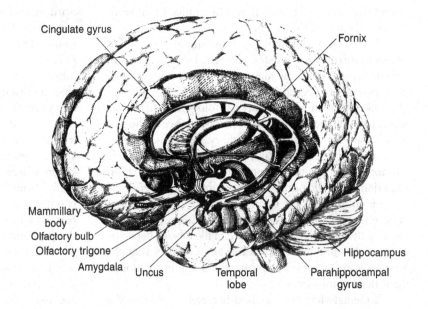

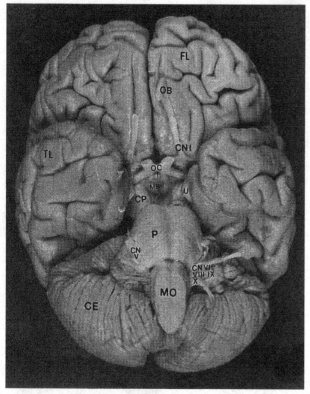

FIGURE 5-19

The brain as seen from beneath.

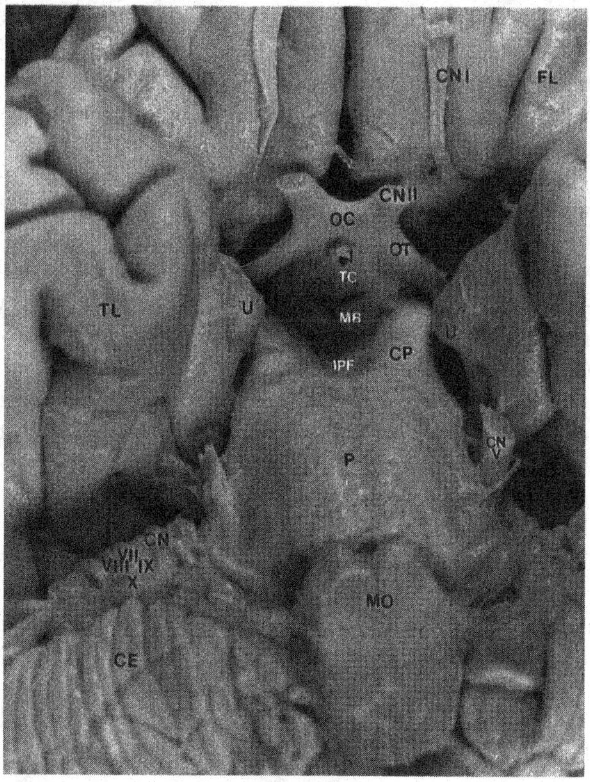

FIGURE 5-20

Base of brain as seen in detail.

Cranial Nerves					
CN **I**	olfactory	**CE**	cerebellum	**OB**	olfactory bulb (19)
CN **II**	optic (20)	**CP**	cerebral peduncle	**OC**	optic chiasm
emergence of		**FL**	frontal lobe	**OT**	optic tract
CN **V**	trigeminal	**I**	infundibulum (broken	**P**	pons
CN **VII**	facial		during dissection)	**TC**	tuber cinereum (20)
CN **VIII**	acoustic	**IPF**	interpeduncular fossa (20)	**TL**	temporal lobe
CN **IX**	glossopharyngeal	**MB**	mammillary bodies	**U**	(uncus) temporal lobe
CN **X**	vagus	**MO**	medulla oblongata		

hemisphere, form three main bundles shown in Figure 5-22A. (1) The **uncinate fasciculus** connects the frontal gyri (of the orbital surface) with the anterior portion of the temporal lobe; (2) the **arcuate fasciculus** flanks the region of the insula and connects the superior and middle frontal gyri with parts of the temporal lobe (those related to speech); and (3) the **cingulum,** located on the medial aspect of the hemisphere, connects parts of the frontal and parietal lobes with the hippocampal region and the cortex of the temporal lobe.

Commissural Fibers. Two bands of commissural fibers interconnect the corresponding cortical regions of the two hemispheres. They are the corpus callosum and the anterior commissure.

The **corpus callosum,** a prominent structure seen in sagittal sections of the cerebrum, reciprocally inter-

connects regions of the cortex in all lobes with corresponding regions of the opposite hemisphere. Note, in Figure 5-17B, that anteriorly the corpus callosum is bent back upon itself to form the **genu.** Behind, the corpus callosum thickens to form the **splenium** (Gk. a bandagelike structure). It overlaps the choroid plexus of the third ventricle, the pineal body, and the mesencephalon.

The **anterior commissure** is small and crosses the midline just beneath the genu of the corpus callosum. Shaped like a bicycle handlebar, it connects the olfactory bulbs and the middle and inferior temporal gyri. The "grips" of the handlebar can be seen in Figure 5-24.

The Ventricles A frontal section through the cerebral hemispheres reveals the cerebral ventricles, part of the adult derivatives of the cavity in the embryonic neural

tube. Not only are the ventricles important from a clinical standpoint, they are very useful as reference landmarks. Each hemisphere contains a lateral cerebral ventricle which communicates with a smaller midline cavity known as the third ventricle.

The **lateral ventricle** is bounded above by the corpus callosum, laterally by part of the basal ganglia, and inferiorly by the thalamus. Each lateral ventricle consists of a **body** and three **horns** (Figure 5-25). The lateral ventricles communicate with the third ventricle by means of an **interventricular foramen** (or foramen of Monro).

The **third ventricle,** which is a rather narrow space between the cerebral hemispheres, is bounded by the structures comprising the diencephalon. It is continuous with the **cerebral aqueduct,** a very narrow canal that courses through the midbrain and in turn is continuous with the fourth ventricle. The **fourth ventricle,**[4] bounded by the cerebellum behind and the pons and medulla oblongata in front, is continued below into the **central canal** of the spinal cord.

A collection of specialized epithelial cells in the ventricles manufactures a lymphlike **cerebrospinal fluid.** These cells constitute the **choroid plexus.**

Cerebrospinal Fluid Circulation   Cerebrospinal fluid begins its circulation in the lateral ventricles, passes into the third and from there to the fourth, where it diffuses, by means of small apertures, into the subarachnoid spaces. It continues to circulate around the brain and is finally absorbed by an elaborate venous system that drains blood from the brain. When the lateral ventricles have filled, the pressure in them will raise a column of water about 100–200 mm. Because of this pressure, the fluid flows into the third ventricle by way of the interventricular foramen, and from there to the fourth ventricle, by way of the cerebral aqueduct. Here, the fluid flows into the subarachnoid space through the **foramen of Magendie** in the roof of the fourth ventricle, and through the **foramina of Lushka** (located at the extreme lateral limits of the fourth ventricle).

Expanded areas of the subarachnoid space are called **cisterns,** and their names indicate their location, as shown in Figure 5-13. The principal cisterns are the cerebellomedullaris, the pontis, the interpeduncularis, and the chiasmatis. Having entered the cisterns, the fluid flows around the brain, which ultimately brings it to the region of the **sagittal sinus** (where the two layers of the dura are separated to form part of the venous system). Small tufts of arachnoid (arachnoid grandulations) pro-

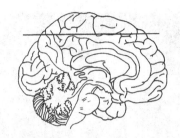

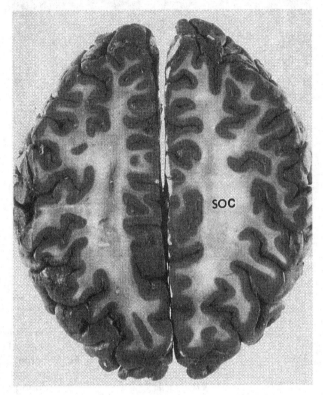

FIGURE 5-21

Projection, association, and commissural fibers all contribute to the semioval center **(SOC)** of the cerebrum.

ject into the sagittal sinus, and through the process of osmosis the fluid passes into the venous bloodstream (Figure 5-26).

CLINICAL NOTE: About 25 milliliters (ml) of cerebrospinal fluid are produced by the choroid plexuses every hour, and since the total quantity of fluid is between 100 and 200 ml, it is completely replaced every six hours. If something such as an acute infection should interfere with either drainage or absorption, elevated cerebrospinal fluid pressures amounting to 500 mm H_2O can develop quite rapidly with symptoms of pressure such as headache, slowed pulse and respiratory rate, loss of consciousness, and in chronic in-

---

[4]The fourth ventricle is not a cerebral ventricle. It is located in the brain stem.

FIGURE 5-22A

Schematic representation of corona radiata (top); association fibers, including the uncinate fasciculus, arcuate fasciculus (sup. long), and the cingulum; and the commissural fibers of the corpus callosum (bottom).

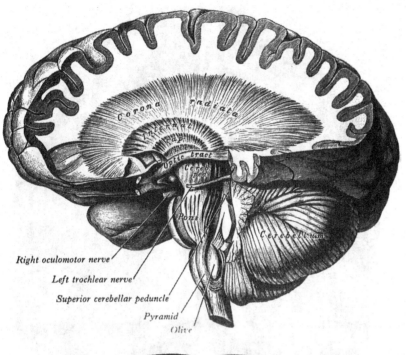

Right oculomotor nerve

Left trochlear nerve

Superior cerebellar peduncle

Pyramid

Olive

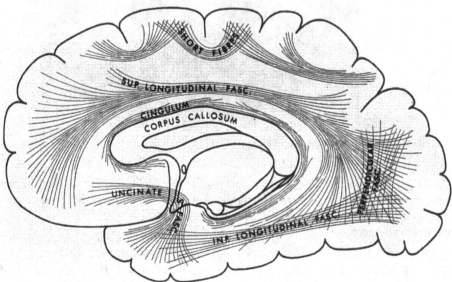

stances, **obstructive** or **communicating hydrocephalus.** In children, prior to fusion of the cranial sutures, hydrocephalus results in an enlargement of the skull and, in some instances, brain damage. Treatment for communicating hydrocephalus is surgical, and a number of techniques have been developed for shunting cerebrospinal fluid into the internal jugular vein.

The Basal Ganglia The term basal ganglia is inconsistently and loosely used to refer to some or all of the masses of **gray matter** within the cerebrum. If defined as just those structures of the telencephalon, the basal ganglia include the **caudate nucleus** and the **lenticular nucleus,** which together with the **internal capsule** form the **striate bodies** (corpus striatum). Some authorities also include the claustrum and the amygdaloid nucleus (a derivative of the diencephalon). And, to complicate matters, because of their anatomical and functional connections, the substantia nigra and red nucleus (in the mesencephalon) are often included. We will adhere to the notion that the basal ganglia are composed of the caudate and lenticular nuclei.

FIGURE 5-22B

Horizontal section through the brain illustrating the corona radiata (CR).

CCS	corpus callosum (splenium)
CCT	corpus callosum (trunk)
CS	calcarine sulcus
FL	frontal lobe
I	insula
LF	longitudinal fissure
LS	lateral sulcus
LV	lateral ventricle
LVAH	(anterior horn)
OL	occipital lobe
SP	septum pellucidum
T	thalamus
TL	temporal lobe

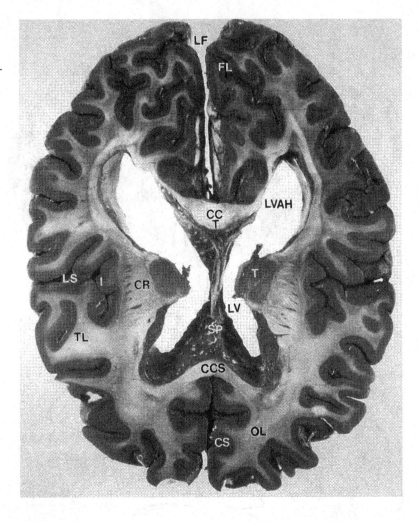

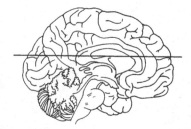

Striate Bodies (Corpus Striatum). The striate bodies are so named because of a striped appearance due to layers of white matter separating parts of the basal ganglia, thus leaving stratified layers of white and gray matter.

Caudate Nucleus. The caudate nucleus (L. having a tail), shown in Figures 5-27A and 5-27B, is an elongated mass of gray matter, which is bent over on itself and conforms throughout its course to the wall of the lateral ventricle. Its swollen rostral extremity or **head** bulges into the anterior horn of the lateral ventricle, as can be seen in Figure 5-28A. Here the head becomes continuous with the lenticular nucleus. The remainder of the caudate nucleus is drawn out into a highly arched tail that turns sharply in a caudal direction and, conforming to the shape of the lateral ventricle, bends sharply again in a rostral direction where it is continuous with the **amygdaloid nucleus** (part of the limbic system). (Because of its curved course, the tail part of the caudate nucleus is cut through twice in frontal sections of the cerebrum.) Throughout much of its extent, the caudate nucleus is separated from the lenticular nu-

cleus by a prominent layer of white matter called the **internal capsule.** Anteriorly (rostrally), the caudate and lenticular nuclei are continuous.

Lenticular Nucleus. The lenticular (L. lens-shaped) nucleus (Figures 5-28A and 5-28B) is located in the midst of the cerebral white matter. It is somewhat similar in size and shape to a Brazil nut. The structure is composed of two separate nuclei, the putamen and the globus pallidus. The **putamen** (L. shell) is a rather thick, convex mass, located lateral to the globus pallidus. The larger portion of the lenticular nucleus, its lateral surface is separated from the cortex of the insula by the interposed claustrum and external capsule (Figure 5-7). The **globus pallidus** is located medial to the putamen and is separated from it by a thin layer of white matter. In addition, the globus pallidus is divided into internal and external parts by an internal layer of white matter **(internal medullary lamina).** Because of its many myelinated fibers, it has a lighter color than the putamen, and so the name—globus pallidus. In addition, due to the medullary laminae and fine myelinated fiber bun-

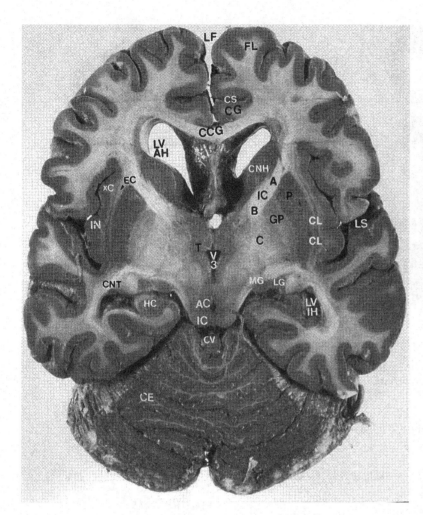

FIGURE 5-23

Horizontal section through the brain showing the internal capsule **(IC)**, anterior limb **(A)**, genu **(B)**, posterior limb **(C)** of internal capsule, and third ventricle **(V3)**.

AC	aquaduct cerebri
CCG	corpus callosum (genu)
CE	cerebellum (CV) vermis of
CNH	caudate nucleus (head)
CNT	caudate nucleus (tail)
CG	cingulate gyrus
CL	claustrum
CS	cingulate sulcus
EC	external capsule
FL	frontal lobe
GP	globus pallidus of lentiform nucleus
HC	hippocampus
IC	inferior colliculus
IN	insula
LF	longitudinal fissure
LG	lateral geniculate body
LVAH	lateral ventricle anterior horns
LVIH	lateral ventricle inferior horns
MG	medial geniculate body
P	putamen
XC	extreme capsule

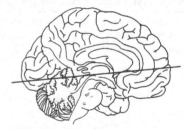

dles, the lenticular nucleus takes on a somewhat striated appearance; hence the term **corpus striatum.**[5]

Claustrum. The claustrum (L. a barrier) is a thin layer of gray matter located between the lateral margin of the putamen and the cortex of the insula. It is bounded laterally and medially by a tract of white matter known as the **external capsule.** The claustrum is sometimes regarded as a detached portion of the gray matter of the insula. Its cellular structure resembles that of the deepest layer of cerebral cortex. Aside from that, not much is known about the claustrum. It is identified in Figures 5-23 and 5-28A.

Amygdaloid Nucleus. The amygdaloid nucleus is located in the roof of the anterior (rostral) limits of the inferior ventricular horn, where it is continuous with the anteriorly directed tail of the caudate nucleus. The amygdala of the two sides are interconnected by means of the anterior commissure. Part of the limbic system, they receive fibers from the olfactory bulb and project fibers to the hypothalamus.

Electrical stimulation of the amygdaloid region in humans produces feelings of fear, confusion, disturbances of awareness, and amnesia for immediate events taking place. The amygdaloid complex also plays an important role in food and water intake.

Internal Capsule. The internal capsule is a rather broad band of white matter that separates the lenticular nucleus from the caudate nucleus and from the thalamus (Figure 5-28). The fan-shaped projection fibers from the cerebral cortex converge toward the basal ganglia region as the **corona radiata.** These fibers enter the basal ganglia as the **internal capsule** and leave, coursing toward the mesencephalon as the **crus cerebri.** *The same fibers that form the major motor projection pathway from the cerebral cortex are known by three different terms.*

---

[5]**Confusion Note:** The caudate nucleus and putamen are often referred to collectively as the *striatum,* and because of its phylogenetic age it is also known as the *neostriatum.* The globus pallidus is referred to as the *paleostriatum,* and the amygdaloid, even though it is olfactory and limbic in function, the *archistriatum.*

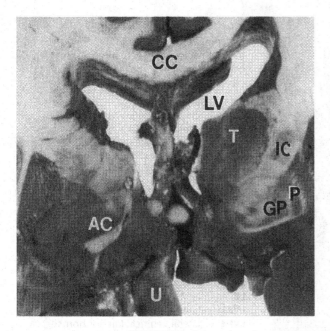

FIGURE 5-24

A frontal section through the brain to illustrate the location of the anterior commissure **(AC)**. Just part of it is visible.

CC	corpus callosum	**P**	putamen
GP	globus pallidus	**T**	thalamus
LV	lateral ventricle	**U**	uncus (temporal lobe)

Initially, the corona radiata, then, the internal capsule, and finally, the crus cerebri.

When seen in a horizontal (transverse) section of the brain, the internal capsule appears **V**-shaped, with the apex of the **V** directed medially, as shown in Figure 5-28A. From the **genu** (or apex), the anterior limb extends in a lateral and rostral direction, while the posterior limb is directed in a lateral and caudal direction. Some of the fibers of the internal capsule connect the medial and lateral groups of the basal ganglia. Some of the fibers in the anterior limb are projections from the thalamus to the cortex of the frontal lobe **(thalamocortical)**, from the cortex of the frontal lobe to the thalamus **(corticothalamic)**, from the frontal lobe to nuclei in the pons **(frontopontine)**. The genu and posterior limb contain efferent fibers from the motor cortex and are an important part of the common motor pathway to the cranial nerves **(corticobulbar)** and to the skeletal muscles of posture and locomotion **(corticospinal)**.

Function. The basal ganglia receive input from nearly all parts of the cerebral cortex, but especially from the motor area. They also receive radiation fibers from the thalamus in addition to important afferent fibers from dopamine-synthesizing cells in the substantia nigra of the mesencephalon. **Dopamine** is an important neurotransmitter (more about this later).

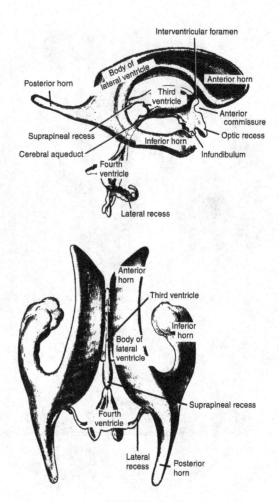

FIGURE 5-25

Drawings of a casting of the ventricles as seen from the side (top figure) and from above (bottom figure). (From *Gray's Anatomy*, 29th ed., 1973. Courtesy Lea & Febiger, Philadelphia.)

These cells project to dopamine-sensitive cells in the striatum. A deficiency of dopamine results in motor disorders, among them Parkinsonism.

The basal ganglia are important components in regulation of complex motor functions such as posture, locomotion, balance, and such activities as arm swinging during walking. Another important function is inhibitory in nature, and the basal ganglia are instrumental in decreasing muscle tone and aid in coordinating the motor behavior of muscle groups.

CLINICAL NOTE: Lesions of the basal ganglia result in involuntary movement, increased muscle tone **(rigidity)**, and **resting tremor** (which disappears during volitional movement). In particular, lesions of the caudate nucleus and putamen result in:

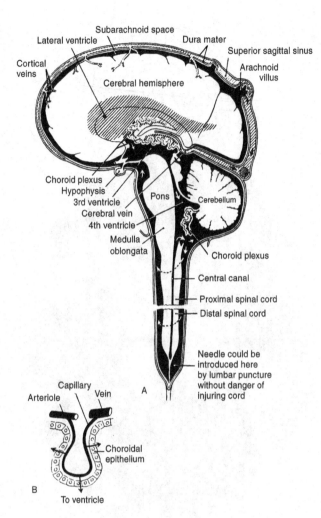

FIGURE 5-26

(A) Circulation of cerebrospinal fluid (in black); arrows indicate the direction of circulation. The drawing represents a median section of the nervous system and therefore shows third ventricle, cerebral aqueduct, fourth ventricle, and central canal, with the approximate size and location of one of the lateral ventricles indicated by oblique lines. Note aperture in the fourth ventricle by which fluid reaches the subarachnoid space. Note also one of the arachnoid villi through which fluid enters venous blood in dural sinus. (B) Fundamental plan of choroid plexuses. Cerebrospinal fluid is formed from blood plasma and passes through choroidal epithelium into the ventricular space. (From Gardner, 1975.)

1. **Athetosis** (involuntary movement, slow, writhing snakelike movements, especially of the fingers and wrists).
2. **Chorea** (sudden jerky and purposeless movements. Chorea can result from rheumatic fever, or it may be inherited as in Huntington's chorea.)

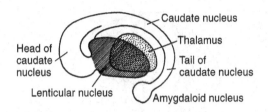

FIGURE 5-27A

The caudate nucleus shown schematically.

3. **Parkinsonism** (rigidity, resting tremor, masklike face, shuffling gait).
4. **Ballismus** (sudden wild flailing movements) or **hemiballismus** (affecting only one side of the body).

The Diencephalon

The diencephalon, which stems embryologically from the prosencephalon, is so completely surrounded by the cerebral hemispheres it appears to be a part of them, and only its ventral surface can be observed in the intact brain. In spite of its small size, the number of nuclei and their connections are incredibly complex and have far-reaching consequences. The diencephalon consists of the **thalamus, epithalamus, subthalamus,** and **hypothalamus.**

Thalamus When observed from above, following removal of the cerebral hemispheres and corpus callosum, the thalami are seen to consist of oval masses, about the size of a walnut on either side of the third ventricle. Each thalamus is greatly expanded caudally, and the expansion is called the **pulvinar,** a Latin word for cushion. The largest of the dorsal nuclei of the thalamus, it overhangs the midbrain.

The pulvinar is continued laterally into an oval swelling known as the **lateral geniculate body,** and, together with the **medial geniculate body,** was once called the **metathalamus.** The geniculate bodies are now considered part of the thalamus proper. The medial geniculate body, which receives fibers from the auditory pathway, is located beneath the pulvinar. The paired **lateral geniculate bodies,** which receive fibers from the optic tract, are connected across the midline through the optic chiasma.

The dorsal and lateral surfaces of the thalamus are covered by thin layers of white matter that are continuous with the **internal medullary lamina,** a Y-shaped layer of white matter that extends into the thalamus and divides it into medial, lateral, and anterior parts (Figure 5-29). *The substance of the thalamus is largely gray matter, which is composed of 26 pairs of nuclei.* One of these, the

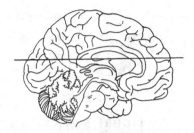

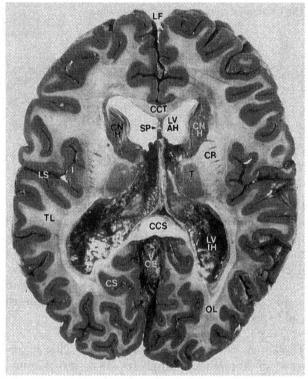

FIGURE 5-27B

Horizontal section through the brain illustrating how the head of the caudate nucleus **(CNH)** projects into the anterior horn of the lateral ventricle **(LVAH).**

CCS	corpus callosum (splenium)	**OL**	occipital lobe
CCT	corpus callosum (trunk)	**SP**	septum pellucidum
CR	corona radiata	**T**	thalamus
CS	calcarine sulcus	**TL**	temporal lobe
LS	lateral sulcus	**V**	vermis of
LVIH	lateral ventricle (inferior horn)	**CE**	cerebellum

midline nucleus, usually bridges the third ventricle and connects the thalami of the two sides. It contains mostly glial tissue.

A schematic of thalamic nuclei and their cortical projections is shown in Figure 5-29. The term **thalamic radiation** is used in reference to the tracts emerging from the lateral surface of the thalamus that then enter the internal capsule and terminate in the cerebral cortex.

The thalamus is very important because it receives all neural impulses, either directly or indirectly, from all parts of the body, except for olfaction. It also receives impulses from

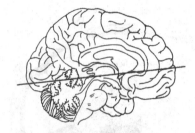

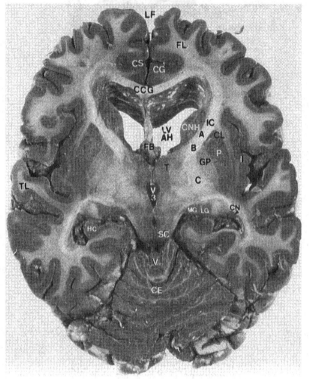

FIGURE 5-28A

Horizontal section through the brain showing the relationship of the internal capsule **(IC)** to adjacent structures. **A** (anterior limb)   **B** (genu)   **C** (posterior limb) of **IC.**

CL	claustrum	**HC**	hippocampus
CCG	corpus callosum (genu)	**I**	insula
CE	cerebellum	**LF**	longitudinal fissure
V	vermis of CE	**LG**	lateral geniculate body of thalamus
CG	cingulate gyrus		
CN	caudate nucleus (tail)	**LVAH**	lateral ventricle anterior horn
CNH	caudate nucleus (head)		
CS	cingulate sulcus	**MG**	medial geniculate body of thalamus
FB	fornix (body of)		
FL	frontal lobe	**P**	putamen
GP	globus pallidus of lentiform nucleus	**SC**	superior colliculus
		T	thalamus

the cerebellum, cerebral cortex, and many adjacent nuclei. A detailed discussion of the functions of the individual thalamic nuclei is simply beyond the scope of this text. Briefly, the role of the thalamic nuclei can be summarized as five basic functions:

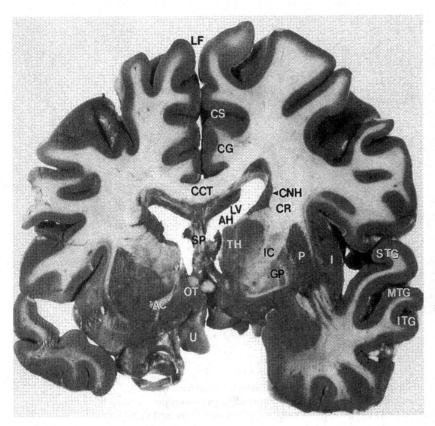

FIGURE 5-28B

Frontal section through the brain showing relationship of the internal capsule **(IC)** to adjacent structures.

AC	anterior commisure
CCT	corpus callosum
CG	cingulate gyrus
CNH	caudate nucleus head
CR	corona radiata
CS	cingulate sulcus
GP	globus pallidus of lentiform nucleus
I	insula
ITG	inferior temporal gyrus
LF	longitudinal fissure
LVAH	lateral ventricle anterior horn
MTG	middle temporal gyrus
P	putamen
OT	optical tract
SP	septum pellucidum
STG	superior temporal gyrus
TH	thalamus
U	uncus of temporal lobe

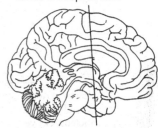

1. Relaying and processing of all the sensory input except olfaction to the cerebral cortex for conscious awareness.[6]

2. Perception of crude aspects of pain, temperature, and touch sensations, but not of accurate localization.

3. Imparting pleasantness or noxiousness to sensations, thus influencing emotional responses to them. Certain smells and visual experiences, for example, may make us ill.

4. Maintaining cortical activity that influences arousal, attention, and sleep-wake cycles.

5. Relay and integration station for input from the cerebellum and globus pallidus to the motor cortex.

The thalamic nuclei can also be grouped on a functional basis into (1) sensory relay nuclei, (2) motor relay nuclei, (3) association nuclei, (4) the limbic relay nucleus, and (5) the reticular nucleus.

In spite of its comparatively large size, widespread connections, and obvious importance, many of the functions of the thalamus remain unknown. The **motor relay** nuclei are known to be important in the control of muscular activity by the cerebellum and basal ganglia, and the effect of thalamic lesions on the limbic system is known to some extent, but beyond that one can only speculate.

Epithalamus The epithalamus consists of the trigonum habenulae, the pineal body, and the posterior commissure. These structures are located at the posterior limits of the third ventricle and can be seen in a sagittal section of the brain stem, as in Figure 5-30. The **trigonum habenulae** (a triangular region adjacent to the pineal body) contains nuclei that receive olfactory fibers and have extensive projections to the brain stem. They are instrumental in olfactory reflexes.

The **pineal** (shaped like a pine cone) **body** is a small, midline, cone-shaped structure located in a depression between the superior colliculi (structures of the mesencephalon). Actually a gland, the pineal body functions in gonad development. It often calcifies after puberty and so serves as a valuable reference landmark in x-ray examination of the brain. The **posterior commissure,** tucked under the pineal body, is a rounded band of white fibers that connect the two superior colliculi (part of the optic tract) of the mesencephalon. It is instrumental in optic reflexes (eye blinking).

Subthalamus The subthalamus is a structure of the diencephalon, which is sometimes included with the basal

---

[6] The fact that olfactory input is not relayed through the thalamus explains why smoke detectors are so essential. People are not awakened by even very strong odors of smoke.

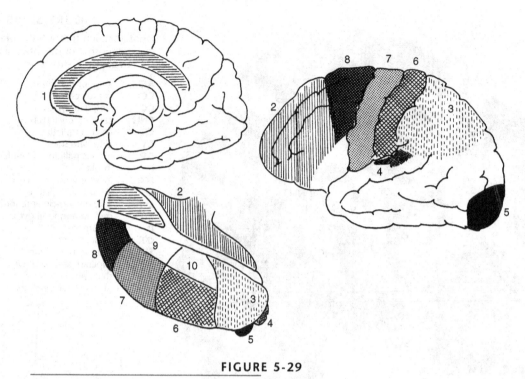

FIGURE 5-29

Thalamic nuclei and their cortical projections. (1) Anterior nucleus, (2) medial nucleus, (3) pulvinar, (4) medial geniculate body, (5) lateral geniculate body, (6) ventroposterolateral nucleus, (7) ventrolateral nucleus, (8) ventroanterior nucleus, (9) dorsolateral and (10) posterolateral nucleus.

ganglia. It is located on the ventrolateral aspect of the thalamus and separates it from the internal capsule. The red nucleus and substantia nigra from the mesencephalon extend into it. The principal nucleus is the **subthalamic nucleus.** It is located on the dorsal surface of the transition between the internal capsule and the crus cerebri. This nucleus receives fibers from the globus pallidus and from the motor and premotor cortex of the cerebrum and is instrumental in regulation and coordination of motor functions.

Hypothalamus The structures constituting the hypothalamus form much of the floor of the third ventricle. They include the mammillary bodies, tuber cinereum, infundibulum, neurohypophysis (neural part of the pituitary), and the optic chiasma, all of which are identifiable in a view of the base of the brain, as in Figure 5-30. Other hypothalamic structures occupy the *paraventricular region* of the third ventricle, outlined in Figure 5-30.

The **mammillary bodies,** part of the limbic system, are two rounded masses on either side of the midline, just beneath the floor of the third ventricle. The **tuber cinereum,** located immediately rostral to the mammillary bodies, is a hollow eminence of gray matter. Laterally it is bounded by the optic tracts (Figure 5-30) and the crus cerebri. Anteriorly it is continuous with a hollow stalk, the **infundibulum,** which projects down and

forward to join the **neurohypophysis** (posterior lobe). The **optic chiasma** is an X-shaped structure located just rostral to the tuber cinereum. It receives fibers from the optic nerve, about half of which decussate at the chiasma and continue to the lateral geniculate body and from there to the occipital lobe of the cerebrum.

The functions of the hypothalamus are so diverse and interwoven with endocrine and autonomic nervous systems that a complete presentation is simply beyond the scope of this chapter. Because the hypothalamus, on each side of the third ventricle, is traversed by the fornix as it courses toward its termination in the mammillary body (Figure 5-22), each half of the hypothalamus is divided into a medial and lateral zone of nuclei that have both afferent and efferent connections, many of them associated with body regulatory functions such as:

Metabolism and water balance. Certain cells in the medial zone nuclei secrete an *antidiuretic hormone* (*ADH*), which acts upon the neurohypophysis to control the reabsorption of water by the kidneys. Carbohydrate and fat metabolism are also regulated by hypothalamic nuclei.

Autonomic nervous system control. The hypothalamus is probably the principal regulator and integrator of the autonomic nervous system. It also mediates expressions of emotional behavior (rage).

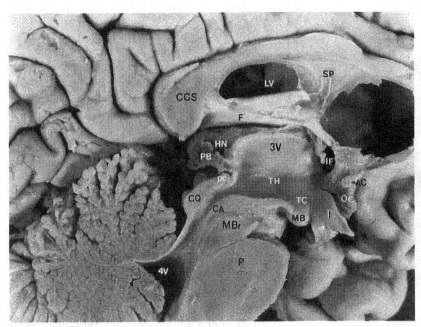

FIGURE 5-30A

A sagittal section through the brain reveals some of the structures of the epithalamus, including the pineal body **(PB)**, the posterior commissure **(PC)**, and the habenular nuclei **(HB)**.

CA	cerebral aqueduct
CCS	corpus callosum (splenium)
CQ	corpora quadrigemina
F	fornix
IF	intervertebral foramen
LV	lateral ventricle
MBr	mid brain
P	pons
PC	posterior commissure
SP	septum pellucidum
4V	fourth venricle
3V	third ventricle—removal of lining reveals thalamus **(TH)**

Hypothalamus includes infundibulum **(I)**, mammillary bodies **(MB)**, optic chiasm **(OC)**, tuber cinereum **(TC)**.

Sleep and wake mechanisms. Radiations from the hypothalamus to the thalamus and to the cerebral cortex are instrumental in controlling states of sleep, wakefulness, and consciousness.

Regulation of body temperature. A body exposed to extreme cold or heat for prolonged periods will exhibit very little change in its internal temperature. Reciprocal stimulation of the sympathetic division of the autonomic nervous system for cold and the parasympathetic division for excessive heat, regulates blood flow and therefore heat dissipation with remarkable accuracy. These autonomic mechanisms maintain body heat at 37° C.

Food intake regulation and the development of **secondary sex characteristics** are other functions attributed to hypothalamic activity.

The Mesencephalon (Midbrain)

The mesencephalon is a short, constricted segment connecting the pons and cerebellum (structures of the hindbrain) with the diencephalon and telencephalon. It consists of two lateroventral **cerebral peduncles** and a dorsal portion the **tectum** (L. rooflike) which contains the paired **superior** and **inferior colliculi (corpora quadrigemina)**. The mesencephalon is pierced by the cerebral aqueduct, which connects the third with the fourth ventricle (Figure 5-30A).

Cerebral Peduncles The cerebral peduncles, which are ventral to the cerebral aqueduct, emerge from the base of the brain as continuations of the internal capsule, converge toward the midline, and enter the upper part of the pons (Figure 5-31). The space between the peduncles is called the **interpeduncular fossa,** and it is

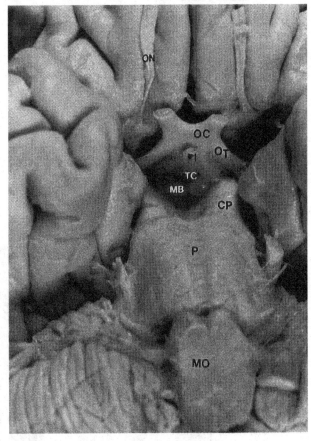

FIGURE 5-30B

The brainstem, as seen from beneath, reveals some structures of the hypothalamus, and the optic tract **(OT)**.

I	infundibulum	**CP**	cerebral peduncles
MB	mammillary bodies	**MO**	medulla oblongata
OC	optic chiasm	**ON**	olfactory nerve (CN I)
TC	tuber cinereum	**P**	pons

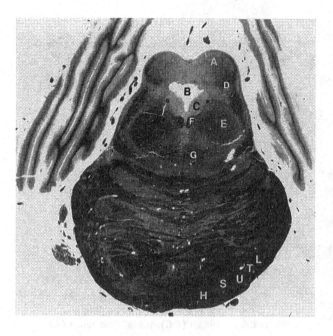

FIGURE 5-31A

Transverse section through the inferior colliculi.

A. Inferior colliculus
B. Cerebral aqueduct
C. Central gray substance
D. Lateral lemniscus
E. Reticular formation
F. Trochlear nucleus
G. Decussation of superior cerebellar peduncles
H. Frontopontine tract
S. Corticobulbar fibers to speech musculature
U. Corticobulbar fibers to upper limb
T. Corticobular fibers to trunk
L. Corticobular fibers to lower limb

FIGURE 5-31B

Transverse section through red nucleus-substantia nigra.

A. Superior colliculus
B. Cerebral aqueduct
C. Central gray substance
D. Nucleus of oculomotor nerve (III)
E. Medial geniculate body
F. Red nucleus
G. Fibers of oculomotor nerve (III)
H. Substantia nigra
I. Crus cerebri
J. Frontopontine tract
K. Corticobular fibers of pyramidal tract to face, head, and neck
L. Corticospinal fibers to upper limb
M. Corticospinal fibers of pyramidal tract to trunk and lower limb
N. Temporoparietooccipitopontine tract
O. Interpeduncular fossa

the site of one of the subarachnoid cisterns. The cerebral peduncles are flanked above by the optic tracts.

Each peduncle consists of a dorsal part called the **tegmentum** and a ventral part called the **crus cerebri.** These two parts are separated by a layer of dark gray matter called the **substantia nigra.** The cells in this region, which project to the striate bodies, contain a pigment called **melanin,** and they synthesize a neurotransmitter called **dopamine.** Destruction of dopamine-synthesizing cells results in serious motor disorders, one of them Parkinsonism.

The **tegmentum,** the dorsal portion of the cerebral peduncle, contains a number of important nuclei and nerve tracts. The gray matter of the tegmentum also contains nuclei of origin for some cranial nerves. As seen in Figure 5-31, a layer of gray matter surrounds the cerebral aqueduct. It contains nuclei for the oculomotor (III) and trochlear (IV) nerves, both of which supply extrinsic muscles of the eye.

The **red nuclei** are conspicuous, on either side of the midline, just ventral to the cerebral aqueduct. They are important structures in the motor (extrapyramidal) system and receive fibers from the cerebellum. They project to the opposite side of the spinal cord as the **rubrospinal tract.** In addition, the two **superior cerebellar peduncles** (brachia conjunctiva) ascend through the tegmentum, decussating at about the level of the inferior colliculus as they do.

Tectum The tectum, the dorsal part of the midbrain, presents the **superior** and **inferior colliculi** (little hills), which together constitute the **corpora quadrigemina.** The colliculi are paired structures, placed one above the

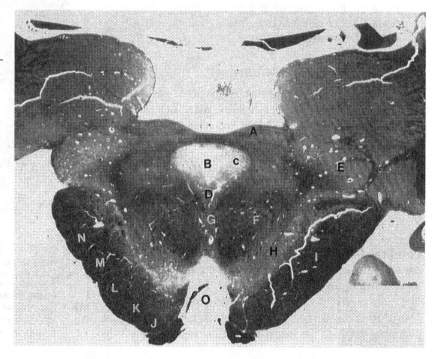

other, on either side of the midline. Normally, they are not visible in the intact brain because they are tucked in between the occipital lobe of the cerebrum and the upper surface of the cerebellum. They can be seen in Figure 5-30, a sagittal section through the brain, labeled as the corpora quadrigemina (CQ). They are also visible in Figures 5-31A and 5-31B, which are transerve sections through the mesencephalon.

The **superior colliculi** are important visual centers. The cells project fibers to the oculomotor, trochlear, and abducent nuclei (all motor nerves to the muscles of the eyes); to other motor nuclei; and to the cerebellum. Many cells in the superior colliculi respond only to movement in the visual fields. The superior colliculi are also integrating centers for certain types of voluntary eye movements, in addition to being reflex centers. *The superior colliculi are responsible for integration of auditory and visual information.*

The **inferior colliculi** are composed of compact masses of nuclei that are important elements of the auditory pathway. They are also important reflex and integrating centers, projecting fibers to the superior colliculi, cerebellum, spinal cord, and medial geniculate body. The inferior colliculi are instrumental in such reflexes as turning of the eyes or head toward the source of a sound, startle responses to sudden noises, and blinking of the eyes in response to sudden, unexpected noise.

The Rhombencephalon (Hindbrain)

The rhombencephalon is divided into the **myelencephalon** or **medulla oblongata** and the **metencephalon,** which consists of the **pons** and **cerebellum.** The medulla oblongata is often referred to as the **bulb,** especially in combined names such as *bulbar polio* and *corticobulbar.*

Myelencephalon (Medulla Oblongata) The medulla oblongata, which is about an inch in length and has a diameter about the same as an ordinary lead pencil, is continuous with the spinal cord and is limited caudally at the level of the upper surface of the first cervical vertebra. This boundary also designates the level of emergence of the first pair of cervical nerves. Above, the medulla is continuous with the pons, but the boundary between these two structures is defined by the **foramen cecum,** a small triangular expansion of the **anterior median fissure** which extends the full length of the spinal cord. On the medulla, this fissure is interrupted by bundles of efferent nerve fibers which cross over the midline and continue down on the opposite side (Figure 5-32A).

This region constitutes an important landmark called the **pyramids,** or **pyramidal decussation.** It contains descending motor fibers from the cerebral cortex on their way to the ventral horns of the spinal cord. This is our *major motor pathway.* About 60 percent of the motor fibers cross over the midline at the pyramids. They con-

tinue into the spinal cord as the **crossed pyramidal tract** (or lateral cerebrospinal fasciculus). The remaining uncrossed (direct) fibers form the **direct pyramidal tract** (or anterior cerebrospinal fasciculus).

On either side of the pyramids in the upper part of the medulla are the **inferior olives,** which are *relay nuclei for proprioceptive impulses* on their way to the cerebellum. An ill-defined **posterior median fissure,** which also courses the full length of the spinal cord together with the anterior median fissure, divides the medulla into symmetrical halves. Between them lie the central canal and fourth ventricle. The lateral surface is further divided by an **anterolateral** and a **posterolateral sulcus,** also continuous with the spinal cord. The inferior olive is located between these sulci, at the level of the upper limit of the pyramids.

The anterolateral and posterolateral sulci are sites of emergence for some of the cranial nerves. The hypoglossal nerve, which supplies motor fibers to the tongue, emerges from the anterolateral sulcus (at the level of the olive) and the glossopharyngeal and vagus nerves emerge on the same level, but from the posterolateral sulcus.

The portion of the medulla dorsal to the posterolateral sulcus contains a number of *ascending nerve tracts,* including the **fasciculus gracilis** and the **fasciculus cuneatus** and their nuclei (Figure 5-32B). These tracts are the continuation of fibers in the spinal cord that terminate in the nuclei. They act as relay stations for ascending sensory data to the thalamus and are important for *locomotion.* The tracts are visible in a dorsal view of the medulla, as two vertical columns flanking the posterior median sulcus. They terminate as bulges (the nuclei), one placed slightly above and lateral to the other.

The upper limit of the posterior portion of the medulla oblongata is continued to the cerebellum by means of a pair of stalks, the **inferior cerebellar peduncles** (or **restiform bodies**). They carry fibers from the spinal cord and medulla oblongata to the cerebellum. In addition to the important motor and sensory nerve tracts, the medulla oblongata also contains the nuclei of other cranial nerves. They are shown in Figure 5-33.

Much of the central portion of the medulla consists of the **reticular formation,** which is composed of three longitudinal columns of nuclei that can be found throughout the entire core of the brain stem. The **nucleus ambiguous,** an inconspicuous nucleus located within the reticular formation, contributes to the vagus, glossopharyngeal, and accessory nerves. Just above the nucleus ambiguous can be found the two small **salivatory nuclei,** which supply, by way of the facial and glossopharyngeal nerves, the submandibular, sublingual, and parotid salivary glands. The nucleus of the **tractus solitarius** extends the length of the medulla oblongata. It is sensory and receives fibers from the facial, glossopharyngeal, and vagus nerves. And finally, the **dorsal** and

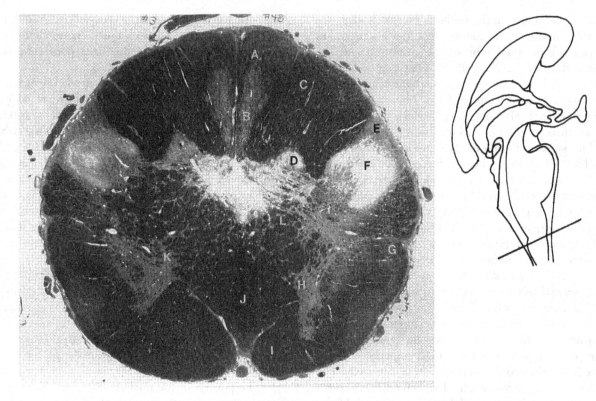

FIGURE 5-32A

Transverse section of the medulla passing through the decussation of the pyramidal tracts.

A. Fasciculus gracilis	G. Spinocerebellar tract
B. Nucleus gracilis	H. Anterior horn of spinal cord
C. Fasciculus cuneatus	I. Anterior corticospinal tract
D. Nucleus cuneatus	J. Pyramidal decussation
E. Spinal tract of trigeminal nerve (V)	K. Reticular formation
F. Nucleus of spinal tract of trigeminal nerve (V)	L. Lateral corticospinal tract

ventral cochlear nuclei are located just beneath the inferior cerebellar peduncle, near the level of the pons. They are very important for us because they receive fibers from the hearing mechanism.

The medulla oblongata also contains the following centers for the regulation of respiration and circulation:

Cardiac inhibitor center—controls heart rate.

Vasoconstrictor center—sends fibers down the spinal cord to emerge at various levels as part of the autonomic nervous system. Some fibers cause peripheral dilation of the blood vessels; others cause vasoconstriction.

Respiratory center—automatically modifies respiratory rate depending upon emotion and physical demands.

In addition, many reflexes are mediated through the medulla. They include coughing, sneezing, vomiting, blinking, and even movements of the alimentary canal.

Metencephalon (Pons) When viewed from the side, as in Figure 5-5, the hindbrain presents a rounded, anteriorly directed eminence known as the **pons.** It is located ventral to the cerebellum, between the mesencephalon above and the medulla oblongata below. The substance of the pons consists of interlaced transverse and longitudinal white fibers, intermixed with gray matter. Much of the internal pons is made up of reticular formation that is continuous with that of the medulla oblongata.

The transverse fibers bridge the midline and collect on either side to form the **middle cerebellar peduncles (brachia pontis).** They serve in part as a commissure and join the two halves of the cerebellum. The **tegmentum,** the dorsal portion of the pons, is continuous with the tegmentum of the cerebral peduncles, while the ventral portion, consisting of longitudinal fibers, is continuous with the crus cerebri of the peduncles. The cerebral peduncles continue to the pyramids of the medulla oblongata. The ventral portion of the pons also contains a cluster of **pontine nuclei** that act

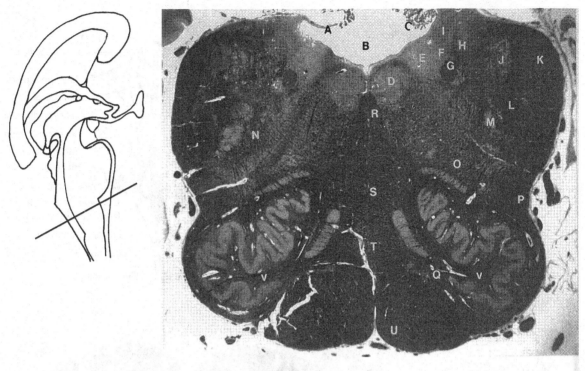

FIGURE 5-32B

Transverse section of the medulla through the middle of the olive.

A. Inferior medullary velum
B. Fourth ventricle
C. Choroid plexus
D. Hypoglossal nucleus (XII)
E. Dorsal motor nucleus of vagus nerve (X)
F. Nucleus of solitary tract
G. Solitary tract
H. Inferior vestibular nucleus
I. Medial vestibular nucleus
J. Accessory cuneate nucleus
K. Inferior cerebellar peduncle
L. Spinal tract of trigeminal nerve (V)

M. Nucleus of spinal tract of trigeminal nerve (V)
N. Nucleus ambiguous
O. Reticular formation
P. Anterior spinocerebellar tract and anterior and lateral spinothalamic tracts.
Q. Fibers of the hypoglossal nerve (XII)
R. Medial longitudinal fasciculus
S. Medial lemniscus-cuneate part
T. Medial lemniscus-gracile part
U. Pyramidal tract
V. Inferior olivary nucleus

as relay centers for impulses from the cerebrum on their way to the cerebellum.

The tegmentum of the pons is similar to that part of the medulla which is dorsal to the pyramids. The tegmentum contains ascending and descending sensory and motor tracts, a continuation of the reticular formation, and nuclei (or parts of the nuclei) for the trigeminal (V), abducens (VI), facial (VII), and acoustic (VIII) nerves (Figure 5-33).

Metencephalon (Cerebellum) The cerebellum (or little brain) makes up the greater part of the hindbrain. Resting on the floor of the posterior cranial fossa, it is somewhat oval in shape, somewhat flattened, with a pronounced constriction at the midline, and its surface is marked by numerous transversely directed ridges, which give the cerebellum a laminated or foliated appearance. In fact, the parallel ridges are called **folia cerebelli,** and they are separated by fissures that cut deeply into the substance of the cerebellum. When seen in a frontal section, as in Figure 5-34, the white matter just deep to the cortex can be seen to take on the appearance of branches. It is called the **arbor vitae** (L. *tree of life*), also shown in Figure 5-34B.

External Structure. Grossly, the cerebellum consists of a narrow median portion called the **vermis,** which is partially covered by the two **cerebellar hemispheres.** They project laterally and posteriorly. Fissures on the surface divide the cerebellum into lobes, which are grouped on a phylogenetic basis into an **archicerebellum** (first), a **paleocerebellum** (old), and a **neocerebellum**

FIGURE 5-33

Nuclei of rhombencephalon, including motor and sensory nuclei of the medulla oblongata as viewed from behind. (Adapted from numerous sources.)

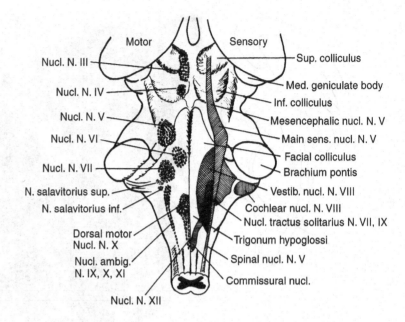

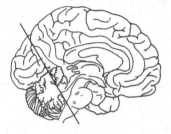

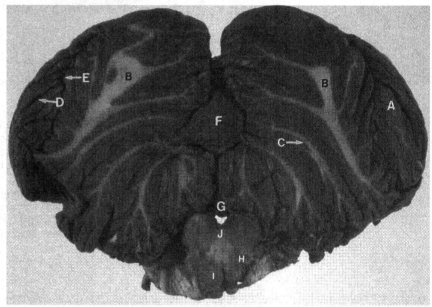

FIGURE 5-34A

Frontal section through the cerebellum illustrating how white matter combined with the foliated nature of the cortex has been likened to branches on a tree, i.e., arbor vitae.

A. Cerebellar cortex (grey matter)
B. Medullary body (white matter)
C. Cerebellar arbor vitae
D. Cerebellar folia (equivalent to gyri in cerebrum)
E. Cerebellar fissures (equivalent to sulci in cerebrum)

F. Vermis of cerebellum
G. Fourth ventricle
H. Inferior olivary nucleus (pons)
I. Pyramidal tract
J. Tegmentum of pons

(new). These divisions reflect a topographical and functional organization.

The archicerebellum, which consists of the **flocculus** (L. a flock of wool) and the **nodulus,** is the most primitive part of the cerebellum and is the first part to de-

velop embryologically. It is closely associated with the vestibular nerve and the sense of *body position* and *equilibrium*. The archicerebellum is separated from the remainder of the cerebellum by the **posterolateral fissure.** The paleocerebellum is primarily associated with control of

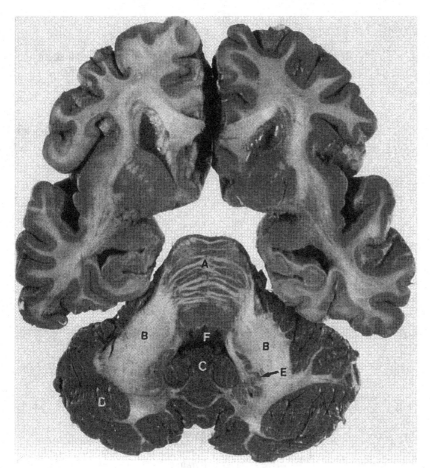

FIGURE 5-34B

The central white matter in this horizontal section through the cerebellum can be seen to arborize.

A. Pons
B. Central white matter
C. Vermis
D. Cerebellar hemisphere
E. Dentate nucleus
F. Fourth ventricle

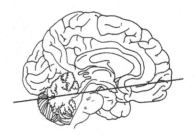

the limbs, and the neocerebellum is associated with the cortex of the cerebrum.

Each cerebellar hemisphere is divided on a functional basis into three lobes: the **anterior, posterior,** and **flocculonodular lobes.** When seen in a sagittal section, the anterior lobe is located on top of the cerebellum and is separated from the posterior lobe by the primary fissure. The flocculonodular node is separated from the posterior lobe by the posterolateral fissure (Figure 5-35). Illustrations of the lobes of the cerebellum are invariably a source of confusion or frustration. How is it that the anterior lobe, which is located above the flocculonodular lobe, appears *behind* the posterior lobe? By convention, neuroscientists have shown the cerebellum as if it had been "unfolded" in much the same manner a book is opened. In the case of the cerebellum, imagine the book binding to be at the back, so when the book is opened, the anterior lobe ends up behind the posterior and flocculonodular lobes.

The **vermis** has been divided into a number of components as shown in Figure 5-36. Beginning anteriorly, the superior aspect of the vermis is divided into the **lingula, central lobule, culmen** (L. summit), **declive** (L. sloping), and **folium** (L. leaflike).

Again, beginning from the front, the structures on either side of the vermis (the cerebellar hemispheres) are

as follows: the **wing of the central lobe** (*ala lobus centralis*), the **anterior quadrangular lobule,** the **posterior quadrangular lobule,** and the **superior semilunar lobule.** Three fissures facilitate these divisions. They are the **postcentral, primary,** and **posterior superior fissures.**

When seen from beneath, the inferior vermis is divided into (beginning from behind) the **tuber, pyramid, uvula,** and **nodulus.** The hemispheres when seen from beneath, are divided into the **inferior semilunar lobule, biventral lobule, tonsil, flocculus,** and **peduncle of the flocculus.** Fissures on the under surface include the **postpyramidal, prepyramidal,** and **postlateral.**

Internal Structure. The cerebellum consists of an extensive surface of gray matter (cerebellar cortex), four paired subcortical nuclei, and white matter.

The **cortex** of the cerebellum consists of an outer molecular layer and an inner granular (or nuclear) layer. The **molecular layer** (Figure 5-37) contains some small nerve cells, the **basket, Golgi,** and **stellate cells.** It also contains the elaborate dendritic extensions of a layer of **Purkinje cells,** which are arranged side by side in a single row. They occupy the deepest part of the molecular layer and form a transition between the molecular and granular layers. Their dendrites extend into the molecular layer while their axons course through

FIGURE 5-35

Principal lobes and fissures of the cerebellum.

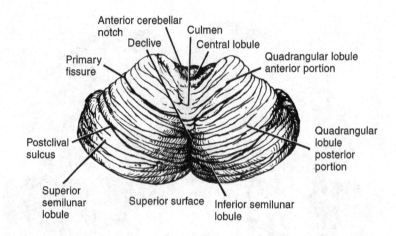

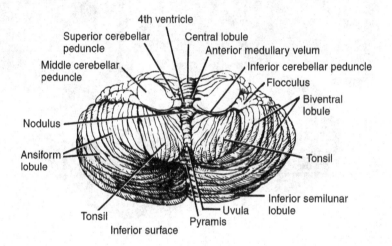

FIGURE 5-36

Sagittal section of cerebellum showing the divisions of the vermis.

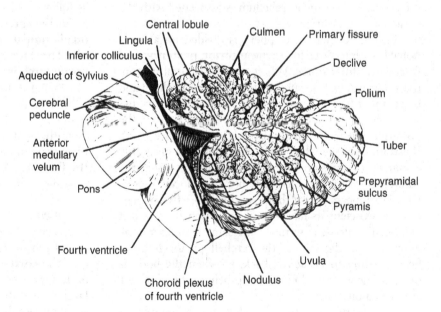

the granular layer into the white matter of the cerebellum. These axons give off recurrent collaterals to other Purkinje cells of the same and neighboring folia, but ultimately the Purkinje cell axons terminate in the cerebellar nuclei.

The **granular layer** is composed of densely packed **granular cells** (the smallest of all neurons), the axons of which penetrate into the molecular layer. Their function is to excite the Purkinje cells. The granular cells, in turn, are excited by way of **mossy fibers** which are the

FIGURE 5-37

A schematic of cortex of cerebellum showing types of cells (top) (from Gray, 1973), and a microphotograph of cortex of cerebellum (bottom).

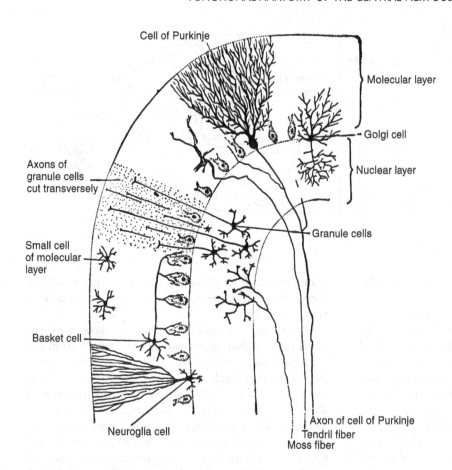

Cell of Purkinje

Molecular layer

Golgi cell

Nuclear layer

Axons of granule cells cut transversely

Granule cells

Small cell of molecular layer

Basket cell

Axon of cell of Purkinje

Tendril fiber

Moss fiber

Neuroglia cell

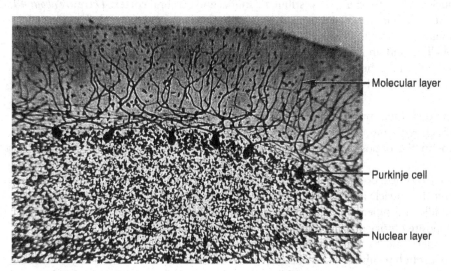

Molecular layer

Purkinje cell

Nuclear layer

terminal branches of afferent fibers entering the cerebellum by way of the cerebellar peduncles. These fibers originate from the inferior olive in the medulla. **Climbing fibers** also enter the cerebellum. They are axons from pontine, vestibular, reticular, and trigeminal nuclei and from the spinocerebellar tract.

The **Purkinje cells** are the final pathway out of the cortex. Their axons terminate in the deep nuclei. They are excited directly through the mossy fibers and granule cells and can be inhibited indirectly through basket, stel-

late, and Golgi cells. This means that *impulses entering the cerebellum activate both inhibitory and excitatory mechanisms, but output from the Purkinje cells is strictly inhibitory.*

Four pairs of nuclei, shown in Figure 5-38, are located within the central white matter of the cerebellum. The largest and most lateral of them is the **dentate nucleus,** so named because of its wrinkled or serrated appearance. Next to it is the **emboliform** (Gk. *emblos,* plug) **nucleus,** then the **globose** (L. globe). On either side of the midline are the **fastigial** (L. to slope up) **nuclei.**

FIGURE 5-38

Nuclei of cerebellum.

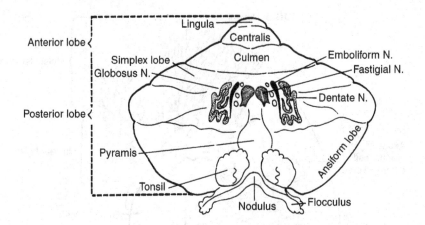

These nuclei receive fibers almost exclusively from the Purkinje cells.

The **white matter** of the cerebellum consists of **afferent, efferent,** and **intrinsic fibers.** Most of the intrinsic fibers are axons from the Purkinje cells, all of which terminate in the cerebellar nuclei, and there are also association and commissural fibers within the white matter. The efferent fibers are projections of the cerebellar nuclei. *All the efferent and afferent fibers leave and enter the cerebellum by three pairs of stalks or cerebellar peduncles.*

The **superior cerebellar peduncle** (brachium conjunctivum) carries **dentaterubral** fibers from the dentate nucleus to the opposite red nucleus and to the thalamus. It also carries **ventral spinocerebellar** fibers that enter the cerebellum from the spinal cord and terminate in the cortex of the paleocerebellum and, in addition, the **uncinate fasciculus,** fibers of which hook around the superior peduncle to terminate in the vestibular nucleus.

The **middle cerebellar peduncle** (brachium pontis), the largest of the peduncles, carries fibers from nuclei in the pons to their terminations in the opposite (contralateral) neocerebellum (Figure 5-39).

The **inferior cerebellar peduncle** (restiform body) ascends along the lateral walls of the fourth ventricle and enters the cerebellum between the middle and superior peduncles. It carries fibers from the opposite olivary nucleus directly to the cerebellar hemisphere and to the vermis. It also carries **dorsal spinocerebellar** fibers coming from the spinal cord and continuing to the anterior lobe and the paleocerebellum. In addition, it carries fibers from the vestibular nuclei to their terminations in the flocculonodular lobe (archicerebellum). Some of the principal connections are shown in Figure 5-39.

Function. The cerebellum receives input about the length and tension of virtually every skeletal muscle in the body. Its role is to make compensations for cortically induced movements so they are smoothly coordinated patterns that require little or nothing in the way of con-

scious effort. *It is a highly integrated motor-regulating system, capable of continuous tracking of muscle and limb movements.*

The cerebellum can be likened to a *comparator* capable of rapid analysis of a variety of input information and whose output coordinates the timing and extent of muscle contraction, limb movement, and so forth. These functions require a substantial amount of information about the body—body position, motion, limb movement, extent and rapidity of muscle contractions and their effects upon joints, autonomic activity, and the extent of the activity of the basal ganglia, pontine ganglia, vestibular ganglia, and cerebral cortex. *There are about 40 times more afferent fibers entering the cerebellum than efferent fibers leaving it.*

The functions of the cerebellum are not under voluntary control. In other words, we are not directly aware of the functions of the cerebellum, nor do we voluntarily modify cerebellar functions to any great extent. The keystone to cerebellar functions seems to lie in the **Purkinje cells** that are excited by way of climbing fibers, mossy fibers, and granule cells. They, in turn, regulate discharge from the four deep cerebellar nuclei by projecting only inhibitory impulses to them. The output from the nuclei to the motor pathway is indirect by way of the thalamus and brain-stem nuclei (vestibular, reticular, and red). The circuit, summarized in Figure 5-40, initially involves the motor and premotor cortexes for voluntary movements.

Motor impulses reach the pontine nuclei and are relayed to the cerebellar cortex. From there, by way of Purkinje cells, to the deep nuclei and on to the thalamus. The thalamus projects to the motor cortex, and the circuit has been completed. During the completion of the circuit, the cerebellum has been receiving information about muscle contractions, limb movement, and posture, from its afferent input. It compares what is happening to what the cerebral cortex has "decided" should happen and, if necessary, relays corrective information back to the cerebral cortex.

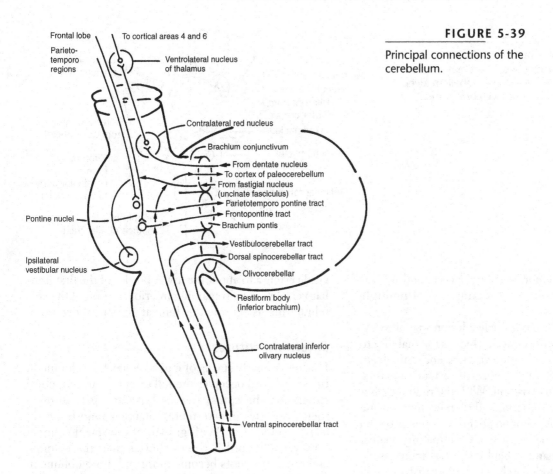

Frontal lobe
Parieto-temporo regions
To cortical areas 4 and 6
Ventrolateral nucleus of thalamus
Contralateral red nucleus
Brachium conjunctivum
From dentate nucleus
To cortex of paleocerebellum
From fastigial nucleus (uncinate fasciculus)
Parietotemporo pontine tract
Frontopontine tract
Pontine nuclei
Brachium pontis
Vestibulocerebellar tract
Dorsal spinocerebellar tract
Ipsilateral vestibular nucleus
Olivocerebellar
Restiform body (inferior brachium)
Contralateral inferior olivary nucleus
Ventral spinocerebellar tract

FIGURE 5-39

Principal connections of the cerebellum.

Cerebellar functions have been shown to be **ipsilateral.** Activity of the right cerebellar hemisphere affects the right side of the body, whereas motor functions of the cerebral cortex are **contralateral.** Activity of the right motor cortex affects the left side of the body.

Because the cerebellum can be "compartmentalized" phylogenetically, its functions are often described in terms of the archi-, paleo-, and neocerebellum. The functions assigned to the various sections of the cerebellum are largely based on clinical signs and comparative physiological experimentation.

Lesions of the **archicerebellum** result in disturbances of maintenance of equilibrium, often to the extent that gait is affected. A person with a lesion of the archicerebellum may attempt to compensate by walking with the feet wide apart (wide base gait). Individuals with acute intoxication show much the same type of gait disturbances that might be caused by archicerebellar lesions. *The swaying, staggering, and trunk ataxia (incoordination) resulting from cerebellar dysfunction will not worsen when the eyes are closed, as they will in the case of vestibular dysfunction.*

The archicerebellum receives input from the vestibular nerve and nuclei regarding muscle tone, equilibrium, and posture of muscles, mainly of the trunk. Its efferent fibers project back to the vestibular nuclei and to the reticular formation by way of the inferior peduncle.

In animals, electrical stimulation of the **paleocerebellum** causes an inhibition of the antigravity muscles on the ipsilateral side. Lesions of the anterior lobe result in facilitations of the motoneurons supplying the extensor musculature and *rigidity*, a condition often seen in cerebral palsy. Tonotopic representation of the paleocerebellum has shown that the caudal regions of the body are represented on the most anterior part, and the cephalic regions of the body are represented on the posterior part.

Afferent impulses from the antigravity muscles enter the cerebellum by way of the dorsal and ventral spinocerebellar tracts that go directly to the culmen of the vermis and to the paleocerebellum. Impulses are then relayed to the deep nuclei, and from there, by way of the superior peduncle, to the red nucleus, the thalamus, and finally to the motor and premotor cerebral cortexes.

The role of the **neocerebellum** seems to be chiefly *synergistic*, and lesions result in the inability to control the range of voluntary motor acts. Movements may be undershot or overshot, and they may be accompanied by tremors associated with voluntary motor acts (**intention tremor**) and the inability to perform rapidly changing movements (**dysdiadochokinesia**). Speech may be slurred with inappropriate blending of sounds (**scanning speech**). Rapid, uncontrolled side-to-side eye movements (**lateral nystagmus**) may also result from neocerebellar

FIGURE 5-40

Neural connections of cerebellum. Note feedback between cerebral cortex–pontine nuclei–neocerebellum–deep nuclei–thalamus–cerebral cortex.

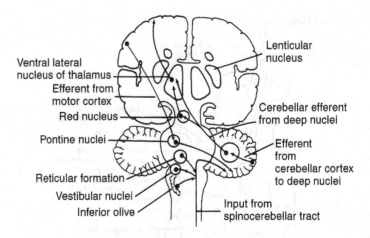

lesions. Intension tremor, scanning speech, and nystagmus comprise the *classic triad* of symptoms of **multiple sclerosis.**

A person with a neocerebellar lesion may also exhibit a **rebound phenomenon,** which is the inability to regulate reciprocal innervation circuits. For example, in the familiar knee jerk, the leg normally extends and then returns to its previous position. With the rebound phenomenon, the lower leg jerks, and then begins to swing like a pendulum. The rebound phenomenon is also seen when the elbow flexors are actively contracting against resistance and the hand is held just a few inches away from the face. A sudden release of the resistance will cause the hand to hit the face. Normally, the cerebellum would inhibit the flexors and stimulate the extensors (triceps) to prevent the hand from hitting the face.

Impulses from the motor cortex reach the cerebellum by way of the pontine nuclei and the middle cerebellar peduncle. The impulses are then relayed to the deep nuclei where they are transmitted out of the cerebellum, by way of the superior peduncle, to the red nucleus, the thalamus, and back again to the motor and premotor cerebral cortexes. This loop arrangement is similar to electronic "servosystems," which are self-regulatory.

The cerebellum is not less resistant to disease and trauma than is the remainder of the nervous system. Depending on the region involved, cerebellar damage results in fairly specific symptoms. We must realize, however, that many cerebellar *symptoms* may result from lesions outside the cerebellum. Dysfunctions that interfere with normal cerebellar input may result in symptoms suggesting cerebellar lesions. Because of the comparatively large cortex in the neocerebellum, it has a high compensatory potential. This partly explains why symptoms caused by certain acute lesions may gradually disappear.

The Spinal Cord

The lower end of the medulla oblongata is prolonged into, and is continuous with, the spinal cord, which extends from the level of the upper border of the first cer-

vical vertebra to about the lower border of the first lumbar vertebra. The remaining inferior portion of the vertebral canal is occupied by lumbar and sacral nerves.

External Features

During the early stages of embryological development, the spinal cord occupies the full extent of the **vertebral canal,** and the **spinal nerves** leave and pass through their respective intervertebral foramina almost at right angles to the cord. With growth of the spinal column, however, the cord becomes shorter than the column, and the nerve roots become more and more oblique in the direction they take when leaving the cord. Beginning at about the first thoracic spinal nerve, the nerves must course downward to exit. The lumbar and sacral nerves descend almost vertically to reach their points of exit from the spinal column (Figure 5-41). The location

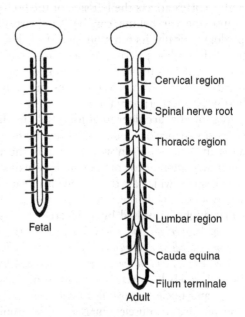

FIGURE 5-41

The course of the spinal nerves in the spinal columns of a fetal and an adult nervous system.

of the lower limit of the spinal cord is somewhat variable among individuals, and it also varies with movements of the vertebral column. For example, it is drawn slightly upward when the spinal column is flexed.

The spinal cord does not end abruptly, but rather, it gradually tapers to a blunt point, the **conus medullaris,** the tip of which is prolonged into a fine filament of fibrous tissue (a continuation of the dura). This filament, known as the **filum terminale,** continues to the coccyx. Below the conus medullaris, the spinal nerves give the appearance of a horse's tail and are called the **cauda equina.**[7] The full extent of the spinal cord is pierced by a **central canal,** which is a remnant of the lumen of the embryonic neural tube. In the adult, however, the central canal is frequently obliterated.

Thirty-one or 32 pairs of **spinal nerves** emerge from the spinal cord, eight in the cervical region, twelve thoracic, five lumbar, and five sacral. One or two coccygeal nerves also emerge from the lower extremity of the spinal cord. Although no segmentation of the cord is visible, it is often regarded as being built of a series of spinal segments, each of which occupies a length equivalent to the extent of the attachment of a pair of spinal nerves.

The spinal cord is described as being roughly cylindrical in shape; however, its transverse diameter is slightly greater than the anteroposterior diameter. It is about 13 mm across, except at the level from the third cervical to the second thoracic and from the ninth through the twelfth thoracic vertebra, where increased nerve tissue associated with the extremities results in **cervical** and **lumbar enlargements.** The cervical enlargement is the more pronounced.

Like the medulla oblongata, the spinal cord is incompletely divided into right and left halves by an **anterior** and **posterior median sulcus.** The anterior median sulcus (or fissure) is the deeper of the two, and its floor is formed by a transverse band of white matter, the **anterior white commissure.** Although the posterior median sulcus is shallow, a septum of neuroglial tissue extends from it more than halfway into the cord. An additional longitudinal sulcus, the **posterior lateral sulcus,** further divides the spinal cord, and as shown in Figure 5-42, the portion of the spinal cord that lies between it and the **posterior median sulcus** is termed the **posterior funiculus.** In the upper two-thirds of the cord, a shallow furrow, the **posterior-intermediate sulcus,** divides the posterior funiculus into a medial **fasciculus gracilis** and a lateral **fasciculus cuneatus.** The portion of the cord anterior to the posterolateral sulcus is termed the **anterolateral region,** and it is further

divided, by the emergence of the anterior roots of the spinal nerves, into a **lateral fasciculus** and an **anterior fasciculus** (Figure 5-42).

Internal Structure

A transverse section of the spinal cord reveals a central core of gray matter surrounded by white matter.

Gray Matter The gray matter consists of two crescent-shaped bodies joined across the midline by a **transverse commissure** of gray matter, giving the gray matter the appearance of the letter **H** or the shape of a butterfly. A frontal plane through the transverse commissure divides each crescent into a **ventral** (or anterior) **horn** and a **dorsal** (or posterior) **horn.** Since they extend the full length of the spinal cord, they are also called the **ventral** and **dorsal columns.**

The ventral columns contain motor nerve cells, the axons of which leave the spinal cord as the **motor roots** of the spinal nerves. In the upper cervical, thoracic, and midsacral regions, the gray matter in the region of the transverse commissure is extended laterally as the **lateral horn** or **column.** It contains cells of the autonomic nervous system. The dorsal columns contain large numbers of sensory cells.

In a region between the anterior and posterior columns, about opposite the transverse commissure, the gray matter extends into the white matter as a net-like series of processes that forms the **spinal reticular formation.**

As we have seen, *the cells in the ventral and lateral columns are associated with motor functions, while those of the dorsal columns are associated with receptor and coordinating functions.* The gray matter has also been organized into specific **nuclei** and **laminae.** They can be thought of as longitudinal columns of neuron cell bodies, many of which extend the full length of the cord, with a specific function (or in the case of laminae, structure).

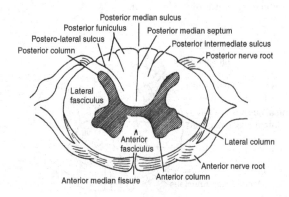

FIGURE 5-42

A transverse section of the spinal cord showing the posterior, lateral, and anterior fasciculus, in relation to the fissures and sulci.

---

[7]In the region of the **cauda equina,** a needle can be inserted between vertebrae L-4 and L-5 to withdraw cerebrospinal fluid without danger of puncturing the spinal cord or damaging the nerves of the cauda equina. This procedure is known as a **lumbar puncture** or a **spinal tap.**

In the 1950s a Swedish neurophysiologist, Bror Rexed, divided the gray matter of the spinal column cord into 10 laminae, based on the cytoarchitecture of the various regions within the ventral and dorsal columns (Figure 5-43). The dorsal horn is composed of laminae I through VI. The dorsal root entry region lies just outside lamina I. The lateral horn contains lamina VII, and the ventral horn contains laminae VIII and IX. Lamina I is called the marginal zone, and its significance is not known. Lamina II and III are known collectively as the **substantia gelatinosa.** It contains internuncial neurons that process sensory information. Lamina IV, the **nucleus proprius,** receives sensory (cutaneous) information which ascends by way of the **spinothalamic tract.** Lamina V receives input from lamina IV, and its cells are continuous with the reticular formation in the brain stem. Lamina VI receives input from proprioceptors and exteroceptors. Lamina VII, also known as the **nucleus dorsalis** (or Clarke's column), receives input from corticospinal fibers, and it also contains preganglionic autonomic cells. Lamina IX contains clusters of **lower motor neurons** that give rise to the ventral (motor) roots of the spinal nerves. Lamina X consists of the cells immediately surrounding the central canal.

White Matter The white matter of the cord is divided into three pairs of **funiculi** (ventral, lateral, and dorsal) in addition to a commissural region. Each funiculus contains (1) ascending fiber tracts that transmit visceral and proprioceptive[8] information to the subcortical motor centers, (2) descending tracts from the higher motor centers, and (3) short intersegmental fibers that mediate reflexive behavior (Figure 5-44).

---

[8]**Proprioception** (L. *proprius,* one's own; L. *perceptio;* pertaining to perception) concerns an appreciation of position, balance, and changes in equilibrium on the part of the muscular system, especially during locomotion. Proprioceptive impulses originate in specialized receptors located in muscles, tendons, joints, and the vestibular apparatus of the inner ear.

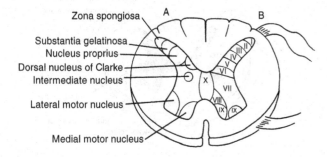

FIGURE 5-43

Transverse section of spinal cord showing division of gray matter into nuclei (A) and laminae (B).

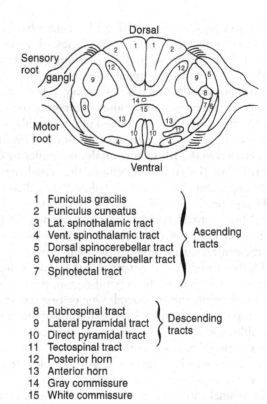

1. Funiculus gracilis
2. Funiculus cuneatus
3. Lat. spinothalamic tract
4. Vent. spinothalamic tract   } Ascending tracts
5. Dorsal spinocerebellar tract
6. Ventral spinocerebellar tract
7. Spinotectal tract

8. Rubrospinal tract
9. Lateral pyramidal tract   } Descending tracts
10. Direct pyramidal tract
11. Tectospinal tract
12. Posterior horn
13. Anterior horn
14. Gray commissure
15. White commissure

FIGURE 5-44

Schematic transverse section of the spinal cord illustrating major ascending and descending tracts within the white matter.

The tracts in each of the funiculi are as follows:

Tracts of the Ventral Funiculus

1. Motor tracts from the vestibular nuclei, the reticular formation, and tectum for regulation of posture and muscle tone.

2. A small uncrossed motor tract for voluntary movements.

3. A sensory tract for awareness of touch, tickle, and itch from the opposite side of the body. This tract is also thought to transmit the sensations of sexual orgasm.

4. An intersegmental **propriospinal tract** for spinal level reflexes.

Tracts of the Dorsal Funiculus

1. The **fasciculus gracilis,** an ascending sensory pathway, transmits sensations of pressure, touch, vibration, and kinesthesia from the lower extremities and from the trunk.

2. The **fasciculus cuneatus,** also an ascending sensory pathway, conveys the same sensations from the upper extremities, and they all reach consciousness.

Tracts of the Lateral Funiculus

1. The **pyramidal** (corticospinal) **tract,** a large crossed motor tract from the motor cortex for voluntary movement.

2. The **rubrospinal tract,** a tract from the red nucleus for muscle tone.

3. The **spinocerebellar tracts,** one direct and one crossed, for transmitting muscle and tendon tension data to the cerebellum.

4. The **lateral spinothalamic tract** conveying pain and temperature from the opposite side of the body.

5. A tract, primarily cervical, transmitting unconscious proprioceptive data to the inferior olive.

6. An intersegmental tract for reflexive activities.

Table 5-1 contains a summary of the major ascending and descending tracts of the spinal cord.

The various tracts within the white matter exhibit **topographical distribution,** as shown in Figure 5-45. Note that in the anterolateral columns, the sacral regions are outermost and the cervical innermost. The arrangement is reversed in the dorsal columns. This in-

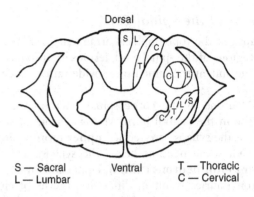

S — Sacral   Ventral   T — Thoracic
L — Lumbar   C — Cervical

FIGURE 5-45

Topographical arrangements of the ascending tracts of the spinal cord. Note that in the anterolateral columns the sacral regions are outermost and the cervical innermost. The arrangement is reversed in the dorsal columns.

formation can be extremely important in diagnoses. A lesion in the dorsal funiculus, just lateral to the midline, for example, will interrupt sensations from the lower limbs, and a person cannot tell what the legs are doing or where they are.

TABLE 5-1

Summary of major ascending and descending tracts of the spinal cord

Anterior White Column	
Descending tracts	*Function*
Ventral corticospinal (direct pyramidal)	Voluntary Motor
Vestibulospinal	Balance-reflex
Tectospinal	Audio-visual reflex
Reticulospinal	Muscle tone
Ascending tracts	*Function*
Ventral spinothalamic	Light touch
Spino-olivary	Proprioception-reflex
Lateral White Column	
Descending tracts	*Function*
Lateral corticospinal (pyramidal)	Voluntary motor
Rubrospinal	Muscle tone-synergy
Olivospinal	Reflex
Ascending tracts	*Function*
Dorsal spinocerebellar	Proprioception-reflex
Ventral spinocerebellar	Proprioception-reflex
Lateral spinothalamic	Pain-temperature
Spinotectal	Reflex
Posterior White Column	
Descending tracts	*Function*
Fasciculus interfascicularis and septomarginal fascicularis	Association and integration
Ascending tracts	*Function*
Fasciculus gracilis and fasciculus cuneatus	Vibration, motion, joint sensations, and two-point discrimination

Lesions of the Spinal Cord

Because of the topographical arrangement of the various regions of the spinal cord, lesions can produce very specific and, at the same time, a wide variety of clinical signs.

Neurons of the corticospinal tract (motor tract) synapse in the ventral horn. Motor neurons above the level of the synapse are termed **upper motor neurons (UMN)**, while neurons below the synapse are called **lower motor neurons (LMN).** Upper and lower motor neuron injuries result in different patterns of clinical signs. At the same time, it is important to realize that damage to the spinal cord can produce signs of both upper and lower motor neuron involvement.

Generally, both upper and lower motor neuron damage result in paralysis and anesthesia below the level of injury, but clinical signs include

UMN Injury	LMN Injury
spastic paralysis	flaccid paralysis
no muscle atrophy	muscle atrophy
no fasciculations or fibrillations	fasciculations and fibrillations
increased deep tendon reflexes	loss of deep tendon reflexes

Disturbances of sexual function and loss of bowel and bladder control may also be part of the clinical picture in spinal cord injuries.

The Cerebral Cortex (Pallium)

The cerebral cortex forms a closely fitting cap for the cerebral hemispheres. Only about a third of its surface area is visible; the walls of the sulci and fissures form the unexposed area. If the cortex were removed it would weigh about 600 gm (1 lb), cover a flat surface area of about 0.75 sq m (2.5 sq ft) and vary in thickness from about 1.5 mm to 4.5 mm. It contains an estimated 15 billion nerve cells and about 50 billion glial cells.

The cerebral cortex can be divided, on a phylogenetic basis, into three functionally distinct parts. The **archipallium,** an ancient cortex associated with the limbic system, is located in the medialmost parts of the frontal, parietal, and temporal lobes. The **paleopallium** includes that part of the cortex associated with the olfactory system. The **neocortex** is the remaining 90 percent of the cerebral cortex.

Microscopic views of the cortex reveals five types of nerve cells, organized in a stratified fashion into six layers (Campbell, 1905; Cajal, 1906; and Brodmann, 1909). As shown in Figure 5-46, they are molecular, external granular, external pyramidal, internal granular, internal pyramidal, and polymorphic layers, comprised of the five cell types: pyramidal, granular, Martinotti's, horizontal, and polymorphous.

The most conspicuous cells are known as **pyramidal cells,** and they can be classified as small, medium, large, and giant pyramidal cells. When seen microscopically, as in Figure 5-47, the cell body appears pyramidal in shape. Its axons extend into the subjacent white matter, while its dendrites are directed toward the surface of the cortex.

Giant pyramidal cells of Betz can be found in the fifth cortical layer, especially in the motor cortex. These cells give rise to the pyramidal (corticospinal) tract which supplies the striated muscles of the body. Small **granule** (or **stellate**) cells can be found throughout the cortex, although they are located in definite layers. They are characterized by short branching axons. Figure 5-46 shows a schematic representation of the six cortical layers. The appearance of the cortex depends upon the stain used in preparation of the microscope slide. Each stain reveals something distinctive about the cytoarchitecture of the cerebral cortex. A Golgi stain shows the more conspicuous neurons, while a Nissl stain shows neuron cell bodies. Other stains reveal just the myelinated fiber patterns.

Just as the thickness of the cerebral cortex varies from region to region, so does the arrangement and distribution of the layers of the various types of cells. Cortical areas differ, for example, in the relative thickness of the various layers, in the number of afferent and efferent fibers, and so forth. The most superficial layers of cortical cells are afferent as well as efferent. They are the **association neurons** which course to other parts of the cortex. The fourth layer contains nerve endings from radiations of the thalamus, while the fifth layer contains motor cells, the giant pyramidal cells of Betz, which are responsible for the initiation of motor nerve impulses.

In the past, the areas of the cortex manifesting histological homogeneity have been described as having specific functional characteristics. A number of experimental and clinical approaches have been used over the years in an attempt to relate **cytoarchitectonics** (cellular architecture) and **myeloarchitectonics** (nerve fiber distribution) to function. They include extirpation of nerve tissue during surgery, the study of disease processes, electrical stimulation of cortical regions under local anaesthesia, and comparative physiology. Countless experiments, both acute and chronic, have been conducted with experimental animals, but, because so much of neurophysiology seems to be species specific, the results must be interpreted with some caution. In other words, extrapolation from one species (dogs, for example) to another (humans) may be hazardous.

The individual regions of the cerebral cortex are not completely autonomous. They are influenced by

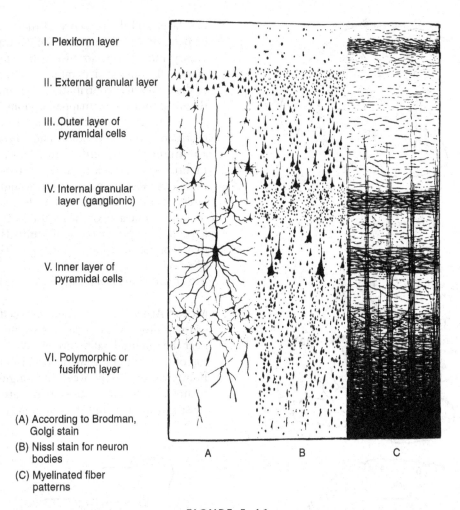

I. Plexiform layer

II. External granular layer

III. Outer layer of
      pyramidal cells

IV. Internal granular
      layer (ganglionic)

V. Inner layer of
      pyramidal cells

VI. Polymorphic or
      fusiform layer

(A) According to Brodman,
      Golgi stain
(B) Nissl stain for neuron
      bodies
(C) Myelinated fiber
      patterns

A   B   C

FIGURE 5-46

Schematic representation of the six cortical cell layers. (1) molecular or plexiform layer, (2) external granular layer, (3) external pyramidal layer, (4) internal granular layer, (5) pyramidal layer, (6) polymorphic layer. (A) The cortex as seen by Brodmann (1909), using a Golgi stain, (B) as seen using a Nissl stain for neuron bodies, and (C) as seen with a stain for myelin.

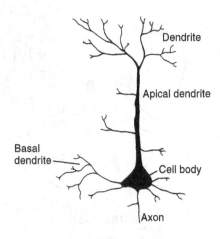

Dendrite

Apical dendrite

Basal dendrite

Cell body

Axon

FIGURE 5-47

A drawing of a microscopic view of a pyramidal cell from the fifth cortical layer.

other regions, or perhaps by the entire hemisphere. Even though the interrelationships between the various regions of the cortex have not been completely documented, we know that certain regions are related to specific functions. The cerebral cortex and some areas which have had functions assigned to them are shown in Figure 5-48.

Cortical Mapping

A significant cortical map, or **architectonic chart** was developed by Brodmann in 1909. He assigned numbers, as shown in Figure 5-49, to 47 various areas of the cerebral cortex on the basis of **cytoarchitecture,** using the Nissl stain for cells. In addition, by electrically stimulating areas of the surgically exposed cortex, researchers have succeeded in mapping some of the *functionally*

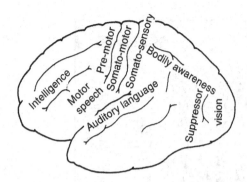

FIGURE 5-48

Schematic localization of cerebral cortex functions.

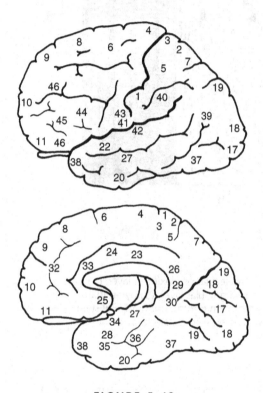

FIGURE 5-49

Brodmann's areas.

homogeneous regions of the brain (Penfield and Roberts, 1959).

The archipallium and paleopallium are composed of Brodmann's areas 24 through 36. The remaining areas are found in the neopallium, and they can, for the most part, be divided into four types: (1) **afferent** (sensory), (2) **integrative** (association), (3) **efferent** (motor), and (4) **suppressor.**

The **motor cortex** of the brain includes all of the precentral gyrus and the posterior parts of the frontal gyri. It corresponds to Brodmann's areas 4 and 6. The motor cortex is characterized by an absence of the gran-

ular layer and the presence of the giant pyramidal cells of Betz. At one time, all pyramidal tract control of voluntary motor behavior was attributed solely to these giant cells, but other pyramidal cells and other regions of the cortex also contribute. The motor cortex is one of the most thoroughly mapped regions of the brain.

A semigraphic technique used to schematize body representation in the motor (and sensory) cortex is called a **homunculus** (L. little man). An example is shown in Figure 5-50. As seen from the distribution of the body, there is almost an inverse relationship between the volume or area of the body and its degree of cortical representation. The area of the motor cortex that supplies the legs, for example, is not significantly larger than the area that supplies the tongue. *The implication is that there is a direct relationship between the amount of cortical representation of a structure and the extent of its nerve supply.*

Motor Areas If a surgically exposed precentral gyrus of the motor cortex (area 4) is stimulated in the region near the longitudinal fissure, in other words right at the top of the brain, movements occur in the hip and trunk. If an area midway between the longitudinal and lateral fissure is stimulated, movements are produced in the wrist and fingers, and if an area near the lateral fissure

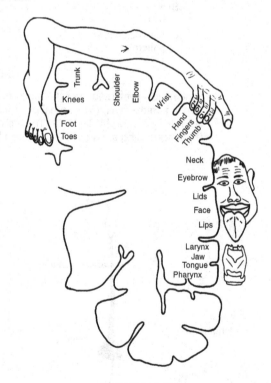

FIGURE 5-50

A motor homunculus. Distortion of body shows extent of cortical representation, and its importance. The hands and tongue have more motor (and sensory) cortical representation than the elbow or trunk.

is stimulated, movements are produced in the facial region. Because of the decussation of the motor fibers at the level of the medulla oblongata (the pyramids), stimulation of the left motor cortex produces movements on the right side of the body. This is especially true of the limbs. Muscles near the median plane of the body are under bilateral cerebral control. The principal input to area 4 is from the cerebellum, by way of the thalamus.

Premotor Areas The premotor or precentral area (area 6) is much like the motor area, except for an absence of the giant pyramidal cells. Motor responses elicited by stimulation of this area are produced by transmission through area 4, the motor area.

Movements produced involve larger groups of muscles in more complex behavior. The region just in front of area 6 is area 8. Stimulation of this region evokes conjugate movements of the eyes, or of the eyes and head. Normally, the eyes move together in the same direction. If the eyes are turned to the left, the movement is caused by contraction of the left rectus lateralis muscle, supplied by the abducent nerve, and the right rectus medialis muscle, which is supplied by the oculomotor nerve. Fibers from the premotor area contribute to an important motor control system called the **extrapyramidal tract.**

Broca's Area A *motor speech area* can be located in the region of the **frontal operculum,** areas 44 and 45, at the junction of the lateral and central fissures. These regions are responsible for the motor movements required for the production of speech. Even though these areas in both hemispheres supply the speech musculature, it is from a person's dominant hemisphere, usually the left, that speech movements are produced. Areas 44 and 45 are larger and more highly convoluted in the left hemisphere than the right, and lesions result in the inability to produce speech.

Supplemental Motor Area This area, not numbered by Brodmann, is located on the medial surface of the frontal lobe, between areas 4 and 6. Movements elicited are bilateral, and consist of raising of the arms, postural changes, and contractions of the leg and trunk musculature.

Primary Sensory Areas These areas are involved in the perception of sensations, their quality, intensity, and localization.

Somatic Sensory Area. The **postcentral gyrus** (areas 1, 2, and 3) receives exteroceptive and proprioceptive afferent fibers from the brain stem by way of the thalamus. The topographical projection of the sensory area is approximately the same as that of the motor area. Other sensations, such as pain, temperature, and crude touch involve both the postcentral gyrus and the thalamus.

Auditory Sensory Area. Areas 41 and 42 are located on the superior border of the transverse temporal gyrus, and they also occupy part of the superior temporal gyrus. This region receives fibers from both medial geniculate bodies. Area 22, sometimes called **Wernicke's area,** surrounds areas 41 and 42. It is involved in relating past auditory experiences to present sensations, and is an *auditory association area.* These auditory areas transmit to Broca's area by way of the **arcuate fasciculus,** one of the major association tracts.

Visual Sensory (or Striate) Area. Area 17 is located in the walls of the **calcarine sulcus,** extending into both the cuneus and the lingual gyri. It is called striate because of its laminated appearance. The optical fibers that enter this region terminate in the fourth cell layer, where they are so concentrated that they form a white band that is visible to the naked eye. This strip, sometimes called the **stria of Gennari,** is the cortical center for vision, and it receives fibers from the lateral geniculate body. Visual sensations such as color, size, form, motion, light, and transparency are all recognized in this area. Areas 18 and 19 are **visual association areas.** Also called the **parastriate area,** it is responsible for elaboration of visual impressions and association of them with past experience, for recognition and identification. It also relates eye movements to visual impressions.

The **parietal area** (areas 5, 7, 39, and 40) is located between the visual, auditory, and somatic sensory areas. This region correlates and integrates sensory impressions from the surrounding areas.

Vestibular Area. Area 43, for recognition of **vertigo,**[9] and for the sensation of **nausea,** is located in the parietal lobe at the junction of the central and lateral fissures.

Suppressor Regions. Electrical stimulation of areas 6, 8, 12, 19, and 24 results in inhibited cortical activity in that region, spreading slowly over the entire cortex, a process requiring up to half an hour. Symptoms produced by cortical lesions may be the result, not only of the loss of specific functions, but the failure of suppressor functions. For example, if the suppressor area just in front of area 4 is damaged, *spasticity* and *hypertonicity* may result.

Hemispheric Dominance

In the second century, Galen, who was physician to the gladiators in Pergamon, discovered that pressure applied to the brain results in paralysis, proof enough, he

---

[9]**Vertigo,** sometimes erroneously equated with dizziness, is actually an illusory sensation of movement. **Objective vertigo** is characterized by the feeling that the world is revolving around you, whereas in **subjective vertigo,** you feel as though you yourself are revolving in space.

wrote, to shatter the tenets of the philosopher Aristotle, who believed the heart was the center for human thoughts. Galen's observations went unheeded, and little progress in understanding the brain was made during the ensuing thousand years.

In the early 1500s, artist Leonardo da Vinci, who claimed to have dissected over one hundred bodies, declared the ventricles were responsible for the functions of the brain. Memory, for example, took place in the third ventricle, and imagination and common sense in the first.

By the mid seventeenth century the architecture of the brain was fairly well outlined, and its blood supply was documented in detail.

In the late eighteenth century, neuroscientist Franz Josef Gall asserted that personality traits such as creativity, intelligence, and almost all attributes of the brain could be determined by feeling the bumps on a person's skull. Thus was born the pseudoscience of **phrenology,** a tragic chapter in the history of science.

In 1871, Santiago Ramon y Cajal discovered a silver staining technique that would, for the first time, outline an individual neuron, a finding that opened new chapters in neuroscience. Shortly after Cajal's discovery, Camillo Golgi provided neurology with the concept of a **synapse** between nerve cells. In 1906 Cajal and Golgi shared the Nobel Prize in Medicine. This was the age of enlightenment in neuroscience.

During this same period, a conflict was taking place between two camps of neuroscientists. One camp held that the two hemispheres were mirrored images of each other and that the hemispheres shared similar functions. The opposition held that the hemispheres were specialized and that certain functions such as speech and language were localized in one hemisphere. Both camps agreed that the left hemisphere controls movement and sensations on the right side of the body and the right hemisphere controls movement and sensations on the left side. This means that a person who suffers an injury to the motor area of the right hemisphere might be partially or totally paralyzed on the left side of the body. Both camps were also aware that neural tissue, once damaged, does not repair itself,

In 1861, at a meeting of the Paris Anthropological Society, Paul Broca, a surgeon and neuroanatomist, presented the brain of a former patient who had been unable to speak. He had understood language and communicated with gestures, but could not talk. Broca argued that a lesion in the left cerebral hemisphere caused the **aphasia.** Broca made a second major discovery. *A similar lesion in the right hemisphere (in 90 percent of the population) did not result in aphasia.* Ten years later, a German neurologist, Karl Wernicke, reported a different type of aphasia. Wernicke's patients were perfectly capable of speech, but what they said was incomprehensible or totally nonsense. Wernicke found damage in the **left temporoparietal region,** at the posterior limits of the lateral fissure (Figure 5-51) in his patients.

Speech recognition and linguistic expression are dependent upon the integrity of **Wernicke's area.** In their cortical mapping research Penfield and Roberts (1959) found that electrical stimulation of Wernicke's area interfered profoundly with the ability of their patients to speak. *Wernicke's area is responsible for the integration of auditory and visual stimuli and for generating input to Broca's area.* Information is transmitted by way of the **arcuate fasciculus,** and damage to this important association tract may also disrupt speech production. A person may be able to understand words, either spoken or written, but is unable to repeat them.

Comprehension of written language and visual recognition requires connections from the visual areas of the cortex to Wernicke's area. The **angular gyrus,** located just behind Wernicke's area, is an important part of the visual recognition integration system. Damage to the left angular gyrus may result in an inability to read or write **(alexia** and **agraphia),** although the person may retain the ability to speak and to understand speech. Similar lesions in the right hemisphere usually have no effect upon language.

Interestingly, and fortunately, lesions in the language areas of children under 8 years of age may result in severe aphasias, but often almost complete recovery occurs.

For about 90 percent of the right-handed population, the left cerebral hemisphere is specialized for lan-

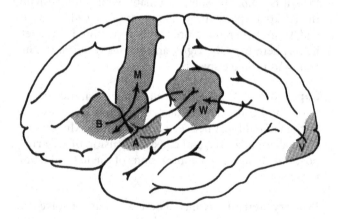

FIGURE 5-51

The left cerebral hemisphere showing areas of specialization for speech production. They include the auditory area (A), Broca's area (B), the motor cortex (M), the visual cortex (V), and Wernicke's area (W). For verbal responses to visual or auditory stimuli, some representation of the response is transmitted from Wernicke's area (where auditory and visual perception are integrated) to Broca's area. The pathway is the arcuate fasciculus.

guage, handedness, analytic thought processes, and certain types of memory. The left hemisphere is dominant in about 64 percent of left-handed people, with a right-dominant hemisphere in about 20 percent. The left hemisphere is also dominant in about 60 percent of ambidextrous people, with both hemispheres equally dominant in 30 percent (Restak, 1984).

We might reasonably ask, if the left hemisphere has such specific functions, what is the function of the right hemisphere? Indeed, aside from the motor and sensory cortexes, is a right hemisphere necessary?

One characteristic of much of the body is the backup system. We have two lungs, and the body can get along with just one. The same is true with the kidneys, and although the loss of an eye or an ear is definitely handicapping, it is not life threatening. At one time neuroscientists (at least some of them) wondered if the two hemispheres constituted a backup system for the nervous system. This question could be answered if the hemispheres could be anatomically separated from one another.

In the 1940s, as a last-ditch effort to save a patient with severe epilepsy (the seizures were being transmitted across the corpus callosum), Dr. Van Wagenen separated the two hemispheres by cutting through the corpus callosum. The seizures were arrested, and the surgery produced no apparent negative effects. Subsequent research showed that each hemisphere operates independently and in instances of **commissurotomies,** the right brain literally does not know what the left brain is doing. A person can touch an object with the right hand (referred to the left brain) and name it. The same person can identify verbally an object presented to the left visual field. When the object is presented to the left hand (right brain), the person cannot identify it verbally. These same people may have difficulty with recent memory. Each hemisphere is an independent brain, with its own specific perception, memory, comprehension, and thoughts.

For about 90 percent of the population, the left hemisphere functions in most aspects of language (writing, reading, and speech), handedness, calculation, and memory. The right hemisphere specializes in **stereognosis** (perception by the sense of touch), in spatial conceptualization, and in nonverbal language. The right hemisphere is also instrumental in the way we listen to music and see works of art. Gardner (1975) states that the right hemisphere deals with holistic processes.

Although gross anatomical differences between the hemispheres can be seen, it is generally acknowledged that until about two years of age, neither hemisphere is dominant. Support for this is found in children who have sustained left hemispheric damage but nevertheless acquire language (and become left handed). The left frontal lobe is usually larger and more heavily convo-

luted than the right, but whether this has any bearing on cerebral dominance is uncertain. These anatomical differences can be found in fetal brains and in brains of animals that do not have language, at least as we know it (Figure 5-52).

Additional information about functions of the left and right hemispheres has been obtained by injecting a short-acting anesthetic, **amobarbital** (Amytol), into one of the internal carotid arteries (which supply the brain). Very quickly one hemisphere ceases to function while the other is unaffected. The results are similar to those obtained from split-brain patients. The dominant (left) hemisphere functions in the comprehension and production of spoken and written language, mathematical calculation, and analytic thought processes. The right hemisphere perceives tactual, visual, and auditory information (which normally is transmitted to the left hemisphere) and is that part of the brain instrumental in artistic creativity. But the right brain does have a very

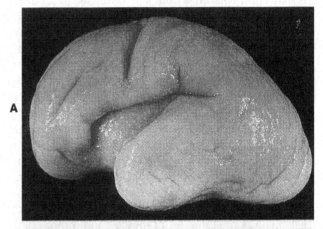

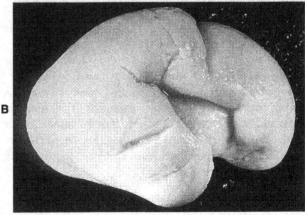

FIGURE 5-52

(A) Lateral view of left hemisphere of a 4-month fetal brain. Note the insular lobe, which has not been covered by the growing frontal and temporal lobes. Note, also, the beginnings of convolutions in the frontal lobe. (B) The right frontal lobe is still smooth. (Dissection by Patty Gauper.)

limited capacity for generating verbal expression of what it is perceiving or thinking (Restak, 1984).

Cerebrocortical Lesions

Lesions of the cerebral cortex produce symptoms that are not only the result of a loss of a specific area, but also the result of adjacent suppressor areas that act as sources of cortical inhibition. Lesions of area 4, the motor cortex, may result in paralyses or partial paralyses that are very specific. Hypotonia and a loss of deep-tendon reflexes may also occur on the contralateral side. These symptoms may improve with time, until only skilled and highly coordinated movements are affected. If, however, the suppressor region in front of area 4 is included, **hypertonicity** and **spasticity** may result. Lesions of area 8 may result in a loss of motor control of the eyes (conjugate deviation).

We have seen that lesions in area 44 in the dominant hemisphere may result in a language-processing disorder called **aphasia.** The person with Broca's aphasia may know what to say but may be unable to produce the words. A distinction must be made between aphasia and **verbal apraxia,** which is a speech disorder resulting from an impairment of motor programming of articulatory movements. The control over learned sequences of motor behavior is a function of an association cortex, and not the motor cortex. Apraxia does not involve paralysis, but rather the inability to perform a voluntary movement due to a lesion of an association cortex in the dominant hemisphere. Interestingly, there does not seem to be a relationship between the part of an association cortex damaged and the type of apraxia produced. Some patients may simply have lost the concept of production of a certain motor act and yet retain a motor act that involves the same set of muscles and motor commands. A differential diagnosis between aphasia and apraxia may be difficult, and requires a considerable amount of expertise on the part of the clinician.

Dysarthria is a speech disorder in which motor control of the speech musculature is impaired due to lesions of the central or the peripheral nervous system. A lesion may involve lower motor neurons that result in a flaccid paralysis **(hypotonicity),** or an upper motor neuron that is characterized by rigidity **(hypertonicity).** Dysarthria may be characterized by slow, labored, and imprecise articulation.

The Reticular Formation

The reticular formation is part of a vital "consciousness system" that extends throughout the central nervous system. This formation regulates cortical activity reaching the cerebral cortex by way of the thalamus.

Anatomically, the reticular formation consists of three columns of diffusely organized nuclei extending from the upper limits of the spinal cord to the thalamus. The reticular formation receives multisensory input from ascending afferent pathways, which is transmitted to the ventral and medial "nonspecific" nuclei of the thalamus. The organization of the reticular formation is such that a single neuron is capable of activating large areas of the thalamus and, in turn, the cerebral cortex. It is important to understand that no single cortical region is responsible for **consciousness** (an awareness of the environment and of one's self). All areas of the cortex are considered to be part of the consciousness system.

Functionally, the reticular formation can be divided into an afferent (receiving) system and an efferent system. During the awake state, sensory information from both the external and internal environments is projected by way of the **ascending reticular activating system (ARAS)** to the thalamus, and finally, by global radiations to all parts of the cerebral cortex. In addition, efferent cortical activity is fed back to the cortex, again, by way of the thalamus. This results in elevated cortical activity that is correlated with the degree of alertness (Figure 5-53).

Consciousness may be altered by two principal factors. The reticular formation can regulate or govern the **ascending exterosensory input** that reaches the cortex, and it can regulate the **endogenous sensory input** that is generated within the body. As input to the cortex is diminished, the level of consciousness decreases, until the level of sleep is reached. Sleep is not just a state of unconsciousness, however, and is described as consisting of **rapid eye movement (REM) sleep,** and **nonrapid eye**

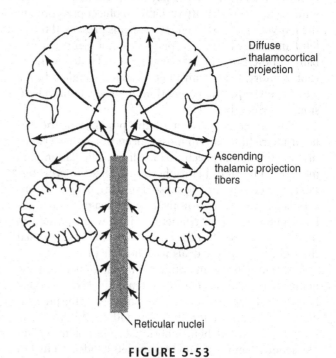

Diffuse thalamocortical projection

Ascending thalamic projection fibers

Reticular nuclei

FIGURE 5-53

Schematic of the ascending reticular activating system.

movement (non-REM) sleep. During non-REM sleep, which precedes REM sleep, no rapid eye movement takes place, and vital signs are stable. Dreaming occurs during REM sleep, and we might say that the body is sleeping but the brain is awake. The condition we call sleep can be quickly reversed by the reticular system, usually after about eight hours.

The reticular formation receives impulses from a variety of sources. They include the ascending somatic and visceral sensory pathways from the spinal cord and from the cranial nerves; motor impulses from the cerebral cortex, basal ganglia, and cerebellum; and impulses from the autonomic nervous system. It has been estimated that a single neuron in the reticular system can activate upwards of 25,000 other neurons. The result of this divergence or spreading out is that *input to the reticular formation can either suppress or excite large numbers of other neurons.*

FUNCTIONAL ANATOMY OF THE PERIPHERAL NERVOUS SYSTEM

The peripheral nervous system is by definition *any neuron or nerve cell process located outside the bony confines of the skull and vertebral column.* It includes the cranial nerves, spinal nerves with their ventral and dorsal roots, dorsal root ganglia and peripheral branches, plus portions of the autonomic nervous system. A **nerve** may be defined as a collection of nerve fibers. A single nerve fiber is so small it cannot be seen without the aid of a microscope, while nerves may reach the diameter of an ordinary lead pencil. Earlier we learned that **neurons** that carry impulses away from the central nervous system are called **efferent** (or motor) neurons, and those that carry impulses toward the central nervous system are **afferent** (or sensory). Almost all nerves are **mixed**; that is, they contain both efferent and afferent fibers. Some cranial nerves, however, are exclusively sensory or motor in function.

On the basis of the tissues supplied, seven types of nerve fibers can be identified. They are

1. General somatic afferent fibers, present in all spinal and some cranial nerves. They conduct impulses to the central nervous system from receptors in the integument, muscles, and connective tissues.

2. Special somatic afferent fibers, found only in the optic and auditory nerves.

3. General visceral afferent fibers, present in both cranial and spinal nerves and distributed to the viscera of the neck, thorax, abdomen, and pelvis and to blood vessels and glands throughout the body.

4. Special visceral afferent fibers, restricted to the special senses of smell and taste and carried, therefore, only by the olfactory, glossopharyngeal, and vagus nerves.

5. Somatic efferent fibers, distributed to the striated muscles in the body and found in some cranial and in all spinal nerves.

6. General visceral efferent fibers, found in both cranial and spinal nerves and distributed to the peripheral ganglia of the autonomic nervous system. In general, these fibers supply the smooth muscles and glands throughout the body.

7. Special visceral efferent fibers are also recognized. Unfortunately, the name is misleading because they supply the striated muscles of the larynx, pharnyx, soft palate, muscles of mastication, and facial expression. The fibers are found only in the cranial nerves.

The Cranial Nerves

Twelve pairs of cranial nerves are usually recognized and are referred to by Roman numerals and by names. They are numbered according to their emergence from the brain stem. Accordingly, the rostralmost nerve is designated as cranial nerve I (olfactory), and the caudalmost nerve is designated as cranial nerve XII (hypoglossal). The names of the cranial nerves reflect *function* (e.g., optic and olfactory), *structure* (e.g., trigeminal), or *distribution* (e.g., facial and vagus). Because they are referred to by number in some instances and by name in others, the student should become familiar with both the names and their associated numbers. The mnemonic device on page 368 may be helpful.

The area of the brain where a cranial nerve appears or attaches is known as its **superficial origin.** The origins of the 12 pairs of cranial nerves, as seen in a view of the base of the brain are shown in Figure 5-54.

Cranial nerves, or branches of cranial nerves that have a motor function, arise from **motor nuclei** within the brain stem. Since these nuclei develop from the embryonic basal plate they are closely analogous to ventral horn cells of the spinal cord. The sensory cranial nerves (or sensory branches) arise from **ganglia** located outside the brain stem, and they may be considered to be analogous to the dorsal root ganglia of the spinal nerves. Upon entering the brain stem, the sensory nerves course to sensory nerve nuclei, which develop from the alar plate of the neural tube. The locations of cranial nerve nuclei are shown in Figures 5-33 and 5-55.

Except for nerves I and II, the olfactory and optic, all of the cranial nerves leave the bony confines of the brain case to supply their respective structures.

Not all cranial nerves are directly associated with speech production or speech reception. The olfactory (cranial nerve I) nerve, for example, is associated with

FIGURE 5-54

Base of brain showing emergence of
cranial nerves.

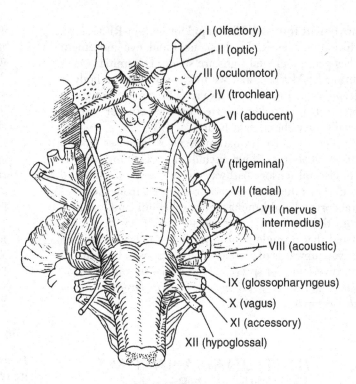

I (olfactory)
II (optic)
III (oculomotor)
IV (trochlear)
VI (abducent)
V (trigeminal)
VII (facial)
VII (nervus intermedius)
VIII (acoustic)
IX (glossopharyngeus)
X (vagus)
XI (accessory)
XII (hypoglossal)

THE CRANIAL NERVES

I.	on—Olfactory	Sensory (smell)
II.	old—Optic	Sensory (vision)
III.	Olympus—Oculomotor	Motor (visual convergence and accommodation)
IV.	towering—Trochlear	Motor (rotates eye down and outwards)
V.	tops—Trigeminal	Sensory and Motor (sensations to eye, nose, and face: meninges) (muscles of mastication and tongue)
VI.	A—Abducent	Motor (supplies lateral eye muscles)
VII.	Finn—Facial	Sensory and Motor (sensations to tongue and soft palate) (muscles of the face and the stapedius)
VIII.	and—Acoustic	Sensory (hearing and balance)
IX.	German—Glossopharyngeal	Sensory and Motor (sensation to tonsils, pharynx, and soft palate) (muscles of pharynx, and stylopharyngeus)
X.	vended—Vagus	Sensory and Motor (sensation to ear, pharynx, larynx, viscera) (muscles of pharynx, larynx, tongue, and smooth muscles of the viscera)
XI.	at—Accessory (spinal)	Motor (muscles of pharynx, larynx, soft palate, and neck)
XII.	hopps—Hypoglossal	Motor (strap muscles of neck, extrinsic, and intrinsic muscles of the tongue)

smell. It may facilitate communication but not speech production per se. The gross functions of the cranial nerves are shown schematically in Figure 5-56; the brief descriptions that follow may enhance an understanding of their functions.

Cranial Nerve I (Olfactory)

The olfactory nerve is, in a sense, not an actual nerve, but an elongated extension of the brain. Olfactory fibers are distributed over the mucous membrane of the superior nasal concha and adjacent nasal septum. About twenty branches of the nerve penetrate the **cribriform plate** of the ethmoid bone, where they enter the **olfactory bulb.** The nasal mucous membrane in which the receptors are located is, like all mucous membranes, secretory. The receptor cells are neurons, each bearing a tuft of filaments that reaches the free surface of the mucous membrane. The central processes of these receptor cells form the olfactory nerve fibers. They ascend in fasciculi to enter

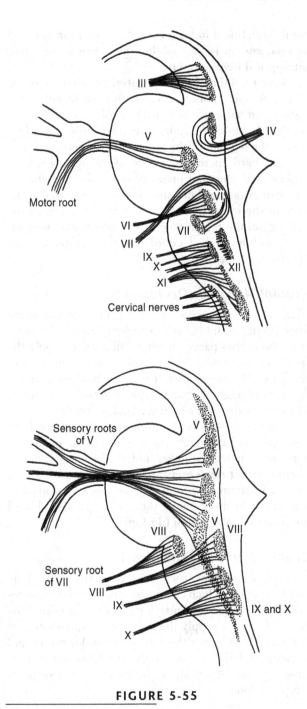

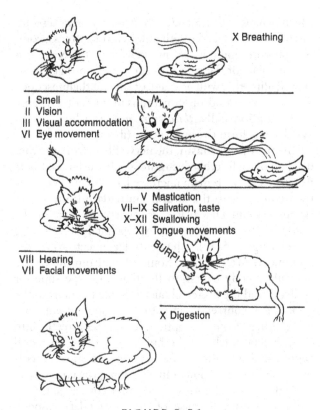

X Breathing

I Smell
II Vision
III Visual accommodation
VI Eye movement

V Mastication
VII–IX Salivation, taste
X–XII Swallowing
XII Tongue movements

VIII Hearing
VII Facial movements

BURP!

X Digestion

FIGURE 5-56

Illustration of cranial nerve functions.

FIGURE 5-55

Schematic of brain stem showing location of nuclei for the motor nerves (top) and the sensory nerves (bottom).

through the cribriform plate and terminate in the gray matter of the olfactory bulbs. The bulbs are what we see when we examine the base of the brain. Axons from cells in the bulb enter the brain at the olfactory tract and travel to the cerebral cortex just lateral to the optic chiasm (pyriform cortex) and the hippocampus.

Some association fibers go directly to the dorsal portion of the midbrain and to the pons, and indirectly by way of the hippocampus. These association fibers are responsible for certain powerful reflexes such as sudden

nausea caused by an offensive odor, or mouth watering (salivation) and a sudden "I'm hungry" sensation due to the pleasant smell of food. The olfactory sense, even in humans, is incredibly sensitive and selective. Substances that we smell release minute quantities of gas, oils, esters, acids, and so forth into the air. Upon reaching the nasal mucosa, they go into solution, migrate to the end brushes of the receptor cells, and stimulate them. The olfactory sense is far more discriminating than the sense of taste, which is confined to sweet (sugar), sour (acid), bitter (quinine), and salty. Other sensations such as temperature, texture, and even pain contribute to what we ordinarily experience as taste. From a clinical standpoint, the olfactory system is not very important; however, loss of smell, especially unilaterally, can have diagnostic significance.

CLINICAL NOTE: The sense of smell complements taste, and that poses problems for persons who have had a laryngectomy. They no longer breathe through the nose and often complain that food is lacking in taste.

Cranial Nerve II (Optic)

The optic nerve is also regarded as an elongated extension of the brain rather than a true cranial nerve. The **rods** and **cones** of the retina form *first-order neurons* which synapse with *second-order bipolar neurons* also located in the retina. The **retina,** which constitutes a complex photoreceptor, is also an extension of the brain. It is the only part of the central nervous system that can be viewed directly (with the aid of an ophthalmoscope). The bipolar second-order neurons in the retina synapse with **ganglion cells,** *third-order neurons* whose myelinated axons form the optic nerve fibers.

At the **optic chiasm,** the nerve fibers from the medial half of each retina decussate, while the lateral fibers from each retina remain uncrossed, or direct. The optic tract continues to the **lateral geniculate body** where synapses again take place, giving rise to *fourth-order neurons.* They continue to the occipital or calcarine cortex (Figure 5-57). The central connections of the optic nerve are complex. Some fibers from the lateral geniculate body course to the thalamus, the superior colliculi, and the pretectal nuclei. Some fibers from the optic tract course directly to the superior colliculi, while others from the optic tract course directly into the pretectal nuclei of the brain stem. (The **pretectal region** is a transition zone between the superior colliculus and the thalamus.) In addition, projection fibers from the occipital cortex go to other cortical and subcortical regions. Because of these secondary associations, the many and varied reflexes associated with vision are possible.

Lesions of the **optic nerve** can cause varying degrees of loss of vision in one eye, while lesions of the **optic chiasm** can cause loss of vision in the lateral (temporal) visual field in both eyes. Loss of vision is called **anopia,** and so lesions of the optic chiasm can cause **bitemporal hemianopia.**

Lesions of the **optic tract, lateral geniculate body,** or the **occipital lobe** can cause the loss of either the right or left halves of the visual field of each eye. For example, a lesion of the right optic tract causes loss of vision in the left half of the visual field of each eye.

The hard sclerotic covering of the eyeball is continuous with the dura mater of the brain, and any increase in intracranial pressure may be transmitted to the back of the eyeball, causing an inward bulging of the **optic disc,** the region where the optic nerve emerges. This condition, called a **choked disc,** is visible with an ophthalmoscope.

Cranial Nerve III (Oculomotor)

The oculomotor nerve, which supplies motor nerve fibers to the eyelid (levator palpebrae) and ocular muscles, also carries parasympathetic fibers that supply the sphincter muscles of the **iris** and the ciliary muscles of the **lens.** The fibers arise from their nucleus near the floor of the cerebral aqueduct, pass forward, and emerge from the medial side of the cerebral peduncle.

Lesions of the oculomotor nerve interrupt both conjugate and convergent eye movements. In **conjugate movement,** both eyes look to the same side, and in **convergent movement,** both eyes look medially (as when you attempt to look at your nose). Lesions also may result in drooping of the eyelid **(ptosis),** dilated pupils, and double vision **(diplopia).**

Cranial Nerve IV (Trochlear)

From its origin at the trochlear nucleus, the fibers of the trochlear nerve, which are motor, wind around the cerebral peduncles prior to entering the superior orbital fissure. The fibers supply the superior oblique muscle of the eye, which moves the axis of vision downward and outward. A lesion of one of the trochlear nerves may cause *diplopia,* especially apparent when a person attempts to look down or to the side.

Cranial Nerve V (Trigeminal)

The trigeminal, the largest of the cranial nerves, is important in speech production. It emerges from the side of the pons by a large sensory and a smaller motor root. Grossly, the **sensory portion** serves the superficial and deep structures in the face, mouth, and lower jaw, while the **motor portion** serves the muscles of mastication, the soft palate, and the mylohyoid and anterior belly of the digastric muscles. The motor root leaves the cranium by way of the foramen ovale, where it immediately joins the mandibular branch of the sensory portion of

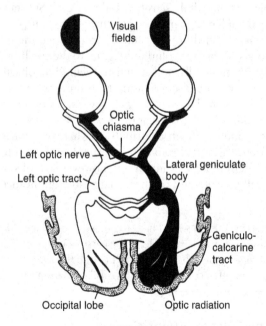

FIGURE 5-57

Schematic of the optic tract.

Visual fields

Optic chiasma

Left optic nerve

Left optic tract

Lateral geniculate body

Geniculo-calcarine tract

Occipital lobe

Optic radiation

the trigeminal. Thus, the **mandibular branch** contains both sensory and motor fibers. The **motor root** of the trigeminal supplies the internal and external pterygoids, the masseter, and the buccinator muscles. The motor root also supplies the tensor tympani (middle ear) and the tensor veli palatini muscles. The **inferior alveolar nerve,** which is largely sensory, does contain a few motor fibers. They supply the mylohyoid and anterior belly of the digastric muscle.

The distribution of the fibers of the **sensory root** is extremely complex, and only a partial description will be permitted. The fibers of the sensory root arise from the **semilunar ganglion** located near the apex of the petrous portion of the temporal bone. From there they pass into the pons and terminate in the sensory nucleus of the trigeminal nerve. As shown in Figure 5-58, the semilunar ganglion gives rise to three large branch nerves (whence the term trigeminal) called the **ophthalmic, maxillary,** and **mandibular nerves.**

The **ophthalmic branch** is sensory. It leaves the cranium by way of the superior orbital fissure, and its branches supply the lacrimal gland, eyelid, cornea, and iris of the eye, as well as the mucous membrane of the nasal cavity, paranasal sinuses, and the skin in the upper facial region and anterior scalp.

The **maxillary branch** supplies part of the dura, the lower eyelid, skin of the upper part of the face, mucous membrane of the upper mouth, nose, upper part of the pharynx, the sinuses, the gums and teeth of the upper jaw, and the palate.

The **mandibular branch,** the largest branch of the trigeminal, contains both sensory and motor fibers. It supplies the lower teeth and gums, the muscles of mastication, the skin of the ear and adjacent temporal regions, the lower facial region, and the mucous membrane of the anterior two-thirds of the tongue.

Just after leaving the semilunar ganglion, it divides into two large branches, the anterior and posterior divisions, and a single small branch, the **nervous spinosus.** It supplies the dura mater and mastoid air cells. The **anterior division** is primarily motor, and as mentioned earlier, it supplies the muscles of mastication. Sensory fibers supply the skin and mucous membrane of the cheek, the ear, the lining of the external auditory meatus (ear canal), and the tympanic (drum) membrane, in addition to the temporomandibular joint, the parotid gland, and the skin in the temporal region.

A **lingual branch,** which supplies the sublingual gland, mucous membrane of the anterior two-thirds of the tongue, and the mucous membrane of the mouth

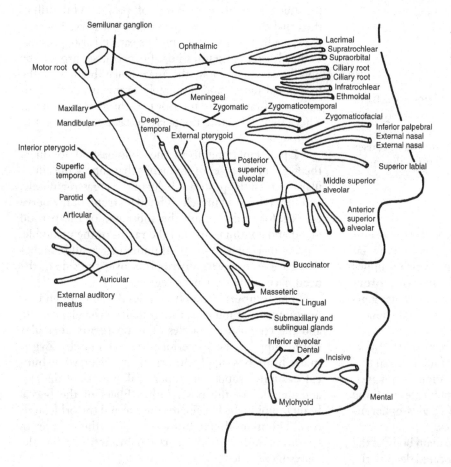

FIGURE 5-58

Schematic of the distribution of the trigeminal nerve.

and gums, communicates with the facial nerve by way of the **chorda tympani,** a nerve carrying fibers for taste. It passes through the tympanic (middle ear) cavity.

The **posterior division** of the mandibular branch is primarily sensory, but it does carry a few motor fibers.

Lesions of the trigeminal nerve can cause a number of symptoms, some of which are

1.   Numbness on the side of the lesion.

2.   Difficulty in chewing as a result of paralysis of the muscles of mastication.

3.   Loss of the **corneal reflex.** Touching the eye with a thread will normally cause an eye blink.

4.   Loss of muscle tone in the floor of the mouth (mylohyoid and anterior belly of digastric muscles).

5.   **Trigeminal neuralgia** or **tic douloureux** (sharp intense pain in the facial region).

6.   Increased sensitivity to sounds because of the paralysis of the tensor tympani muscle.

CLINICAL NOTE: Since the trigeminal also supplies the tensor palati muscle, we might reasonably expect that a lesion of the motor fibers would affect the integrity of the soft palate. This does not seem to be the case, however.

Cranial Nerve VI (Abducent)

The abducent, a motor nerve whose fibers arise from the abducent nucleus, enters the orbit through the superior orbital fissure and terminates in the lateral rectus muscle of the eye. A *lesion* of the abducent nerve causes **internal strabismus** (the eye pulls toward the nasal side), and double vision may result.

Cranial Nerve VII (Facial)

The facial nerve, which is large, complex, and important in speech production, is actually two nerves: the **facial nerve proper** (special visceral efferent), which supplies the muscles of facial expression, and the **nervous intermedius,** which carries general visceral efferents, general and special visceral afferents, and general somatic afferents.

A striking characteristic of the facial nerve is that it communicates with other cranial nerves. The functional significance of the branches of communication is not well understood, but the facial nerve communicates with the acoustic (VIII), trigeminal (V), vagus (X), glossopharyngeal (IX), and even with cervical nerves.

The **motor root,** which forms the main body of the nerve, arises from its motor nucleus located deep in the substance of the pons. Initially the motor root courses backward and medialward; it then makes a complete bend (around the nucleus of the abducent nerve) and emerges at the lower border of the pons, between the olive and inferior cerebellar peduncle, in the immediate vicinity of the acoustic nerve.

The nervous intermedius arises from the **genicular ganglion,** located at the external genu of the facial nerve (Figure 5-59). The central processes of the ganglion cells leave the trunk of the facial nerve while still in the internal auditory meatus. This root enters the pons near the motor root and terminates in a nucleus called the **tractus solitarius.** From their superficial points of origin, the two roots course (in the company of the acoustic nerve) into the facial nerve canal located at the bottom of the meatus. The facial nerve canal takes a complex course through the petrous portion of the temporal bone, at first coursing lateralward, then bending abruptly, it courses back and down where it emerges at the stylomastoid foramen. The point where the facial nerve canal changes course is known as the **geniculum,** and it contains the genicular ganglion, from which the nervous intermedius arises.

Other nerves emerge from the genicular ganglion, one of them being the **greater superficial petrosal nerve.** It is mainly sensory (special visceral) and supplies the mucous membrane of the soft palate. While still in the canal the facial nerve gives off motor nerve fibers to the stapedius muscle of the middle ear, and also gives rise to the **chorda tympani,** whose fibers course through the middle ear cavity, join the mandibular branch of the trigeminal nerve, and ultimately terminate in the mucous membrane of the anterior two-thirds of the tongue, where they constitute the nerve of taste for that part of the tongue.

Upon emerging from the stylomastoid foramen, the facial nerve gives off branches that supply the auricular muscles, the posterior belly of the digastric muscle, and the stylohyoid muscle. The main trunk of the nerve courses forward through the substance of the parotid gland and continues behind the ramus of the mandible. During its course, it gives off numerous small branches that have an extensive distribution over the side of the head, face, and upper neck region.

The **temporal branch** supplies the anterior and superior auricular muscles, the frontalis, orbicularis oculi, and the corrugator muscles. The **posterior auricular nerve** supplies the posterior auricular muscle. **Zygomatic branches** supply the orbicularis oculi, while **buccal branches** supply the superficial muscles of the face and muscles of the nose. Other fibers of the buccal branch supply the buccinator muscle and the orbicularis oris. The **mandibular branch** supplies the muscles of the lower lip, while the **cervical branch** supplies the platysma muscle.

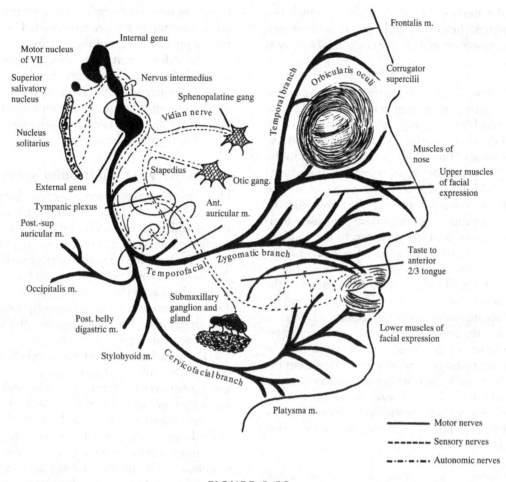

FIGURE 5-59

Schematic of the distribution of the facial nerve.

The nervous intermedius carries fibers of the parasympathetic division of the autonomic nervous system. These fibers arise from the **superior salivatory nucleus** and are carried to glands and mucous membranes of the pharynx, palate, nasal cavity, and paranasal sinuses. The sublingual and submandibular salivary glands are also supplied by a branch of the nervous intermedius.

Lesions of the facial nerve can produce a variety of symptoms. The most frequently encountered lesion is the result of edema of the facial nerve within the canal of the petrosal portion of the temporal bone.

The complex of symptoms, called **Bell's palsy**, usually subsides within three weeks. It includes

1. Paralysis of the ipsilateral facial muscles with drooping of the corner of the mouth and a flattening of the nasolabial fold.

2. Inability to close the eyelid and an increase in size of the palpebral fissure.

3. Loss of the corneal reflex.

4. Sensitivity to low-frequency sounds because of paralysis of the stapedius muscle in the middle ear.

5. Lack of tear production, decreased saliva production, and loss of taste on the ipsilateral two-thirds of the tongue (chorda tympani functions).

The facial nerve motor nucleus is divided into two parts, one serving the facial muscles above the eye, and the other serving the lower facial muscles. The *upper facial motoneurons receive bilateral cortical input*, while the *lower motoneurons receive contralateral cortical input*. A cortical lesion results in paralysis of the contralateral facial muscles but will not affect the frontalis muscle. The facial muscles receive their innervation from the contralateral motor cortex, but the frontalis muscle receives bilateral cortical innervation.

Cranial Nerve VIII (Vestibulocochlear)

The eighth cranial nerve is a composite sensory nerve, consisting of two separate parts known as the **cochlear** and **vestibular nerves.** These nerves differ in their peripheral endings, functions, and central connections. *They form a common trunk only when entering the internal auditory meatus.*

Cochlear Nerve The cochlear nerve, which *conveys the impulses for hearing,* arises from cells in the spiral ganglion of the cochlea. The peripheral fibers pass to the hair cells of the cochlea, while the central fibers course through the canal of the modiolus and continue into the internal auditory meatus. Its fibers end in the ventral and dorsal cochlear nuclei, and from there, by way of second-order neurons, pass through the trapezoid bodies and lateral leminiscus to the medial geniculate bodies. Auditory fibers are then projected to the auditory cortex of the temporal lobe. Some reflex fibers pass to motor nuclei of the eye musculature and other motor nerve nuclei of cranial and spinal nerves by means of the tectospinal and tectobulbar tracts. The superior and inferior colliculi are the nuclei of the tectum.

A lesion of the cochlear nerve can result in deafness or partial deafness of the ipsilateral ear, and in the case of **acoustic neuroma** (a benign tumor arising from the auditory nerve and located within the auditory canal), symptoms will depend on the size and location of the tumor. They may include, in addition to hearing problems, facial pain or numbness, headache, and **tinnitus** (ringing in the ear).

Vestibular Nerve The vestibular nerve *conveys impressions of equilibrium and orientation* in three-dimensional space. It arises from cells in the vestibular ganglion (of Scarpa). Three peripheral branches supply the **utricle, ampullae,** and the **saccule,** in the vestibular part of the labyrinthine apparatus of the inner ear. The central fibers follow the course of the cochlear nerve and terminate in the vestibular nucleus which is located on the lateral floor and wall of the fourth ventricle in the pons and medulla oblongata. Some central fibers pass directly to the cerebellum. Fibers from the vestibular nuclei are also carried to the cerebellum, and other fibers are projected to various spinal and cranial nerve nuclei (in particular to eye muscle nuclei). These fibers establish important reflex pathways.

Vestibular irritation or disease can result in vertigo, postural deviations, unsteady walking and standing, deviations of the eyes, and nystagmus. **Vertigo** is characterized by a sense of rotation, either of the person or the surrounding environment. The most obvious objective sign of vertigo is **nystagmus,** an involuntary spasmodic oscillation of the eyeball. Nystagmus can be induced by using a rotary chair **(Barany chair).** Following a period of rotation, the chair is stopped suddenly, but the endolymphatic fluid (in the vestibular apparatus) remains in motion for a time. The slow phase of the nystagmus

(as well as postural deviation and past-pointing) are all in the direction of the prior rotation. The sense of vertigo is opposite to that of the rotation.

The **caloric test** may also be used to evaluate vestibular function. The external auditory canal is irrigated with water at a temperature that will produce convection currents in the endolymphatic fluids. If the labyrinth of the inner ear is normal, nystagmus will develop, but there will be no nystagmus if it is diseased.

Cranial Nerve IX (Glossopharyngeal)

The glossopharyngeal nerve contains both motor and sensory fibers which, as its name implies, supply the tongue and pharynx. It also carries fibers of the autonomic nervous system. From its superficial origin in a groove between the olive and inferior cerebellar peduncles, the nerve courses lateralward and emerges from the cranium by way of the jugular foramen. In the foramen, the nerve presents two enlargements, the **superior** and **inferior ganglia.** For our purposes, the superior ganglion may be disregarded.

The **inferior ganglion** contains cell bodies for the sensory fibers of the glossopharyngeal nerve, although motor fibers course through it. The glossopharyngeal nerve gives off several branches, some of which are directly associated with the speech mechanism. The **tympanic branch,** for example, supplies parasympathetic fibers to the parotid gland and also supplies the mucous membrane of the middle ear cavity and the auditory (Eustachian) tube. The **carotid sinus nerve** supplies the internal carotid artery with sensory fibers for the blood pressure receptors. The **pharyngeal branches** supply the mucous membrane of the pharynx, while a single **motor branch** supplies the stylopharyngeal muscle. A complex system of **tonsillar** and **lingual branches** supplies the mucous membrane of the palatine tonsils, the fauces, soft palate, and posterior portion of the tongue. In addition, special visceral sensory fibers innervate the taste buds on the posterior third of the tongue. The glossopharyngeal, along with fibers of the vagus nerve (X), supply motor fibers to the **pharyngeal plexus,** which innervates the upper pharyngeal constrictor muscles.

Lesions of the glossopharyngeal nerve may result in a loss of sensation and taste from the posterior third of the tongue, unilateral loss of the gag reflex (if the person ever had one), and deviation of the uvula to the uninvolved side. A person with the ninth nerve lesion may also have difficulty in the initial stages of swallowing. Disturbance of the carotid sinus may result in **tachycardia,** a very rapid heartbeat.

Cranial Nerve X (Vagus)

The vagus nerve, so named because of its *wandering course,* has an extensive distribution through the neck and thorax and extends into the abdominal cavity. Many of its fibers originate from the **nucleus ambiguous,** which also gives rise to fibers of the glossopharyngeal and spinal accessory nerves. The superficial origin of the vagus nerve consists of a number of small rootlets that emerge between the olive and inferior cerebellar peduncle, just beneath the roots of the glossopharyngeal nerve. Both the vagus and glossopharyngeal nerves leave the cranium by way of the jugular foramen, where the vagus presents two enlargements, the **jugular** and **nodose** (knotty) **ganglia.** They contain cells for the sensory portion of the nerve. Some of the branches from the ganglia join several of the cranial nerves, and others supply sensory fibers to the dura mater and the skin on the posterior part of the external ear and external auditory canal.

The vagus also gives off several branches in the neck region, some directly serving the speech mechanism. In addition, the vagus receives fibers from other cranial nerves. Motor fibers from the spinal accessory nerve, for example, enter the vagus and emerge as the **recurrent nerve.** Thus, although many of the nerve fibers that supply the larynx emerge from the vagus nerve, they actually arise from the spinal accessory (XII) nerve.

The **pharyngeal branch** of the vagus contains both sensory and motor fibers that supply the muscles and mucous membrane of the pharynx and soft palate (except the tensor veli palatini). The **superior laryngeal branch** divides into external and internal branches. The **external branch** is motor and supplies the cricothyroid muscle and part of the inferior pharyngeal constrictor. The **internal branch** is sensory. It supplies the mucous membrane of the base of the tongue and also pierces the thyrohyoid membrane to supply the mucous membrane of the supraglottal portion of the larynx.

The **recurrent** (or **recurrent laryngeal**) **nerve** is so named because it arises from a point on the vagus considerably below the larynx. It ascends to terminate at the larynx, where it supplies the subglottal laryngeal mucosa and all the intrinsic muscles of the larynx, except the cricothyroid. The **right recurrent nerve** loops behind the right common carotid and subclavian arteries at their junction and courses vertically to the larynx. The **left recurrent nerve** leaves the vagus at a lower level than does the right. It loops under and behind the aortic arch and ascends in a groove located between the trachea and esophagus to enter the larynx through the cricothyroid membrane. It is also distributed to the subglottal laryngeal mucosa and all the intrinsic laryngeal muscles, excepting, as noted before, the cricothyroid muscle. The course of the recurrent laryngeal nerve is shown in Figure 5-60. Small branches leave the recurrent nerve and supply the mucous membrane and muscles of the esophagus and trachea. As the vagus continues on its downward course, it gives off branches that supply

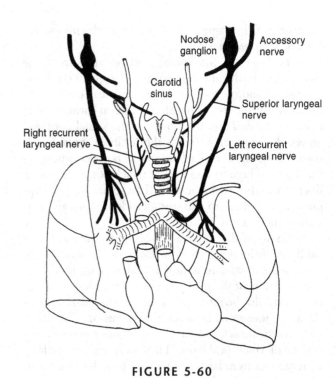

FIGURE 5-60

Schematic of partial distribution of the vagus nerve, showing the course of the recurrent laryngeal branch.

such structures as the pericardium, stomach, pancreas, spleen, kidneys, intestines, and liver.

Lesions of the vagus are varied and include a paralysis of the soft palate (resulting in nasality), difficulty in swallowing, and deviation of the uvula to the uninvolved side (during phonation, for example). Lesions of the recurrent nerve may result in a wide variety of voice problems, including aphonia, breathiness, or if unilateral, roughness of the voice.

The glossopharyngeal and vagus nerves are functionally very closely related, and tachycardia may be due to a lesion of either nerve (or both). The two nerves also blend to form the **pharyngeal plexus** which supplies the upper pharyngeal musculature.

Cranial Nerve XI
(Accessory or Spinal Accessory)

The accessory is a motor nerve consisting of a cranial and a spinal portion. The fibers of the **cranial part** arise from the nucleus ambiguous and emerge from the side of the medulla oblongata by means of four or five small rootlets. They then course laterally, passing through the jugular foramen. Branches from the accessory connect with the jugular ganglion of the vagus. The remainder of the fibers are distributed to the pharyngeal and superior branches of the vagus nerve. The cranial portion of the accessory nerve supplies the uvula and levator veli palatini. Other fibers of the cranial portion continue into the trunk of the vagus and are distributed with the recurrent laryngeal nerve.

The fibers of the **spinal portion** arise from the motor cells in the anterior horn of the spinal cord and emerge as motor roots from the cervical nerves one through four or five. The fibers unite to form a single nerve trunk that ascends alongside the spinal cord and enters the cranium through the foramen magnum. It then follows the course of the cranial portion, emerging through the jugular foramen, at which point it receives fibers from the cranial portion. The spinal portion supplies motor fibers to the sternocleidomastoid and trapezius muscles.

Lesions of the spinal accessory nerve may result in paralysis of the sternocleidomastoid muscle, inability to turn the head away from the side of the lesion, and a general weakness of the neck. A person with a lesion of this nerve may also be unable to shrug the shoulders or raise the arm above shoulder level. Since accessory fibers supply intrinsic muscles of the larynx, lesions can result in a variety of voice problems. They were discussed along with the recurrent laryngeal nerve, a branch of the vagus that carries fibers of the spinal accessory nerve.

Cranial Nerve XII (Hypoglossal)

The hypoglossal is primarily a motor nerve and, as the name implies, *supplies the musculature of the tongue.* The fibers arise from the hypoglossal nucleus and emerge from the brain between the pyramid and olive. The nerve leaves the skull by way of the **hypoglossal canal,** located just lateral to the foramen magnum. The nerve then descends, coursing between the internal carotid artery and jugular vein and, at the same time, giving off communicating branches to other cranial nerves and to the first cervical nerve. Its motor fibers are distributed to extrinsic muscles of the tongue and to some strap muscles of the neck, including the sternohyoid, sternothyroid, thyrohyoid, styloglossus, hyoglossus, genioglossus, geniohyoid, mylohyoid, and the anterior belly of the omohyoid muscle. *The main trunk of the muscle supplies all the intrinsic muscles of the tongue.* The hypoglossal nerve also carries special visceral afferent fibers from stretch receptors in the tongue.

Ansa Hypoglossi (Ansa Cervicalis) As the hypoglossal nerve descends from its origin, it gives off a branch that follows the course taken by the vagus nerve. This branch unites with branches of cervical nerves C-1 or C-2, and then begins a sharp ascent. An abrupt change of course of a nerve is called an **ansa,** and the ascending nerve, which contains fibers of the hypoglossal and C-1 or C-2, is known as the ansa hypoglossi or ansa cervicalis. It supplies the infrahyoid muscles and extrinsic muscles of the tongue listed in the previous paragraph.

Lesions A lesion of the twelfth nerve results in ipsilateral paralysis of the tongue. Upon protrusion, the tip of the tongue deviates to the side of the lesion (due to the unopposed contraction of the opposite genioglossus muscle). Because so many tongue muscles cross the midline, there is usually little in the way of functional disturbance, but articulation could be affected. Unilateral upper motor neuron lesions usually cause the tongue to deviate away from the side of the lesion. Fasciculations may also appear on the affected side of the tongue. A **fasciculation,** a small localized quivering of muscle fibers visible through the skin or mucosa, usually involves the fibers of a single motor unit.

Differences in the size of the two halves of the tongue are not a reliable indication of hypoglossal damage. Most people are left- or right-tongued when they swallow, and the musculature of one side or the other is more highly developed. After some time following a lesion, however, the musculature of the affected side will atrophy.

The Spinal Nerves

Ordinarily thirty-one pairs of nerves arise from the spinal cord. They leave the vertebral canal by way of intervertebral foramina. The spinal nerves emerge in the form of **dorsal** (afferent) and **ventral** (efferent) **roots.** For the most part, the ventral root arises from the ventral and lateral regions of spinal gray matter, while the dorsal root arises from the dorsal and medial gray matter. Near or within each intervertebral foramen is an oval-shaped swelling of the dorsal root, the **spinal ganglion.** It contains the cell bodies of the somatic and visceral afferent neurons in the nerve root. As shown in Figure 5-8, the dorsal and ventral roots join just beyond the spinal ganglion to form a completed spinal nerve, which then makes its exit through the intervertebral foramen. The spinal nerves are divided, on a topographical basis, into eight **cervical** pairs, twelve **thoracic,** five **lumbar,** five **sacral,** and one **coccygeal.** Conventionally, they are referred to in abbreviated form. The third cervical appears as C-3, while the first lumbar is L-1.

The first pair of cervical nerves leaves between the first cervical vertebra and the occipital bone, and the remaining cervical nerves leave above their corresponding vertebrae, with the exception of the eighth cervical nerve, which leaves above the first thoracic vertebra. The remainder of the spinal nerves leave below their numerically corresponding vertebrae.

Because of the relationship of the spinal nerves with the segmented vertebral column, the spinal cord is often divided into segments, one for each pair of nerves. Although there is no visual evidence of actual segmentation of the cord, a certain segmental characteristic is retained in the ultimate *cutaneous distribution* of the sensory fibers known as a **dermatome.** The distribution of spinal and cervical nerves is shown by the cutaneous areas served by the sensory fibers of each nerve in Figure 5-61. Because some muscles, in their embryonic development, migrate considerably and carry their motor nerve supply along, the distribution of the motor fibers is not necessarily reflected in the dermatomes.

Due to the comparatively slow growth rate of the spinal cord in relation to the spinal column, the mature spinal cord extends only to about the lower border of the first lumbar vertebra. Consequently, successive roots take an increasingly vertical course toward their respective foramina. The roots of the cervical nerves run horizontally, those of the thoracic nerves course obliquely downward, and those of the lumbar and sacral nerves course vertically, as shown schematically in Figure 5-41. The collection of vertically directed lumbar and sacral nerve roots is known as the **cauda equina** (L. horse's tail).

Immediately after leaving the intervertebral foramen, each spinal nerve divides into a **posterior** (or dorsal) and an **anterior** (or ventral) **ramus** (Figure 5-8). Each ramus carries fibers from both the ventral and dorsal roots; that is, *each ramus carries both sensory and motor fibers.*

The **posterior rami** are distributed to the deep and superficial muscles of the back and to the skin of the back. The muscles supplied by the posterior rami are, for the most part, postural.

The **anterior rami** of the first four cervical nerves join by communicating branches to form the **cervical plexus,** and bundles of fibers from the cervical plexus, in turn, communicate with some of the cranial nerves, especially those that supply the facial and anterior neck regions. An important branch of the cervical plexus is the **phrenic nerve.** It contains both sensory and motor fibers, and is distributed to the diaphragm. The word **plexus** stems from the Latin expression for a twining, and pertains to an interlacing network of nerves or anastomosing blood vessels or lymphatics.

The anterior rami of the lower four cervical nerves, plus the first thoracic, unite to form the **brachial plexus.** It supplies muscles and skin of the chest and upper limb. The anterior rami of the upper eleven thoracic nerves course between the ribs and are known appropriately as **intercostal nerves.** Unlike the cervical nerves, they follow independent courses. These nerves supply the sacrospinalis and intercostal muscles and the skin of the thorax. Sensory branches also supply the parietal pleura. The lower six thoracic nerves also supply the muscles of the abdominal wall.

The anterior rami of the lumbar, sacral, and coccygeal nerves join to form the **lumbosacral plexus.** It is a very elaborate network and for descriptive purposes is usually divided into the **lumbar, sacral,** and **pudendal plexuses,** which together supply the trunk and lower limbs.

The Autonomic Nervous System

Although the autonomic nervous system is very complex, it can be defined simply as a division of the peripheral nervous system that supplies the smooth muscle and glands throughout the body. Because of the nature and functions of the structures supplied by it, the autonomic

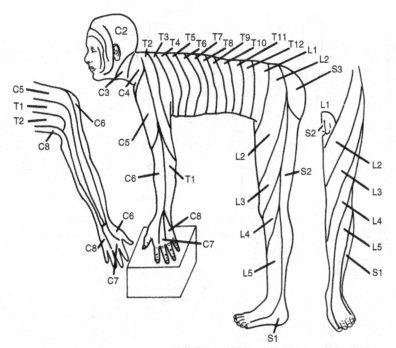

FIGURE 5-61

Schematic of the distribution of typical spinal and cervical nerves. The cutaneous distribution is known as a dermatome.

nervous system is also known as the **visceral efferent** or the **involuntary system.**

　　There is not a great deal of difference between the somatic efferent and the visceral efferent systems, but there is an interesting morphological difference between the two. *Two neurons are required to carry an impulse from the central nervous system to an effector in the viscera, while only a single neuron is required to carry an impulse from the central nervous system to a skeletal effector.*

The autonomic nervous system, which is efferent, can be divided on both a morphological and a physiological basis into the **sympathetic** (or **thoracolumbar**) and the **parasympathetic** (or **craniosacral**) **systems.** The sympathetic division receives outflow from the thoracic and lumbar segments of the spinal cord, and its ganglia are located near the spinal column (Figure 5-62). The parasympathetic division receives outflow from the cranial and sacral portions of the central nervous system,

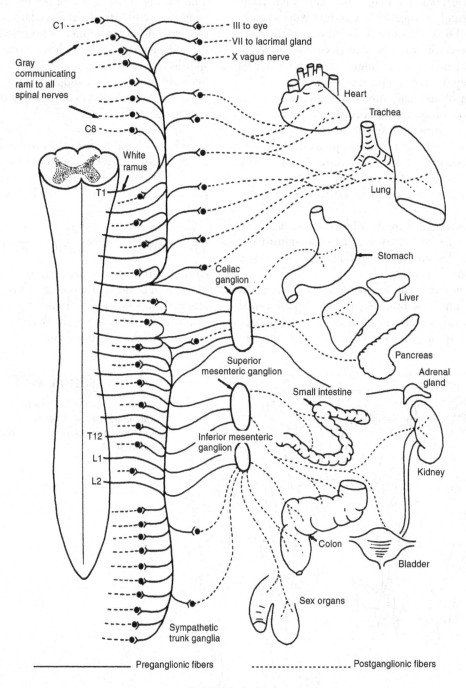

FIGURE 5-62

The sympathetic (thoracolumbar) division of the autonomic nervous system.

and its ganglia tend to be located peripherally near the structures that are supplied (Figure 5-63).

Together, the sympathetic and parasympathetic divisions constitute a highly integrated system that helps to maintain a relatively constant internal body environment. As shown in Figures 5-62 and 5-63, many visceral structures are supplied by both divisions. In certain situations the sympathetic division may dominate the function of these structures and prepare the body to cope with emergencies or periods of excitement. In other situations the parasympathetic division may dominate the functions of the same structures and act in antagonism to the effects of the sympathetic division. Generally speaking, the sympathetic system mobilizes the body for emergency or threatening situations, while the parasympathetic system acts to conserve body resources.

Imagine you are deeply engrossed in reading or studying at your desk. It's quite late and the world about you is very still and quiet, when suddenly someone begins to scream hysterically just outside your window, and then you hear a frenzied banging on your door. Your heart begins to pound, your eyes dilate, your skin gets "goose-bumps," your hair stands on end, your blood vessels dilate, your muscles become tense, and in an instant your entire body is alerted to and prepared for an emergency situation. At the same time that your body is being prepared to do battle, digestion slows, activity of the sex organs is inhibited, the musculature of the bladder relaxes, and the sphincters constrict (good thing).

The sympathetic system is responsible for internal adjustments to stress or crises, while the parasympathetic reduces internal activity.

FIGURE 5-63

The parasympathetic (craniosacral) division of the autonomic nervous system.

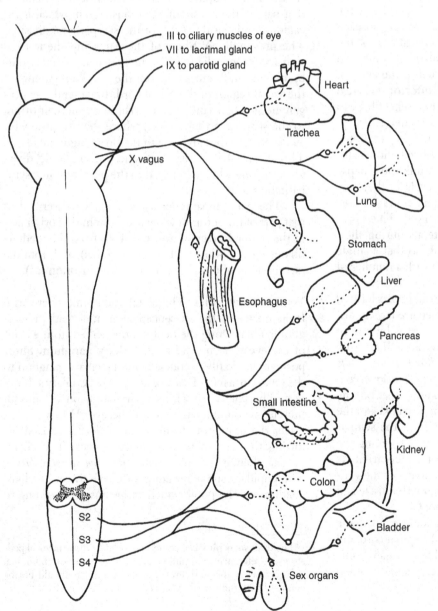

Sympathetic or Thoracolumbar Division

In addition to the dorsal and ventral rami, spinal nerves in the region between the first thoracic and third lumbar segments give rise to additional branches known as the **white rami communicantes.** These branches contain myelinated (white) fibers whose cell bodies are located in the **lateral column** or **horn** of the gray matter of the spinal cord. The axons of these lateral horn cells constitute the **preganglionic fibers** of the sympathetic division of the autonomic nervous system.

On either side of the vertebral column, extending from the first cervical vertebra to the coccyx, is a chain of ganglia, connected together by bundles of nerve fibers. These chains are known collectively as the **sympathetic trunk,** and the ganglia are called **trunk** (or chain) **ganglia.** As illustrated in Figure 5-62, the preganglionic fibers leave the spinal cord as part of the ventral root and continue to the paravertebral trunk ganglia of the sympathetic trunk. There are 21 or 22 ganglia in each trunk, three or four associated with cervical nerves, ten or eleven with thoracic, four with lumbar, and four with sacral nerves. Three ganglia are located in the cervical region, the **superior, middle,** and **inferior cervical ganglia.** As shown in Figure 5-62, they send fibers to the eye, the lacrimal gland, and the vagus nerve.

Upon entering the trunk ganglia, the preganglionic fibers may synapse with a number of ganglion cells, course up or down in the sympathetic trunk and synapse with ganglion cells at higher or lower levels, or they may continue through the trunk ganglia and course to collateral ganglia located deep within the body. These preganglionic fibers may give off collaterals during their course through the sympathetic trunk, so that a single preganglionic fiber may communicate with a number of postganglionic neurons.

Postganglionic fibers have their cell bodies located in the trunk ganglia. Their axons, which are largely unmyelinated, course back to the spinal nerves by way of delicate nerve bundles called the **gray rami.** *While each spinal nerve receives a gray ramus, the distribution of white rami is limited to the thoracic and first four lumbar nerves.* Thus, the white rami carry preganglionic fibers from the central nervous system to the sympathetic trunk, and the gray rami carry postganglionic fibers from the sympathetic trunk back to the spinal nerves. After joining the spinal nerves, the postganglionic (visceral efferent) fibers are distributed along with the somatic fibers of the ventral ramus, and ultimately supply the smooth muscle and the glandular tissue throughout the body.

As shown in Figure 5-62, preganglionic sympathetic fibers from T-1 to T-5 emerge from the spinal cord and synapse in the sympathetic ganglia. The postganglionic axons are then distributed to the heart and to blood vessels.

Fibers from T-6 to T-12 form the **splanchnic nerves.** Their preganglionic fibers pass through the trunk ganglia, emerging as the splanchnic nerves, which terminate in the **celiac ganglia** (Figure 5-62). The postganglionic fibers from the celiac ganglia are then distributed to the esophagus, stomach, part of the intestines, the liver, pancreas, and gallbladder. The celiac ganglia and the many nerves radiating from them have been likened to the sun and sun rays, so the entire complex is often referred to as the **solar plexus.**[10]

The fibers from L-1 to L-3 form preganglionic fibers that terminate in the **mesenteric ganglia.** The postganglionic fibers are distributed to the colon, rectum, and genitourinary organs.

Parasympathetic or Craniosacral Division

As the name implies, the parasympathetic division is that part of the autonomic nervous system which is located on either side (*para*) of the sympathetic division. The preganglionic fibers of the parasympathetic division arise from cell bodies in the gray matter of the midbrain and hindbrain, and from the middle segments of the sacral region of the spinal cord. In general, the preganglionic fibers course uninterrupted from their origin to the structures they supply, where they synapse with ganglion cells that give rise to the postganglionic fibers. This means that parasympathetic preganglionic fibers are very long when compared to the preganglionic sympathetic fibers.

The parasympathetic division can be described as that part of the autonomic nervous system that originates in the midbrain **(tectal autonomics),** from the medulla oblongata and pons **(bulbar autonomics),** and from the sacral region of the spinal cord **(sacral autonomics).**

Tectal Autonomics The tectal autonomic fibers arise from nuclei in the mesencephalon and send preganglionic fibers along the oculomotor nerve into the orbit of the eye to terminate in the **ciliary ganglion.** Short postganglionic fibers course from the ciliary ganglion to the **ciliary muscle** of the eye and to the pupillary sphincters. The ciliary muscle is a circular band of smooth muscle surrounding the iris of the eye. When it contracts, the suspensory ligament of the lens is relaxed, allowing the lens to become more convex. The ciliary muscle, then, is the chief agent for *visual accommodation.* The pupillary sphincter adjusts the eye to various light conditions. The pupil, which varies in size according to

---

[10]The term **solar plexus** is sometimes used by those in vocal pedagogy in reference to a midline area on the anterior abdominal wall just below the sternum (the epigastrium). It should not be confused with the *solar* or *celiac plexus* found in neurology.

the degree of light striking the eye, is surrounded by the **iris,** so named because of its many colors.

Bulbar Autonomics The bulbar autonomics arise from nuclei in the medulla and in the pons and emerge with cranial nerves VIII (facial), IX (glossopharyngeal), and X (vagus). Preganglionic fibers from the glossopalatine branch of the facial nerve terminate in the **sphenopalatine (pterygopalatine) ganglion** and from there are distributed to the lacrimal glands and glands in the mucous membrane of the nose, soft palate, tonsils, lips, and gums.

A branch of the facial nerve, the **chorda tympani** follows a much different course. It terminates in the **submaxillary ganglion,** and the postganglionic fibers supply taste to the anterior two-thirds of the tongue; they also supply the sublingual and submaxillary salivary glands. Parasympathetic fibers in the glossopharyngeal nerve course to the **otic ganglion** where they terminate by synapses with postganglionic neurons, whose axons supply the parotid gland.

The preganglionic fibers of the **vagus nerve** have a very extensive distribution throughout the neck and torso, as can be seen in Figure 5-63. Structures supplied include the heart, lungs, esophagus, stomach, small intestine, part of the colon, the liver, gallbladder, and pancreas. The vagus nerve also carries sensory nerve fibers from pressure receptors in arteries and from stretch receptors in the lungs. Earlier we learned that fibers of the vagus nerve (actually spinal accessory) are distributed to the skeletal muscles of the larynx and pharynx.

Sacral Autonomics The sacral autonomics are those preganglionic fibers that emerge from the sacral portion of the spinal cord. Fibers from S-2 to S-4 merge to form the **pelvic nerve.** Postganglionic fibers are distributed to the pelvic viscera. Efferent fibers are distributed to the descending colon, rectum, anus, bladder, and the reproductive system. In addition, vasodilator fibers are distributed to the reproductive organs and to the external genitalia.

Visceral Afferent Fibers Autonomic nerves carrying visceral afferent (sensory) fibers are found in the facial, glossopharyngeal, and vagus nerves. Their cell bodies are located in the dorsal root, geniculate, and inferior cervical ganglia. These fibers, mainly unmyelinated, carry visceral sensations such as pain. They are also instrumental in mediating respiratory and cardiac reflexes; the peristaltic rate of the digestive system; and bowel, bladder, vomiting, and coughing reflexes. These reflexes are modified by input from higher centers, such as the hypothalamus, cerebral cortex, thalamus, and basal ganglia, by way of the reticular formation.

THE STRUCTURAL AND FUNCTIONAL ASPECTS OF NEURONS

Imagine two persons, each faced with the task of describing a city. One sees it at night from the window of a plane and describes a wide, multicolored expanse characterized by orderly rows of tiny lights, elaborate systems of freeways, and an orderly flow of traffic that suggest pleasant suburban living, away from the pace and congestion of the metropolis. The other person sees the city in early morning from the window of a train and describes junkyards, sagging back porches, dust and rubbish blowing about tall, gray buildings, and almost never-ending streams of people, facing a biting wind and always in a hurry to get somewhere without ever quite knowing why. Both persons may produce accurate, vivid descriptions that are representative of the city as they viewed it, yet both are aware that neither description is truly characteristic of the city when seen in all its aspects.

A person bent on describing the nervous system or, indeed, a single nerve cell is faced with problems that are not unlike those encountered by our two sightseers. Structures revealed in the study of a neuron are largely dependent upon the techniques used to view it and equally dependent upon the method of preparation of the specimen. A microscopic view of a fresh neuron is completely different from a view of a fixed and stained specimen, mounted on a glass slide. In addition, ordinary tissue-staining techniques reveal little of a neuron, except its nucleus and cell body, while special (silver) stains reveal many of the intricate details of nerve fibers and the shapes of the cell bodies. Other stains may produce certain artifacts, structures that do not even exist in the living neuron, but which nevertheless, are valuable.

The Structure of Neurons

A **neuron,** the functional unit of the nervous system, consists of a nucleated **cell body** (or soma) and cytoplasmic extensions or **processes** that are classified as either **axons** or **dendrites** (sometimes called dendrons).

Neurons have many of the morphological characteristics of other cells in the body. A nerve cell body consists of an outer cell membrane, the **plasma membrane,** which surrounds the cytoplasm. The cell membranes are less than 200 Å in thickness[11] and are composed of alternating layers of protein and lipids (fatlike substance). **Lipids** have the property of insolubility in water and

---

[11]**Ångstrom (Å)** is a unit used in measuring the length of light waves. One Å is equal to one-hundred millionth of a centimeter.

probably provide an effective barrier to diffusion of water through the cell membrane. Small **pores** in the membrane (3 Å) are large enough to permit diffusion of certain ions, a point to be considered in some detail later.

Structures of the Cytoplasm

When properly fixed and stained, the cytoplasm of a neuron reveals:

1. A **nucleus** and **nucleolus.** They contain **deoxyribonucleic acid (DNA)** and **ribonucleic acid (RNA),** which function in the transmission of hereditary characteristics, in protein synthesis, and in cellular repair after injury.

2. **Mitochondria.** They are responsible for the synthesis of **adenosine triphosphate (ATP),** which is vital for the formation of nerve action potentials.

3. **Golgi complex.** They form temporary storage for RNA derived proteins, which are necessary for the production of new cytoplasm.

4. **Endoplasmic reticulum.** An elaborate network of a tubular system that is continuous with the nuclear membrane, Golgi complex, and the plasma membrane. Proteins and synthesized enzymes are transported throughout the neuron by way of this network.

5. **Nissl bodies.** Especially characteristic of neurons, they are found in cell bodies and dendrites, but only rarely in axons. Nissl bodies consist of parts of the endoplasmic reticulum that are coated by tiny granules or flakes on the outer surface. The granules are called **ribosomes** and contain RNA. They are instrumental in production of neurotransmitters. Nissl substance apparently is in a state of solution or suspension in living cells, and it is precipitated in the form of granules either by death or by the fixing process, and as such represents a fixation artifact. A peculiar characteristic of Nissl substance is valuable in the study of neurons. When a cell body is injured, it demonstrates a phenomenon called **chromatolysis** (a disintegration of Nissl substance), and the cytoplasm appears lightly stained and without granules after preparation. Thus, the status of Nissl substance (in fixed and stained specimens) seems to be a fairly valid index of the functional integrity of a neuron.

6. **Neurofibrils.** Depending upon the staining techniques, neurofibrillae may appear to be fine, filament-like fibers which are unevenly distributed throughout the neuron, or they may appear (probably correctly) as fibers which anastomose to form a true network. Neurofibrillae extend into the nerve processes and can be traced to the terminal endings of both axons and dendrites and may function in the metabolism of the neuron. They may also lend support to the delicate axons and dendrites and contribute to the transmission of nerve impulses. Neurofibrillae stain differentially and help to distinguish nerve tissue from surrounding supportive tissue.

Pigment granules are also found in the cytoplasm of nerve cell bodies. In certain areas of the brain, for example, the substantia nigra, the cells contain large amounts of melanin (a black pigment). This accounts for the appearance of the nucleus. In addition, yellow granules appear and accumulate with advancing age, but no significance has been assigned to this pigmentation.

Derivation of Neurons

Neurons vary widely in the complexity of their forms, depending on the shape of the cell body and on the number and shapes of their processes. Earlier we learned that neurons are classified as **unipolar, bipolar,** or **multipolar,** although variations of these classes are commonly encountered, particularly of the multipolar neurons. A word about the derivation of neurons may be helpful.

Early in the development of the embryo, many **neuroblasts** in the neural crest develop two processes that extend in opposite directions from the poles of the cell body. These cells are called **bipolar.** Later, rapid growth of the cell body causes the poles of the cell to move together, until the nerve processes fuse at their point of emergence from the cell body. The resultant neuron is now called **unipolar,** and its single short process is abruptly divided into a central and a peripheral branch. The **peripheral process** normally conducts an impulse toward the cell body and functions as a dendrite, while the **central process** conducts the impulse away from the cell body and functions as an axon. On a histological basis, the two processes are identical. In a few selected regions, particularly the spiral and vestibular ganglia, the bipolar cells retain their embryonic structure.

Axons and Dendrites

The duties of a **dendrite** are always to conduct impulses toward the cell body, while the duties of **axons** are to conduct impulses away from the cell body. The pyramidal cells of the motor cortex and primary motoneurons provide adequate examples of **multipolar neurons.** They are characterized by numerous, short, branching dendrites and a single, rather long axon, which may be as much as a meter in length. Dendrites are characterized by "spines" that are the sites of synapses. Axons conduct the nerve impulse from the cell body to another neuron, muscle cell, or gland. The junction of the axon and the cell body is known as the **axon hillock,** which is the site of origin of the efferent nerve impulse.

Axons usually do not branch until they reach their termination, although some motoneurons branch a short distance from the cell body giving rise to a **recurrent collateral.** The termination of an axon is characterized by numerous branches called **telodendria** or collectively the **end brush.** Each branch is tipped by **synaptic knobs** or **boutons.** The synaptic knobs contain a **neurotransmitter** substance that is essential to synaptic activity. Transport of the enzymes and chemicals used to synthesize the neurotransmitter is by way of the **neurotubules** that are found in the plasma of the axon. They are thought to be continuations of the endoplasmic reticulum. In this way, substances produced by the Nissl bodies are transported to the extreme limits of the telodendria. Aside from neurotubules, the only other structures found in axons are **neurofilaments,** which provide support for the axon, and **mitochondria,** which synthesize adenosine triphosphate, or ATP, essential for the production of the nerve action potential.

Inasmuch as axons constitute the major communicating pathways from the central nervous system to effectors, from receptors to the central nervous system, and from one part of the central nervous system to another, it is understandable that *the bulk of the nervous system is axonal.* The transmission pathways are axonal and may be myelinated or unmyelinated. **Myelin** on the axon extends from the region of the end brush to the axon hillock, which is never myelinated.

Neuroglial (Supportive) Cells

Glial cells are more numerous than neurons, by a factor of about 10, and account for about half the bulk of the central nervous system. *Glial cells offer support to the neurons and their processes, electrically insulate neurons from one another, and help maintain balance in the fluid environment of the neurons.*

The glioblasts which form in the embryonic neural tube develop into oligodendrocytes and astrocytes. **Oligodendrocytes** are found around the cell body and provide support. They also surround nerve fibers, supporting them and providing an insulating sheath of myelin. **Astrocytes,** which are also found around the cell body and have a supportive function, isolate the synaptic areas so that synaptic activity is confined to a specific region. Astrocytes also regulate extracellular fluid.

Another type of glial cell found in the central nervous system is called a **microglial cell.** Because, unlike other structures of the nervous system, it is mesodermal rather than ectodermal in origin, it may not be considered a true neuroglial cell. The cells act as scavengers and *phagocytize* (devour) damaged neurons.

Development of Glial Cells

Glioblasts in the neural crest develop into satellite cells and Schwann cells. **Satellite cells** are supportive cells for the peripheral nervous system, and many of them remain in the neural crest with the unipolar neurons and contribute to the dorsal root ganglia. Others migrate out with autonomic neurons to form other ganglia.

Schwann cells migrate out of the dorsal root ganglia along with the unipolar cell processes and the axons from the lower motor neurons of the neural tube. Schwann cells form an insulating layer of myelin around many of these nerve processes. Thus, *oligodendrocytes form myelin in the central nervous system, and Schwann cells form myelin in the peripheral system.* In the peripheral nervous system, the Schwann cell is also known as a **neurilemma cell.** All axons of the peripheral nervous system, myelinated or not, possess a neurilemma. In addition to forming myelin, neurilemma also plays an important role in the regeneration of damaged nerve fibers.

Neuroglial Cells and Nerve Processes

In some instances these neuroglial cells surround the nerve process on three sides, leaving part of the axon or long dendrite exposed. Each neuroglial cell may partially envelop a number of nerve processes (Figure 5-64) that are regarded as *unmyelinated.* In other instances these neuroglial cells completely wrap around a neuron process like a "jelly roll" and form *myelinated neurons.*

Each neuroglial cell membrane occupies about a millimeter of the length of the axon or dendrite, so that an individual nerve process resembles a miniature string of sausages. In these myelinated fibers the junction between neuroglial cells leaves the nerve process exposed to extracellular fluid. The junctions, known as the **nodes of Ranvier,** have an important role in the conduction velocity of nerve impulses.

The relationship between nerve processes and neuroglial cells is complex. Many nerve fibers are ensheathed by either myelin or neurilemma, or by both. Other fibers are devoid of covering and are called **naked fibers.** They are particularly common in gray matter and in some pathways in the brain and spinal cord. **Remak fibers,** unmyelinated fibers with a thin neurilemma, are abundant in the autonomic nervous system. Many afferent fibers of the cerebrospinal nerves are also unmyelinated, but possess a neurilemma. These fibers tend to occur in groups with a single, common **neurilemmal** (Schwann cell) **sheath.** Myelinated (medullated, white) fibers without a neurilemma are found in the brain and spinal cord. In all probability, the myelin sheaths in the central nervous system are formed by oligodendrocytes.

Myelin does not form simultaneously with the nerve fibers, but makes its appearance after the nerve processes have reached a rather advanced stage of development. Myelinization of some nerve fibers is not

FIGURE 5-64

FIGURE 5-64

Relationship of axon to its neuroglial cell. Each axon, whether myelinated or not, is at least partially surrounded by neuroglial cells. Note that the only part of an axon (or unipolar dendrite) exposed to extracellular fluids is at the node of Ranvier.

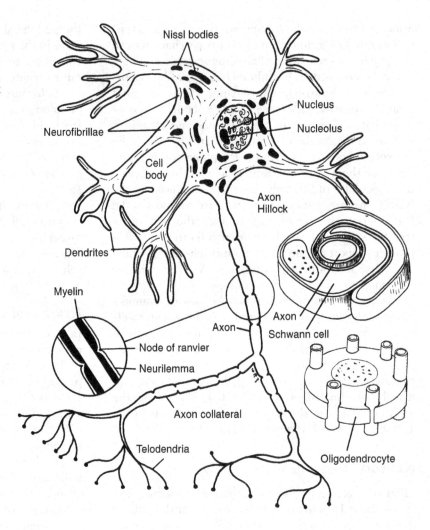

completed until late childhood. Myelin forms a segmented covering around the nerve fiber, but does not continue to the final termination of the fiber or, in most cases, beyond the axon hillock. The cell bodies of the spiral and vestibular ganglia are exceptional in that they are covered by myelin.

Connective Tissue Coverings of Neural Tissue

In the peripheral nervous system, the Schwann cells are surrounded by three layers of connective tissue which function to protect the nerve processes and to help form the cranial, spinal, and peripheral nerves. The neurilemma (Schwann cell) that envelops one or more nerve processes is surrounded by a layer of connective tissue called the **endoneurium.** In turn, the neuron processes with their neurilemma and endoneurium are grouped into *bundles* by a second layer of connective tissue called the **perineurium.** These bundles are further grouped into *nerve trunks* by a third layer of connective tissue called the **epineurium.** A nerve is much more than a

cluster of axons and long dendrites. It includes neurilemma and myelin (usually) and a complex arrangement of connective tissue (Figure 5-65).

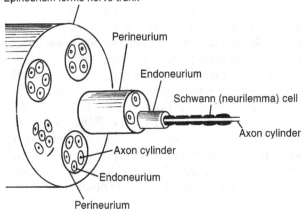

FIGURE 5-65

Connective tissue coverings of neuron processes in peripheral nerves.

Degeneration and Regeneration of Peripheral Nerve Fibers

When a peripheral nerve fiber is *cut* or *severely injured*, it cannot be replaced by mitotic cell division. Permanent loss of the nerve fibers, however, is not inevitable, for under favorable conditions it may regenerate. At first the distal portion of the severed axon begins to degenerate slowly **(Wallerian degeneration)**, a process that may require several days. The axis cylinder and myelin sheath disintegrate, forming small fat droplets along the course of the nerve fiber. The degeneration begins distally and progresses proximally toward the cell body, but usually does not involve the next neuron. The neurilemmal sheath, however, does not degenerate, but rather, its cells near the site of injury proliferate to form a scar tissue. At this stage, the situation may become rather static. The remaining distal portion of the neurilemmal tube may persist for months, but if development of a new axon fails to occur, the tube may slowly shrink.

Changes also occur in the proximal portion of the neuron. It may undergo a limited **retrograde degeneration,** usually to the first node of Ranvier, or the entire proximal portion of the process may completely degenerate—in that event the entire cell soon dies and will be consumed by microglial (phagocytic) cells. If, however, the cell should survive the trauma, the stump of its axis cylinder will begin to grow distally. Fine filaments or sprouts begin to find their way through the scar tissue. Usually their path is tortuous, and may be misdirected, until eventually a few sprouts find their way into the distal part of the neurilemmal tube. Some sprouts may never cross the scar tissue, and they may even turn back and course for a short distance toward the cell body. Sprouts which fail to cross the scar tissue barrier may form a painful **neuroma,** a small cluster of afferent pain fibers.

A *crushed peripheral nerve* will show good recovery because the regenerating sprouts are confined to the original tunnel formed by the myelin and neurilemma. Unlike the peripheral nerve fibers, fibers of the central nervous system do not possess a neurilemma and are not able to regenerate. The neurilemma seems to provide the pathway for the growth of the new sprouts and, in addition, may provide nutrition to the developing axon. New axons tend to become myelinated shortly after their development. Recovery is slow, and can take 12 to 18 months. All during this period, muscles that have lost their nerve supply must be kept active. A muscle that has atrophied may not return to a viable condition even if it is reinnervated.

Neuron Excitation and Conduction

Every sensation we experience, every thought we have, every movement we execute is dependent upon the gen-eration and transmission of electrical energy called an **action potential (AP).** Action potentials can be produced only by neurons, sensory receptors, and muscle cells. An appreciation of nerve action potentials demands an understanding of some basic principles of electricity.

Charged Particles and the Resting Membrane Potential

It has long been recognized that living tissue, plant and animal, is capable of developing electrical potentials. These potentials, which rarely exceed 100 mV (0.1 volts), are of special interest to the physiologist. Although these bioelectrical potentials are of a small magnitude (a flashlight cell produces 1.5 volts), they are easily measured and recorded. In a state of rest, any two points on the surface of a cell membrane exhibit the same electrical potential (Figure 5-66). If, however, a suitable electrode is placed on the surface of a cell and a specially constructed microelectrode is thrust into the cytoplasm of the cell, an electrical potential amounting to –50 to –90 mV will be detected.

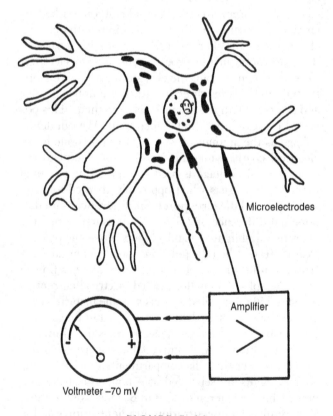

Microelectrodes

Amplifier

Voltmeter –70 mV

FIGURE 5-66

Method of recording a resting membrane potential. Any two points on the surface of a neuron exhibit the same electrical potential. Measurements across the cell membrane reveal an electrical potential amounting to –50 to –90 mV, due to unequal ion distribution.

These potential differences are due to an unequal ion concentration across the plasma membrane of the cell. An **ion** is an atom that has either gained or lost an orbital electron and as a consequence has acquired an electrical charge. An **atom** is normally in a state of electrical equilibrium and has no charge. This is because the negatively charged electrons just balance the positively charged protons in the nucleus. A **chlorine atom,** for example, normally contains seven electrons in its outer orbital ring; if it accepts a free electron to make up a full complement of eight in the outer ring, it assumes a negative charge and is no longer known as an atom, but a negatively charged chloride ion (Cl^-). **Potassium (K)** and **sodium (Na) atoms** contain a single electron in their outer ring, and the next outermost ring contains eight electrons. If these atoms lose an electron, they assume a positive charge and are known as positive ions (Na^+), (K^+).

When ordinary table salt (NaCl) is dissolved in water, it dissociates into its separate ions (Na^+) and (Cl^-). As everyone who has taken high school chemistry knows, an exchange of ions across a membrane constitutes a flow of electrical current, and, by the same token, current flow causes ions to move.

It is important to keep in mind that ions with similar charges repel each other and that ions with opposite charges attract. When opposite charges are separated, the work done in the process generates an electrical force that tends to pull the charges together. This **potential force** varies directly with the number of ions and inversely with the distance between them. This potential is measured in units called **volts.** We can define voltage as the amount of work that can be done by an electrical charge when moving from one point to another. Usually voltage is used to express the potential for work that exists when oppositely charged ions are separated, and the term **potential difference** is used. A potential difference of 1.5 volts is measured across the poles of a flashlight cell and 12 volts across the poles of a car battery. When the poles are connected by an **electrical conductor** (a copper wire, for example), a flow of ions takes place. This flow, called electrical current, is measured in units called **amperes.** Some materials conduct electricity better than others. The unit for expressing resistance to the flow of electricity is the **ohm.**

In Figure 5-67A, ordinary table salt has been dissolved in water that fills compartments I and II. These compartments are separated by a nonpermeable membrane which, when removed as in B, allows ions to move as a result of **concentration gradients** (forces). Ion movement continues until an electrical equilibrium is established in the fluid (now an electrolyte). Movement results in an expenditure of energy. Suppose that the membrane, rather than being nonpermeable, contained small pores which allowed it to be selectively permeable

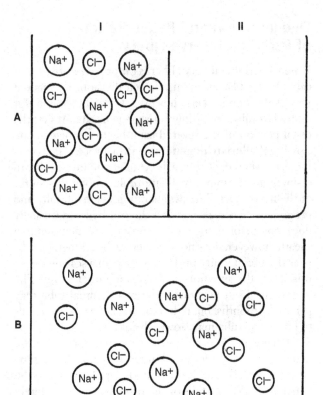

FIGURE 5-67

Diffusion of ions from regions of high concentration to regions of low concentration. In A, salt (NaCl) is placed in compartment I and water is added to both I and II, allowing salt to dissolve into its separate ions. In B, nonpermeable membrane is removed, allowing ions to move as a result of concentration gradients (forces). This ion movement represents work done. (From D. R. Brown, *Neurosciences for Allied Health Sciences,* 1980, The C. V. Mosby Co., Pub.)

to Cl^- ions and not to the larger Na^+ ions (Figures 5-68A and B). Because of the concentration gradient, Cl^- ions will diffuse into compartment II and a positive **voltage gradient** will be generated in compartment I due to its loss of negative ions (Figure 5-68). The Cl^- ions will continue to diffuse into compartment II until electrical equilibrium is reached. That is, the concentration gradient causing the negative ions to flow out of compartment I will be balanced by the electrical gradient that tends to hold them in. A voltmeter will register a positive reading. If the membrane were now made permeable to both the Cl^- and the Na^+ ions, there would be an initial flow of Na^+ ions because of the concentration and voltage gradients.

In the body, the **plasma membrane** of the cell separates the intracellular and extracellular fluids. Both of these fluids contain **electrolytes,** salts in solution that are good conductors. The cell membrane is a poor con-

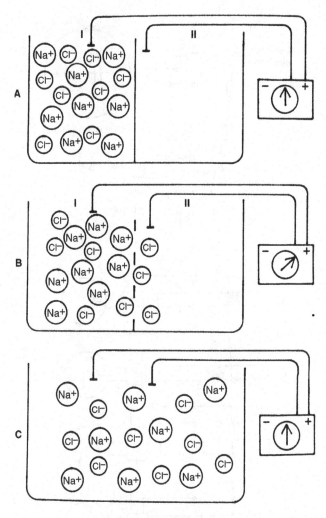

FIGURE 5-68

Factors influencing diffusion of ions. In A, NaCl has been added to compartment I. Compartments I and II are filled with water and are separated by a nonpermeable membrane. Voltmeter will record zero voltage gradient (potential difference). In B, the membrane is permeable only to chloride ions, and some chloride ions diffuse into II as a result of the concentration gradient, leaving I more positive. This creates a voltage gradient that will balance the flow of the chloride ions out of I. In C, the membrane is removed, permitting all ions to flow. Sodium ions will move as a result of both concentration and voltage gradients. Voltmeter will show zero voltage gradient after ion concentration has reached equilibrium.

ductor because one of its layers is lipids (fat). Chemical analysis of cytoplasm of nerve cells reveals a concentration of potassium ions (K^+), which may be 20 to 50 times higher than that in the extracellular fluid. The cytoplasm also contains a high concentration of negative protein ions (A^-). Thus, although both the intracellular cytoplasm and extracellular fluids contain positive ions, the concentration outside the cell is so much higher than inside the cell that *the cytoplasm is negative*

relative to the outside of the membrane. This bioelectrical voltage, the **resting membrane potential,** is due to the polarization of the cell membrane. If electrodes are placed one on either side of the cell membrane, a continuous steady or resting potential amounting to as much as 100 mV is recorded. *This resting membrane potential can be attributed to the selective permeability of the plasma membrane.*

Potassium (K^+) and chloride (Cl^-) ions are small and can pass through the membrane, but sodium ions (Na^+) are hydrated (contain water) and are too large to diffuse through the membrane without difficulty. In a resting state, potassium ions (K^+), being attracted by the negative protein ions (A^-) in the cell, diffuse inward through the cell membrane. At the same time potassium ions within the cell, being attracted by a lower external concentration gradient, diffuse outward through the cell membrane. This two-way diffusion is nearly a balancing process, but there is also a steady but slight diffusion of sodium ions (Na^+) from a region of high concentration (inside the cell membrane). If it were not for some additional mechanism, positive sodium ions (Na^+) would ultimately equalize inside and outside the cell membrane, and the resting potential would diminish to zero.

The Sodium-Potassium Pump

There is, however, an active process that extrudes sodium ions as fast as they enter the cell, so that the sodium ion concentration is always kept to about one-tenth of that outside the cell. This active mechanism, which is due to the expenditure of energy by the cell membrane, acts on both potassium and sodium ions. Called the sodium-potassium pump, it is an enzyme system powered by adenosine triphosphate (ATP), a product of the mitochondria in the cytoplasm.

This sodium-potassium pump simultaneously ejects any excessive Na^+ ions that may diffuse into the cell and brings back K^+ ions that may have left the cell (Figure 5-69). In this way, *the pump continuously maintains the concentration and voltage gradients.*

If a neuron retained its resting potential indefinitely, it would be of little use to the nervous system. Many forms of stimuli may produce a sudden change in the resting potential of a neuron. Once stimulated, the only function a neuron has to perform is to conduct impulses, either afferent from peripheral sense organs to the central nervous system or efferent from the central nervous system to muscles or other effectors.

The Action Potential

Electricity is the most often used source of artificial stimulation for neurons. It can easily be controlled and measured and can be applied to either muscle or nerve tissue without causing damage. One method of stimulating a

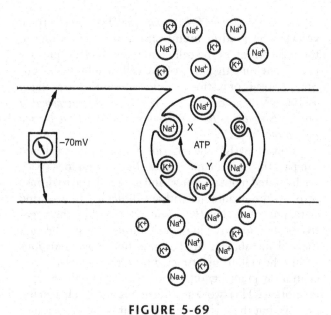

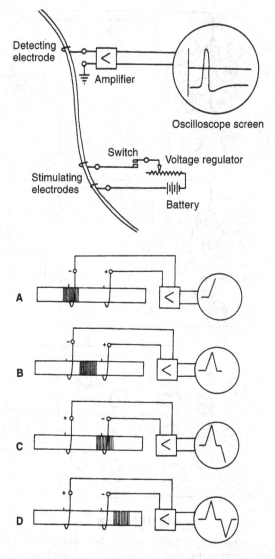

FIGURE 5-69

Model of sodium-potassium pump, which is a property of excitable cell membrane that enables the cell to maintain its resting membrane potential. The pump retrieves potassium ions lost from the cell and removes sodium ions that have leaked in. The pump is powered by ATP and involves two ion carrier molecules X and Y that facilitate the diffusion of sodium and potassium across the cell membrane.

nerve fiber and of detecting a nerve impulse is shown in Figure 5-70.

Initially, the resting nerve fiber has a voltage gradient of –70 mV. Negative ions are located inside of the cell membrane and positive ions on the outside. Current flow is prevented because of the poor conductive properties of the cell membrane, but the ions are nevertheless attracted to one another.

A negative pole **(cathode)** from the stimulator serves as the active electrode. As stimulus intensity is increased, positive ions in the immediate region begin to flow toward the cathode, producing a **local current flow.** The amount of this flow varies directly with the stimulus intensity and effects a decrease of the voltage gradient. In other words, the loss of positive ions from outside the cell membrane makes that region less positive, and the voltage difference across the membrane is reduced. This loss of polarity, called **depolarization,** is directly reflected in a decrease in the resting membrane potential. If stimulation is increased to the extent that the membrane potential reaches –50 mV **(critical firing level),** a sudden change in the membrane permeability occurs, particularly for Na⁺ ions. The reason for this change is unknown. The sudden flow of Na⁺ ions reaches a maximum within 1 msec and results in a **reversal of polarity** of the cell membrane. Sufficient Na⁺ ions enter the cell to cause the inside to become positive (+30 mV) relative to the outside. The cell membrane immediately

FIGURE 5-70

Method of stimulating a nerve fiber and of detecting a nerve impulse. In the top figure, a battery, voltage regulator, switch, and electrodes comprise the stimulator. Closing the switch briefly initiates a nerve impulse that is sensed by the detecting electrode and passed through an amplifier to be displayed on an oscilloscope screen. In the lower figure, A, the propagating depolarization has reached the first electrode, and the oscilloscope registers a negative charge. In B, the impulse is between the two electrodes, and no voltage is registered. In C, the impulse has reached the second electrode, and the oscilloscope registers a voltage that is negative relative to the first electrode, but current flows through the instrument in the opposite direction so the deflection of the oscilloscope is downward. When the impulse has passed the second electrode (D), the voltage difference between the electrodes is zero, and the oscilloscope tracing returns to the base line.

enters a recovery phase that lasts several milliseconds. The conductance of Na⁺ decreases, and at the same time the conductance of K⁺ increases. This results in removal of positive ions from the cell and a repolarization from +30 mV to a resting membrane potential of –70 mV, due to the action of the sodium-potassium pump. The minimal strength of current, which, when left on for an indefinite period of time, produces a nerve stimulation, is called the **rheobase.** Clinically, it has become common practice to select a current strength that is twice that of rheobase and to determine the current duration required for excitation at that strength. This is known as **chronaxie** or **excitation time,** and it has a very real use in the clinical and laboratory setting (Figure 5-71).

Once the critical firing level has been reached, further stimulation of the neuron will have no effect. During the 1 msec of polarity reversal, which is the **action potential,** the membrane cannot be excited no matter how intense a stimulus is. This period is known as the **absolute refractory period.** The cell cannot depolarize until it has restored its resting membrane potential to a level of about –50 mV. When that has happened, it is possible to reexcite the neuron, provided a stronger stimulus is used. During this period, known as the **relative refractory period,** the concentration and electrical gradients are still recovering from the period of the action potential.

The conduction of the action potential along the cell membrane is self-propagating. Regions immediately adjacent to the disturbed region react to the current (ion) flow, and the process of cell membrane disturbance and current flow spreads rapidly over the cell membrane. In Figure 5-72, arrows represent ion flow inward through

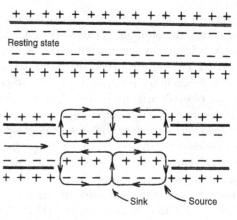

FIGURE 5-72

Illustration of the direction of current flow during the passage of an impulse.

the depolarized membrane. They also indicate that within the fiber, current flows longitudinally, reaching polarized membrane on either side of the depolarized region. Current flow in the polarized region is outward. The point where inward current flow occurs is referred to as the **sink,** and the point where outward flow occurs is called the **source.** We see that the source acts as a stimulus to propagate the breakdown of the cell membrane. This means that *once the impulse has been initiated by the stimulus, it becomes self-propagating* and is no longer dependent upon the presence of the stimulus.

The most conspicuous electrical change that is evident in a recording of a nerve impulse is the **action** (or **spike) potential** (Figure 5-73). As we have seen, *the cell membrane is completely depolarized during the spike potential and is rendered physiologically incapable of further*

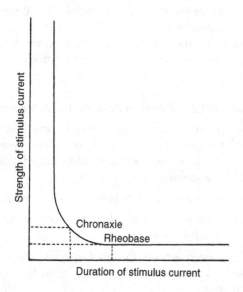

FIGURE 5-71

Illustration of the relationship between current strength and duration of stimulus. The minimal strength of current, which, when left on for an indefinite period of time, produces a nerve stimulation, is called the rheobase. A current strength twice that of rheobase is known as chronaxie.

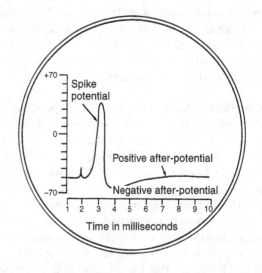

FIGURE 5-73

Illustration of a nerve impulse when displayed on an oscilloscope.

depolarization or of being receptive to another stimulus. In motor nerves, this absolute refractory period, which lasts for about 0.5 msec, is continued into the relative refractory period. During this period the threshold of excitability is less than in the resting state, and impulses, if they occur, are of small magnitude. The duration of the relative refractory period is about 3 or 4 msec in motor fibers.

Because repolarization of cell membrane is not complete during the relative refractory period, a stronger than usual stimulus is required to initiate an impulse, and for the same reason the magnitude of response is reduced. This period of diminished excitability is continuous with one during which the nerve fiber is more excitable than during the resting state. It is called the **supernormal phase,** which may last 10 msec or longer, and it corresponds in time to the duration of the **negative after-potential.** Finally the nerve fiber enters a **subnormal phase** during which excitability is less than normal. It lasts up to 70 msec and corresponds in time to the **positive after-potential.**

When a nerve fiber has been subjected to several rapid and successive stimuli, the duration of the supernormal phase and negative after-potential may become sharply reduced, with a proportionate increase in the duration of the subnormal phase and positive after-potential.

Because a nerve fiber is refractory to stimuli during the passage of a spike potential, the frequency of the number of impulses is limited. If the **total refractory period** amounts to 1 msec, the maximum frequency of impulses could not exceed 1000 per second. In addition, the refractory period has been shown to lengthen during continuous transmission at high frequencies.

A stronger stimulus may stimulate a larger number of neurons, but the magnitude and duration of the individual nerve impulse will remain unchanged. An increase in sensation or response is due solely to an increase in frequency of nerve impulses, and not to any changes in the characteristics of the individual impulses. If a motor nerve is stimulated by a succession of stimuli, the resulting contractions tend to become fused into a single sustained contraction, or **tetanus.**

Conduction Velocity On the basis of velocity of conduction, mammalian nerve fibers have been divided into types A, B, and C, and the type A fibers are further divided into **alpha** (α), **beta** (β), **gamma** (γ), and **delta** (δ) fibers. **Type A** consists of the typical somatic, myelinated fibers, both sensory and motor. They are large fibers, having the shortest chronaxies and a conduction velocity of up to 120 meters per second. Collaterals of type A fibers, such as the beta or gamma fibers, conduct at much lower velocities, and they are also much smaller in diameter. This means that the different fiber components of a single neuron may have different conduction velocities. **Type B** consists of the myelinated fibers, such as the preganglionic fibers of the autonomic nervous sys-

tem. They are smaller in diameter than type A alpha fibers and have longer chronaxies. Their conduction velocities range from 3 to 14 meters per second. **Type C** fibers consist of fine, unmyelinated fibers, such as those found in the dorsal roots of spinal nerves and in the postganglionic autonomic fibers. They have conduction velocities in the vicinity of 0.2 to 2.0 meters per second.

There is a definite relationship between nerve fiber diameter and conduction velocity. The product of nerve fiber diameter in microns and a constant factor of 6 gives the approximate conduction velocity in meters per second. An axon with a diameter of 15 microns has a conduction velocity of about 90 meters per second. The velocity of conduction seems to be due in part to the presence of myelin. It acts as an electrical insulator and prevents the outward flow of ions, except at the **nodes of Ranvier.** Consequently, conduction in myelinated fibers is characterized by outward current flow only at the nodes and jumps from node to node. Called **saltatory conduction,** it is unlike the continuous type of conduction characteristic of the unmyelinated fibers.

The properties of the various types of mammalian nerve fibers are summarized in Table 5-2.

The All-or-None Principle Once a nerve fiber is stimulated to the extent that cell depolarization is initiated, the process is complete. If a single weak, but nevertheless adequate, stimulus initiates a nerve impulse, its characteristics (magnitude of spike potential and duration of after-potentials) will be much the same as an impulse initiated from a much stronger stimulus. This characteristic is referred to as the all-or-none principle. The flushing of a toilet is a good analogy. Once flushed, a toilet cannot be reflushed until the tank has at least partially refilled. Toilets, like neurons, have absolute and relative refractory periods.

Characteristics of Action Potentials—A Summary

1. Action potentials require a minimal length of stimulus intensity and duration. A very intense stimulus, of a short duration, will not sufficiently depolarize a cell membrane.

2. An action potential is initiated at the axon hillock.

3. An action potential is either produced or not produced—all or nothing.

4. For a given neuron, the amplitude and duration of the spike potential is constant, regardless of the stimulus.

5. The maximum frequency of action potentials is limited by the absolute refractory period.

6. Action potentials are self-propagating and do not deteriorate with distance. (An electrical impulse on a wire will deteriorate.)

TABLE 5-2

Properties of different mammalian nerve fibers

Type of Fiber	Diameter of Fiber (μ)	Velocity of Conduction (meters/sec)	Duration of Spike (msec)	Duration of Negative After-potential (msec)	Duration of Positive After-potential (msec)	Function
A (α)	13–22	70–120	0.4–0.5	12–20	40–60	Motor, muscle proprioceptors
A (β)	8–13	40–70	0.4–0.6	(?)	(?)	Touch, kinesthesia
A (γ)	4–8	15–40	0.5–0.7	(?)	(?)	Touch, excitation of muscle spindles, pressure
A (δ)	1–4	5–15	0.6–1.0	(?)	(?)	Pain, heat, cold, pressure
B	1–3	3–14	1.2	None	100–300	Preganglionic autonomic
C	0.2–1.0	0.2–2	2.0	50–80	300–1000	Pain, heat(?), cold, pressure, postganglionic autonomic, smell

7. An action potential produced naturally in the body will be unidirectional. The absolute refractory period of the previously excited region will prevent reexcitation. Action potentials produced in the laboratory will be bidirectional. One action potential will travel peripherally, the other centrally.

8. Action potentials cannot "add up" or be summated.

The Neural Synapse

In order for the nervous system to function as a highly integrated, behavior-controlling mechanism, excited neurons must initiate impulses in adjacent neurons. Dorsal root fibers, for example, enter the spinal cord and branch repeatedly. Some branches ascend in the dorsal columns of the spinal cord and terminate at the level of the medulla oblongata, while others terminate in the gray matter of the dorsal horn, either at or below the level of entrance. As these fibers terminate, they form *functional connections* with other nerve cells, and their axons, in turn, travel to other nerve cells (or effectors), establishing additional functional connections. In this manner, long and intricate pathways are created in the nervous system. The functional connections between neurons are known as **synapses.** It is important to keep in mind that *there is no cytoplasmic continuity of neurons at the synapse.*

Although it has long been suspected that individual neurons in a pathway retain their anatomic identity, only recently has the electron microscope revealed the structural details of the synapse. A schematic of a **pre-** and **postsynaptic neuron** is shown in Figure 5-74, and a schematic of a synapse is shown in Figure 5-75. As an axon approaches another nerve cell, its telodendria terminate at the surface of a dendrite or at the surface of the body of the postsynaptic cell. Each telodendron terminates as a small swelling or loop where it makes synaptic contact with the postsynaptic cell. These endings are called **boutons terminaux** (terminal buttons). Telodendria may also make a synaptic junction by means of a **bouton de passage** and then continue on to synapse with a number of additional nerve cells. A single axon may have a small number of boutons, or as many as 50,000. The average is about 1000. Any single cell may form synaptic junctions with many other cells (up to 100,000).

Synapses vary in size, complexity, and arrangement, but most have certain characteristics in common. As shown in Figure 5-75, a slight indentation occurs at the point where the dendrite or cell body meets the terminal bouton. Electron microscopy reveals a **synaptic cleft** of only about 0.01 microns between the two cell membranes.

Mitochondria, especially numerous in the terminal bouton, supply the cell with the energy (ATP) required for synaptic transmission. In addition, the bouton has a high concentration of **synaptic vesicles** containing a vital chemical transmitter that depolarizes the cell membrane below the synaptic cleft. The bouton not only has the same concentration and voltage gradients as the cell body, but it also has a sodium-potassium pump, and like the axon, responds by depolarization.

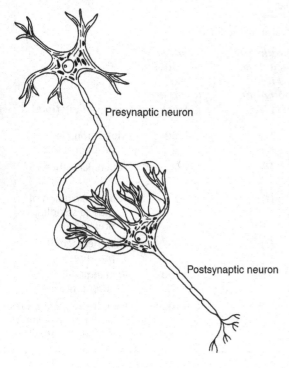

FIGURE 5-74

Schematic of a synapse between two neurons.

Presynaptic neuron

Postsynaptic neuron

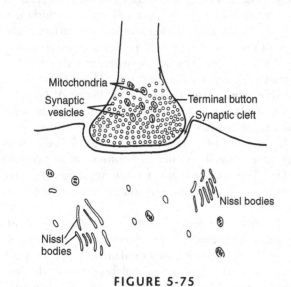

Mitochondria

Synaptic vesicles

Terminal button

Synaptic cleft

Nissl bodies

Nissl bodies

FIGURE 5-75

Schematic of an electron micrograph of a synapse.

Neurotransmitters

Although the anatomical arrangements between the axon and postsynaptic neuron may vary considerably in different regions throughout the body, *nerve impulses are conducted in just one direction*. This is due to the properties of the synapse. When action potentials reach the bouton of a presynaptic neuron, the ion flow causes the synaptic vesicles to release a neurotransmitter through the cell membrane into the synaptic cleft. This neurotransmitter produces a small, localized ion flow through the postsynaptic cell membrane, for about a millisecond, and then the transmitter substance becomes ineffective, either by diffusion or by the effect of localized enzymes.

It has been shown that the neurotransmitter **acetylcholine** is destroyed by an enzyme called **acetylcholinesterase.** During the short duration the neurotransmitter is effective, it produces a localized depolarization known as the **excitatory postsynaptic potential,** abbreviated **EPSP.** This local effect may not be adequate and may fail to reach threshold; in that event, the nerve impulse simply terminates. The total time required for the generation of an EPSP, even though it may be inadequate, is only a few microseconds. The EPSP is a local nonpropagating depolarization that can be summated. In other words, the effect of subsequent (by a very short time interval) or simultaneous impulses from other boutons may alter the magnitude of the EPSP. Should it ultimately prove adequate, the postsynaptic action potential appears at the axon hillock (the part of a neuron with the lowest threshold to excitation). The cell fires, and the message is on its way.

Another neurotransmitter response is to increase K^+ diffusion into the synaptic cleft. This results in an **inhibitory postsynaptic potential (IPSP),** a hyperpolarization of the postsynaptic membrane. If enough inhibitory transmitter substance is released, the IPSP causes the spread of positive ion flow to the axon hillock, and it becomes hyperpolarized. Some boutons which reach a cell body or a dendrite may be inhibitory, others excitatory. The effect on the axon hillock of thousands of excitatory and inhibitory synapses is the algebraic sum of their effect.

There are a number of neurotransmitter substances. They include acetylcholine, norepinephrine, serotonin, dopamine, gamma-amino-butyric acid (GABA), glycerine, glutamic acid, and others. They increase membrane permeability by the release of either Na^+ or of K^+ into the synaptic cleft. Sodium ions cause a local depolarization we earlier identified as the EPSP, while potassium ions result in the IPSP.

In the ganglia of the autonomic nervous system, the transmitter substance is **acetylcholine,** and such a synapse is called **cholinergic.** Most of the parasympathetic postganglionic axons and the sympathetic postganglionic axons to sweat glands and the blood vessels of skeletal muscle release acetylcholine. All the remaining sympathetic postganglionic axons release **norepinephrine,** and their synapses are called **adrenergic.** These two types of synapses are divided into two subtypes on the basis of their sensitivity to various drugs.

The sensitivities are the result of what happens at the receptor site on the postsynaptic membrane. The sites contain large protein molecules that have varying responses to the neurotransmitter depending upon the type of molecule. Cholinergic synapses are typed as either **nicotinic** or **muscarinic.** Nicotinic receptors that are found at the neuromuscular junction and in the autonomic ganglia are excited by nicotine. Muscarinic receptors, which are found at the synapses of smooth and cardiac muscle and in glands, are excited by muscarine, a derivative of mushrooms.

Adrenergic synapses are classified as **alpha** or **beta.** Alpha receptor sites have an affinity for norepinephrine and epinephrine. Alpha receptors are excitatory for smooth muscle contraction and glandular secretion, except for the gut where the effect is inhibitory. Epinephrine is released by the medulla of the adrenal gland during sympathetic activity. Beta receptors have an even higher sensitivity for epinephrine, and their effect is a relaxation of the smooth muscles of the viscera and blood vessels, and an excitation of the muscles of the heart.

The synapse is the most sensitive region in the nervous system to the lack of oxygen. Synaptic transmission will begin to fail after just 45 seconds of anoxia. This sometimes happens when a person stands up very quickly, and then feels faint.

Summation

We have seen that the arrival of a nerve impulse at a synapse may fail to excite the postsynaptic neuron. But if two or more closely successive impulses should arrive, synaptic transmission is more likely to occur. This summation of impulses is referred to as **temporal summation,** and it is shown schematically in Figure 5-76. On the other hand, terminal boutons from one or more axons may impinge on a single dendritic ending or cell body; in the event a single impulse from one axon should fail to accomplish the synaptic event, the simultaneous or near-simultaneous arrival of impulses from a number of axons may result in synaptic transmission. This is called **spatial summation,** and it is illustrated in Figure 5-77.

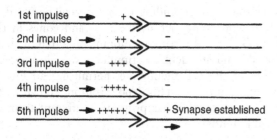

FIGURE 5-76

The arrival of a single nerve impulse may fail to excite the postsynaptic neuron, but if two or more closely successive impulses should arrive, synaptic transmission is more likely to occur. This is referred to as temporal summation.

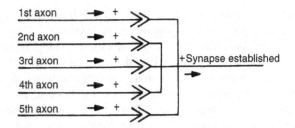

FIGURE 5-77

Should a single impulse from one axon fail to accomplish the synaptic event, the simultaneous or near-simultaneous arrival of impulses from a number of axons may result in synaptic transmission. This is called spatial summation.

The Neuromuscular Synapse (or Junction)

The structure of the neuromuscular synapse is very similar to that of the neural synapse. The bouton terminates on a region of the muscle cell that functions as a postsynaptic membrane. The membrane of the synaptic region is known as the **motor end plate** (Figure 5-78).

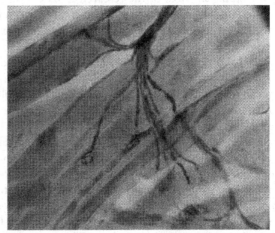

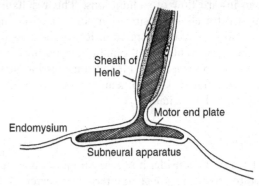

FIGURE 5-78

Photograph of an axon and motor end plates (top) and schematic myoneural junction (bottom).

There is also a synaptic cleft, and the boutons on all alpha motor neurons liberate acetylcholine.

The chemistry for producing a muscle cell potential (**muscle action potential**) is the same as that for producing a nerve action potential. The nerve action potential on the motor axon depolarizes the bouton, and it allows calcium ions to enter. The calcium causes a release of the neurotransmitter that increases the permeability of Na^+ ions. Local depolarization produces an action potential that is propagated along the sarcolemma of the muscle cell to the T system. The **T** or **transverse system** conducts the action potential to the myosin and actin filaments in the cell.

Most normal muscle functions involve two groups of muscles, one acting as a **flexor** and the other as an **extensor.** *In order that even the simplest reflex response may occur, relaxation of an antagonistic muscle usually takes place.* This relaxation is due to an important regulatory activity called **nervous inhibition.**

According to Wilson (1966), inhibition affecting voluntary muscles must reside in the central nervous system, and it can take one of two possible forms. *Inhibition of a response may be the result of a reduction of the excitability of a motor neuron, or a reduction of the excitatory input reaching it.* Most of the research to date has been centered on the mechanism in which the receptiveness of the postsynaptic neuron is reduced—in other words, **postsynaptic inhibition.**

Sir John Eccles (1965) and his colleagues, pioneers in the study of inhibitory synapses, propose a synapse that can inhibit the firing of a neuron in spite of a volley of excitatory impulses. They further suggest that because the inhibitory synapse causes the postsynaptic cell to become more negative than it is during the resting state, it is less likely to be stimulated by excitatory stimuli. One explanation of the inhibitory mechanism proposes that the transmitter substance released at the inhibitory synapse affects the selective permeability of the membrane, permitting an outward flow of potassium ions but not an inward flow of sodium ions. This results in increased extracellular positive-ion concentration and in greater negativity of the neuron. Researchers also suggest that a given nerve cell cannot have both excitatory and inhibitory properties. Neural transmission may require two different kinds of neurons, one for inhibition and another for excitation.

Receptors

We have yet to consider how nerve impulses may be initiated to effect a response to internal and external environmental changes. An organism must be able to detect environmental changes and respond appropriately if it is to survive. These receptors, which respond to changes in our environments, *can be classified by function, by the type of tissue with which they are associated, by their shape, and by whether they are free or encapsulated.*

Types of Receptors

There are basically five types of receptors in the body:

1. **Mechanoreceptors,** which respond to mechanical pressure or deformation of the receptor and adjacent tissues.
2. **Thermoreceptors,** which respond to changes in temperature.
3. **Nociceptors** (L. *nocere*, to hurt), which respond to tissue damage.
4. **Photoreceptors,** which detect light directed on the retina of the eye.
5. **Chemoreceptors,** which are responsible for taste and smell.

The sensations mediated by these various receptors are all initiated as a series of more or less rapid impulses. An obvious question is, how can different nerve fibers transmit the various modalities of sensation? Why does stimulation of the optic nerve, whether by chemicals, light, or electricity, always produce a sensation that is one of light, rather than of taste or pain? The nerve tracts for each of the sense modalities terminate in their own specific region in the central nervous system—a region that elicits a specific sensation in our consciousness. This is called the **doctrine of specific nerve energies** given to us by Johannes Müller in the mideighteenth century.

Receptor Potentials

A receptor will usually respond to just one type of stimulus. A touch receptor around a hair follicle will not respond well to heat or cold, but is sensitive to mechanical movement of the hair. The term **adequate stimulus** implies a specific stimulus which will activate a particular receptor. The receptor potential begins at either the terminal ending of an afferent nerve fiber, or a receptor cell such as the rods and cones in the retina. There is a resting membrane potential of about −70 mV, and an adequate stimulus results in depolarization of the cell membrane, permitting an inward flow of sodium ions. This depolarization, known as the **receptor potential,** has properties different from an action potential.

1. The magnitude of the receptor potential varies directly with the strength of the stimulus and with the rate of stimulation.
2. The receptor potential does not propagate, but spreads over the membrane.

3. Most receptors have no refractory period, and the receptor potential continues as long as the stimulus is applied.

4. Receptor potentials can be summated.

The receptor potential attracts positive ions from the afferent nerve fiber to depolarize it to the critical firing level. This means that a weak receptor potential may not produce an action potential or that a train of action potentials may be generated.

Once action potentials are initiated in the afferent fiber, they are always the same, regardless of the magnitude of the stimulus. The frequency of the action potentials will increase with an increase of the adequate stimulus. If a strong stimulus is applied at a receptor, the initial train of nerve impulses will persist for a short duration, and then gradually diminish in frequency, until there is only an occasional nerve impulse. This decrement of nerve-impulse frequency is known as **adaptation.** There is a cessation or decrement of nerve-impulse frequency in spite of continuous stimulation. It happens, for example, when we initially jump into a pool of cold water. Gradually, the sensation of cold diminishes. Adaptation is a characteristic of the nervous system that relieves us of many of the conscious consequences of body position that would otherwise be purely redundant. Once a limb has been moved to a certain resting position, there is no need for the receptors continuously to "remind" us where it is. We only need new information when the limb is moved to a new position, or when continuous movements are involved.

Form and Function

Although you cannot always tell the function of a receptor by its structure, there is a certain relationship between form and function. The sensation of light touch, for example, is initiated by receptors that are responsive to deformation. The nerve endings, which may take the form of small expanded lamellas (tactile discs), are primarily responsive to deformation and not to other stimuli such as heat. Structurally, receptors are specialized dendrites or neurons that, combined with nonnervous tissue, are particularly sensitive to certain types of stimuli. Some receptors consist of a neuron body with a specialized dendrite—such as the bipolar neurons in the olfactory epithelium, or the rods and cones of the retina. Many of our receptors are imbedded in capsules of connective tissue and are said to be *encapsulated.* The relatively large unmyelinated nerve fiber lies within a gelatinous substance that is surrounded by the connective tissues. The neurofibrils form a delicate network within the capsule, bearing numerous swellings or *varicosities.*

Specialized Receptors

Environmental changes are detected by highly specialized receptors called **exteroceptors;** some examples are shown in Figure 5-79. They are sensitive to touch (mechanoreceptors) and to temperature (thermoreceptors). Touch receptors called **Meissner's corpuscles** are elliptical encapsulated structures that can be found in groups on the skin of the fingertips, lips, the nipples, and orifices of the body. Meissner's corpuscles, which permit us to recognize the texture of objects touched, are stimulated mechanically and adapt quickly. This means they are particularly sensitive to movements of light objects over the skin.

Free nerve endings, which are found in the skin throughout the body, are also sensitive to light touch and pressure.

A tactile receptor, called **Merkel's disc,** differs from Meissner's corpuscles because it transmits long, continuous signals and does not adapt rapidly.

A fourth type of tactile receptor is widely distributed as the **hair end organs.** Consisting of a hair and a basal nerve fiber, it responds to the slightest movement, adapts quickly, and therefore detects movement on the surface of the body.

A fifth type of mechanoreceptor or tactile receptor, **Ruffini's end organ,** appears as tufted nerve endings located in the deeper layers of the skin. These structures do not adapt rapidly, but rather report continuous states of pressure and deformation of the deeper tissue.

A sixth type of pressure receptor is the **Pacinian corpuscle.** They are large and have a lamellated structure which gives them the appearance of an onion slice. Pacinian corpuscles are found in subcutaneous tissues and are particularly abundant around joints and tendons. They respond to pressure and adapt quickly, within a fraction of a second. Thus, they can detect vibrations and extremely rapid changes in the mechanical states of the tissues. The Pacinian corpuscles may tell us that our legs or arms are in motion, but once the extremities get to where we want them to be, the corpuscles cease to report, which is just as well.

These specialized tactile and pressure receptors, such as Meissner's corpuscles, expanded tip endings, and Ruffini's endings, all transmit their signals along **beta type A nerve fibers,** which have transmission velocities of from 40 to 70 meters per second. The free nerve endings and hair end organs transmit their information over the small **delta type A nerve fibers** that conduct at very low velocities, in the neighborhood of 5 to 15 meters per second. Crucial information such as excessive pressure or rapid changes in environment is transmitted by way of the rapidly conducting sensory nerve fibers. Other information of a less acute nature is delivered to the central nervous

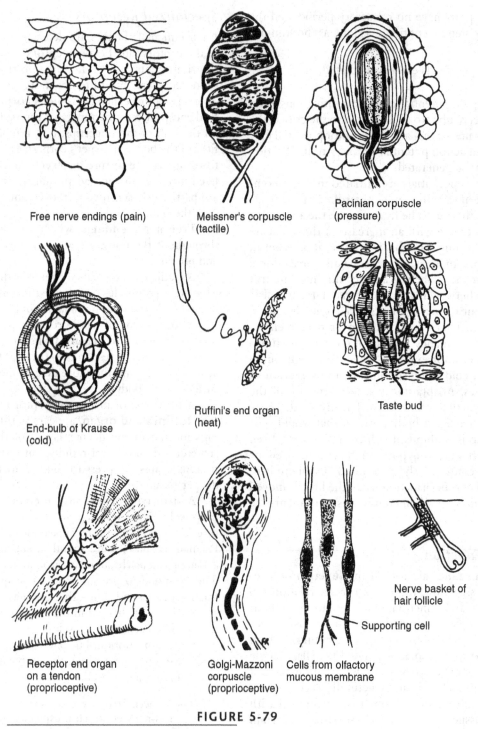

Free nerve endings (pain)

Meissner's corpuscle
(tactile)

Pacinian corpuscle
(pressure)

End-bulb of Krause
(cold)

Ruffini's end organ
(heat)

Taste bud

Receptor end organ
on a tendon
(proprioceptive)

Golgi-Mazzoni
corpuscle
(proprioceptive)

Cells from olfactory
mucous membrane

Supporting cell

Nerve basket of
hair follicle

FIGURE 5-79

Examples of some specialized receptors. (From Kimber, et al., 1966.)

system by much slower nerve fibers, fibers that also require less space in the nerve.

The detection of vibration involves all the various
tactile receptors, some responding to low-frequency,
others to high-frequency vibrations. Low-frequency
events, up to about 100 per second, can be detected by
the Meissner's corpuscles and by the Ruffini endings
in the deeper tissue of the skin. Pacinian corpuscles,

on the other hand, are capable of responding to vibrations as high as 700 per second. These signals are carried by **beta type A nerve fibers,** which can transmit
in excess of 1000 impulses per second.

The **kinesthetic receptors** are very important because they provide us with sensations that generate a
conscious recognition of the orientation of the body and

its position, as well as movements of the head, trunk, and extremities. These receptors are located in the joint capsules and in ligaments. The most common kinesthetic receptor, a **spray ending,** is a type of Ruffini's end organ (Figure 5-79). These endings transmit vigorous signals when a joint is in motion, adapt somewhat, but then continue to transmit a steady signal. Receptors are also found in the ligaments of joints. Their properties are very similar to those of the Ruffini end organs. We learned earlier that Pacinian corpuscles are found in tissues around the joints. Because they are such rapidly adapting receptors, they are thought to transmit information about the rate of movement at a joint.

Thermoreceptors respond to changes in temperature and are located in the skin. Cold receptors are known as the **end bulbs of Krause.** In structure they resemble tactile receptors, but they are more spherical and their afferent fibers are heavily myelinated. Both Ruffini type and free nerve endings are probably heat receptors.

The sensation of pain is probably mediated by the activation of specific free nerve endings that function as **nociceptors.** Tissue injury may be accompanied by damage to free nerve endings, or the injury may result in the release of chemicals that stimulate the nerve endings. These receptors are slow to adapt, and nerve impulses from them are transmitted by way of type A delta and type C fibers, which are very slow conductors.

Photoreceptors consist of the rods and cones of the retina, while **chemoreceptors** consist of the olfactory receptors and the taste buds of the tongue and month which are stimulated by molecules in solution.

Muscle and Tendon Receptors

The receptors we have discussed thus far transmit signals to the central nervous system that ultimately reach conscious levels. Muscles and tendons, however, are liberally supplied with receptors that operate entirely on a subconscious level and generate no sensory awareness at all. This is called **unconscious proprioception,** and although it may alter the output of the motor cortex, the information does not reach consciousness. These receptors are muscle spindles and Golgi tendon organs. **Muscle spindles** respond to the length of muscle fibers and to the rate of change of muscle fiber length. **Golgi tendon organs** detect tension generated in tendon fibers as a consequence of muscle contraction. The information transmitted by these receptors may terminate at motor control mechanisms at the spinal level, or it may terminate in the cerebellum. Either way, these receptors are responsible for reflexes associated with fine control of muscle movement, with equilibrium, and with posture.

The Muscle Spindle The muscle spindle was described in some detail by Sherrington in 1894, and by Ruffini in 1897. It is an exquisite structure, the most thoroughly investigated of the proprioceptors.

Muscle Fibers. Each muscle spindle is composed of from two to twelve thin specialized muscle fibers, called **intrafusal muscle fibers.** These fibers, which are surrounded by regular **extrafusal muscle fibers,** are distinctive, not only because they are found exclusively in muscle spindles, but also because of their structure and function. *Extrafusal fibers constitute the contractile substance of muscle tissue.*

As shown in Figure 5-80, the intrafusal fibers of the spindle are encased throughout much of their length by a fairly thick connective tissue capsule. At its center, called the **equatorial region,** this capsule is expanded into a fluid-filled sac. The connective tissue sheath and the expanded sac give the entire muscle spindle its fusiform shape and its name, and the small cluster of specialized muscle fibers contained within the capsule are appropriately called **intrafusal.** A muscle spindle may have a total length of 7 to 8 mm, with the connective tissue sheath encasing the middle 5 mm. This means that the intrafusal fibers project beyond the capsule somewhat, as shown in Figure 5-80. The intrafusal muscle fibers are also fusiform (spindle-shaped), and as they come to a taper, they attach to the immediately adjacent extrafusal fibers. The intrafusal and extrafusal fibers are therefore aligned parallel with one another, which means that contraction of the extrafusal fibers will shorten or relax the intrafusal fibers, and stretching of the extrafusal fibers will also cause the intrafusal fibers to be stretched.

Microscopic views of muscle spindles reveal *two types of intrafusal muscle fibers*; the difference is most apparent in the region of the capsular sac. One of the most obvious differences is in the diameter of the fibers. The larger-diameter fibers are characterized by clusters of nuclei, especially in the equatorial (sac) region of the spindle. Because of these clusters of nuclei, the large-diameter intrafusal fibers are called **nuclear bag fibers.** The nuclei of the smaller-diameter intrafusal fibers are distributed end to end along the axis of the fibers, and they are called **nuclear chain fibers.**

Both nuclear bag and nuclear chain fibers are striated, but the density of striations gradually diminishes from the polar extremes of the spindle, so that the fibers in the equatorial (sac) region are almost completely devoid of striations. Because the muscle fibers in this midregion lack the myosin and actin complex, only the ends (poles) of intrafusal fibers are contractile. The fibers in the equatorial region, being noncontractile, are stretched by an increase in length of the extrafusal fibers or by contraction of the ends of the intrafusal fibers.

Nerve Fibers. As shown in Figure 5-80, both nuclear bag and nuclear chain fibers receive a large alpha type A afferent nerve fiber. It is wound around the muscle fibers

FIGURE 5-80

An illustration of a muscle spindle.

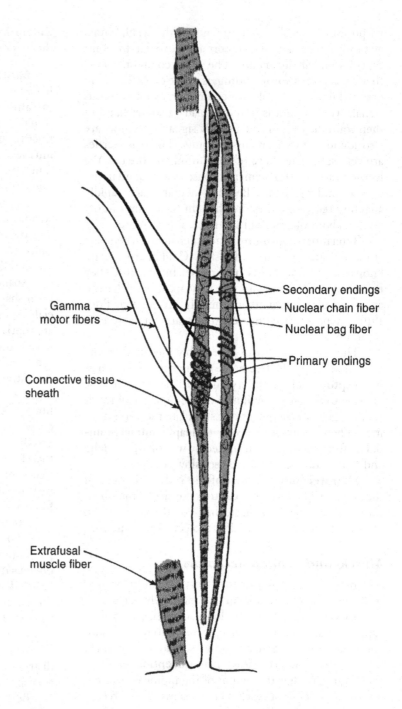

Gamma
motor fibers

Secondary endings

Nuclear chain fiber

Nuclear bag fiber

Primary endings

Connective tissue
sheath

Extrafusal
muscle fiber

so as to form an **annulospiral** or a **primary ending.**
These spiral endings, found on the noncontractile portion of the intrafusal fibers, form the actual **stretch receptor.** On either side of the primary endings can be
found **flower spray** or **secondary receptors.** They excite beta type A nerve fibers. The extrafusal fibers in a
muscle are supplied by alpha type A efferent nerve fibers.

The actual mechanical events that occur in muscle
spindles (often called stretch receptors) are almost self-
explanatory. The primary and secondary endings are
stimulated by stretching of the equatorial or noncontractile regions of the intrafusal fibers. This stretching
occurs when the stretch of an entire muscle belly
stretches the muscle spindle, or when contractions of the
ends of intrafusal fibers stretch the equatorial region.

The sensitivity and adaptability of the primary and
secondary receptors are quite different. The **primary
receptors** are very sensitive, responding almost instantly
to any stretching by transmitting a barrage of impulses
and shortly thereafter firing at a slower, but steady, rate.
The initial burst of impulses tells the central nervous system about the rate of change of the receptor's length,
while the steady-state impulse train transmits information about the actual length of the receptor. **Secondary**

receptors are much slower in response and seem to react to the actual length of the receptors.

Gamma Excitation. Stimulation of the gamma fibers causes contraction of the polar regions of the intrafusal fibers, thus decreasing the overall length of the muscle spindle. If extrafusal fibers fail to contract simultaneously, contraction of the extreme ends of the intrafusal fibers must necessarily stretch the equatorial regions, thereby stimulating the primary and secondary receptors. A reduction in gamma excitation will slacken the muscle spindle and reduce receptor stimulation.

In this manner, the muscle spindle functions as a *comparator*, comparing the length of the spindle with the length of the skeletal muscle fibers that surround it. If the relative length of the extrafusal fibers exceeds the length of the intrafusal fibers, the spindle receptors are excited. On the other hand, if the length of the extrafusal fibers is less than that of the intrafusal fibers, excitation of the primary and secondary receptors is diminished. And, as we have seen, when the spindle is shortened because of gamma efferent excitation, the spindle receptors are again stimulated because the spindle is shorter in length than the surrounding extrafusal fibers. The process is illustrated in Figure 5-81.

Suppose a resting muscle and spindle complex is stimulated, but only by gamma efferents (which supply the intrafusal fibers). Contraction of the spindle, located within the resting extrafusal fibers, results in a stretch-

ing of the primary and secondary receptors. These impulses, carried by the alpha and beta afferent fibers to the spinal cord, excite the ventral horn motor neurons supplying the muscle, and contraction begins. As a consequence of the shortening of the extrafusal muscle fibers, the primary and secondary receptors are restored to their normal length, and they stop transmitting impulses to the alpha efferent fibers supplying the extrafusal fibers. All of this takes place on a subconscious level, and is an important part of the control mechanism over postural musculature.

Summary of Gamma Excitation

1. Excitation of gamma efferents
2. Contraction of intrafusal muscle fibers in spindle
3. Shortening of spindle overall
4. Stretching of receptors in midregion of spindle
5. Stimulation of lower motor neurons supplying same muscle
6. Contraction of muscle; muscle and spindle shorten
7. Cessation of stimulation of receptors
8. Cessation of contraction of extrafusal fibers

The muscle spindle and muscle complex are brought into equilibrium, and the entire process never enters our minds.

Golgi Tendon Organs These receptors are sensitive to tension generated within a tendon due to contraction of a muscle. They are encapsulated and are located within the tendon of a muscle, or in the muscle near the musculotendinous junction. Approximately 10 to 15 muscle fibers are associated with each receptor. *The major difference between the Golgi tendon organ and the muscle spindle is that the spindle is responsive to muscle length and the Golgi tendon organ is responsive to tension.* A Golgi tendon organ is activated by tension produced in the tendon during contraction of the muscle fibers related to that particular tendon organ, by contraction of the entire muscle, or by passive stretching of a muscle.

These sensitive receptors act very rapidly, responding with a burst of impulses initially, followed by a slower but constant rate of discharge. The Golgi tendon organ transmits information to the central nervous system about the degree of muscle tension in each muscle segment. The impulses are transmitted by the rapidly conducting alpha type A fibers. In the central nervous system, fibers of the **spinocerebellar tract** conduct Golgi tendon organ impulses to the cerebellum. These signals also generate inhibitory reflex behavior in the same muscle. When tension on the muscle-tendon complex becomes extreme, the **inhibitory reflex** can be so powerful that it causes a sudden and complete relaxation of

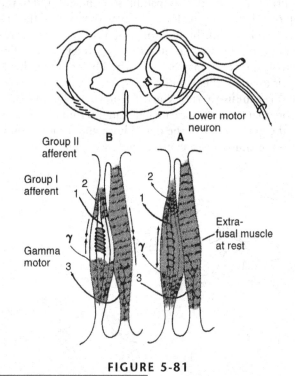

FIGURE 5-81

Reflexive contraction mediated by the gamma system.

the muscle. The effect is just the opposite to that produced by a muscle spindle.

At the spinal level, Golgi tendon organ signals excite a single inhibitory **internuncial neuron** which in turn inhibits the activity of the respective **ventral motor neuron.** Inhibitory internuncial neurons are found at the base of the dorsal horn and in the ventral horn, and are distributed diffusely between the two. They are small, extremely excitable cells responsible for many of the integrative functions of the spinal cord. Hardly any activity takes place at the spinal cord level without involving these extremely important internuncials. As in the case with muscle spindle impulses, Golgi tendon organ effects take place entirely on a subconscious level.

The Stretch Reflex

Skeletal muscle is dependent upon a nerve supply if it is to function normally. Smooth muscle and glands are somewhat independent of a nerve supply. Their activity may be initiated by chemical stimulation.

If electrodes are placed over a normal muscle and a pulse of electrical current applied, the resultant contractions are due to stimulation of the motor nerve supply to the muscle, and the motor impulses initiate the muscle contraction. **Strength-duration curves** may be obtained for muscle-nerve preparations, and the curves are very similar to those obtained from nerve fibers. If a muscle is denervated, the electric stimulation, when intense enough, may cause the muscle to contract. The chronaxie, however, will be many times normal.

Muscles are usually in a state of slight, constant contraction (**muscle tone**). If the peripheral nerve supply for a muscle is destroyed, the muscle simply becomes limp, and the usual tone is lost. If the tendon of a denervated muscle is pulled, it offers only passive resistance and is easily stretched. If the damage is such that the organism is decerebrate, at least for a particular muscle, and the peripheral nerve supply left intact, the stretched muscle offers more than passive resistance. It

returns, pull for pull, and actively contracts in opposition to stretching forces. The response is called a **stretch reflex.** If the afferent fibers from the muscle are destroyed (by cutting the dorsal nerve root, for example), the stretch reflex disappears completely.

When a muscle is stretched, the muscle spindle initiates a train of impulses. They reach the spinal cord by way of afferent fibers, which synapse with the large lower motor neurons. The transmitted impulses then travel out of the spinal cord, by way of the ventral roots of the spinal nerve to the muscle originally stretched, which then contracts. As stretching is increased, impulses follow each other more frequently and along an increasing number of fibers. As a result, the muscle contracts more and more forcefully.

The Reflex Arc

The paths taken by the afferent and efferent nerve impulses constitute what is called the reflex arc. The example just cited is known as the **two-neuron arc,** illustrated in Figure 5-82. The reflex arc, sometimes called the functional unit of behavior, is probably an oversimplification, but it does illustrate a basic form of behavior, seen in the familiar knee jerk, for example.

Another basic form of behavior is seen in the withdrawal of the hand from a painful stimulus. The afferent nerve fibers enter the dorsal horn of the spinal gray matter and may synapse with a number of internuncial neurons, which in turn activate a large number of motor neurons. For this reason, painful stimuli delivered to the tip of a finger may be followed by withdrawal of the entire hand or arm. In addition, impulses reach the cerebral cortex by way of an ascending tract. The reflex activity, however, may have occurred before the individual is aware of the painful consequences of the stimulus. A **three-neuron reflex arc** is shown in Figure 5-83. Note that this reflex arc includes an internuncial neuron in the gray matter of the dorsal horn and information is also transmitted to a contralateral ascending tract.

FIGURE 5-82

Schematic of a two-neuron reflex arc.

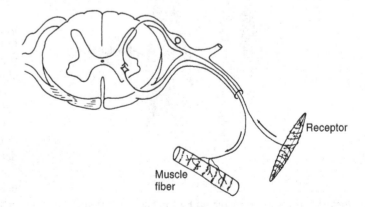

Receptor

Muscle
fiber

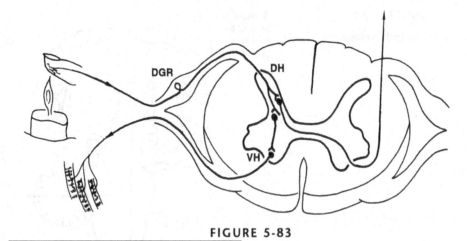

FIGURE 5-83

A three-neuron reflex arc: dorsal root ganglion (**DGR**), dorsal horn (**DH**), and ventral horn (**VH**).

NEURAL PATHWAYS

Pathway for Pain and Temperature

The receptors for pain and temperature are located in the dermal and epidermal layers of the skin. Afferent fibers have their cell bodies in the dorsal root ganglia. Fibers enter the spinal cord through the dorsal root of the spinal nerve and course to the dorsal horn of the gray matter (Figure 5-84). The neuron synapses with a second-order neuron that crosses to the contralateral side of the cord, enters the lateral white column, and ascends as the **lateral spinothalamic tract** to the thalamus (ventral posterolateral nucleus).

Here the axons synapse with third-order neurons that leave the thalamus and ascend through the internal capsule to the **postcentral gyrus** (areas 3, 1, 2), which is the somatic sensory area of the brain.

The pain and thermal pathway from the head has first-order neurons with cell bodies located in the semilunar ganglion of the trigeminal nerve (V). The cell bodies of the second-order neurons are located in the spinal nucleus of the trigeminal nerve and project to the contralateral thalamus (ventral posteromedial nucleus). Third-order neurons project from the thalamus to the somatic sensory area of the cortex by way of the posterior limb of the internal capsule.

Crude pain and temperature sensations are perceived at the level of the thalamus and emotional reactions may be initiated. The sensory information receives interpretation at the cortical level.

CLINICAL NOTE: Visceral pain is not well localized and in certain instances is not felt at the injured or diseased organ, but is experienced at the surface of the body. This is known as **referred pain.** A person suffering from a heart attack often experiences a sharp radiating pain along the inner aspect of the left arm, for example, and pain from the lungs and diaphragm may be felt in the shoulders, near the base of the neck.

Following amputation of a limb, a person may experience excruciating pain from a body part that no longer exists. This phenomenon, known as **phantom limb,** occurs because a stimulus applied anywhere along a nerve fiber is interpreted as coming from the area supplied by the nerve and not from the site of the stimulation. Nerve fibers at the stump of a limb are frequently disturbed by scar tissue, and this pain stimulus is interpreted by the sensory cortex as coming not from the stump area but from the skin area of the missing limb.

Pathway for Pressure and Crude Touch

The receptors for pressure and crude touch are located in the dermal layer of the skin, and the cell bodies of the afferent neurons are located in the dorsal root ganglia. Axons enter the spinal cord through the dorsal root of the spinal nerve and pass to the ipsilateral dorsal white column (see Figure 5-85). Here, they bifurcate with one branch entering the dorsal horn gray matter to synapse with a second-order neuron. The other branch ascends in the ipsilateral dorsal white column for as many as ten spinal segments and then enters the dorsal horn gray matter to synapse with second-order neurons.

In both instances the second-order neurons decussate to the opposite side and then enter the ventral white column and ascend as the **ventral spinothalamic tract.** This tract ascends to the thalamus (ventral posterolateral

FIGURE 5-84

Pathway for pain and temperature.

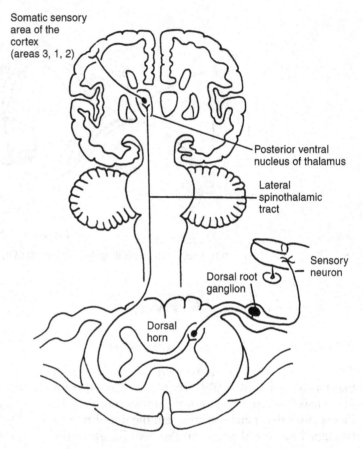

Somatic sensory area of the cortex (areas 3, 1, 2)

Posterior ventral nucleus of thalamus

Lateral spinothalamic tract

Sensory neuron

Dorsal root ganglion

Dorsal horn

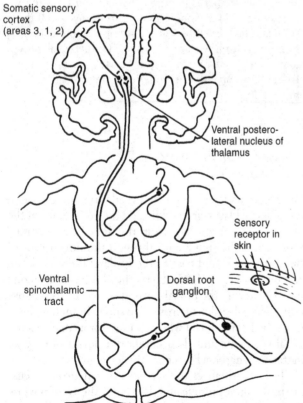

Somatic sensory cortex (areas 3, 1, 2)

Ventral postero-lateral nucleus of thalamus

Sensory receptor in skin

Ventral spinothalamic tract

Dorsal root ganglion

FIGURE 5-85

Pathway for pressure and crude touch.

nucleus) where a synapse with third-order neurons occurs. The sensations are then conducted to the postcentral gyrus of the cortex (areas 3, 1, 2).

> **CLINICAL NOTE:**   Because one branch of the first-order neuron synapses immediately with a second-order neuron while the second branch ascends the spinal cord for quite some distance, sensations of pressure and crude touch may be preserved in spite of localized spinal cord injury.

Pathway for Proprioception, Fine Touch, and Vibration

Proprioception, fine touch, and vibration are all carried by the same pathway. **Proprioception** is the sense of awareness of the position of the body and its parts. **Fine touch** enables a person to identify objects by touch and gives us the property of **stereognosis.** Fine touch also gives the sensation of **two-point discrimination,** which is most sensitive in the fingertips and lips and least sensitive on the back.

The cell bodies for the afferent nerves are located in the dorsal root ganglia. Axons that enter the spinal cord pass into the ipsilateral dorsal white column and ascend to the level of the medulla (see Figure 5-86).

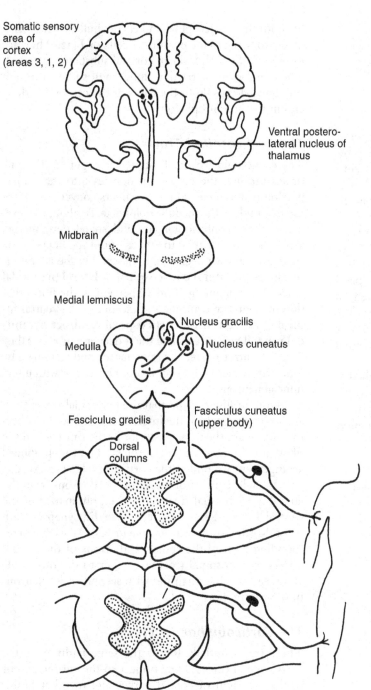

Somatic sensory area of cortex (areas 3, 1, 2)

Ventral postero-lateral nucleus of thalamus

Midbrain

Medial lemniscus

Nucleus gracilis

Medulla

Nucleus cuneatus

Fasciculus gracilis

Fasciculus cuneatus (upper body)

Dorsal columns

FIGURE 5-86

Pathway for proprioception, fine touch, and vibration.

Axons entering the sacral and lumbar levels of the spinal cord are carried by the **fasciculus gracilis,** the medial part of the dorsal column. Axons that enter the spinal cord from the thoracic and cervical levels are carried by the **fasciculus cuneatus,** the lateral part of the dorsal column. Each fasciculus terminates at nuclei in the medulla by synapsing with second-order neurons and then decussating and ascending as a trunk known as the **medial lemniscus.** It ascends to the thalamus (ventral posterolateral nucleus), where synapses with third-order neurons occur. They course, by way of the internal capsule, to the sensory cortex.

CLINICAL NOTE: Damage to the medial lemniscus, fasciculus cuneatus, fasciculus gracilis, or dorsal root ganglia results in one of several clinical signs. They include the loss of stereognosis, loss of vibratory sense, loss of two-point discrimination, and loss of proprioception.

In the latter, a person does not know what the arms and legs are doing without watching them. Such a person will be unable to stand upright with the eyes closed without swaying. (Swaying is a positive **Romberg sign.**)

The Pyramidal (Corticospinal, Voluntary Motor) Pathway

All of the motor impulses that originate at the cortical level travel through an important motor tract commonly referred to as the pyramidal tract (Figure 5-87). It is the **direct motor pathway** from the cerebral cortex to the spinal cord and brain stem, and its function is primarily excitatory. The pyramidal system, which is responsible for all voluntary movements, primarily supplies the voluntary muscles of the head, neck, and limbs. It also supplies the nuclei of the cranial nerves that innervate the musculature of the speech mechanism.

As we saw earlier, the coordination and timing of fine, skilled movements are due in large part to the cerebellum, while inhibitory functions related to skilled voluntary movements are mediated through the basal ganglia. We also saw that the body, as represented on the cerebral motor cortex, is upside down. Whereas the head, neck, and trunk are all represented by the motor cortex of both hemispheres, the limbs are represented only contralaterally.

The pyramidal system is probably best described as consisting of **corticospinal** and **corticobulbar** tracts, and although they actually comprise a single system, it is simpler to treat them separately. The motor impulses

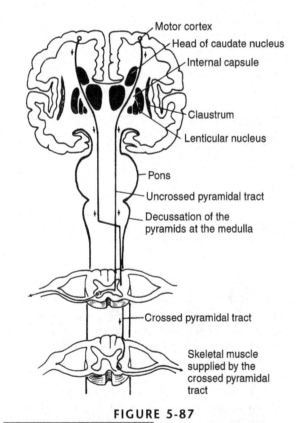

Motor cortex
Head of caudate nucleus
Internal capsule

Claustrum

Lenticular nucleus

Pons
Uncrossed pyramidal tract
Decussation of the pyramids at the medulla

Crossed pyramidal tract

Skeletal muscle supplied by the crossed pyramidal tract

FIGURE 5-87

The pathway for voluntary motor activity (pyramidal system).

for both the corticospinal and corticobulbar tracts originate from the giant pyramidal cells of Betz. They are located in the fifth layer of cortical substance in area 4. The impulses are carried by upper motor fibers through the internal capsule to the roots of the cerebral peduncles in the mesencephalon.

The Corticospinal Tracts

The corticospinal tract, illustrated in Figure 5-87, continues through the cerebral peduncles into the ventral portion of the pons. The nerve fibers converge to form the pyramids of the medulla oblongata. At about the level where the medulla oblongata and spinal cord merge, somewhere between 70 to 90 percent of the fibers of the corticospinal tract decussate to descend in the lateral funiculus as the **lateral corticospinal** or **lateral pyramidal tract.** The remaining 10 to 30 percent of the fibers that do not decussate continue to descend, in the ventral funiculus, as the **ventral corticospinal** or **direct pyramidal tract.** The corticospinal tracts decrease in size as they descend, turn to enter the gray matter, and terminate by synapsing either with lower motor neurons or with internuncial neurons.

Note in Figure 5-88 that the pyramidal fibers twist as they course toward the internal capsule, so that fibers for the leg are the most posterior in the capsule and the fibers for the face are anteriormost. The topographical arrangement we find at the cortical level is preserved.

At each segment of the spinal cord, axons from the lateral corticospinal tract enter the gray matter of the ventral horn where they terminate by synapses with second-order or lower motoneurons. At each corresponding level of the spinal cord, axons of the ventral (direct) corticospinal tract cross over to the other side and terminate by synapsing with second-order neurons in the ventral horn.

The Corticobulbar Tracts

These tracts initially follow the same pathway as the corticospinal tracts. They project to the various motor nuclei of origin of cranial nerves and to other brainstem nuclei, where they terminate. Even though the tracts do not descend to the level of the pyramids, they are still part of the pyramidal pathway.

Brain-stem nuclei supplied by the corticobulbar fibers are those of the oculomotor (III), trochlear (IV), abducent (VI), and hypoglossal (XII) nerves. Each half of the tongue is innervated by a hypoglossal nerve, and the nuclei are bilaterally controlled (usually). The musculature of the face, pharynx, larynx, and soft palate is, for the most part, bilaterally supplied by the cerebral cortex. These structures are all important to us because of their contributions to speech production, in addition to such functions as chewing and swallowing. The nuclei

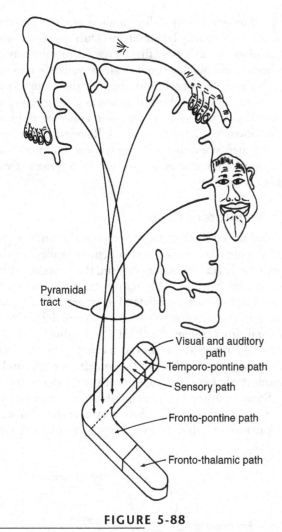

FIGURE 5-88

Topographical arrangement of motor fibers in the internal capsule.

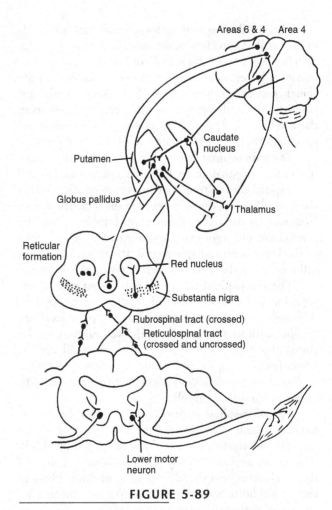

FIGURE 5-89

The extrapyramidal system.

for the facial nerves receive bilateral cortical representation for some muscles and unilateral representation for others. *The facial region that is bearded in the adult male is represented from the contralateral motor cortex, while the remainder (the upper face) has bilateral representation.*

Some of the axons of the pyramidal tract originate from the **suppressor part** of the cortex, which is located just in front of the motor cortex (area 4). These inhibitory fibers prevent lower motor neurons from overreacting in reflexive contractions. Damage to suppressor fibers results in **hyperreflexion** and **spasticity.**

The Extrapyramidal Pathway

We might define the extrapyramidal system (Figure 5-89) as all of the descending pathways except the pyramidal tracts. The extrapyramidal pathways have a diffuse origin in the cerebral cortex, but especially from the motor cortex of the precentral gyrus of the frontal lobe, where they descend through the internal capsule and cerebral peduncles to synapse with nuclei in the pons and cerebellum. The projections are to both inhibitory and excitatory centers in the brain stem. The extrapyramidal impulses that terminate at the pontine level, in pontine nuclei, are relayed to the cortex of the contralateral cerebellar hemispheres by way of the middle cerebellar peduncle. Some extrapyramidal fibers of cortical origin descend to the basal ganglia, and from this level projections are sent again to inhibitory and excitatory centers in the brain stem.

The principal function of the extrapyramidal system is to act as a coordinating mechanism for the control of the final motor pathways. Purkinje cells of the cerebellar cortex send axons to the dentate nucleus of the ipsilateral hemisphere, where they are relayed via the branchium conjunctiva to the red nucleus. At this level the fibers decussate and descend as the rubrospinal tract. In all, there are four descending pathways associated with the extrapyramidal system.

The **vestibulospinal pathway** originates from cells in the vestibular nucleus of the medulla oblongata. It descends uncrossed in the spinal cord, and the fibers terminate at lower motor neurons in the ventral horn of the spinal cord. In addition to fibers from the vestibular apparatus, the vestibular nucleus also receives fibers from the cerebellum. The vestibulospinal tract has an influence on muscles that maintain equilibrium and posture.

The **rubrospinal tract** originates in the red nucleus of the mesencephalon. Its fibers decussate and descend in the spinal cord to terminate by synapsing with cells in the ventral horn of the spinal cord in the thoracic region. Inasmuch as the red nucleus relays impulses from the cerebellum and vestibular apparatus to the motor nuclei of the brain stem and spinal cord, the rubrospinal tract influences coordination of reflexive postural behavior.

The **tectospinal tract** originates from cells in the superior and inferior colliculi in the mesencephalon. The fibers decussate and descend to the spinal level and synapse with motor neurons in the ventral horn of the spinal gray matter. The colliculi, you will recall, receive fibers from the optic and auditory nerves, and so the tectospinal tract mediates reflexive action in response to visual and auditory stimuli.

The **olivospinal pathways** originate in the olivary nucleus, which is located on the lateral aspect of the medulla oblongata, at about the level of the pyramids. The olivary nucleus is a relay center for fibers to and from the cerebellum, and the olivospinal tract sends fibers to the ventral horn gray matter for purposes of integrating and coordinating voluntary motor activity.

The **reticular substance** of the brain stem also receives cortical fibers. The cranial portion of the reticular substance seems to be excitatory in nature, while the caudal portion has primarily an inhibitory influence over the ventral horn motor neurons.

The extrapyramidal system is indirectly associated with voluntary movements, equilibrium, and posture. It forms, along with the pyramidal tract, an inordinately complex but nevertheless beautiful integrating network that makes possible the fine, smooth voluntary motor activities in which most of us effortlessly engage. The extrapyramidal system, sometimes described as an alternate pathway for motor impulses, definitely functions as a *coordinating pathway*.

NERVOUS CONTROL OF THE SPEECH MECHANISM

Respiration

The depth and rate of breathing can be controlled at the voluntary level or may be regulated reflexively at the involuntary level. Depending upon a person's activity, one or the other may be dominant. During exercise and other physical activities, the increased metabolism of the body could quickly result in an oxygen deficit in the bloodstream. In speech and singing, the inspiratory-expiratory duration ratio is dramatically altered, and so the tendency to build up excessive concentrations of carbon dioxide (CO_2) is increased. Regulation of respiration is necessary, then, to supply increased quantities of oxygen to the tissues and to remove increased accumulations of CO_2.

The Respiratory Center

Located in the brain stem, the respiratory center regulates the alveolar ventilation so that, regardless of the level of body activity or metabolism, the concentrations of blood oxygen and CO_2 remain relatively constant. This center consists of bilateral aggregates of neurons located in the reticular substance of the medulla oblongata and pons (Figure 5-90). It can be divided into a **medullary respiratory center,** located in the medulla oblongata, near the floor of the fourth ventricle, and a **pneumotaxic center,** located near the subthalamus.

Some neurons in the respiratory center discharge during inspiration, others during expiration. Although these neurons seem to be intermingled, respiratory reg-

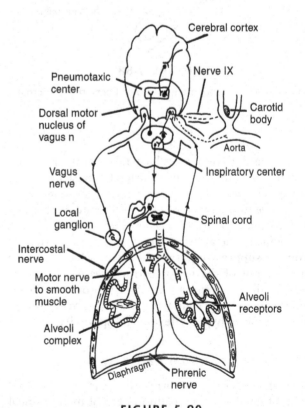

FIGURE 5-90

The control of respiration.

ulation is said to be under the control of an **inspiratory** and **expiratory center.** Together, they comprise the **respiratory center.**

Stimuli Regulating Respiration

Three principal stimuli are effective in respiratory regulation. They are (1) **carbon dioxide** in the blood that stimulates the respiratory center directly, (2) the response of **chemoreceptors** to the chemical composition of the bloodstream, and (3) the activity of **stretch receptors** that are located in the lungs.

Carbon Dioxide in the Blood The respiratory center can be stimulated directly by relative concentrations of carbon dioxide and oxygen in the arterial blood. An oxygen deficit will excite the neurons of the inspiratory center, but they are more sensitive to excessive carbon dioxide.

Response of the Chemoreceptors The role of the chemoreceptors seems to be especially important in regulating respiration. These chemoreceptors are found concentrated in two regions: the carotid and aortic bodies. The **carotid bodies** are located bilaterally, just where the common carotid bifurcates into the internal and external carotid arteries. Their afferent fibers are transmitted by way of the glossopharyngeal nerve to the upper part of the nucleus solitarius in the medulla oblongata. The **aortic bodies** are distributed along the aortic arch, as illustrated in Figure 5-90, and their afferent fibers are carried by the vagus nerve to the lower part of the nucleus solitarious.

These chemoreceptors respond to the chemistry of the blood supplied by special, minute arteries that are branches of the immediately adjacent main trunks. The receptors are sensitive to hydrogen ion concentration, oxygen, and carbon dioxide. The chemoreceptors are relatively insensitive to oxygen concentrations within normal limits, but become extremely active when the oxygen level falls to below normal. In most instances, carbon dioxide is the major chemical factor regulating alveolar ventilation.

When carbon dioxide levels in the blood become excessive, afferent impulses from the carotid and aortic bodies enter the nucleus solitarius, which in turn projects to the inspiratory center in the medulla oblongata. Impulses are then relayed from the inspiratory center to motor fibers of the phrenic nerve, which is a composite cervical nerve that arises from the anterior rami of C-3, C-4, and C-5 and innervates the diaphragm. In addition, motor impulses are relayed to supplementary muscles of inhalation such as the intercostals. Once inspiration is completed, the oxygen level is raised in the blood, the inspiratory musculature becomes inhibited, and the passive forces of expiration expel the carbon dioxide–laden alveolar air. This is a sketch of the quiet, unconscious process that takes place about 12 times a minute, all through our lives; it is quickened or slackened only with heightened or depressed physical activity.

Impulses from Stretch Receptors The lung tissue, visceral pleura, and part of the bronchial tree are liberally supplied with stretch receptors, and they too have an important role in respiratory regulation. In addition, they are the mediators of some very important reflexive behavior. When the lungs are deflated, impulses from stretch receptors, which are carried by vagus nerves to the solitary nucleus, have a low frequency of discharge. These impulses are relayed by way of the reticulospinal tract to the motor neurons in the spinal cord and to the inspiratory center that sends impulses to the phrenic nerve. When the lung is distended, the high-frequency impulses are transmitted to the solitary nucleus, where the impulses are relayed to the expiratory center. This center inhibits the contraction of the inspiratory muscles, thus allowing the passive expiratory forces to assume their role.

Out goes the bad air.

If the receptors that respond to stretch are stimulated, some significant reflexive behavior takes place. When the lungs are inflated to a certain point, stretch receptors located mostly in the bronchioles become active, transmitting impulses to the nucleus solitarius via the vagus, where they inhibit further inspiration thereby preventing overdistention of the lungs. On the other hand, when the receptors are relaxed, their impulses diminish in frequency, and that signals the onset of inspiration.

Impulses from Compression Receptors Compression receptors have been postulated, especially in the alveoli, and they are thought to transmit impulses that inhibit expiration, just as stretch receptors inhibit inspiration. This mechanism, called the **Hering-Breuer reflex,** is instrumental in maintaining normal respiratory rates and depth on the one hand, and preventing inflation and deflation on the other. The role of the **pneumotaxic center,** shown in Figure 5-90, is not known for certain. It receives afferent impulses from the inspiratory center and relays efferent impulses to the expiratory center. Stimulation of the pneumotaxic center can change the rate of respiration. It probably serves as a buffer to maintain normal respiration. Its name implies a reaction to stimulation by carbon dioxide in solution.

Proprioceptive Impulses Inhalation for speech purposes is controlled not only by the same mechanism responsible for involuntary breathing but by proprioceptive impulses from the muscles of exhalation and from the lungs. The amount of air we inhale and the rate of inhalation are also dependent upon the speech task in which the individual is engaged. The muscles required when breathing for speech purposes include those involved in involuntary breathing and, in addition, supplementary muscles of inhalation and the muscles of active exhalation.

Plexuses

As the spinal nerves emerge from the spinal cord, certain of them merge to form large bundles called **plexuses.** They include the **cervical** plexus, which is formed by the cervical nerves C-1, C-2, C-3, and C-4. The **phrenic** plexus is formed by the anterior rami of cervical nerves C-3, C-4, and C-5, and the **anterior thoracic** plexus is formed by cervical nerves C-5, C-6, and C-7, plus some fibers from T-1. The **long thoracic** plexus is formed by cervical nerves C-5, C-6, and C-7, while the **thoracodorsal** plexus is formed by cervical nerves C-6, C-7, and C-8. These plexuses are largely responsible for innervation of the muscles of respiration and the muscles of the ventral thoracic wall. The sequence of muscle action for speech purposes was dis-

cussed in the chapter on breathing. Table 5-3 lists muscles, with their nerve supply, to which a breathing function has often been assigned. The contributions of some of those muscles are open to question. However, they may contribute to breathing under abnormal circumstances and are therefore included in the table.

The Tongue

The intrinsic and extrinsic muscles of each half of the tongue are supplied by a **hypoglossal nerve,** the nucleus of which is usually bilaterally supplied by input from the motor cortex. For most of us, each hypoglossal nucleus of origin receives fibers from the precentral gyrus of both cerebral hemispheres. The **palatoglossus** probably receives its motor fibers from the nucleus of the bulbar portion of the accessory nerve, which reaches the muscle by way of the pharyngeal plexus. For this reason, the palatoglossus can be regarded as a muscle of the soft palate and not of the tongue.

Primate tongues have been found to contain muscle spindles, and they probably play an important role in the execution of the finely coordinated movements

TABLE 5-3

Motor nerve supply for the muscles of breathing

Muscles of Inhalation	Innervation Plexus and Nerves
Diaphragm	Phrenic nerve (C-3, C-4, and C-5)
Pectoralis Major	Medial and lateral anterior thoracic (C-5, C-6, C-7, C-8, and T-1)
Pectoralis Minor	Brachial (C-5, C-6)
Subclavius	Brachial (C-5, C-6)
Serratus Anterior	Long thoracic (C-5, C-6, C-7)
External Intercostals	Intercostal nerves (Anterior rami of T-2 through T-12)
Costal Elevators	Intercostal nerves (Anterior rami of T-2 through T-12)
Serratus Posterior Superior	T-1 through T-4
Sternomastoid	Accessory (XI)
Scalenes	C-2, C-3 (Anterior rami)
Latissimus Dorsi	Thoracodorsal (C-6, C-7, C-8)
Sacrospinalis	Thoracic nerves (Posterior rami)
Muscles of Exhalation	
Triangularis Sterni	T-6 through T-12 (Anterior ramus)
Internal Intercostals	T-2 through T-12 (Anterior ramus)
External Oblique	T-6 through T-12 (Anterior ramus)
Internal Oblique	T-6 through T-12 (Anterior ramus)
Transversus Abdominis	T-6 through T-12 (Anterior ramus)
Rectus Abdominis	T-6 through T-12 (Anterior ramus)

As noted in Chapter 2, the contributions of some of the above muscles are open to question. They are included here because they may in fact contribute to respiration in a compensatory role.

required in the articulation of speech (Bowman, 1971). The afferent fibers are probably carried by the hypoglossal nerve, even though it is almost always described as exclusively motor.

As the hypoglossal nerve descends from its origin, it gives off a descending branch, or ramus, which follows the course taken by the vagus nerve. This branch unites with branches of the cervical nerves C-2 and C-3, and then begins a sharp ascent. An abrupt change of course of a nerve is called an **ansa.** Thus, the ascending nerve, which contains fibers of the hypoglossal and cervical nerves C-2 and C-3, is known as the **ansa hypoglossi** or **ansa cervicalis.** It supplies the omohyoid, sternohyoid, and sternothyroid muscles. Table 5-4 lists the muscles of the tongue and their nerve supply.

By way of review, the sensory nerves of the tongue are the **facial, glossopharyngeal,** and **vagus.** The pathway of the taste fibers is a complex one. The cell bodies, located in the geniculate ganglion, most often send their peripheral fibers by way of the chorda tympani to the lingual nerve of the mandibular branch of the **trigeminal** nerve (V). It supplies the anterior two-thirds of the tongue. This explains why the trigeminal is sometimes said to supply the tongue with sensory fibers. The posterior third of the tongue (circumvallate papillae) is supplied by the glossopharyngeal nerve, while the root is supplied by diffuse fibers from the vagus nerve.

The Muscles of Mastication

The muscles of mastication are all pharyngeal arch derivatives embryologically. *The nuclei of the nerves supplying these muscles are all bilaterally supplied by the cerebral cortex.* These nuclei and their pathways are very important to us, not only because of their role in chewing, swallowing, breathing, and facial expression, but because they mediate movements of the articulators during speech produc-

tion. As is the case with most of the descending cortical fibers, the course is through the internal capsule and cerebral peduncles to the nuclei of origins of the trigeminal, glossopharyngeus, vagus, and accessory nerves.

The facial nuclei are important exceptions to bilateral cortical representation. The motor cells supplying the facial structures important for speech production on one side of the face receive cortical representation from the opposite cerebral hemisphere. As stated earlier, that part of the face which is unbearded in the adult male receives bilateral cortical representation.

The jaw depressors are supplied by branches of the mandibular division of the trigeminal nerve and by the hypoglossal nerve. The elevators are supplied by the anterior trunk of the mandibular branch of the trigeminal nerve. Sensory fibers to the lower teeth and adjacent structures are also supplied by the posterior trunk of the mandibular branch. Table 5-5 lists the muscles of mastication and their nerve supply.

The Pharynx

As it courses inferiorly, the vagus sends off two rami. They originate from the nodose ganglion and form the motor branch of the **pharyngeal plexus.** These fibers and others, not well understood, supply the pharyngeal constrictor muscles. Sensory fibers from the glossopharyngeal nerve, for example, are also contained in the pharyngeal plexus. They supply the mucous membrane of the pharynx, the faucial pillars, the pharyngeal orifice of the auditory (Eustachian) tube, and the soft palate. Fibers from the accessory nerve are also thought to contribute to the pharyngeal plexus.

The Soft Palate

The motor fibers for the muscles of the soft palate are derived from the mandibular branch of the trigeminal and accessory nerves. The latter supplies motor fibers to

TABLE 5-4

Nerve supply for muscles of the tongue

Intrinsic Muscles	Innervation Nerves
Superior longitudinal	Hypoglossal (XII)
Inferior longitudinal	Hypoglossal
Transversus	Hypoglossal
Verticalis	Hypoglossal
Extrinsic Muscles	
Styloglossus	Hypoglossal (XII)
Palatoglossus	Accessory (XI)
Hyoglossus	Hypoglossal
Genioglossus	Hypoglossal

TABLE 5-5

Nerve supply for the muscles of mastication

Muscle	Innervation Nerve
Masseter	Trigeminal, anterior trunk of mandibular branch
Temporalis	Trigeminal, anterior trunk of mandibular branch
Internal pterygoid	Trigeminal, anterior trunk of mandibular branch
External pterygoid	Trigeminal, mandibular branch
Depressors of mandible	See extrinsic laryngeal muscles (Table 5-6)

the uvula. The nerves that supply the palate with both sensory and motor fibers are contained in the pharyngeal plexus and arise from the **sphenopalatine ganglion** located in the pteropalatine fossa. The sphenopalatine ganglion receives sensory fibers from the facial nerve and from the maxillary branch of the trigeminal nerve. It sends off numerous branches, some of which descend to enter the hard palate through the incisive foramina. They are called the **nasopalatine nerves.** Others course forward to innervate the mucosa of the nasal cavities, while some enter the posterior portion of the hard palate by way of the greater and lesser palatine foramina, located just medial to the third molars. The mucosa of the hard palate and of the entire soft palate is supplied by the lesser palatine nerves.

The Larynx

We have seen how the intrinsic muscles of the larynx are supplied by the accessory fibers carried by the vagus nerve. Other muscles associated with phonation include the laryngeal elevators and depressors. These muscles are supplied by the cranial nerves and by the nerves contained in the cervical plexus. A sensory branch of the superior laryngeal nerve, called the internal branch, supplies the laryngeal mucosa, the base of the tongue, and the epiglottis. Table 5-6 lists the muscles of phonation,

TABLE 5-6

Nerve supply for the muscles of phonation

Extrinsic Muscles	Innervation
Digastricus, anterior belly	Trigeminal, mylohyoid branch
Digastricus, posterior belly	Facial, digastric branch
Stylohyoid	Facial, stylohyoid branch
Mylohyoid	Trigeminal, mylohyoid branch
Geniohyoid	Hypoglossal, geniohyoid branch
Sternohyoid	Hypoglossal, C-1, C-2, and C-3
Omohyoid	Hypoglossal, C-1, C-2, and C-3
Thyrohyoid	Hypoglossal, C-1, and C-2
Stenohyoid	Hypoglossal, C-1, C-2, and C-3
Intrinsic Muscles	
Thyroarytenoid	Vagus, inferior recurrent branch
Lateral cricoarytenoid	Vagus, inferior recurrent branch
Posterior cricoarytenoid	Vagus, inferior recurrent branch
Arytenoid muscles	Vagus, inferior recurrent branch
Cricothyroid	Vagus, superior recurrent branch

extrinsic muscles of the larynx, and their nerve supply. The nerve supply is shown schematically in Figure 5-60.

The content of the chapter has been restricted to some specific topics and was but an introduction to the nervous system. It can only point the way for further study. Although we have examined the nervous system in a piecemeal fashion, in retrospect a very valuable concept seems to emerge: the function of the nervous system is far more than the combined separate functions of all its components. A fitting close to this chapter has been given to us by Sir John Eccles: "the task of understanding in a comprehensive way how the human brain operates staggers its own imagination."

AN INTRODUCTION TO THE ENDOCRINE SYSTEM

The endocrine system is largely glandular, but the endocrine glands should be distinguished from those glands that discharge to the surface of the body (e.g., lacrimal, mammary, and sweat glands) and those that discharge their secretions into the alimentary tract (e.g., salivary, gastric, and intestinal glands). *Secretions of the endocrine glands are delivered directly into the bloodstream and are then carried to the various tissues of the body.*

Endocrine systems, which evolved later than nervous systems, are found in the more highly specialized animals whose nervous systems were apparently inadequate in certain respects. Vertebrates have seven clearly recognized endocrine glands: the **thyroid, parathyroids, adrenals, pituitary, gonads, pancreas,** and the **thymus.** An eighth structure, the **pineal body,** is sometimes recognized as an endocrine gland. The location of the endocrine glands is shown in Figure 5-91.

The Thyroid Gland

The thyroid gland consists of two **lobes,** placed one on either side of the lower larynx and connected by a strip of thyroid tissue called the **isthmus.** When seen under the microscope, the glandular tissue appears to be composed of a mass of alveoli or follicles, each of which is lined by a single layer of cuboidal epithelial cells. The follicles contain a viscous material called **colloid.** This substance, which contains the thyroid hormone **thyroxin,** is secreted by the epithelial cells. If an animal is deprived of a thyroid gland, stark metabolic changes occur which, if prolonged, may result in death. If thyroxin is administered, however, the animal will remain perfectly healthy and normal in every respect.

Deficiencies in thyroxin may produce **cretinism** in children and **myxedema** in adults. A child remains small and becomes badly formed, with puffy skin and a

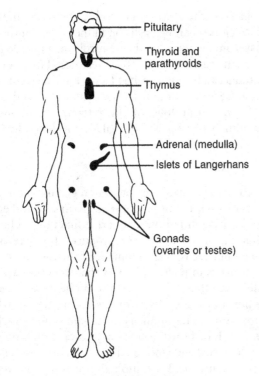

FIGURE 5-91

Illustration of the location of the endocrine glands.

tongue that seems much too large for the mouth. Mental development is at a standstill, and deafness is frequent. If given thyroxin at an early age, a child usually responds well and develops into a normal adult. Usual symptoms of myxedema include a general lethargy, both mental and physical, an increase in weight, and thickening of the skin. The entire mechanism of the body seems to slow down. The administration of thyroxin (or thyroid extracts) restores metabolism to its normal level, and subsequently all symptoms disappear.

In the early part of the century an enlarged thyroid gland was quite commonplace in areas of the world where there was a deficiency of iodine in the water and soil (in the United States, the Midwest). Adding iodine to diets (e.g., iodized salt) prevented the development of enlarged thyroid glands or **goiters.** Iodine is an important constituent of thyroxin.

Occasionally the thyroid gland begins to produce more thyroxin than the body needs, and this condition **(hyperthyroidism)** may also be accompanied by a slight enlargement of the gland. Excessive thyroxin increases metabolism and speeds up the entire mechanism of the body. Along with nervousness and tremor and rapid action of the heart, the eyeballs may also become protruded, a condition called **exophthalmos.** Control of thyroxin secretion is mediated through the hypothalamus and the anterior lobe of the pituitary gland. The controlling mechanism is very complicated due to the reciprocal

effects of a thyroid-stimulating hormone secreted by the pituitary and the level of thyroxin in the blood. A decrease in thyroxin stimulates the pituitary mechanism, and more thyroid-stimulating hormone is released. Exophthalmos seems to be caused, not by an excess of thyroxin, but by the thyroid-stimulating (thyrotrophic) hormone of the anterior lobe of the pituitary gland.

The Parathyroid Glands

The parathyroid glands are two pairs of pea-sized structures. One pair is located just behind the upper poles of the thyroid gland, and the other is located just behind the lower poles. In animals, removal of the parathyroids results in increased excitability of the neuromuscular tissues, which eventually culminates in a severe and usually fatal convulsive disorder called **tetany.** Death is due either to exhaustion or asphyxia resulting from a spasm of the larynx.

The parathyroids function to maintain the proper levels of phosphorus and calcium in the blood. When the glands are removed, blood calcium level falls off rapidly, which correlates with the symptoms of the disease. In the event the parathyroids become overactive, the calcium level in the blood rises too high. If prolonged, the calcium of the bones is sacrificed, resulting in a weak and twisted skeleton. In addition, the excessive blood calcium is brought to the kidneys for excretion, which may result in deposition of calcium, or **kidney stones.**

The Adrenal Glands

As the name implies, the adrenal glands are located on the upper surface of the kidneys. Each gland is composed of two parts, a central, dark-colored mass called the **medulla** and an outer covering called the **cortex.** The medulla and cortex have different embryonic origins, and there is little evidence that their functions are very closely related. The cortex is derived from the tissue that gives rise to the sex glands, whereas the medulla is a derivative of the neural crest. The medulla produces a hormone called **adrenalin,** sometimes called adrenin or **epinephrine.** Destruction of the medullary portion of the adrenal glands does not result in very great changes in an animal's behavior. If, however, adrenalin is administered to an animal, heart action becomes stronger, the spleen contracts, forcing its reserve into the bloodstream, the skin blanches, the pupils dilate, and the hair "stands on end." The entire picture is very similar to that due to excitation of the sympathetic division of the autonomic nervous system.

The cortex of the adrenal gland is essential for life. Animals die in about two weeks following complete removal of both adrenal glands. Numerous compounds have been isolated from the cortex, and their functions seem to be complicated. If the cortex should fail, carbohydrate metabolism is affected, and the blood sugar level drops drastically. Sodium chloride is lost from the blood and other tissues, and blood pressure falls. Overactivity of the cortex produces changes of a different kind. In children, precocious development of the sex organs and of the secondary sex characteristics is seen. In female children, a tendency toward virilism also occurs. In adult males, overactivity of the adrenal cortex may produce excessive hair growth, and a generalized increase in "maleness." Adult females fare even worse. The changes are toward maleness; facial hair may begin to appear, the body becomes muscular, and often the voice deepens in pitch. Even the sex organs may show signs of atrophy and become nonfunctional.

The Pituitary Gland

The pituitary or **hypophysis** is a very complex and important gland. It lies tucked in the sella turcica of the sphenoid bone and is continuous with the base of the brain by means of the infundibulum. It is a double gland, composed of an **anterior lobe,** which develops from the roof of the embryonic pharynx, and a **posterior lobe,** which is a direct outgrowth of the floor of the brain. Because of its location in humans, research has been difficult. The gland is easily removed in some lower vertebrates, however, and the effects of removal, especially in young animals, are profound. Growth is immediately inhibited, and sexual maturity never occurs. In addition, atrophy of the entire adrenal gland also takes place. *Clearly the pituitary is an important gland that regulates the functions of other endocrine glands and the growth and development of the entire mechanism of the body.*

The effect of overactivity of the pituitary gives some clues as to its function. The somatic effects usually include abnormal growth of the entire body, which, in spite of awesome dimensions, remains rather well proportioned. On the other hand, gland failure may result in dwarfism. These effects only occur when the gland malfunctions in the young child. If the pituitary should become overactive after maturity, a person may develop a syndrome known as **acromegaly.** It includes enlarged hands, a protruding lower jaw, and massive brows.

The effects of the pituitary on the thyroid gland have already been mentioned. A hormone from the pituitary probably initiates or stimulates the thyroid to produce thyroxin. The pituitary also regulates the adrenal cortex and its production of the hormone called **cortisone.** It seems to facilitate the body's potential for regenerating new tissue and also prevents shock and other symptoms associated with severe trauma.

We have briefly encountered the effects of the pituitary on sexual development. It produces at least two gonad-stimulating hormones, one that affects the Graafian follicles in the ovaries and another that causes the follicles to release their egg cells or, in the male, to produce **testosterone,** a hormone that controls the physiological status of the secondary sex characteristics. The pituitary also produces a hormone called **lactogen,** which controls lactation (secretion of milk by the mammary glands).

The posterior lobe of the pituitary functions in maintaining the proper water balance in the body.

The Gonads

The testes and ovaries are compound glands whose primary function is the production of sperm cells and eggs. They also have important endocrine functions. The interstitial tissue of the testes produces **testosterone,** which stimulates the development of the secondary sex characteristics in males. The fact that the testes are associated with these characteristics can be demonstrated by removal of these glands or castration, which, when performed in young humans, results in a high-pitched voice, a lack of beard, a tendency toward obesity, and few of the sexual and emotional characteristics associated with the adult male. Castration after maturity, however, results in few of these changes.

The onset of interstitial tissue activity and the production of testosterone are associated with puberty, when pubic hair appears and when growth of the larynx, change of voice, and increased development of the genitalia occur. Occasionally the testes fail to descend into the scrotal sac during the latter part of gestation. This condition, known as **cryptorchidism,** results in impairment in the production of live sperm cells but does not affect the secretion of testosterone. As a result, these males are perfectly virile in every respect, except fertility.

The ovary produces a complex battery of hormones, many of which are associated with care of the embryo, before and after birth. As an egg matures in the ovary, a fluid-filled space develops around it. The egg and the space together form a **Graafian follicle,** which produces **estrogen.** It is the counterpart of testosterone in the male. Estrogen stimulates the onset of puberty and the development of the female secondary sex characteristics. Another hormone, **progesterone,** is produced by a specialized part of the ovary called the **corpus luteum** (L. yellow body). Subsequent to the release of the mature egg from a Graafian follicle, progesterone initiates the menstrual cycle in humans and the estrus cycle in other mammals.

The Pancreas

The most obvious function of the pancreas is to produce enzymes that aid digestion. An additional function of a small group of cells called the **Islets of Langerhans** is to produce a hormone called **insulin,** which is responsible for the retention and storage of sugar in the body. If these islets are destroyed or become nonfunctional, as in the case of human diabetes, sugar is no longer stored in the liver and other tissues but is carried to the kidney and is excreted along with urine.

The Thymus

The thymus lies behind the upper part of the sternum and extends upward into the root of the neck. It is relatively large in infants and at the time of puberty begins to shrink until at adulthood it is reduced to little more than a vestigial structure. The thymus has been linked to immunoglobulin production, regulation of the level of vitamin B, and in the production of lymphocytes.

BIBLIOGRAPHY AND READING LIST

Abbs, J., and C. Welt, "Lateral Precentral Cortex in Speech Motor Control," in R. Daniloff, ed., *Recent Advances in Speech Science.* San Diego: College-Hill Press, 1985.

Albernaz, J. G., "Nervous System," in L. DiDio, ed., *Synopsis of Anatomy.* St. Louis: C. V. Mosby, 1970.

Arey, L. B., *Developmental Anatomy,* 7th ed. Philadelphia: W. B. Saunders, 1965.

Bowman, J. P., *The Muscle Spindle and Neural Control of the Tongue: Implications for Speech.* Springfield, Ill.: Charles C Thomas, 1971.

Brodal, A., *The Cranial Nerves.* Oxford: Blackwell, 1959.

Brodmann, K., *Vergleichende Localization der Grosshirnrinde.* Leipzig: Barth, 1909.

Cajal, Ramon y Santiago, *Studien uber die Hirnrinde des Menschen.* Aus dem spanischen ubersetz von Johannes Bresler, Leipzig, 1906.

Cajal, S. R., "Histologie du Système Hervoux de L'homme et des Vertébrés," *Maloine,* Paris: 1908.

——, *Studies on the Diencephalon,* compiled and translated by Enrique Ramon Moliner. Springfield, Ill.: Charles C Thomas, 1966.

Campbell, A. W., *Histological Studies on the Localization of Cerebral Function.* Published by aid of a subsidy from the Royal Society of London. Cambridge: Cambridge University Press, 1905.

Chusid, J. G., and J. J. McDonald, *Correlative Neuroanatomy and Functional Neurology,* 10th ed. Los Altos, Calif.: Lange Medical Publications, 1960.

Dickson, D., and W. Maue-Dickson, *Anatomical and Physiological Bases of Speech.* Boston: Little Brown, 1982.

DiDio, L. A., ed., *Synopsis of Anatomy.* St. Louis: C. V. Mosby, 1970.

Eccles, Sir John C., "The Synapse," *Scientific American,* 212, January 1965, 56–69.

Gardner, E., *Fundamentals of Neurology,* 6th ed. Philadelphia: W. B. Saunders, 1975.

Gray, H., *The Anatomy of the Human Body,* 29th ed., C. M. Goss, ed. Philadelphia: Lea & Febiger, 1973.

Gray's Anatomy, Edinburgh: Churchill-Livingston, 1995.

Guyton, A. C., *Textbook of Medical Physiology,* 4th ed. Philadelphia: W. B. Saunders, 1971.

Hathaway, S. R., *Physiological Psychology.* New York: Appleton-Century-Crofts, 1952.

Hodgkin, A. L., *The Conduction of the Nervous Impulse.* Liverpool: University Press, 1964.

Kimber, D. C., C. E. Gray, C. E. Stockpole, L. C. Leavell, and M. A. Miller, *Anatomy and Physiology.* New York: Macmillan, 1966.

Kuehn, D., M. Lemme, and J. Baumgartner, *Neural Bases of Speech, Hearing and Language,* Boston: College Hill Press, 1989.

Larson, C., and B. Pfingst, "Neuroanatomical Bases of Hearing and Speech," in N. Lass, L. McReynolds, J. Northern, and D. Yoder, eds., *Speech. Language, and Hearing,* Vol. I, *Normal Processes.* Philadelphia: Saunders, 1982.

Larson, C., and G. Kempster, "Voice Fundamental Frequency Changes Following Discharge of Laryngeal Motor Units," in I. Titze and R. Sherer, eds., *Vocal Fold Physiology: Biomechanics, Acoustics, and Phonatory Control.* Denver: Denver Center for the Performing Arts, 1983.

Larson, C. R., and M. K. Kistler, "The Relationship of Periaqueductal Gray Neurons to Vocalization and Laryngeal EMG in the Behaving Monkey," *Exp. Brain Res.,* 63, 1986, 596.

Larson, C., K. Wilson, and E. Luscher, "Preliminary Observations on Cortical and Brainstem Mechanisms of Laryngeal Control," in D. Bless and J. Abbs, eds., *Vocal Fold Physiology: Contemporary Research and Clinical Issues.* San Diego: College-Hill Press, 1983.

Love, R., and W. Webb, *Neurology for the Speech-Language Pathologist,* 2nd ed. Boston: Butterworth-Heinemann, 1992.

Netter, F. H., *Nervous System.* Summit, N.J.: Ciba Pharmaceutical Products, 1953.

Nishio, J., T. Matsuya, K. Ibuki, and T. Miyazadu, "The Roles of the Facial, Glossopharyngeal, and Vagus Nerves in Velopharyngeal Movement," *Cleft Palate J.,* 13, 1976, 201.

Penfield, W., and L. Roberts, *Speech and Brain Mechanisms.* Princeton, N.J.: Princeton University Press, 1959.

Pernkopf, E., *Atlas of Topographical and Applied Human Anatomy.* Philadelphia: W. B. Saunders, 1963.

Ranson, S. W., and S. L. Clark, *The Anatomy of the Nervous System,* 10th ed. Philadelphia: W. B. Saunders, 1959.

Restak, R., *The Brain,* Toronto: Bantam Books, 1984.

Sherrington, Sir Charles, *The Integrative Action of the Nervous System.* New Haven, Conn.: Yale University Press, 1906.

Snyder, S. H., "Opiate Receptors and Internal Opiates," *Scientific American,* 236, March 1977, 44–56.

Steward, O., Principles of Cellular, Molecular, and Developmental Neuroscience. New York: Springer-Verlag, 1989.

Weber, C., and A. Smith, "Reflex Responses in Human Jaw, Lip, and Tongue Muscles Elicited by Mechanical Stimulation," *J. Sp. Hrng. Res.,* 30, 1987, 70.

Wilson, V. J., "Inhibition in the Central Nervous System," *Scientific American,* 214, May 1966.

Zealear, D., M. Hast, and Z. Kurago, "The Functional Organization of the Primary Motor Cortex Controlling the Face, Tongue, Jaw, and Larynx in the Monkey," in I. Titze and R. Sherer, eds., *Vocal Fold Physiology: Biomechanics, Acoustics, and Phonatory Control.* Denver: Denver Center for the Performing Arts, 1985.

Zentnay, P. J., "Motor Disorders of the CNS and Their Significance for Speech," *J. SP. Hrng. Dis.,* 2, 1937, 131–138.

Hearing

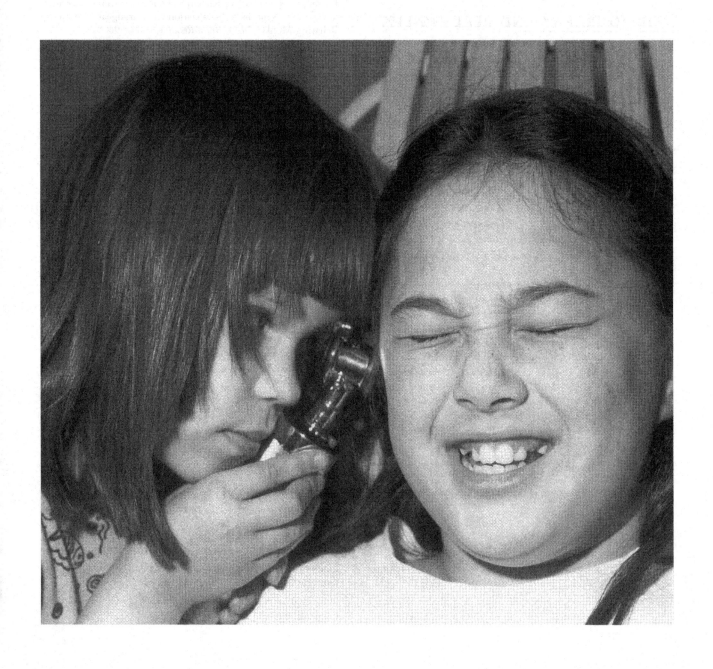

THE NATURE OF SOUND

Sometime during the early 1700s the British philosopher George Berkeley asked if a falling tree makes noise when no one is nearby to hear the sound. Ever since, writers have introduced discussions of sound and hearing by asking that same question. It is raised here only to point out the dual nature of sound. That is, a physicist might say that in falling, the tree dissipated energy, setting up a propagating disturbance in the air, a wave of sound, while the psychologist might reply with the notion that such a propagating disturbance must first be perceived in order to be called sound. In the next few pages we shall concern ourselves with the mechanism that serves as the receptor of sounds and permits us to perceive propagating disturbances of air, such as those produced by falling trees or the rustling of leaves.

Before proceeding to the structure and workings of the hearing mechanism, we may benefit from reviewing briefly some of the basic properties of sound.

The Properties of Sound

Undisturbed air may be said to be in a state of equilibrium; that is, with the exception of the ubiquitous random air particle movement **(Brownian movement)** and atmospheric pressure variations, the density of air particles remains relatively constant over time. When an external force impinges upon them, however, they may move closer together **(compression)** or farther apart **(rarefaction)** than when in a state of equilibrium.

Because air is a **fluid,** it tends to *flow from regions of higher pressure to regions of lower pressure.* In addition, since air has **mass,** it exhibits *inertial properties* and, when once put into motion, tends to remain in motion until the energy imparted has been dissipated. Thus, once a disturbance of the air particles has been initiated, by a sharp clap of the hands, for example, a layer of compressed air will move outward in all directions, compressing the air ahead, with rarefied air trailing behind.

It is important to note that disturbed air particles exhibit a minute forward-and-backward motion, imparting their energy to the air particles ahead, while they return to a state of equilibrium behind. It is the *disturbance,* and *not the air particles, that moves in a wavelike fashion* through the air. For this reason, sound may be thought of as a flow of power or a transfer of energy from one place to another.

Although the sounds with which we are most familiar are almost invariably generated by a vibrating element, it is important to realize that **vibratory motion** and **wave motion** are not the same thing. A vibrating body produces waves when it is immersed in some elastic medium, or coupled to it, and the waves that are generated travel through the medium.

Vibration

Vibratory motion may be defined as motion back and forth along a path in such a manner that there is a **restoring force,** increasing with displacement, and always directed toward the position of rest. The motion is called **periodic** when it occurs in equal time intervals.

Measurable Characteristics of Vibratory Motion

There are five important measurable characteristics of vibratory motion: **displacement, amplitude, frequency, period,** and **phase.** These characteristics or parameters are also useful in describing wave motion.

1. **Displacement** of a vibrating body at any instant is the distance from equilibrium to the position of the body at that instant.

2. **Amplitude** of vibration is the maximum displacement of the body from its position of equilibrium and is equal to half the total extent of vibration. This is also known as the **peak amplitude. Peak-to-peak amplitude** is the maximum displacement in one direction plus the maximum displacement in the other. In a linearly vibrating system, such as a pendulum swinging through a small arc, peak amplitude and displacement have equal values, and peak-to-peak amplitude is twice that of peak amplitude.

3. **Frequency,** f, is the number of complete vibrations or cycles per unit time and is usually measured in vibrations or cycles per second (cps). The symbol Hz is most commonly used to express frequency. It is in honor of Heinrich Hertz, a nineteenth-century German physicist. A vibratory rate of 100 per second is expressed as 100 Hz.

4. The **period,** T, of a vibrating body is the time elapsed during a single complete vibration. Frequency and period are *reciprocals.* If a body makes 60 vibrations per second, its frequency is 60 Hz, and since each vibration occurs in 1/60 seconds, its period is 1/60 seconds, or 16.66 msec. The relation between frequency and period is $T = 1/f$ and $f = 1/T.$

5. **Phase** is a term used in describing vibratory as well as wave motion and is useful in describing the relationship between two or more vibrations or wave motions. Since in a complete vibratory cycle the body moves through its position of equilibrium and back to it again (Figure 6-1), the process may be compared to circular motion. For this reason, phase may be defined as the *portion of a cycle through which a vibrating body has passed up to a given instant;* it is usually *expressed in terms of degrees of a circle.* The phase change in a complete vibratory cycle is 360°. The phase changes of a pendulum swinging through a small arc are shown schematically in Figure 6-1. The point in the displacement cycle at which an object begins its vibration is called its **starting phase** (0°). In the case of a pendulum, the bob is displaced from its position of rest to position B in Figure 6-1 and is then released. In this instance the starting phase is 90°. Its **phase angle** is 90°.

Simple Harmonic Vibration

The simplest form of vibratory motion, that executed by the tines of a tuning fork, by a pendulum swinging through a small arc, or by a weight bobbing up and down on an *ideal* spring, is called **simple harmonic motion,** abbreviated **SHM** (Figure 6-1). It is simple because of

the simple relationship between restoration force and displacement.

In accordance with **Hooke's law** the *restoring force is proportional to the displacement.* In Figure 6-2, if k is the spring constant (force per unit of stretch or compression), the restoring force, F, for a displacement, y, is ky, and k is proportional to F/y. No matter whether the mass, m, is displaced downward or upward, there will always be a restoring force proportional to the displacement, and in addition, since the acceleration of a vibrating body is proportional to the force acting on it, acceleration is also directly proportional to the displacement from equilibrium and is directed toward it.

Simple harmonic motion can be produced only when the foregoing conditions have been satisfied. A pendulum swinging through a small arc also executes simple harmonic motion. As the pendulum reaches maximum displacement, restoring forces also reach maximum, and the mass stops for an instant, to begin its round trip. At that instant, velocity of the mass is zero. As the mass swings through its point of equilibrium (displacement is zero), its velocity is at a maximum, and its restoring force is zero. The relationship between displacement, velocity, and acceleration (restoring force) is shown in Figure 6-2.

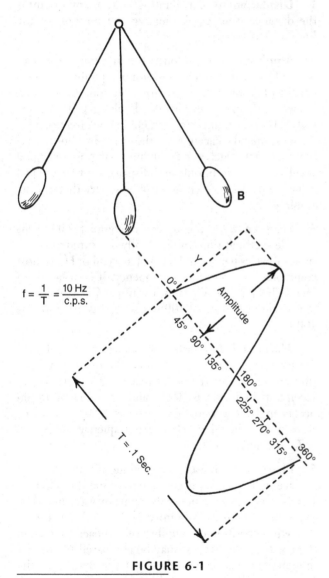

$$f = \frac{1}{T} = \frac{10\ Hz}{c.p.s.}$$

FIGURE 6-1

Illustration of phase changes in a complete cycle of a pendulum swinging through a small arc. Each complete cycle represents 360° of phase change. Simple harmonic motion is compared with circular motion.

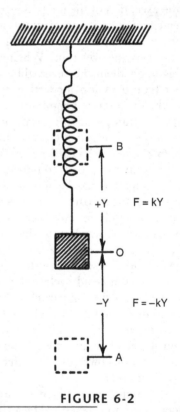

FIGURE 6-2

A mass bobbing on an "ideal" spring complies with Hooke's law. No matter whether the mass, m, is displaced downward or upward, there will always be a restoring force proportional to displacement. Acceleration is also proportional to displacement from equilibrium and is directed toward it.

Projected Uniform Circular Motion Simple harmonic or sinusoidal motion is sometimes defined as projected uniform circular motion. In Figure 6-3, if point P moves around the circle in a clockwise direction, its projection on the vertical axis $y_1 y_2$ is represented by the point R. As point P rotates at constant velocity, R moves along the vertical axis in simple harmonic motion. This motion may be represented graphically by plotting the distance OR against the angle swept by the line OP. Thus, the displacement, y, at any point is proportional to the sine of the angle θ, through which P has rotated on the circle, and the amplitude of the wave at any time can be obtained from the equation of simple harmonic motion:

$$y = A \sin \theta = A \sin \omega t$$

where A is the amplitude (equal to the radius of the generating circle or to the length of the line OP) and ω is the angular velocity (measured in radians per second) of the point P on the generating circle. The number of times P goes around the circle in 1 sec is the frequency, and since there are 2π radians in a complete circle, the relation between frequency, f, and angular velocity is $\omega = 2\pi f$.

If we assign a value of 1 to the line OP, then the vertical distance, or the displacement plotted on the vertical scale ($y_1 y_2$), is the same as the sine of the angle θ, and the resultant graph is referred to as a **sine curve**. The graph in Figure 6-3 shows the extent of the vertical displacement plotted for each $10°$ of rotation of point P on the circle. The graph is referred to as a **sinusoid**. The line OP represents the peak amplitude, and $y_1 y_2$ represents peak-to-peak amplitude. Often, some sort of "average of amplitude" over its entire period is used. Neither peak or peak-to-peak amplitudes will have much value (the arithmetic average of peak-to-peak amplitude is zero).

Expression of the **root-mean-square amplitude** is commonly used. If we obtain the instantaneous amplitude at a number of points along the entire sinusoid, and average them, the result is zero: since half the values are positive in sign, the other half, equal in value, have negative signs—the average is zero. If all the values of instantaneous amplitudes are squared, however, the neg-

ative signs are eliminated. The arithmetic average can then be obtained, and the square root of the average computed. This gives the average amplitude over an entire period. The expression is called **root-mean-square** or, simply, **rms**. In the case of sinusoids, the rms amplitude is 0.707 times the peak amplitude (A .707) or A $1/\sqrt{2}$.

Damping Graphic representations of the displacement of a bobbing mass on a spring, the swinging mass of a pendulum, will yield sinusoidal curves. Because of *friction* in these systems, however, *each cycle of vibration will result in the dissipation of a small amount of energy.* The energy of a moving mass is **kinetic energy (KE),** while the energy of the mass away from its position of equilibrium (energy of displacement) is **potential energy (PE).** Total energy is the product of the two.

For a mass on a spring, $KE = \frac{1}{2}mv^2$ and $PE = \frac{1}{2}Ky^2$. Potential energy is greatest when displacement is at a maximum. This means that acceleration toward equilibrium is also at a maximum. Kinetic energy is at a minimum when displacement is at a maximum. The mass actually stops for an instant, changes direction, and begins moving in the opposite direction. *Simple harmonic motion* can be thought of as representing a *constant exchange of kinetic and potential energies.*

In Figure 6-2 the mass has maximum kinetic energy at point O, the point of equilibrium, and potential energy is zero. At points B and A, potential energy is maximum, kinetic energy is zero. If the mass were displaced and released, the system would go into vibration at a rate dependent upon the stiffness of the spring and the mass of the bob. This is an example of **free vibration,** and with each cycle of vibration, a small amount of work is done to overcome friction. As a result, the *amplitude of vibration will decrease with each vibratory cycle,* but the *frequency of vibration will remain the same,* as illustrated in Figure 6-4. The decrease is amplitude of successive vibrations is called **damping.** The dashed line indicates the change in amplitude, as a function of time. It represents the **decay curve** or **envelope,** and the rate of decrease of amplitude is referred to as the **damping constant.** Note that the amplitude decreases at a constant ratio.

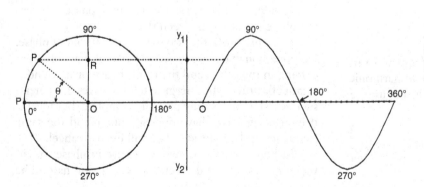

FIGURE 6-3

Simple harmonic motion represented as projected uniform circular motion.

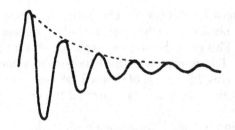

FIGURE 6-4

The decrease in amplitude of successive vibration is called damping. The dashed line represents the decay curve or envelope.

Sound Waves

When a vibrating body is immersed in, or coupled to, a propagating medium, **wave motion** results. Wave motion, for all its complexities and almost infinite diversity, must be either **transverse** or **longitudinal.** Any medium that will support a **shearing stress**[1] will transmit transverse waves. Liquids and gases will not support a shearing stress and therefore cannot transmit transverse waves. Fluids can only be subjected to **compressional stress.**

Any matter that responds to compression and has elasticity will transmit longitudinal waves. *Since all forms of matter exhibit compressional elasticity, they will all transmit longitudinal waves,* some better than others. The most familiar example of longitudinal wave motion is the propagation of sound in air, while examples of transverse waves include waves on a string. A disturbance that is traveling through air is known as a **progressive longitudinal wave,** and its distinctive properties are

1. The direction of movement of each molecule of the medium is parallel to the direction of propagation of the disturbance.

2. Each molecule in the propagating medium executes the same motion as the preceding molecule, but a short interval of time later.

The distinctive characteristic of a **transverse wave** is that the *displacement of the individual particles is perpendicular to the direction of the propagation of the wave.*

Compression and Rarefaction of Air Particles

It is possible to demonstrate visually what happens to air particles when a sound generated by simple harmonic motion passes through the air. The dots in Figure 6-5

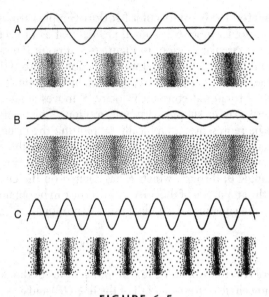

FIGURE 6-5

Illustration of the compression and rarefaction of air particles in a sinusoidal wave.

represent air particle movement. In a state of rest or equilibrium, air particles will be evenly distributed. In Figure 6-5A, the particles are alternately compressed and rarefied. Graphic representations also can be used to picture differences in wave motion. Note that the frequency in A and B is the same but that the extent of compression and rarefaction in wave A is approximately twice that of B. The amplitude in A is twice that of B, and since the air particles in A must move a greater distance but at the same frequency as those in B, they must move with greater velocity. Thus, a *sine curve can represent the velocity of air particle movement as well as the extent and frequency of movement.* The sine curve of C has the same amplitude as that in A; however, the frequency of wave C is twice that of either wave A or B.

Phase Relationships of Sound Waves

Sine waves may differ in *amplitude, starting phase,* and/or *frequency.* Consider the two waves in Figure 6-6A, for example. Both have the same frequency and amplitude, but whereas the starting phase for one is 0°, the other begins at 90°. These waves are 90° out of phase, or there is a phase lag of 90° between them.

In Figure 6-6B, the two tones are 180° out of phase. Compression in one wave occurs when rarefaction is occurring in the other, and the result in airborne sound is a **cancellation** of the energies in both waves. In general such interference is only partially complete, but ideally, if interfering waves have opposite phase and the same frequency and amplitude, they will exactly cancel.

In Figure 6-6C the two waves are in phase. In air, the compressions and rarefactions will summate. The

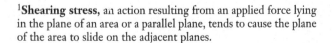

[1] **Shearing stress,** an action resulting from an applied force lying in the plane of an area or a parallel plane, tends to cause the plane of the area to slide on the adjacent planes.

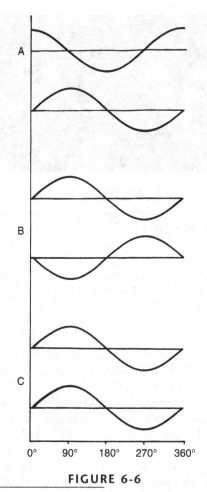

FIGURE 6-6

Oscillographic recordings of various phase relationships between sinusoidal sound waves. A = 90° out. B = 180° out. C in.

amplitudes obtained by *superposition* of two sine waves with the same frequency and various phase relationships are given in Table 6-1.

Types of Vibration

Sound vibrators generally fall into one of three categories, those exhibiting **free, forced,** or **maintained** vibrations.

Free Vibration Examples of free vibrators include tuning forks, pendulums, and vibrating strings. Once they have had energy imparted to them, they continue to

vibrate periodically until the energy has been dissipated. It is characteristic of a free vibrator to vibrate at its own **natural frequency.** In the case of the pendulum, the natural frequency or period is determined by its length. The period is the same regardless of amplitude, and regardless of the mass of the bob (gravity cancels out in the equation). Strings vibrate at various frequencies depending upon their tension, length, and mass, as expressed by the formula

$$f = \frac{1}{2L} \sqrt{\frac{T}{M}}$$

No matter whether a string is plucked, struck, or bowed, its rate of vibration is the same. The rate of vibration of tuning forks is dependent upon the mass and stiffness of their tines.

It is also characteristic of a free vibrator to absorb sound energy best when the energy source has a frequency rate exactly the same as the vibrator. This characteristic is known as **resonance,** which is easily demonstrated with the aid of three tuning forks, two of which have the same natural frequency. If one fork is struck and held in the vicinity of another fork matched in frequency, some of the energy radiated by the vibrating fork will be absorbed by the second fork, which will soon go into vibration on its own. There has been a transference of energy from one fork to the other. This transference of energy can be facilitated by touching the handles of the forks together. Whereas in the first instance the forks were *loosely coupled*, they are now *closely coupled*, and the transference of energy is more efficient.

Forced Vibration If two forks with different natural or resonant frequencies are used, there will be little or no transference of energy, especially if they are loosely coupled. If, however, they are tightly coupled for a few seconds, and then separated, the second fork may vibrate, not at the frequency of the first fork but rather at its own natural frequency. This is an example of **forced vibration,** where *vibratory or sound energy is imparted to a structure at a frequency rate other than its own natural frequency.*

If the stem of a struck tuning fork is held firmly against a table top, the whole table will be set into vibration at the same rate as the tuning fork. There is a transference of energy, but it is very inefficient. If the vibrating fork is removed from the table, the vibrations

TABLE 6-1

Amplitude of resultant obtained by superposition of two simple harmonic motions with the same frequency

Phase difference	0	45°	90°	135°	180°	270°
Amplitude of resultant	$A + B$	$\sqrt{A^2 + B^2 + 1.4AB}$	$\sqrt{A^2 + B^2}$	$\sqrt{A^2 + B^2 - 1.4AB}$	$A - B$	$\sqrt{A^2 + B^2}$

of the table cease almost instantly. This is because the table offers a great deal of resistance to vibrations at the rate of the fork, and the vibrations are *highly damped.* Oscillograms of free and damped vibrations are shown in Figure 6-7. An extreme example of damping occurs when a *displaced body returns to its position of equilibrium without passing through it.* Such a condition is known as **critical damping,** and no free vibrations can occur. Critical or nearly critical damping can be demonstrated by releasing a displaced pendulum weight that is immersed in water. The human ear is highly, but not quite critically, damped. Imagine the state of confusion if the structures of the ear continued to vibrate for some time after a sound had ceased.

Maintained Vibration Maintained vibration is not very different from free vibration. *A constant quantity of energy is applied to the vibrator at an integral multiple of the natural frequency of the vibrator,* and any damping effects can be overcome, permitting the vibrator to maintain a constant amplitude of vibration. When the driving force is removed from a system in maintained vibration, it will continue to vibrate for a while at the same frequency.

Common examples of maintained vibration include a child "pumping" on a swing and the weight-driven pendulum of a clock.

Wavelength, Frequency, and Velocity

In Figure 6-8, the distance between crests has been designated by the Greek letter λ (lambda). This symbol is used to represent **wavelength.** We have seen that a complete cycle of simple harmonic motion represents a phase change of 360°; for this reason, wavelength can be measured from any two points that represent a 360° phase change.

The **velocity** with which sound waves travel through air is about 1130 feet per second at room temperature.

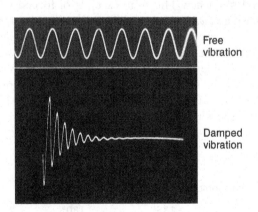

FIGURE 6-7

Oscillograms of free and damped vibrations.

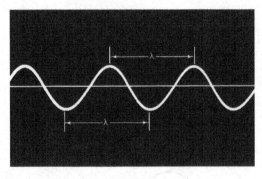

FIGURE 6-8

Illustration of wavelength. The distance between any two points that represent a 360° phase change is 1 wavelength.

If the frequency of the sound wave is known, the wavelength in feet can be determined by

$$\lambda = v/f$$

where v is velocity in feet per second and f is the frequency in Hz. On the other hand, if the wavelength is known, the frequency is $f = v/\lambda$.

The **frequency** of a sound wave is determined by the frequency of vibration of the source of the sound. A tuning fork when struck may vibrate at 440 Hz, and the air particles surrounding the fork are set into vibration at the same rate. The result is a sinusoidal note, often called a **pure tone,** with a frequency of 440 Hz, or A_4 on the musical scale.

Energy of Sound Waves

One might at first expect the energy of a sound wave to be directly proportional to its amplitude; actually it is *proportional to the square of the amplitude.* In other words, a wave in which the amplitude of vibration is twice that of another, actually represents four times as much energy. When an elastic medium such as air is deformed, the potential energy is given by the product of the average force and the distance through which it acts. We have seen that the value of the average force depends upon the distance through which the medium is displaced **(Hooke's law).** As a result, the work done, or energy of the wave, depends on the product of the two, or the square of the amplitude.

Sounds in Air

Sounds consist of propagating regions of compression, followed by regions of rarefaction of the molecules in the medium. A model for demonstrating propagation of a compressional wave is shown in Figure 6-9. It consists of a string of metal balls all coupled together by springs. If ball A were suddenly displaced to the right, a distur-

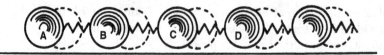

FIGURE 6-9

A ball and spring model for demonstrating propagation of a compressional wave.

bance would quickly pass down the string as the compression is transmitted from ball to spring to ball, and so on. In this model, the elasticity of the transmitting medium is provided by the springs and the density of the medium by the mass of the balls.

Sounds propagating through air generate regions of compressed air molecules, followed by regions of rarefied air. The rapid back and forth movement of the air particles constitutes work being done. The relationship between particle displacement, particle velocity, and the instantaneous pressure exerted by the air particles is shown in Figure 6-10. Referring back to our swinging pendulum, recall that at maximum displacement, velocity falls to zero for an instant, while the direction of swing reverses. Here, potential energy is

maximum, and kinetic energy is zero. As the pendulum swings through its position of equilibrium, velocity is at a maximum (potential energy is zero). The same holds for air particles in a sound wave. *At maximum displacement* (either compression or rarefaction), *air particle velocity is zero, but as the air particles pass through their position of equilibrium, velocity is maximum*, and it is here (at maximum kinetic energy) that the instantaneous pressure exerted by the air particles is at a maximum.

Spherical Radiation and Plane Waves

Because a **compressional wave** constitutes a region of increased air pressure, it will exert a force on adjacent particles equally and in all directions so that the propagated

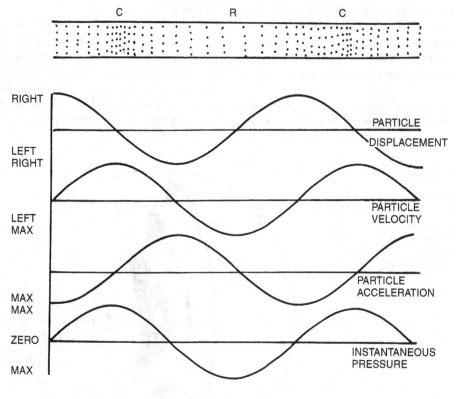

FIGURE 6-10

Illustration of relationship of particle velocity, particle acceleration, particle displacement, and instantaneous pressure in a propagating compressional wave, all shown in relation to the compressions (C) and rarefactions (R) of the air particles.

wave actually takes on the shape of an ever-expanding sphere. A tuning fork, a light source, or indeed, any energy source radiates its energy in the form of a sphere.

An example is shown in Figure 6-11, in the form of "shells" of compressions and rarefactions radiating in all directions. Any one of the many possible directions in which this wave travels is called a **ray of sound,** just as we call the direction of the path of light a *ray of light.* The outermost ring in the schematic is called the **wave front.** When the radius of the sphere is small, a segment of the wave front will be sharply curved, but as the sphere becomes larger, the curvature becomes less pronounced, until at some distance from the sound source it is called a **plane wave front.**

Since **intensity** is the rate of energy flow per unit of area of surface receiving the flow, it follows that, *as the distance from the sound source increases, the distribution of energy flow must necessarily decrease.* The wave front of a spherical sound wave, as it advances, is a sphere of increasing area, $4\pi r^2$, where r is the radius (equal to the distance from the sound source). If the total quantity of energy at the sound source is P, the energy crossing a unit of area of surface would be $P/4\pi r^2$. From this it is apparent that the intensity of a sound wave varies inversely as the square of the distance from the source, or $I = 1/d^2$. A sound with an intensity, I, at a certain distance from the source will have one-fourth the intensity at twice the distance and one-sixteenth the intensity at four times the distance. This relationship, known as the **inverse square law,** is one of the fundamental laws of physics and is illustrated in Figure 6-12.

We must keep in mind that the *inverse square law only applies where the sound encounters no obstacles.* When there are obstacles, the sound reflects, and the law no longer holds.

Reflection

Sound is reflected when it encounters an **interface,** a boundary between two propagating mediums that have different physical properties. Anyone who has experienced hearing their voice returned by an echo can appreciate the reflection of sound.

For an explanation of reflection we can turn to our ball and spring model employed earlier. Suppose, in the model shown in Figure 6-13A, ball B_1 is suddenly displaced to the right; it in turn will compress spring S_2, and so on, until ball B_6 is displaced to the right. The last ball, however, will encounter no resistance because of *discontinuity,* and so by virtue of its momentum, it will continue to move to the right until the tension of spring S_5 brings it to rest. The spring can be thought of as being in a rarefied state, and this tension or rarefied force will travel back down the series of springs and balls until ball B_1 is reached, and since it has no resistance in front of it to provide compression or tension forces, it will move to the right under the influence of the first spring and will continue to do so until the first spring has been compressed, and the entire series of events is repeated.

In Figure 6-13B, a similar model is shown, except that the last ball is rigidly fastened to a wall which acts as a *fixed barrier.* A wave of compression traveling along the series of balls will be reflected as a compression when the last spring is compressed, and the compression will move back along the series of balls to the left until the first ball is subjected to a compression force

FIGURE 6-11

Illustration of spherical radiation from a point source. Energy radiates in all directions in the form of "shells" of compressions and rarefactions. The outermost ring in the schematic represents the wave front.

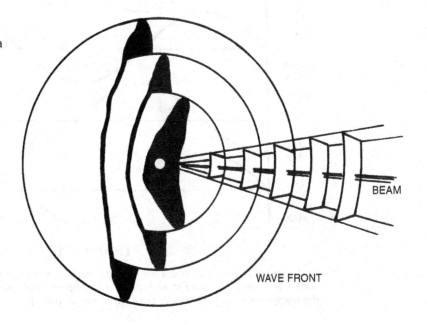

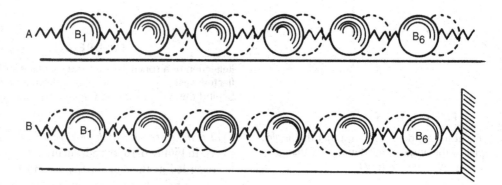

FIGURE 6-12

Schematic illustration of the principle of the inverse square law. Ideally, sound intensity is inversely proportional to the square of the distance from the source. The law only applies where the sound encounters no obstacles.

$$I = \frac{1}{r^2}$$

A = area   r = radius

FIGURE 6-13

Ball and spring model to explain reflection with (A) and without (B) a change in phase of pressure. See text for explanation.

from spring S_1. This force will cause the first ball to move to the left, but since it encounters no resistance, its momentum will carry it to the left to generate a tension force in spring S_1, and the tension force in turn will pull ball B_2 to the left as tensions in the springs are transmitted to the right until the wave is again reflected at the barrier. When this wave reaches the free end at the left, it will be reflected, but this time as a compressional wave, and the process repeats itself until the energy is spent.

We see that a **compression wave** is *reflected as a compression at the barrier, but is reflected as a rarefaction at the free end.* The most commonly encountered interfaces in acoustics are the walls, ceilings, and floors of the rooms we live and work in. In Figure 6-14, the wave initially generated at the source is called the **incident wave,** while the wave that is moving away from the wall is known as the **reflected wave.** If the reflecting barrier is large, sound complies with the **law of reflection** that states that *the angle of incidence is equal to the angle of reflection.* Consider the incident wave shown in Figure 6-14 as solid lines, and the reflected waves shown as dashed lines. The triangles formed by *ADC* and by *ABC* are *congruent.* They coincide exactly when one is placed on the top of the other.

The reflection of a spherical wave at a plane surface is quite different. In Figure 6-15 a point source *S* is located in front of a plane surface. The spherical incident waves radiating from the source strike the wall and are reflected back toward the source. The interesting feature of this type of reflection is that the reflected waves are also spherical, but they appear to be coming from a

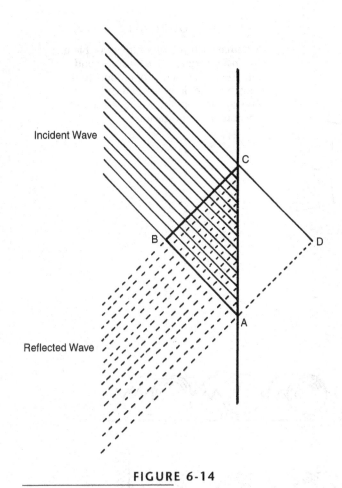

FIGURE 6-14

Reflection of a wave at a wall, demonstrating that the angle of reflection is equal to the angle of incidence. The triangles formed by ADC and by ABC are congruent.

point S_1 located behind the wall. It is called the **image of the source,** and it is located as far behind the wall as the **true source** is in front.

Incident and reflected waves are encountered in rooms and are multiple reflections, which when superposed may result in interference: **destructive interference** if compressions and rarefactions coincide and **constructive interference** if the compressions and compressions coincide.

A person sitting in a classroom or concert hall is literally bombarded by multiple reflections from the ceiling, the walls, and the floor. These multiple reflections, called **reverberation,** reach the ear at slightly different time intervals and phase relationships. Reverberation also results in a sound persisting for a longer interval of time, when compared to the incident sound.

Diffraction

Christian Huygens, a seventeenth-century mathematician and physicist, advanced the notion of **secondary wavelets.** He stated that *every point of an advancing wave*

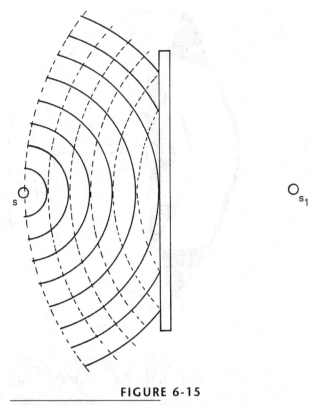

FIGURE 6-15

Reflection of a spherical wave from a plane surface. Reflected waves appear to be coming from a point S_1 located behind the wall. It is called the image of the source.

front is the center of a fresh disturbance and a source of new waves. In Figure 6-16, the advancing wave as a whole may be regarded as the sum of the secondary waves arising from points in the medium already traversed. This principle makes possible a clear understanding of **diffraction,** which means *a change in the direction of propagation of sound waves due to the presence of obstacles in the path of the sound.* Diffraction explains why a sound can go around the corner and down the hallway. Diffraction is also a property of light waves, but because of their extremely short wavelengths, we are seldom aware of the effects of light diffraction. When obstacles appear in the pathway of light, shadows are produced. A **shadow,** then, is a region characterized by the absence of wave energy (light or sound) due to the presence of obstacles in the pathway of the wave. When sound waves diffract, they tend to fill up the space we normally would think of as a **sound shadow.**

In Figure 6-17, an obstacle in the path of a sound wave does not produce a substantial shadow, but rather, the sound waves diffract and fill up the shadow space. This is why we need not be in the direct line of sound in order to hear it. Sound shadows, except in the case of extremely short wave lengths, are usually not a problem in acoustics; on the other hand, sound shadows may be helpful.

Imagine the distress if, in the concert hall, every time people in front of you moved their heads and ob-

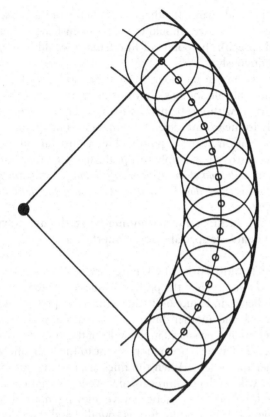

FIGURE 6-16

Huygen's principle of secondary wavelets states that every point on an advancing wave front is the center of a fresh disturbance and a source of a new train of waves.

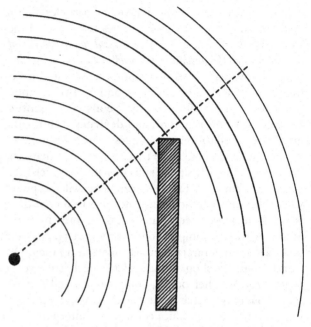

FIGURE 6-17

Diffraction of sound waves around an obstacle to fill up the shadow space behind it. Sounds with a long wavelength diffract better than do those with a short wavelength.

scured the view of the orchestra, they at the same time produced a sound shadow, which would prevent you from hearing the orchestra as well! It is enough that people spend countless nonproductive hours watching television. What if they had to watch radio as well?

Huygen's principle also explains why sound waves diffract when they reach an obstacle with a small opening in it. Neglecting reflection, the schematic in Figure 6-18, shows that the portion of the disturbance that progresses through the opening acts as the source of a new wave front.

Interference

The principle of superposition by Huygens states that if two wave motions are passing simultaneously through the same medium, the displacement of any particle in the medium is the algebraic sum of the displacements due to the individual waves. This means that *any wave passing through a medium will not be affected by any other wave passing through the medium at the same time.*

In the case where sound waves from two different sources exist simultaneously in the same medium, each wave travels as it would if the other wave were not there.

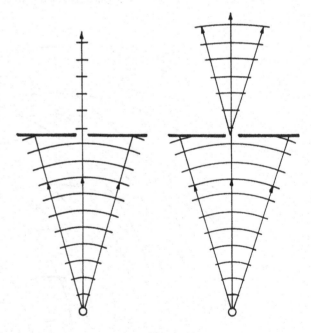

FIGURE 6-18

Diffraction of sound through a small opening in an obstacle. We might think that sound waves would continue through the opening as short segments of the wave front. That is not the case. Waves radiate from the opening as if it were a source of sound itself.

The displacements of the individual particles in the medium cannot have different values at the same time, so *when both waves are present, the resulting displacements are the sum of the displacements produced by the individual waves.* Individual waves may reinforce one another or they may cancel. The result of adding two or more waves is called **interference.** Both **constructive interference** or **reinforcement,** and **destructive interference** or **cancellation** are examples of interference.

If two superposed wave trains are *coherent* (have the same frequency, amplitude, and constant phase relationships), as shown in Figure 6-19, there will be points where the atmospheric disturbance due to one of them is always met by an equal and opposite force from the other. So, when a compression is arriving at a point from one wave train, a rarefaction may arrive from the other. At this point, we should expect silence or destructive interference. At other points, compressions and rarefactions from each source arrive together, so the individual waves reinforce or produce constructive interference.

In Figure 6-19, compressional waves are shown as solid lines marked *A,* while the rarefaction waves are shown as dashed lines, marked *B.* Constructive interference takes place where either the solid or the dashed lines intersect, but destructive interference occurs wherever solid lines from one source intersect the dashed lines from the other source.

In order for interference to take place, the two sources of sound must be coherent (have the same fre-quency and phase). If either the frequency or the phase of one of the sources should vary continuously (as in music and speech), the points of interference would also vary continuously.

When we consider wave trains as a whole, and from multiple sources, they normally pass through one another without being dissipated. They "interfere" only to the extent of reinforcement at some points and cancellation at other points. The acoustical energy is not destroyed; it simply reappears at some other point. *The distribution of energy is modified, but the total amount of the outward flow is equal to the sum of the individual outputs.*

The **tuning fork, standing** or **stationary waves,** and **beats** are special cases of interference.

The Tuning Fork The tuning fork is a *double source of sound waves.* When the prongs or tines move toward one another, as in Figure 6-20, they send a compression wave upward, and another downward, and at the same time a rarefaction is produced in the wake of the inward-moving tines so that one rarefaction is sent to the right and another to the left. When the tines are moving outward, they will send a compressional wave to the right and to the left and a rarefaction wave moving upward and downward. If a tuning fork is sounded and then slowly rotated about an axis passing through the stem of the fork, the sound will be heard to wax and wane. Four relatively silent points will be noticed in each revolution of

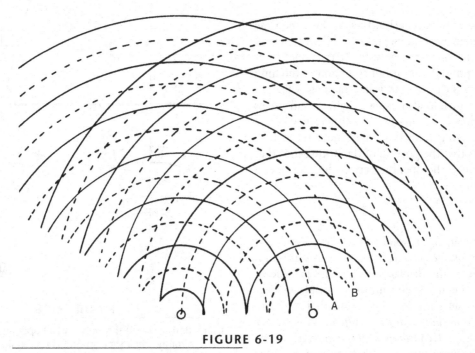

FIGURE 6-19

Interference pattern resulting from the superposition of two trains of waves. Compressional waves are shown as solid lines A, while rarefaction waves are shown as dashed lines B.

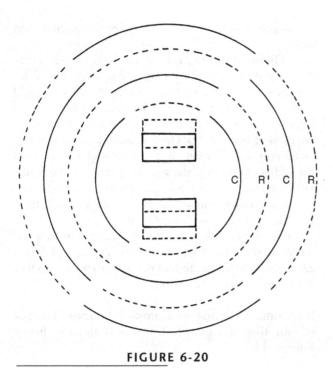

FIGURE 6-20

Interference pattern formed around the tines of a tuning fork.

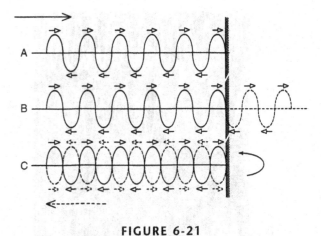

FIGURE 6-21

Illustration of particle movement in a standing or stationary wave. Maximum and minimum particle displacement occurs at half-wavelength intervals, and these regions remain stationary.

the fork, caused by the combinations of compressions and rarefactions.

Stationary (Standing) Waves Stationary waves can form where *two identical trains of simple harmonic waves are following the same path in a medium but going in the opposite direction.* In Figure 6-21, the solid wave represents an incident wave as it strikes the wall. Imagine the wave to pass through the wall as the dotted line indicates, and then in your imagination fold the wave that has passed through the wall over, to represent a superposed reflected wave traveling in a direction opposite to that of the incident. It is shown as a dashed line. The solid arrows indicate the direction of particle movement in the incident wave and the dotted arrows show the movement of the particles in the reflected wave. The ordinate in Figure 6-21 represents displacement of the air molecules. It reaches maxima and minima at points one-quarter wavelength apart, and these points do not change their positions. Thus the term **standing** or **stationary waves.**

Transverse stationary waves can be easily generated by tying a length of rope to a doorknob and flipping the rope up and down at regular intervals. After a few seconds, regions will appear where maximum displacement occurs (**loops**) and where minimum displacement occurs (**nodes**).

Beats A third type of interference is seen when two sound waves, identical in every respect except that they differ in frequency by a small amount, travel in the same medium. Because the velocity of the propagation of the two waves must be the same and because they differ slightly in wavelength, two waves that begin in phase at some point will become increasingly out of phase until they differ by 180°. At that point *destructive interference* results. After a short interval the difference in phase becomes less and less until once more the waves begin to reinforce. *The effect is a periodic rise and fall in amplitude that is heard as a regular increase and decrease in loudness,* called **beats.**

The number of times this increase and decrease occurs in a second is called the **beat frequency,** or $f_b = f_2 - f_1$. Two waves that differ slightly in frequency are shown in Figure 6-22. When they are superposed and displayed on an oscilloscope, the beats become visible. Beats are easily demonstrated by sounding two tuning forks that differ only slightly in frequency, or by wrapping a small rubber band around one tine of a fork (the mass-loaded tine will produce a tone with a slightly longer wavelength than the unloaded tine).

Beats are produced only when the beat frequency is low enough to be detected as individual variations in intensity. In addition, beats can only be heard when the principal sounds are within the frequency limits of audibility. Beats are no more than alterations in the intensity of wave motion. *They are not waves, but are the product of interference of waves,* and for this reason, *the term "beat note" is incorrect.*

Complex Sounds

Thus far we have been dealing with sine waves, which are relatively rare acoustic events in our day-to-day lives. The sounds to which we are most accustomed are

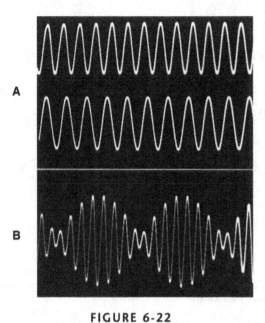

FIGURE 6-22

(A) Two sound waves of slightly different frequencies.
(B) An oscillogram of the interference that is perceived as beats.

usually quite complex; that is, they are *composed of more than one frequency.* This means that the *vibrating elements that generate sound also vibrate in a complex manner or mode.*

Vibratory Characteristics of Complex Sounds A

string, for example, may vibrate as a whole, as in Figure 6-23, or it may vibrate in segments in various ways. Each mode of vibration contributes to the shape of the sound wave, and each separate frequency that is generated contributes to the sound that is heard.

We have seen that when transverse waves are reflected at the fixed end of a string, the reflected and incident waves combine to form **stationary waves.** They have an amplitude that is equal to the combined amplitudes of the reflected and incident waves. Keep in mind that, with stationary waves, **displacement nodes** are located at the fixed ends (they can't vibrate) and at one-half wavelength intervals along the entire length of the string. This means that the simplest mode of vibration a string can execute is one where there is a displacement node at each end, with a single **displacement loop** halfway between. The **wavelength** is twice the distance between the fixed ends of the string **(2L).** If more complex modes of vibration are to occur, they must be located at distances along the string that are integrally related to the wavelength. So, another way of expressing the location of nodes is that they occur at distances, **x,** from the fixed end by the following rela-

tionship, $x = k\lambda/2$, where k is any integer greater than zero.

When both ends of a string are fixed, two sets of reflected and incident waves combine to form sets of stationary waves. If the loops and nodes of each set should coincide, the amplitudes of vibration will build up to large values. Inasmuch as displacement loops or nodes are located one-half wavelength apart, a string can resonate only when its length is some integral multiple of the half-wavelength of the stationary wave on the string. When a stationary wave is generated on a string, any one of a number of modes of vibration is possible, from very simple to extremely complex.

Each value of k in $L = k\lambda/2$ corresponds to a different mode of vibration, and so each value of k in $\lambda = 2L/k$ gives the wavelength of the wave that will produce stationary waves on the string.

Harmonic Structure of Complex Sounds The **law of vibrating strings,** which was introduced earlier, is expressed by

$$f = \frac{1}{2L} \sqrt{\frac{T}{M}}$$

where T is tension, M is mass per unit length, and L is length. By assigning various values to k, a series of modes of vibration will be obtained on a string that has a length L, a mass per unit length of M, and a tension of T.

In Figure 6-23, five modes of vibration are shown, and for each mode a different value of k has been assigned in the formula for vibrating strings. The lowest frequency of vibration is generated with a value of 1 assigned to k. This is the **fundamental frequency** and the tone produced is the **fundamental tone.** By assigning various values to k, a series of modes of vibrations will be generated, each with different frequencies. When a series of vibrations is generated in which the frequencies are whole-numbered multiples of the lowest, or fundamental frequency, it is called a **harmonic series.** Any whole-numbered multiple of the fundamental frequency is a **harmonic.** *Since the fundamental frequency can be multiplied by itself, it forms the first harmonic as well as the fundamental frequency.*

Complex waves can also be considered to consist of parts or **partials.** The fundamental frequency, which is also the first harmonic, is the **first partial.** With a value of 2 assigned to k, the vibratory rate is twice that when a value of 1 is assigned to k. This second frequency is the second harmonic and the second partial. The third tone (a value of 3 assigned to k) is the third harmonic and the third partial. The term **overtone** is also used, denoting any component in a complex tone having a

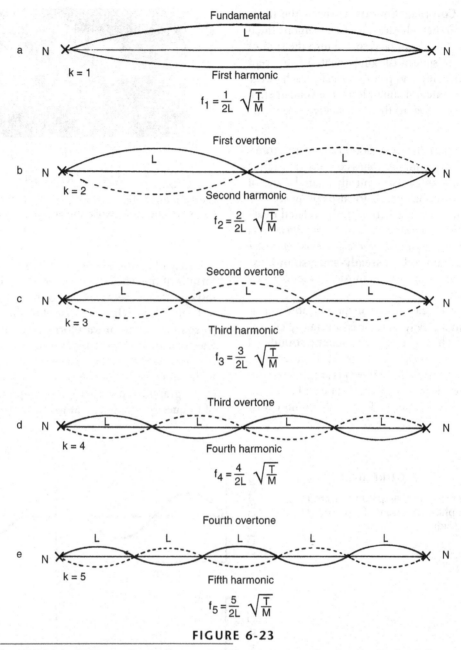

Fundamental
L
a N ✕ ———————————————————— ✕ N
k = 1
First harmonic

$$f_1 = \frac{1}{2L} \sqrt{\frac{T}{M}}$$

First overtone
L   L
b N ✕ ———————————————————— ✕ N
k = 2
Second harmonic

$$f_2 = \frac{2}{2L} \sqrt{\frac{T}{M}}$$

Second overtone
L   L   L
c N ✕ ———————————————————— ✕ N
k = 3
Third harmonic

$$f_3 = \frac{3}{2L} \sqrt{\frac{T}{M}}$$

Third overtone
L   L   L   L
d N ✕ ———————————————————— ✕ N
k = 4
Fourth harmonic

$$f_4 = \frac{4}{2L} \sqrt{\frac{T}{M}}$$

Fourth overtone
L   L   L   L   L
e N ✕ ———————————————————— ✕ N
k = 5
Fifth harmonic

$$f_5 = \frac{5}{2L} \sqrt{\frac{T}{M}}$$

FIGURE 6-23

Five different vibration patterns that can develop on a string. The simplest mode of vibration is one with a loop in the middle and a node at each end. The wavelength of the sound produced is twice the length of the string.

frequency higher than that of the fundamental frequency. By way of definition and by way of summary,

1. The **fundamental frequency** is the lowest-frequency component in a complex vibration or tone.

2. An **overtone** is any component of a complex tone having a frequency higher than that of the fundamental frequency.

3. A **partial** is any component in a complex tone or complex vibration.

4. A **harmonic** is a partial in a complex vibration, or a tone whose frequency is an integral multiple of the fundamental frequency.

5. And, finally, even though the term hasn't been used yet, an **octave** is any interval of two frequencies having a frequency ratio of 2:1.

Waveforms of Complex Sounds Early in the nineteenth century, a French physicist, Fourier, demonstrated that any complex sound can be resolved into the sum of a finite number or sinusoidal components of different amplitudes, frequencies, and phases. Usually, each of the components is an integral multiple of the fundamental (which has a period equal to that of a single cycle of the whole complex tone).

Steady-State and Transient Sounds. Musical tones are, for the most part, complex tones composed of a fundamental frequency and a harmonically related series of overtones. The vowels in speech are also composed of a fundamental frequency and harmonically related overtones. When the *frequency composition, amplitude, and phase relationships of the partials of a tone are constant over time*, the sound is said to be a **steady-state sound,** examples of which are a prolonged musical tone or a sustained vowel sound.

An important characteristic of speech, however, is that it is rarely in a steady state; it is constantly changing. That is, speech is a series of **transient sounds.** *A change in steady state is known as a transient.* Transients are generated, for example, when a vowel is abruptly terminated by the articulators. The steady-state and transient features of a speech sample can be grossly examined by

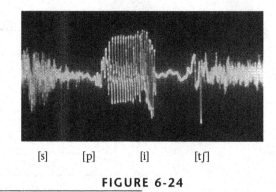

[s]	[p]	[i]	[tʃ]

FIGURE 6-24

Oscillogram of the word speech. The initial and final consonants are aperiodic, while the vowel is periodic.

a display of its **waveform,** as in Figure 6-24. The waveform is of the word *speech* as seen displayed on an oscilloscope. Note the waveform of the [s] phoneme seems to be aperiodic when compared to the waveform of the [i] sound. The term waveform as used here is in reference to a *graphic representation of displacement or amplitude as a function of time.* The waveform of a 100 Hz sinusoid is shown in Figure 6-25A.

A graphic representation of amplitude as a function of frequency is called an **amplitude spectrum,** and the

FIGURE 6-25

The waveform, amplitude spectrum, and phase spectrum of two 100-Hz sinusoids.

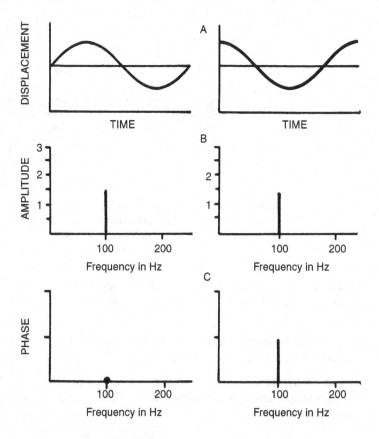

amplitude spectrum of a 100 Hz sinusoid is shown in Figure 6-25B. A representation of the starting phase, in degrees, is called the **phase spectrum,** as shown in Figure 6-25C.

Waveforms, amplitude spectra, and phase spectra of some commonly encountered sounds are shown in Figure 6-26. The waveforms of three sinusoids, which vary in their frequency and amplitude, are shown in Figure 6-27A, their amplitude spectra in 6-27B, and the results of the addition of the three sinusoids, in 6-27C.

Noise. A *sound that has little or no periodicity* is usually called noise. Noise may also mean a *sound with an instantaneous amplitude that varies over time in a random manner.* **Gaussian noise** pertains to a sound that has an instantaneous amplitude that varies in the manner of a **normal** or **Gaussian distribution,** as shown in Figure 6-28.

Noises can be generated in a number of ways, by the turbulence of air as it passes through a constriction or by a body vibrating in an aperiodic manner. Noise is also defined as any undesirable sound. It is apparent that noise is not rigidly defined.

A well-recognized and often-used term is **white noise.** All frequencies within a specified range are present, without regard to phase, and the average power over a frequency range is constant. **Average power** is equal to the product of the frequency range and intensity.

Another type of noise, called **pink noise,** is commonly used in studies of audition. Its amplitude decreases by one-half with each doubling of frequency.

Resonance and Filters

We learned earlier that tuning forks and other vibrating objects absorb energy best at some specific frequency. These objects also radiate energy best at that same frequency. This is an example of **resonance.** *Resonators act as acoustic filters.* They passively reject sounds at frequencies other than their natural frequency.

Returning to our mass-spring system, suppose the spring is attached to a revolving crank that is variable in its rotational rate. In Figure 6-29, let the natural frequency of the spring-mass oscillator be f_0 and the rotational rate of the crank be f. If the rate of rotation is varied slowly, the amplitude of oscillation of the mass will change, reaching a maximum A_{max} when $f = f_0$. The mass is engaged in forced vibration until the rotational rate approximates the natural or resonant frequency of

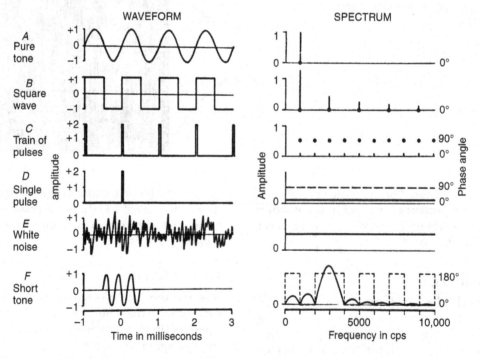

FIGURE 6-26

Waveforms, amplitude spectra, and phase spectra of some commonly encountered laboratory sounds. (From S. S. Stevens, ed., *Handbook of Experimental Psychology,* John Wiley & Sons, Inc., New York, 1951.)

FIGURE 6-27

Waveforms of three sinusoids that vary in their frequency and amplitude (A), their amplitude and phase spectra (B), and the results of their addition (C).

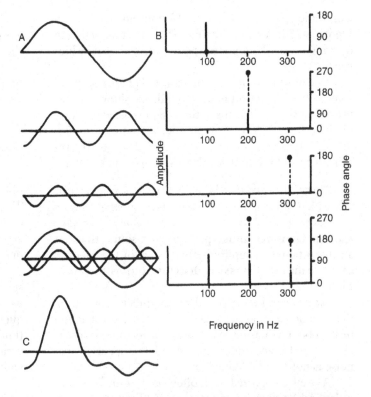

FIGURE 6-28

Gaussian noise has an instantaneous amplitude (A) that varies in the manner of a normal distribution.

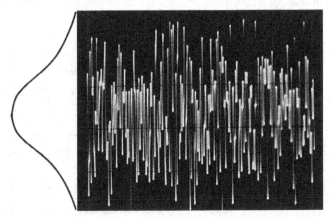

the spring-mass oscillator. The curve that is generated is referred to as a **resonant curve,** and its **linewidth** or **bandwidth** is the range of frequencies that have an amplitude of .707 of A_{max} or A_{max} **$1/\sqrt{2}$**.

Tuned Resonators

Resonators can also be tuned. An ordinary pop bottle can function as a resonator when you blow across its top to produce an **edge tone.** If the bottle is partly full of water, the tone will have a higher frequency. Incidentally, the wavelength of the tone will be four times the length of the air column in the bottle. The air in the neck of the bottle functions as a piston, and the volume

of air in the bottle functions as the spring. This type of oscillator is called a **Helmholtz resonator,** after Hermann von Helmholtz, an early nineteenth-century physician and physicist.

Passive Filters

It is sometimes necessary to filter out parts of a broadband signal in the study of hearing. This is possible with a **passive filter,** an example of which is the tone control on your tape or record player. Generally, just three types

---

[2]**Attenuate:** to decrease the amplitude or energy of a signal; to decrease.

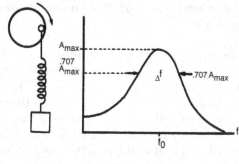

FIGURE 6-29

A spring-mass oscillator connected to a variable-speed crank. Let the natural frequency be f_0 and the rotational rate of the crank be f. If the rate of rotation is varied slowly, the amplitude of oscillation will change, reaching a maximum A_{max} when $f = f_0$. The bandwidth of the resonant curve is the range of frequencies that have an amplitude of .707 of A_{max}.

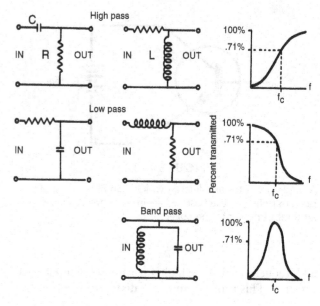

FIGURE 6-30

Simple electrical high-, low-, and band-pass filters. In high-pass filters, the low frequencies are attenuated by the series capacitor (**C**), allowing the high frequencies to pass. The inductor (**L**) acts as a shunt for low frequencies but passes high frequencies. In low-pass filters, high frequencies are shunted by the inductor. A band-pass filter uses a parallel combination of an inductor and capacitor. The characteristics of these filters are also shown.

of filters are used. One attenuates[2] high-frequency energy but passes low-frequency energy (**low-pass filter**), while a second type attenuates low-frequency energy but passes high-frequency energy (**high-pass filter**). *Combining low-pass and high-pass filters results in a filter that will pass signals within a certain frequency band, but attenuate others.* The **cutoff frequency** of a high- or low-pass filter is the frequency at which the output has dropped to 70 percent of the maximum.

Simple electrical high-, low-, and band-pass filters are shown schematically in Figure 6-30. The filters shown are known as **passive filters.** They attenuate a band of high or low frequencies, passing the remaining.

Amplifiers

An active device is an amplifier in which a *small amount of power is used to control a large amount of power.* A water amplifier is shown in Figure 6-31, in which a small amount of power at the valve controls a large flow of water. A single-transistor amplifier is shown in Figure 6-32. A small amount of power applied to the base results in the flow of a large amount of power in the collector.

Ideally, amplifiers increase the power of an electrical signal without the introduction of distortion. Two commonly encountered problems with amplifiers are a *limited frequency range* and *nonlinearity*. For acoustic signals, an audio amplifier should pass energy that falls within the hearing range. Twenty to 20,000 Hz is usually satisfactory.

The frequency response is sometimes given by the bandwidth between the 3dB points. That is the point on the frequency range where the output of the amplifier is

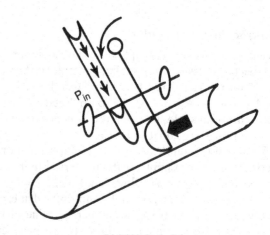

FIGURE 6-31

A water amplifier, in which a small amount of power (P_{in}) controls a large amount of water flow.

70 percent of its midfrequency range (Figure 6-30). If an amplifier is *nonlinear*, the output is not truly representative of the input. A nonlinear amplifier may actually

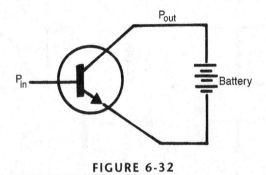

FIGURE 6-32

A single-transistor amplifier in which a small amount of power applied to the base results in the flow of a large amount of power in the collector circuit.

add frequencies that are higher harmonics of input components. This is one example of **distortion.**

The Decibel

In everyday applications of acoustics, the ratios of intensity, pressure, and velocity are often measured. Most often a **ratio scale** is used, but since the intensity ratio of the loudest tolerable sound to the just audible sound is on the order of 100,000,000,000,000 to 1, the ratio scale is far too unwieldy. In order to avoid such cumbersome numbers, the ratio scale has been changed to an **interval scale** by means of logarithms.

Ratio and Interval Scales

Conventionally we count simply by adding a numerical unit to each successive number. For example, if the numerical unit is 1, we count by adding as follows: $1 + 1 = 2, + 1 = 3, + 1 = 4, + 1 = 5$, and so on. Such a scale is called an **interval scale,** in which the intervals between successive values are equal or linear.

We may also count by successive multiplication of a numerical unit. For example, if the numerical unit is 2, the scale would progress as follows: $2 \times 1 = 2, \times 2 = 4, \times 2 = 8, \times 2 = 16, \times 2 = 32$, and so on. It is apparent that each successive product has twice the numerical value of its predecessor, or that the ratio between successive products is always 2:1. Such a scale is called a **ratio scale.** A ratio scale with a base of 2 may be expressed in other ways, as

2 (the base)	$= 2^1 =$	2
2×2	$= 2^2 =$	4
$2 \times 2 \times 2$	$= 2^3 =$	8
$2 \times 2 \times 2 \times 2$	$= 2^4 =$	16
$2 \times 2 \times 2 \times 2 \times 2$	$= 2^5 =$	32
$2 \times 2 \times 2 \times 2 \times 2 \times 2$	$= 2^6 =$	64
$2 \times 2 \times 2 \times 2 \times 2 \times 2 \times 2$	$= 2^7 =$	128

On the other hand, if the multiplying unit is 10, the scale would appear as

10 (the base)	$= 10^1 =$	10
10×10	$= 10^2 =$	100
$10 \times 10 \times 10$	$= 10^3 =$	1,000
$10 \times 10 \times 10 \times 10$	$= 10^4 =$	10,000
$10 \times 10 \times 10 \times 10 \times 10$	$= 10^5 =$	100,000
$10 \times 10 \times 10 \times 10 \times 10 \times 10$	$= 10^6 =$	1,000,000
$10 \times 10 \times 10 \times 10 \times 10 \times 10 \times 10$	$= 10^7 =$	10,000,000

Logarithmic or Exponential Scales

In each scale the multiplying unit is called the **base.** It was 2 in the first scale and 10 in the second. *Any scale whose successive units are multiplied by a specific base* is called a **logarithmic** or **exponential scale.** Each time a unit is multiplied by the base, it has been raised by one power. Thus, 10^6 (read "ten to the sixth power") means that 10 has been multiplied by itself six times. It also means that 10^6 has a numerical value of 1,000,000. If we know the base of a logarithmic scale is 10, we need not write the number 10, because it does not tell us anything. All we need to do is write down the value of the power to which 10 has been raised. Thus, we deal only with the exponent in our mathematical manipulations.

Logarithms are a valuable labor-saving device, especially when large numerical values must be dealt with. Since the exponents of a logarithmic scale in reality form an interval scale, such complex manipulations as multiplication and division are reduced to adding and subtracting exponents.

Suppose we are faced with the problem of multiplying $1,000,000 \times 10,000$. We know that 1,000,000 is the same as 10^6 and that 10,000 is the same as 10^4. To solve the problem we need only add the exponents, to give 10^{10}, which may be expressed as 10,000,000,000.

In order to divide 1,000,000 by 10,000 we need only express their numbers logarithmically and subtract their exponents as follows: $10^6 - 10^4 (6 - 4) = 2 = 10^2 = 100$.

The Bel

The intensity ratio of the loudest to the faintest tone can therefore be represented logarithmically by determining the power to which 10 must be raised to equal 100,000,000,000,000. It turns out to be 10^{14}. The 10 does not carry any information, so just the logarithm of the ratio is used, and it is expressed in units called **bels.** Thus, a ratio of $10^{14} : 1$ may be expressed as 14 bels.

The bel is not satisfactory, however, because the entire intensity range encompassed by human hearing amounts to only 14 bels. In order to specify smaller intensity ratios without using fractions, the term **decibel**

has been introduced. It is one-tenth the power ratio in bels. The bel is rarely used today, being supplanted by the more convenient decibel. Therefore, any power ratio or intensity ratio may be expressed in decibels (dB) by the following formula:

$$dB = 10 \log_{10} I_2/I_1$$

Standard Reference Intensities

Intensity is a measure of energy flow per unit of area per unit of time: cm^2/second. Energy per second is also **power,** measured in watts per square centimeter. Because a logarithmic scale has no true zero, it is a scale of ratios, always comparing two values.

If we are interested in the relationship between two sound intensities or powers, one must become the reference for the other. Certain standard reference intensities have been adopted. The **intensity level (IL)** of any sound is the *ratio of that intensity (expressed in dB) to the standard intensity of* 10^{-16} **watt/cm^2.**

A negative exponent may be thought of as the reciprocal of the same number with a positive exponent. For example, 10^{-2} is $1/10 \times 1/10$, or $1/10^2$, or $1/100$.

Sound Pressure Level Expressed in Decibels

Because the ear is a pressure-sensing device, comparisons between sound pressures are often made, especially in reference to hearing. The **power** of a sound is proportional to pressure multiplied by itself, or in other words, to the square of the pressure. Thus, if pressure is doubled, the power becomes four times as great. To express pressure ratios in decibels, therefore, the formula may be written

$$dB = 10 \log_{10} \frac{(P_2)^2}{(P_1)^2}$$

or

$$dB = 10 \log \left(\frac{P_2}{P_1}\right)^2$$

or

$$dB = 20 \log \frac{P_2}{P_1}$$

Pressure is a familiar term, but it is often used improperly, being equated with force. **Force** may be defined simply as *a push or a pull*, whereas **pressure** is defined as *force per unit area, when the force is at right angles to a surface*: Pressure = Force/Area (**P = F/A**). Force = Pressure × Area (**F = PA**).

Sound pressure is often measured in dynes per square centimeter (dynes/cm^2), and the standard reference pressure that has been adopted is .0002 dynes/cm^2. Any sound pressure when compared to .0002 dynes/cm^2, is known as **sound pressure level,** abbreviated **SPL.** Thus SPL is the *difference in dB between a particular pressure and the standard reference of .0002 dynes/cm^2*. For reference purposes, commonly encountered intensity and pressure ratios and their values expressed in dB are given in Table 6-2.

TABLE 6-2

Commonly encountered pressure and intensity ratios and their values expressed in decibels

A Ratios	B Decibels (dB) for Intensity	C Decibels (dB) for Pressure
1	0	0
2	3.0	6.0
3	4.8	9.6
4	6.0	12.0
5	7.0	14.0
6	7.8	15.6
7	8.45	16.9
8	9.0	18.0
9	9.5	19.0
10	10.0	20.0
20	13.0	26.0
30	14.8	29.6
40	16.0	32.0
50	17.0	34.0
60	17.8	35.6
70	18.5	37.0
80	19.0	38.0
90	19.6	39.2
100	20.0	40.0

THE EAR

Introduction

The ear is an extraordinary sound-detecting device, so sensitive it can almost hear the random Brownian movements of the air particles as they strike the eardrum. Yet, such a sensitive instrument is able to tolerate (and even enjoy) the sound waves generated by an entire symphony orchestra! The ear can also respond to a wide frequency range. It just misses the low-frequency rumblings caused by muscle contractions and by blood rushing through the veins and arteries in the vicinity of the ear mechanism. The ear can also detect shrill whistles with an extremely high frequency. The range of audibility is often stated to be from 15 or 16 Hz to about 20,000 Hz. In most adults, however, the upper limit of the frequency range is in the vicinity of 14,000 or 15,000 Hz, while in some young children the upper limit of hearing exceeds 20,000 Hz.

The ear's power of discrimination is very impressive. Suppose a sinusoidal tone is sounded at a moderate intensity level (comfortable to the listener) to a person with normal hearing. Then suppose we should change, very slightly, the frequency of that tone, sound it again, and ask our listener to tell us when a change in frequency is detected. Our listener, even without special training, could detect at least 1000 different pitches of sound and at frequencies below 1000 Hz could detect a change of only 3 Hz.

In addition to having fine powers of pitch discrimination, the ear can also do well in detecting different levels of sound intensity. Within the total intensity range to which the ear can safely respond, a listener can detect over 250 different intensity levels, which, of course, are perceived as changes in loudness. The number of just noticeable differences within the dynamic range of hearing amounts to about a quarter of a million!

We are privileged to listen to sinusoidal or "pure"[3] tones on very few occasions in our everyday lives. The discrimination powers of the hearing mechanism are not, however, confined to pure tones. Consider the fact that we can usually keep our wits about us and carry on a relatively normal conversation in a room crowded with people all talking at the same time, or almost. In fact, we are quite able to suppress all sorts of sounds about us in an environment and "tune in" on a conversation on the other side of the room. It helps, of course, if we can see the person who is doing the talking.

The hearing mechanism, as viewed by anatomists and physiologists, is often described as consisting of three divisions: the **external, middle,** and **inner ears.** This division is based largely on the *anatomical* relationships between the various structures of the auditory system. On a *functional* basis, however, it may be divided into just an **outer** and **inner ear.** A schematic representation of the hearing mechanism along with the functional roles of the various divisions is shown in Figure 6-33. The **outer ear** is the part of the system that has to do with *protection,* and with *absorption and transformation of the acoustic wave energy into mechanical vibratory*

---

[3] The term **pure** tone is often used synonymously with sinusoidal, and although, strictly speaking, it is incorrect, it is convenient.

FIGURE 6-33

A schematic representation of the anatomical divisions of the hearing mechanism and their functional roles. (Based on Dallos, 1973, and Gray, 1980.)

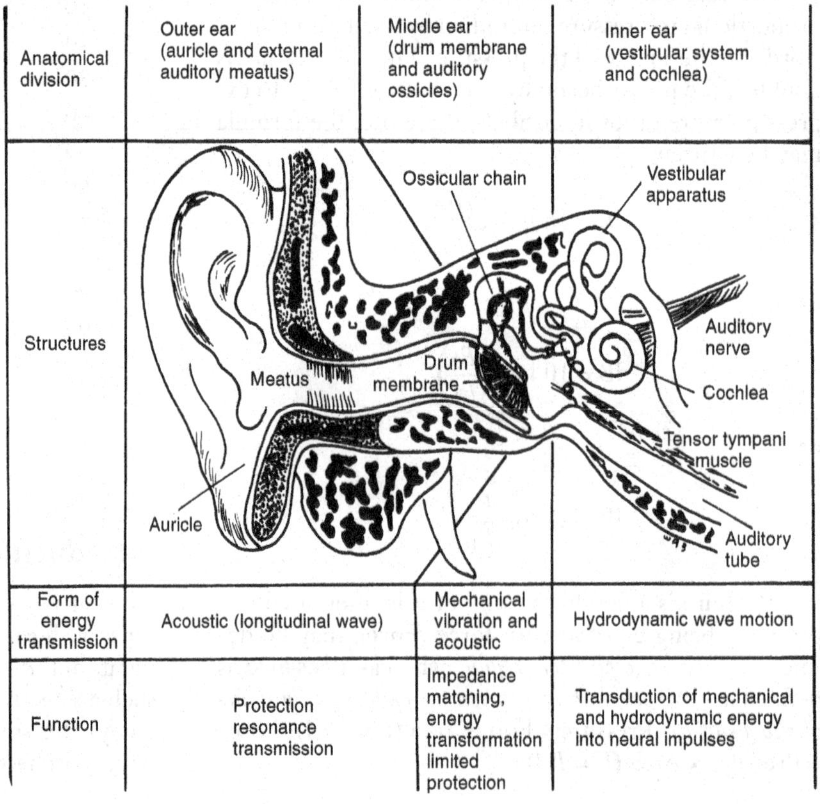

Anatomical division	Outer ear (auricle and external auditory meatus)	Middle ear (drum membrane and auditory ossicles)	Inner ear (vestibular system and cochlea)
Structures			
Form of energy transmission	Acoustic (longitudinal wave)	Mechanical vibration and acoustic	Hydrodynamic wave motion
Function	Protection resonance transmission	Impedance matching, energy transformation limited protection	Transduction of mechanical and hydrodynamic energy into neural impulses

energy. The **inner ear** is the part of the system that has to do with transduction of the mechanical energy; that is, the inner ear must *absorb and transform mechanical energy into a series of neural impulses,* the characteristics of which are somehow analogous to the original energy pattern.

We must also recognize the role of the central auditory neural pathway and the central nervous system.

The External Ear

The Auricle (Pinna)

The auricle or pinna is the visible, flaplike part of the hearing mechanism that is fastened to the side of the head at an angle of about 30 degrees. It is funnel-like and functions, somewhat poorly, to gather and direct sound waves through the **external auditory meatus** or **ear canal,** to the **tympanic membrane** or **eardrum.**

Although the terms auricle and pinna are both used, auricle is the more proper anatomical term; it is related to *aural,* a Latin term pertaining to the ear. *Pinna* is a Latin term for wing or, in other words, the projecting part of the ear lying outside of the head. In animals like the horse, rabbit, and bat, the auricle can be moved in several directions and rotated by means of functional extrinsic muscles. This movement is important in localizing the source of sound. The particularly large ears in some animals double as temperature-regulating mechanisms, since their size and elaborate vascular systems serve as excellent radiators of heat.

In humans, however, the contributions of the auricle are somewhat different, although the sensitivity of hearing (auditory acuity) seems to be about the same in those of us endowed with generous ears as in those with very small ears.

Surface Anatomy   The surface of the auricle is uneven and filled with pits, grooves, and depressions. The deepest of these complex depressions is called the **concha** (Gk. shell), while the rimlike periphery of the auricle is known as the **helix,** which, as shown in Figure 6-34, descends into the concha anteriorly. This part of the helix is called the **arm** or **crus,** and it divides the concha into the **skiff** or **cymba** superiorly, and the **cave** inferiorly.

A frequently found variation of the helix, near the tip posteriorly, is a thickened portion called **Darwin's tubercle.** A second semicircular ridge, just anterior to the helix, is called the **antihelix,** while a depression between the helix and antihelix is called the **scaphoid fossa,** or "boat-shaped ditch." At the level of the ear canal anteriorly is a cartilaginous flap, which partially occludes the opening into the canal. This flap is called the **tragus** (Gk. goat) while just opposite it, forming the inferior bound-

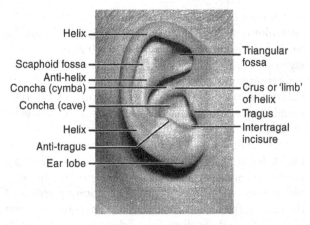

FIGURE 6-34

The auricle or pinna and its major landmarks.

ary of the concha, is a smaller ridge, the **antitragus.** The tragus and antitragus are separated by a notch called the **intertragal incisure.** In some aquatic animals the tragus is modified so as to form a valve that closes to protect the ear from water pressure. The inferior extremity of the ear is the **ear lobe** or **earlap.** It seems to have no biological function, but it is quite vascular.

Internal Structure   The core of the auricle consists of a fibrous cartilage, which has a shape roughly similar to that of the ear. Medially the **auricular cartilage** is continuous with the cartilaginous skeleton of the ear canal. It fastens to the zygomatic arch by a cartilaginous spine and to the mastoid process of the temporal bone by a tail. Although **anterior, superior,** and **posterior auricular muscles** attach to the auricle, they are vestigial and serve little or no function in humans. Some small intrinsic muscles extend from one part of the auricle to the other, but they too are considered nonfunctional.

Variability   Auricles are highly variable in their shape, to the extent they have been used for purposes of identification much as fingerprints have been used. One reason for the variability of the ear can be found in its embryonic development, a topic that is discussed in the following chapter.

The External Auditory Meatus (Ear Canal)

Communication between the middle and inner ears and the external environment is provided by the external auditory meatus or, simply, the ear canal. It has one primary function, and that is to conduct sound to the eardrum. It also has some acoustical properties we should examine.

The external auditory meatus is a curved and irregularly shaped tube, about 25 mm in length and about 8 mm in diameter in the adult. The diameter is largest at the **auricular (external) orifice,** becoming gradually smaller toward the **isthmus,** which is the junction of the cartilaginous framework with the bony framework. The diameter expands again, only to decrease in size just before the meatus terminates medially at the tympanic membrane (eardrum). The meatus is also somewhat oval, having its greatest diameter vertically.

As the drawing in Figure 6-35 reveals, the supporting skeleton of the lateral one-third to one-half of the meatus is cartilaginous, while the skeleton for the medial portion is osseous. Whereas the **bony portion** of the canal is fixed in diameter, the **cartilaginous portion** is variable, and its diameter is dependent upon such things as movements of the mandible. At birth there is no osseous canal, and it does not become fully developed until about the end of the third year. The bony canal develops from an incomplete cartilaginous ring known as the **tympanic annulus.** In children up to four or five years, there is a gap in the anteroinferior wall of the osseous part of the meatus that is known as the *foramen of Huschke.* This gap is filled in by membrane and may persist in the adult (British *Gray's Anatomy,* 1995).

The Course of the Meatus   As shown in Figure 6-35, the axis of the external auditory meatus is directed slightly downward, which means that water and other foreign materials are not liable to collect in the ear canal as they might if the axis of the canal were the other way. The course of the meatus is such that it forms an S-shaped curve. This curvature, which is slightly variable from person to person, may be straightened out by gently pulling the auricle upward and back. With adequate illumination this will afford a view of the tympanic membrane.

The course of the ear canal in infants and small children is less tortuous and more horizontal than in the adult, and there is a tendency for foreign materials to accumulate in it.

The Lining of the Meatus   The skin lining the external auditory meatus is closely adherent to the periosteum and perichondrium of the supportive skeleton and, in fact, forms the outer (lateral) layer of tissue of the drum membrane. The lateral one-third of the canal presents numerous **hairs** or **cilia** and modified sebaceous glands which produce, in conjunction with the ceruminous glands, the waxlike cerumen or "earwax." **Cerumen** protects the ear canal from drying out and, since it is bitter, noxious, and sticky, prevents the intrusion of insects and other foreign bodies.

Acoustical Properties of the External Ear

The meatus and auricle each have acoustical properties of interest to physiologists in hearing. In addition to the outer ear structures, however, *the presence of the head in a sound field has an effect on the sound intensity at the eardrum.* If a constant sound pressure level over a range of

FIGURE 6-35

Coronal section of the human ear. (From Max Brodel, *Three Unpublished Drawings of the Anatomy of the Human Ear,* W. B. Saunders Company, Philadelphia, 1946.)

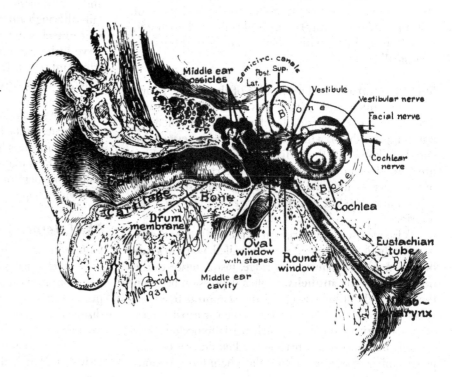

frequencies is generated in a relatively reflection-free environment (free-field), the presence of the head will result in changes in the sound pressure level that existed when the head was not present. The sound shadow it produces is part of the answer to the question of **sound source localization.**

This was demonstrated by Sivian and White (1933), Wiener (1947), and Nordlund (1962). Figure 6-36 shows what happens to sound pressure levels at the entrance to the plugged ear canal when the source of sound is moved in a circle around the head at a constant distance from it. Because of the relationship of the wavelengths of sound and the dimensions of the head, frequencies above 1000 Hz cast a considerable sound shadow, so that the intensity of the sound at the ears is somewhat dependent upon the **azimuth**[4] of the sound source. The effect is variable, dependent upon the size and shape of the head, frequency of the sound, azimuth, and elevation of the sound source.

According to Békésy and Rosenblith (1958), a number of experiments were conducted during the second half of the nineteenth century to determine the contributions of the external ear. The experimenters introduced hollow glass tubes into the ear canal and filled the irregularities with wax or dough. The results were consistent; although the sensitivity for sounds in the middle frequency range was not substantially affected, the ability to localize the source of sounds suffered, especially if the source was directly in front or back of the head. The *acoustic properties of the auricle and meatus augment the*

sound shadow effect and, in addition, *heighten our sensitivity to sounds.*

Resonance Effects of the Outer Ear

The velocity of sound at room temperature is about 350 meters per second. Since the meatus is a tube, essentially closed at one end, we can assume it will resonate best when its length is one-fourth the wavelength of the applied sound, or a frequency of about 4000 Hz. Wiener and Ross (1946) found the average length of the meatus in their subjects to be 2.3 cm. The meatus should resonate to a sound with a wavelength of about 9.2 cm, or a frequency very near 3800 Hz, which is in close agreement with the **resonant frequency** observed. These results are in agreement with earlier ones obtained by Fleming (1939). In Figure 6-37, note the prominent resonant peak near 4000 Hz. We should recognize, however, that the meatus is closed off by a compliant drum membrane that transmits sound energy in addition to reflecting it. This modifies the effective length and generates a **damping effect.** As a consequence, the *meatus resonates over a fairly wide frequency range.* The concha of the auricle also has a resonance effect that complements that of the meatus.

Shaw, in 1966, showed a **resonance peak** attributed to the concha in the frequency range of 5000 Hz and a peak due to the meatus at about 2500 Hz. The combined effect of these two resonances is shown in Figure 6-38. They are in agreement with computations by Békésy (1960), who found about a *15 to 16 dB increase in sound pressure level at the drum membrane due to resonance and head effects.* Note that the resonance extends over a frequency range of from 2000 Hz to 5000 Hz.

---

[4]When pertaining to sound, **azimuth** refers to the angular direction of the sound source in relationship to the listener.

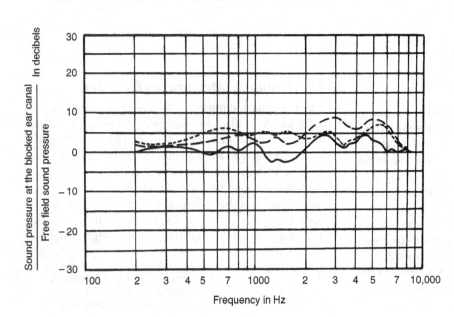

FIGURE 6-36

The effect of the head in a sound field when the angle of incidence of sound is 0° (solid line), 45° (long dashes), and 90° (short dashes). At frequencies above 500 Hz, the effects exceed 5 dB when the azimuth is 90° (sound is looking directly into the ear), which helps to explain why we turn our head toward a faint sound instead of facing it.

FIGURE 6-37

FIGURE 6-37

Resonance effects of the external auditory meatus, shown as the ratio of the sound pressure at the eardrum to the sound pressure at the entrance of the ear canal. In this instance the subjects faced the source of sound (0° azimuth). (After Wiener and Ross, 1946.)

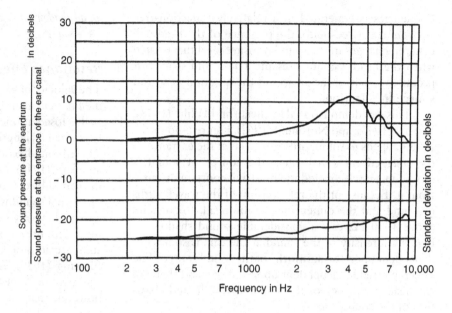

FIGURE 6-38

Combined effects of the presence of the head in a sound field. (After Wiener and Ross, 1946.) The upper solid curve represents 0° azimuth, long dashes represent 45°, and the short dashes represent a 90° azimuth.

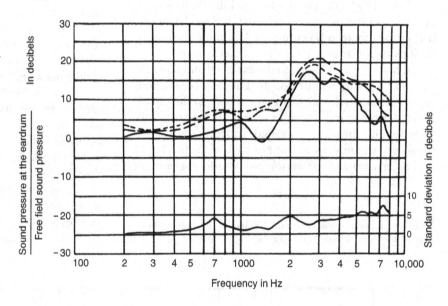

The Middle Ear

The medial limit of the external auditory meatus is formed by the **eardrum** or **tympanic membrane,** which also serves as the boundary for much of the lateral wall of the **tympanic** or **middle ear cavity.** The middle ear was described in some detail in 1561 by Fallopius, who saw in it some resemblance to an army drum or "tympanum," whence the cavity gets its name.

The middle ear is composed of the tympanic membrane, the air-filled middle ear cavity, and the structures contained within it, such as the auditory ossicles (the malleus, incus, and stapes), middle ear muscles, and the highly vascular mucous membrane that invests the structures in the middle ear cavity.

The Tympanic Membrane (Eardrum)

The tympanic membrane, which reaches its full size during fetal life, is placed obliquely in the external auditory meatus in such a manner to form an obtuse angle (140°) with its upper wall and an acute angle (40°) with its lower wall. At birth the drum membrane is set so obliquely that it almost lies upon the meatal floor; it erects gradually as the meatus lengthens. The drum membrane of a newborn human is shown in Figure 6-39. It is very thin (0.1 mm) and very compliant[5] but amazingly tough and

---

[5] **Compliance** pertains to the *ease* with which the membrane may be stretched or deformed. **Stiffness** pertains to the *difficulty* encountered when the membrane is stretched or deformed.

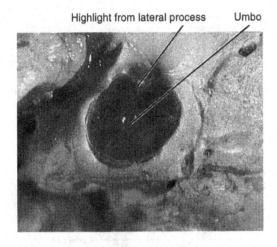

Highlight from lateral process   Umbo

FIGURE 6-39

A newborn human eardrum. Note the absence of a bony external ear canal.

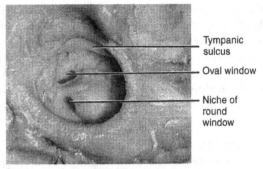

Tympanic sulcus

Oval window

Niche of round window

A. Lateral view showing oval and round windows, and the tympanic sulcus.

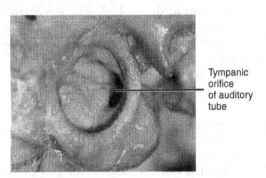

Tympanic orifice of auditory tube

B. Postero-lateral view showing tympanic orifice of auditory tube.

FIGURE 6-40

Two views of the middle ear cavity of a young ape. (A) Lateral view showing oval and round windows and the tympanic sulcus. (B) Posterolateral view showing tympanic orifice of auditory tube.

resistant to breaking. Wever and Lawrence (1954) give a mean breaking strength of 1.61×10^6 dynes/cm^2.

Cone-shaped, like a miniature loudspeaker, the tympanic membrane is displaced inward near its center by about 2 mm. Its very *small mass* (14 milligrams), *compliance*, and *cone shape* make the drum membrane especially suitable for its important task of sound absorption. The periphery of the membrane, except for a small section superiorly, is thickened to form a fibrocartilaginous ring or annulus, which is accommodated by a groove in the bony wall of the meatus called the **tympanic sulcus.** By means of this attachment the membrane is fixed into position at its periphery. The tympanic sulcus is deficient superiorly at the **notch of Rivinus,** and while it is not easily seen in the adult, it is readily visible in lower primates and very young children.

The sulcus shown in Figure 6-40 is in the temporal bone of a young adult ape. The slanted orientation of the membrane results in a larger cross-sectional area than it would have were the membrane perpendicular to the wall of the meatus. As it is, the area of the drum membrane ranges from about 0.5 to 0.9 cm^2, but because it is held rigid at its periphery, the effective, movable area is about 55 mm^2.

The Structure of the Tympanic Membrane Structurally the eardrum consists of three layers of tissue: a *thin outer cutaneous layer,* which is continuous with the lining of the external auditory meatus; a *fibrous middle layer,* which is largely responsible for the compliance of the eardrum; and an *internal layer of serous (mucous) membrane,* which is continuous with the lining of the tympanic cavity.

The fibrous layer actually contains two layers closely connected one with the other. One layer consists of fibers that radiate from the center toward the periphery. These fibers are unevenly distributed throughout most of the eardrum, giving the fibrous layer a fancied resemblance to spokes in a wheel. The other layer is composed of concentric rings of fibrous tissue which also have an uneven distribution. Their density is greatest toward the periphery, and in the center where the membrane attaches to the manubrium of the malleus (the outermost of the middle ear ossicles). A small triangular area, bounded by the notch of Rivinus, contains very few fibers, accounting for the flaccid nature of that portion of the eardrum, which is known as the **pars flaccida,** or by the old term Schrapnell's membrane. The pars flaccida is said to function in a very limited manner in maintaining equalization of the air pressure between the external and middle ears. The remainder of the eardrum is held rather tense and is known as the **pars tensa.**

Examination of the Tympanic Membrane The eardrum may be examined by means of an *otoscope*. It normally appears as a concave, smooth, translucent, pearl-gray membrane. The fact that it is concave is easily derived from a wedge-shaped reflected spot of light, usually seen radiating from the center toward the periphery, as in Figures 6-41 and 6-42. It is called the **cone of light,** and its presence is regarded as the hallmark of a healthy eardrum. In fact, many otologists regard the cone of light as the highlight of an otological examination.

Landmarks. Extending from the center to the periphery of the membrane, at about 1 o'clock in the right ear and about 11 o'clock in the left, is an opaque, whitish streak, the **malleolar stria,** which is formed by the handle of manubrium of the malleus. The manubrium is firmly attached to the medial surface of the eardrum by the network of connective tissue of the middle layer, and by the mucous membrane that invests the middle ear and its structures. The manubrium is firmly attached as far as the center of the drum membrane, which is drawn inward toward the tympanic cavity to form the **umbo.** This is the spot from which the cone of light radiates.[6]

Another highlight may be seen at the upper end of the malleolar stria. It is due to light reflecting from the **malleolar prominence,** which is formed by the attachment of the lateral process of the malleus to the eardrum. Two ligamentous bands, the **anterior** and **posterior malleolar folds,** course from the notch of Rivinus to the lateral process of the malleus. The triangular area contained above these folds is the pars flaccida.

The Tympanic (Middle Ear) Cavity

The student of the anatomy of the ear is faced with the difficult and often frustrating task of acquiring a sense of spatial relationships between the various structures.

---

[6]The term **umbo** is from the Latin, which means "a boss" or "bos." A boss in botany or anatomy is in reference to a rounded projection or eminence.

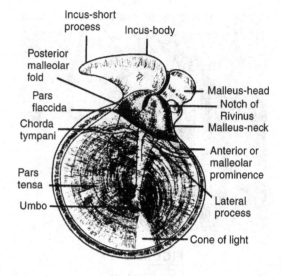

FIGURE 6-41

Schematic of tympanic membrane and some associated structures.

The illustration in Figure 6-43 depicts the middle ear cavity as a rectangular box with each side representing a wall of the tympanic cavity.

The tympanic cavity, shown in Figures 6-44 and 6-45, is an irregular space within the *petrous* (L. rock-like) *portion* of the **temporal bone.** It is narrow, varying in width from 2 to 4 mm, while its vertical dimension is about 15 mm, with a total volume of about 2.0 cubic centimeters. Usually the tympanic cavity is described in two parts, the **attic** or **epitympanic recess,** which is the portion extending upward beyond the superior border of the eardrum, and the **tympanic cavity proper,** which is the portion of the cavity lying medially to the eardrum.

The **epitympanic recess** is largely occupied by the head of the malleus and the bulk of the incus, two of the middle ear ossicles. Its posterior wall is perforated by an orifice, the **tympanic aditus,** which forms the connect-

FIGURE 6-42

Schematic of the divisions of the tympanic membrane into quadrants.

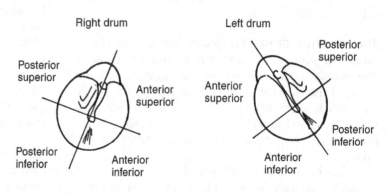

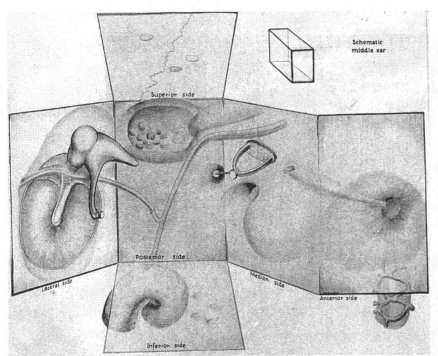

FIGURE 6-43

Schematic representation of the middle
ear cavity and the structures contained
within it. The middle ear is depicted as
a rectangular box with each of the six
sides representing a wall. The lateral
wall is partly bone, but mostly membranous (eardrum). The tympanic
membrane, malleus, incus, and chorda
tympani nerve are shown. The tegmen
tympani with the petrosquamosal suture running through it forms the roof,
and the floor is shown in relation to the
jugular vein. The medial wall forms the
lateral wall of the inner ear and is
shown along with the horizontal portion of the facial nerve, the stapes,
promontory and niche of round window. The posterior wall of the middle
ear cavity contains the descending portion of the facial nerve and the aditus
of the mastoid air spaces, while the anterior wall contains the opening to the
auditory tube, and the proximity to the
carotid artery is shown.

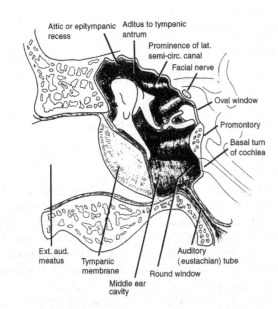

FIGURE 6-44

A schematic of the middle ear as seen from the front.

ing link between the tympanic cavity and the **tympanic
antrum.** Because the tympanic antrum communicates
with the mastoid air cells, there is indirect communication between the middle ear cavity and the mastoid air
cells. In addition, the mucous membrane that lines the
middle ear cavity is continuous with that which lines the
antrum and air cells.

CLINICAL NOTE: This relatively resistance-free
pathway established for the spread of infections from
the middle ear cavity, or indeed from the nasal cavity,
to the mastoid air cells is just one reason earaches and
middle ear infections (otitis media) ought not be taken
lightly. Earache is a common symptom, especially in
children. **Otitis externa** (inflammation of the external
auditory meatus) is one cause. Movement of the tragus
results in increased pain because the cartilage in the
auricle is continuous with that of the external auditory
meatus.

The Roof and the Floor The tympanic cavity is
bounded *superiorly* by a paper-thin plate of bone called
the **tegmental wall** or **tegmen tympani** (roof of the
tympanum). It separates the tympanic cavity from the
cranium and the meningeal coverings of the brain. The
tegmen tympanum is continued posteriorly so that it
forms the roof of the tympanic antrum as well. The
union of the petrous portion of the temporal bone with
the remainder of the temporal bone forms the **petrosquamosal suture** in children. Inflammatory conditions
in the middle ear may spread through the tegmen tympani by way of this suture directly to the meninges of
the brain (Moore, p. 968). The *floor* of the tympanic cavity, somewhat narrower than the roof, is formed by the
tympanic plate of the temporal bone. It separates the

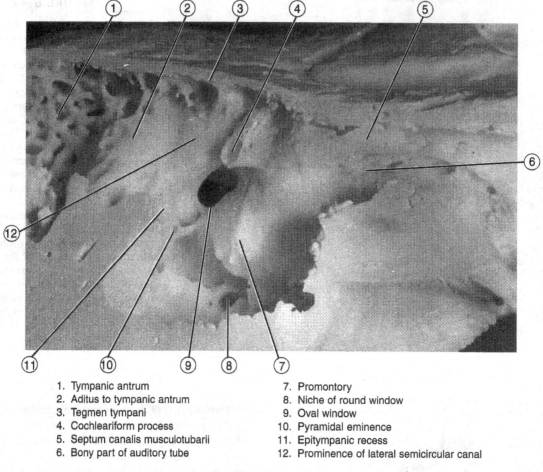

1. Tympanic antrum
2. Aditus to tympanic antrum
3. Tegmen tympani
4. Cochleariform process
5. Septum canalis musculotubarii
6. Bony part of auditory tube

7. Promontory
8. Niche of round window
9. Oval window
10. Pyramidal eminence
11. Epitympanic recess
12. Prominence of lateral semicircular canal

FIGURE 6-45

A lateral view of the medial wall and part of the anterior and posterior walls of the tympanic cavity (human).

tympanic cavity from the jugular fossa, a large groove that accommodates the jugular vein.

The Lateral (Membranous) Wall As stated earlier, most of the lateral wall of the tympanic cavity is formed by the eardrum, and for this reason the terms lateral and membranous wall are often used synonymously. Above the tympanic membrane, however, in the epitympanic recess, the lateral wall is formed by part of the *squamous portion* of the temporal bone.

The Medial (Labyrinthian) Wall The medial or labyrinthian wall, shown in Figure 6-45, is vertically directed and has as its landmarks the **oval window** (fenestra vestibule), the **round window** (fenestra rotunda), the **promontory,** and the **prominence of the facial nerve canal.**

The **oval window** is a somewhat kidney-shaped opening into the vestibule of the inner ear. During life, the oval window is occupied by the **footplate of the stapes,** the periphery of which is fixed into place by an annular ligament.

The **round window** is a circular opening into the basal (lowermost or first) turn of the **scala tympani** of the cochlea (to be discussed later). It is located beneath the oval window in a cone-shaped depression partially hidden from view by the promontory. The round window is closed by a thin membrane, the **secondary tympanic membrane.** The round window and adjacent structures in the middle ear of a cat are shown in Figure 6-46. The round window may also be seen in Figure 6-47. It shows the ossicles and cochlea of a 4-month human fetus.

The **promontory** is a rounded prominence projecting into the middle ear cavity. It is formed by the lateral projection of the basal turn of the cochlea ("P" in Figure 6-46).

Just superior to the oval window is a small prominence, formed by the lateral projection of the canal (aqueduct of Fallopius), through which the facial nerve courses.

The Posterior (Mastoid) Wall The posterior or mastoid wall has as its landmarks the previously described

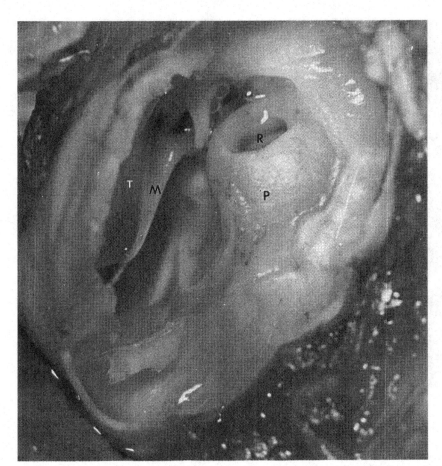

FIGURE 6-46

A view of the middle ear of a cat. The inner surface of the drum membrane (**T**), the manubrium of the malleus (**M**), the promontory (**P**), and round window (**R**) are all clearly seen (new, improved, modified, and labeled, Weber technique).

tympanic aditus, which is the entrance to the tympanic antrum, the **pyramidal eminence,** and the **fossa incudis.**

The **pyramidal eminence** is located just behind the oval window near the prominence of the facial canal. The eminence is hollow and in life contains the **stapedius muscle,** one of the middle ear muscles. The apex of the eminence is pierced by an extremely small aperture through which courses the tendon of the stapedius, as it emerges to enter the middle ear cavity. The **fossa incudis** is a small evacuation in the lower and back part of the epitympanic recess that accommodates the short process of the incus.

At the angle of the junction of the posterior (mastoid) and lateral (membranous) walls of the tympanic cavity, behind the eardrum and on a level with the lateral process of the malleus, is a small aperture through which courses the **chorda tympani nerve,** a small branch of the facial nerve that ultimately joins the lingual branch of the trigeminal nerve. The chorda tympani enters the tympanic cavity, courses just medially to the neck of the malleus, and leaves the cavity by way of the **iter chordae anterius** (*iter* is a general term for passage), which is also known as the canal of Huguier. It opens just above and in front of the tympanic sulcus. The chorda tympani was shown schematically in Figure 6-41.

The Anterior (Carotid) Wall The anterior or carotid wall is somewhat wider at the top than at the bottom. It is separated from the carotid canal (through which courses the internal carotid artery) by a very thin plate of bone. The upper part of the anterior wall is perforated by the tendon for the **tensor tympani** muscle and by the orifice of the **auditory (Eustachian) tube.** The canals for the auditory tube and the tensor tympani are roughly parallel and are separated by a very thin plate of bone called the **septum canalis musculotubarii,** and it is shown in Figure 6-45.

The Auditory (Pharyngotympanic, Eustachian) Tube

The auditory tube was described in some detail by the sixteenth-century anatomist Eustachius and the eponym lingers on. The auditory tube is the canal which *establishes communication between the middle ear and the nasopharynx.* It is about 35 to 38 mm in length and in the adult is directed downward, forward, and medialward. The tube may be divided into four sections: the **osseous, cartilaginous,** and **membranous** portions, and the **isthmus.**

The **osseous portion,** about 12 mm in length, begins in the anterior wall of the tympanic cavity, just beneath the septum canalis musculotubarii. Thus, as seen

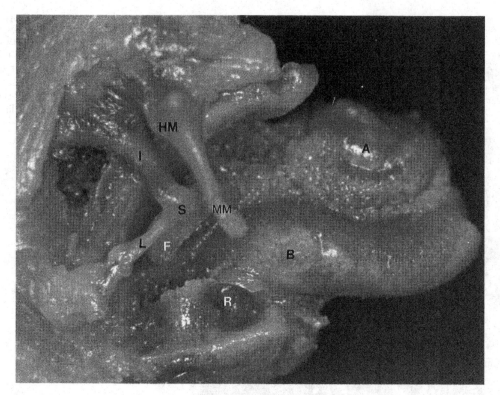

FIGURE 6-47

The ossicles and cochlea of a 4-month human fetus. The apex (**A**) can be seen at the top of the cochlea; the round window (**R**) can be seen at the basal turn (**B**). Also seen are the head of the malleus (**HM**), the manubrium of the malleus (**MM**), the long arm of the incus (**I**), the head of the stapes (**S**) and the footplate of the stapes (**F**), along with the ligament of the stapedius muscle (**L**). (Dissection by Patricia Gauper.)

in Figure 6-45, the tympanic opening of the auditory tube is about 3 mm above the floor of the tympanic cavity.

The **lumen** through the osseous portion is normally patent (open) and varies from about 3 to 6 mm in diameter. It is narrowest at its medial limit where it ends at the junction of the squamous and petrous portions of the temporal bone as a ragged margin, which serves as the attachment for the cartilaginous portion. The junction of the osseous and cartilaginous portions is called the **isthmus.**

The **cartilaginous portion** varies in length from about 18 to 24 mm. It begins as a rounded shelf located above the lumen of the tube and gradually widens to form an incomplete ring whose upper edge is curled upon itself laterally so as to present the appearance of a hook when seen in transverse section. The tube is completed by soft connective tissue.

The Torus Tubarius   At the pharyngeal ostium the cartilage and its coverings form a prominent elevation, the torus tubarius. It is located on a level about the same as the inferior nasal concha. As shown schematically in Fig-

ure 6-48, the anterior elevation of the torus is made by a small muscle sometimes identified as the **salpingopalatine** (Gk. *salpinx*, tube), which arises from the superior-lateral border of the cartilage and courses downward and forward to blend with the muscle tissue of the soft palate. Usually these fibers are regarded as a continuation of the **levator palatini.** The posterior fold of the torus is made by the **salpingopharyngeus,** which arises from the medial superior border of the cartilage and arches downward and lateralward to blend into the lateral wall of the pharynx and with the **palatopharyngeus.**

Two other muscles, the levator palatini and the tensor palatini, also arise from the cartilage. The **levator palatini** originates from the medial surface of the petrous portion of the temporal bone below the junction of the osseous and cartilaginous portions of the tube. A few fibers arise from the medial fold of the cartilage. The course of the muscle is roughly parallel to the cartilage until the fibers radiate and blend into the soft palate. Some fibers of the **tensor palatini** arise from the lateral side of the cartilage, but for the most part the muscle arises from adjacent bone. This muscle converges on the hamulus of the medial pterygoid plate where the

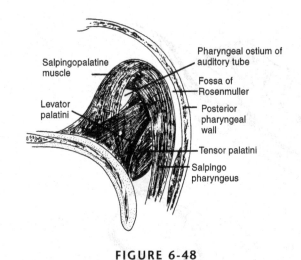

Salpingopalatine muscle
Levator palatini
Pharyngeal ostium of auditory tube
Fossa of Rosenmuller
Posterior pharyngeal wall
Tensor palatini
Salpingo pharyngeus

FIGURE 6-48

Torus tubarius with mucous membrane removed.

tendon courses at right angles to blend with the palatal aponeurosis.

The torus tubarius is liberally covered with ciliated mucous membrane that is continuous with that of the nasopharynx. The mucous membrane is a modified nasal type, and it continues into the tympanic cavity. Near the pharyngeal orifice, especially in children, may be found a mass of **pharyngeal tonsil** (tubal tonsil) tissue, which in many instances may actually penetrate into the lumen of the tube. *This partly accounts for the rapid spread of upper respiratory infections through the auditory tube and into the middle ear.*

Due to its elastic properties, the cartilaginous portion of the tube is normally collapsed, its walls folded parallel with its long axis. Simpkins (1943) has noted, however, that the passive elasticity of the cartilage is supplemented by active contraction of the salpingopalatine and salpingopharyngeus muscles.

Functions of the Auditory Tube The primary biological functions of the auditory tube are (1) to permit middle ear pressure to equalize with the external (ambient) air pressure and (2) to permit drainage of normal and diseased middle ear secretions from the middle ear cavity into the nasopharynx.

Almost all of us have experienced an uncomfortable, dull sensation in our ears just after a rapid descent in an elevator. This is due to a sudden increase in air pressure outside with respect to the pressure in the middle ear, and it may be accompanied by strange, low rumblings and clicking sounds. Such conditions, which may cause temporary hearing loss, can be alleviated simply by yawning, swallowing, or shouting loudly (depending upon your immediate circumstances, of course), all of which will open the normally closed pharyngeal orifice of the auditory tube, allowing air pressures to become

equalized. Swelling (edema) in the lining at the tympanic or at the pharyngeal orifice may also cause the tube to be closed. In chronic cases, air is absorbed by the highly vascular mucous membrane lining of the middle ear cavity, and a negative pressure results. As a consequence, the eardrum may be forced inward and fluid may exude from the mucous membrane. These conditions may increase both the *stiffness* and *damping* of the middle ear structures and result in temporary hearing impairment, with losses confined especially to the lower frequencies (Wever and Lawrence, 1954).

If the eardrum is to absorb the energy in sound waves, it must be equally responsive to inward and outward (positive and negative) pressures. A static pressure differential across the eardrum will bias it to move more easily in one direction than in the other, and the response characteristics become nonlinear. In addition, a constant positive or negative pressure in the middle ear (relative to ambient pressure) will also bias the pressures against the oval and round windows, to change the static inner ear fluid pressures and further complicate matters. *Slight differences in air pressure elevate the threshold for hearing at low frequencies more than at high frequencies.* These results seem to be due to an increase in stiffness of the membrane. Negative middle ear pressure (relative to ambient) produces more of an effect than does positive pressure. Negative pressure may also cause decoupling of the incudostapedial joint.

Fortunately, the auditory tube is frequently dilated temporarily to permit pressure equalization and middle ear drainage. Usually it is thought to be opened by contraction of a small slip of the tensor palatini, the **dilator tubae,** which pulls the membranous lateral wall away from the relatively stationary medial wall, uncurling the cartilage in the process. Evidence has suggested that the levator palatini has no substantial influence on the auditory tube (Sicher and Dubrul, 1975). Subsequently, however, Seif and Dellon (1978) suggest that the levator palatini elevates the cartilage of the auditory tube when it contracts and that action, combined with the contraction of the belly of the tensor tympani, results in a "milking action," as illustrated in Figure 6-49. These authors also suggest that no muscle actively opens the tube in the classical sense of pulling open a lumen. Rood and Doyle (1978), on the other hand, reported that the **dilator tubae** actively draws the membranous wall of the auditory tube laterally and inferiorly and that the muscle should be regarded as the active dilator. They also found muscle fibers of the **tensor palatini** to be continuous with the **tensor tympani** of the middle ear. The mechanism popularly thought to be responsible for dilating the auditory tube is shown schematically in Figure 6-50, but the exact mechanism is not known for certain. Wever and Lawrence (1954) point out that in instances where significant negative pressure has developed in the

FIGURE 6-49

The proposed mechanism of auditory-tube function of Seif and Dellon. The tube is closed at rest. During swallowing and phonation, a "milking" or pumping action is created by contraction of the LVP and TVP muscles. No muscle opens the tube in the classical sense of pulling open a lumen. (From Seif and Dellon, 1978.)

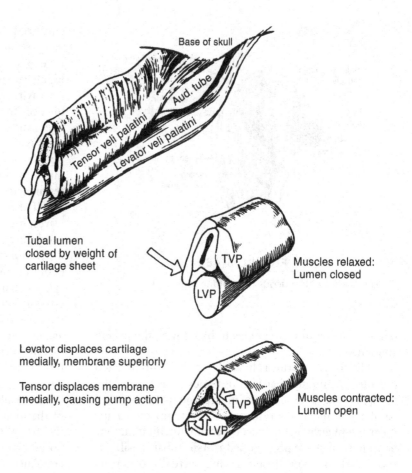

Base of skull

Aud. tube

Tensor veli palatini

Levator veli palatini

Tubal lumen closed by weight of cartilage sheet

TVP

LVP

Muscles relaxed: Lumen closed

Levator displaces cartilage medially, membrane superiorly

Tensor displaces membrane medially, causing pump action

TVP

LVP

Muscles contracted: Lumen open

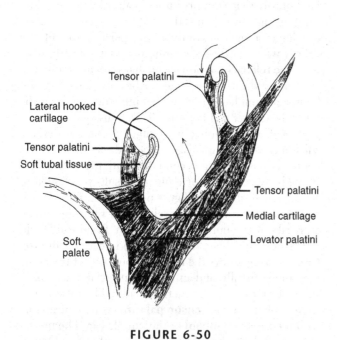

Tensor palatini

Lateral hooked cartilage

Tensor palatini

Soft tubal tissue

Tensor palatini

Medial cartilage

Levator palatini

Soft palate

FIGURE 6-50

The popular concept of the mechanism of dilation of the auditory tube, in which the *dilator tubae* (the tensor palatini) pulls the lateral hooked cartilage away from the membranous wall.

middle ear cavity, the auditory tube may collapse and resist dilation. In these cases prompt medical attention is strongly advised.

> **CLINICAL NOTE:** The auditory tube is about half as long in children as it is in adults, and no bony canal exists at birth. In children the tube lies in a plane almost parallel to the pharyngeal ostium. In addition, it is more horizontal and wider. Because of these structural differences, children are particularly susceptible to the spread of infection from the pharyngeal regions to the middle ear.

The Auditory Ossicles

Most of the space within the middle ear cavity is occupied by the ossicular chain, which consists of the **malleus, incus,** and **stapes.** These three bones, which except for some Wormian bones in the skull are the smallest in the human body, are shown greatly enlarged in Figures 6-51 and 6-52. The ossicles, like the eardrum, reach their adult dimensions late in fetal life, and their overall size and shape do not change substantially. Some idea of the size of the ossicles can be gained from Figure 6-53. The

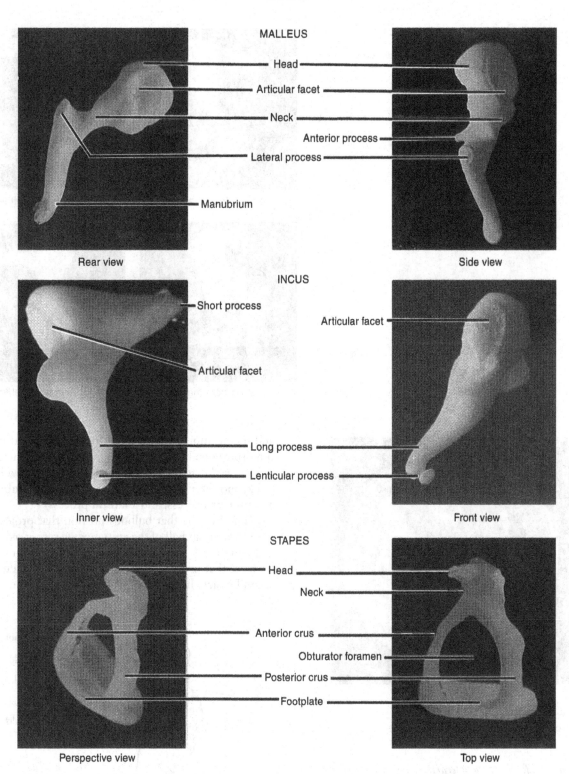

MALLEUS

Head
Articular facet
Neck
Anterior process
Lateral process
Manubrium

Rear view

Head
Articular facet
Neck
Anterior process

Side view

INCUS

Short process
Articular facet
Long process
Lenticular process

Inner view

Articular facet
Long process
Lenticular process

Front view

STAPES

Head
Neck
Anterior crus
Obturator foramen
Posterior crus
Footplate

Perspective view

Head
Neck

Top view

FIGURE 6-51

Various views of disarticulated human auditory ossicles.

malleus is about 9 mm in overall length, and its weight ranges from about 23 to 27 mg, while the weight of the incus ranges from 25 to 32 mg. The tiny stapes ranges in weight from 2.05 to 4.34 mg, with an overall height of about 3 mm. *The ossicles have two main purposes*: (1) *to deliver sound vibrations to the inner ear fluids* and (2) *to help*

Various views of an articulated ossicular chain.

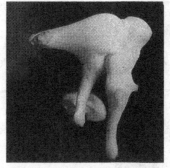

As seen from the side

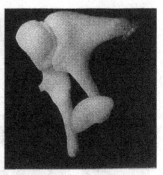

As seen from within

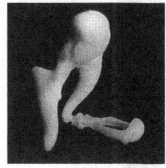

As seen from the front

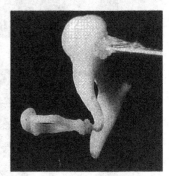

As seen from behind

and the position of the malleus in the middle ear cavity, the drum membrane is pulled inward to take the shape of a cone. Anatomically, the malleus consists of a **head, neck,** and three **processes** (the **handle** or **manubrium,** an **anterior** process, and a **lateral** process).

The **head** is that bulbous portion that projects up to occupy about half of the epitympanic recess, as shown in Figure 6-54. Its posterior surface contains an articular facet that provides an attachment for the **incus,** the second ossicle in the chain. A constriction in the center

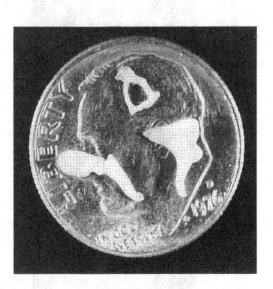

FIGURE 6-53

The size of the ossicles compared to a dime.

the inner ear from being overdriven by excessively strong vibrations.

The Malleus The most lateral of the auditory ossicles is the malleus, which gets its name from the sculptor's mallet it resembles. *The malleus is attached to the connective tissue fibers of the eardrum.* The attachment is most intimate at the middle of the membrane, becoming less so toward the superior border. Because of this attachment

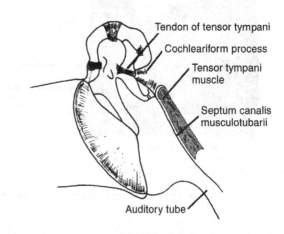

Tendon of tensor tympani

Cochleariform process

Tensor tympani muscle

Septum canalis musculotubarii

Auditory tube

FIGURE 6-54

Schematic of the tensor tympani muscle illustrating its bipennate architecture. The head of the malleus projects up into and occupies much of the epitympanic recess.

divides the articular facet into upper and lower portions, placed nearly at right angles to one another.

The **neck** of the malleus is a constriction between the manubrium and the head. In the earlier discussion of the eardrum, the shadow of the **manubrium** was seen as a long, narrow process directed downward, somewhat backward, and medially. At the point where the manubrium joins the neck, a small projection forms the point of attachment for the tensor tympani, one of the middle ear muscles.

The **anterior process** is a spinelike structure at the junction of the manubrium and the neck, while the **lateral process** is directed laterally from about the same level and is attached to the upper part of the eardrum. In otoscopic views of the tympanic membrane, the lateral process may be seen as a highlight near the pars flaccida.

The Incus The second of the ossicles, the incus, is so named because of its resemblance to an anvil. The incus doesn't resemble the blacksmith's anvil as we know it, but it does look something like a premolar tooth with two diverging roots. It consists of a **body** and two **arms** (crura) or **processes.** The anterior surface of the body presents an articular facet. It joins with the articular facet of the malleus.

The processes of the incus arise from the body at nearly right angles to each other. The **short process,** about 5 mm in length, is directed almost horizontally backward, as shown in Figure 6-54, and occupies the space of the fossa incudis in the epitympanic recess. The **long process,** which is about 7 mm in length, courses vertically, almost parallel to the manubrium of the malleus. Inferiorly, the end of the long process bends sharply medialward and terminates as a rounded projection called the **lenticular process,** which is tipped with cartilage and articulates with the head of the stapes. Occasionally the lenticular process appears almost like a minuscule sesamoid bone (Figure 6-51). The ossicles shown here are devoid of their mucous membrane and do not look the same as they do in the fresh state.

The Stapes So named because of its resemblance to a riding stirrup, the stapes consists of a **head, neck,** two **crura,** and a **footplate.** In life the **footplate,** which is partly osseous and partly cartilaginous, occupies the oval window (Figure 6-55). The footplate is connected to the neck by the **anterior** and **posterior crura,** two delicate but incredibly strong struts, which usually originate from points nearer the inferior than the superior margin of the footplate. The anterior crus is somewhat more slender, shorter, and less curved than is the posterior crus. Each is markedly channeled on its inner surface, which significantly reduces the mass of the stapes.

The crura and footplate enclose a triangular space named the **obturator foramen** (Figure 6-55). The **neck,** which is usually well defined, is simply a constriction between the junction of the crura and the expanded head of the stapes. The **head** presents a concave articular facet for reception of the lenticular process of the incus. The head or neck usually presents a small spine, indicating the attachment of the tendon of the stapedius muscle. A photograph of the eardrum and ossicular chain, as seen from within the tympanic cavity, is shown in Figure 6-56.

The Ligaments and Articulations of the Ossicles

The principal ligaments responsible for the suspension of the ossicular chain within the tympanic cavity are shown in Figure 6-57. There are eight in all, including the tendons of the two middle ear muscles, but these tendons are often referred to as ligaments.

A small **superior malleolar ligament** extends from the head of the malleus to the tegmen tympani. It is complemented by the **lateral malleolar ligament,** which extends from the neck of the malleus to the bony wall near the notch of Rivinus. Another ligament, the **anterior malleolar ligament,** extends from the anterior process of the malleus to the anterior or carotid wall of the middle ear cavity. A single ligament lends support to the incus. It courses from the tip of the short process to the fossa incudis in the tympanic recess. Sometimes a superior incudal ligament is identified, but it is no more than an inconsistent fold of mucous membrane.

Both the vestibular surface and periphery of the oval footplate of the stapes are covered by a thin layer of hyaline cartilage which is fastened to the bony walls of the oval window by means of an elastic **annular ligament.** It is more pronounced anteriorly than it is posteriorly, which means the footplate is more rigidly held in place behind. A section through the stapes showing the annular ligament may be seen in Figure 6-55. This section was made through the temporal bone of a young dog, but the structures closely resemble those of the human. When the stapes is acted upon by the lenticular process of the incus, it executes a motion largely dictated by the characteristics of the attachments of the footplate to the oval window.

The malleus and incus are articulated by a diarthrodial (double saddle) joint. The joint is effected by a typical articular capsule, and the joint cavity is partially divided in two by a wedge-shaped articular disc or meniscus.

While some anatomists consider the **incudostapedial joint** to be of the syndesmosis type (immovable or just slightly movable), it is usually regarded as a true enarthrodial (ball-and-socket) joint.

Because of the way the ossicular chain is suspended by the ligamentous system, its inertia is very small, and its rotational axis is very near the center of gravity (the ossicles are balanced). If this were not the case, the ossicular chain would tend to swing in the manner of a

FIGURE 6-55

FIGURE 6-55

Serial section through temporal bone of a dog, showing the cochlea, stapes, annular ligament, and some associated structures. The crura and footplate enclose a triangular space called the *obturator foramen* (**OF**).

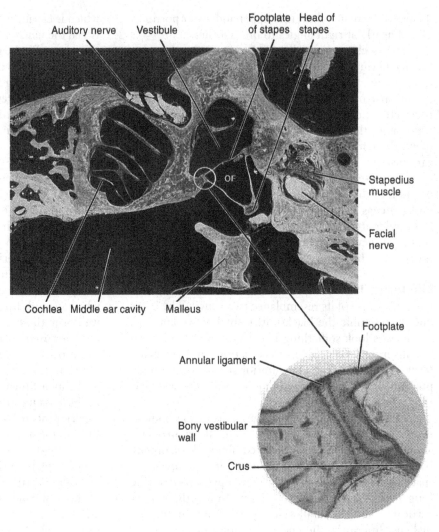

The Tympanic Muscles

As mentioned earlier, the middle ear structures include the **tensor tympani** and the **stapedius,** the smallest striated muscles in the body. They are *pennate muscles*, consisting of many short fibers directed obliquely to impinge on a tendon at the midline (Figure 6-54). The tension exerted by a pennate muscle is the sum of the combined forces from contraction of all the muscle fibers, taking into account the angle at which they exert their force, whereas the total displacement is just the amount per-

pendulum and would continue to vibrate after the vibratory energy had ceased. As it is, the ossicles are suspended so the mass above and below the axis of rotation is about equal (Kirikae, 1960). As a result, *once sound vibrations have ceased, the vibrations of the ossicles also terminate abruptly*, which minimizes a potential source of distortion in the middle ear.

mitted by contraction of the shortest fibers. Pennate muscles can exert a lot of force for small muscles.

The *tendons* of the tympanic muscles differ from usual tendons due to an abundant amount of elastic tissue. According to Jepsen (1963), the elastic properties of the tendons may serve a dual purpose: (1) to damp the vibrations of the ossicles and (2) to render muscular traction slower and less sudden in onset.

A second unique feature of the tympanic muscles is that they are *completely encased in bony canals* and only their tendons (in humans) enter the tympanic cavity. According to Békésy (1936), the arrangement *reduces muscular vibrations* that might interfere with sound transmission by generating subharmonics. The arrangement also *reduces the effective mass of the ossicular chain.*

The Tensor Tympani Muscle The tensor tympani, the larger of the tympanic muscles, is about 25 mm in length, has a cross-sectional area of about 5.85 mm^2,

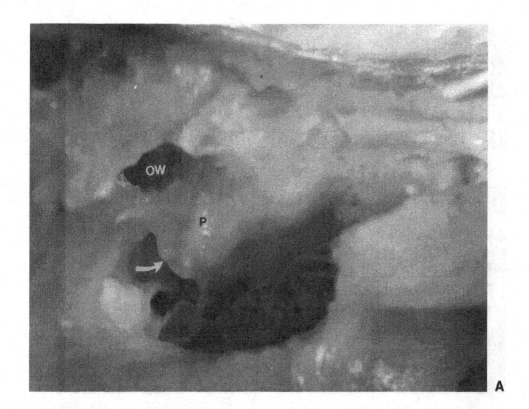

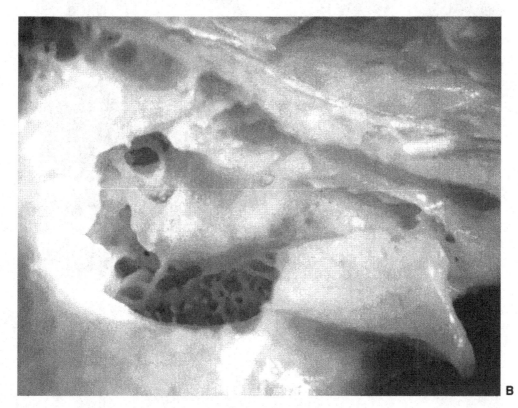

FIGURE 6-56

(A) The middle ear cavity devoid of the ossicles. The oval window (**OW**), and promontory (**P**). The niche of the round window is indicated by an arrow.

(B) Middle ear cavity with the stapes in the oval window.

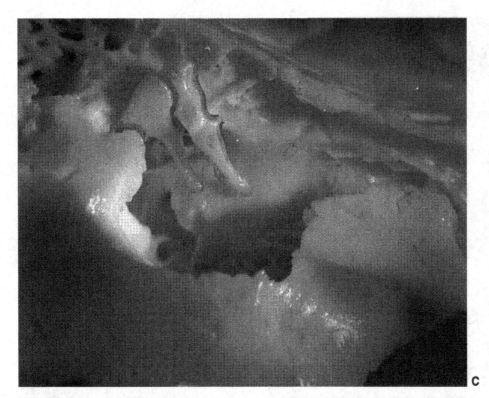

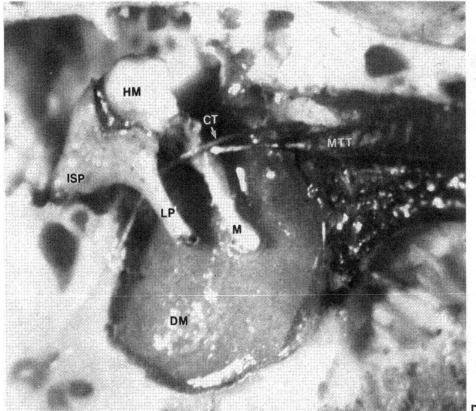

FIGURE 6-56 (continued)

(C) Middle ear cavity with stapes, incus, and malleus in place.

(D) Middle ear structures as seen from within a reconstruction of the tympanic cavity. They include the head of the malleus (**HM**), the chorda tympani (**CT**) (branch of the facial nerve), the tensor tympani muscle (**MTT**), the short process of the incus (**ISP**), the long arm or process of the incus (**LP**), and the drum membrane (**DM**).

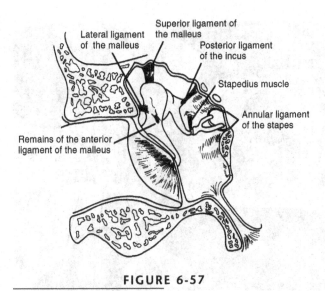

FIGURE 6-57

Schematic illustration of middle ear ligaments and the stapedius muscle.

and is contained within a *bony semicanal* that runs nearly parallel with and superior to the osseous framework of the auditory tube. The muscle fibers are liberally impregnated with fat, an indication that it is an active muscle. In addition, scattered smooth muscle fasciculi have been reported (Gerhardt, et al., 1966). This implies both autonomic (parasympathetic) and voluntary control (trigeminal and glossopharyngeus) over the muscle (Kobrak, 1959).

A thin partition of bone, the **septum canalis musculotubarii**, separates the canal of the tensor tympani from the canal of the auditory tube. The curved lateral terminal of the muscle is called the **cochleariform process** (Figure 6-54). As the tendon emerges from the orifice of the canal, it makes a rather sharp bend, conforming to the curvature of the cochleariform process, and is then directed to its insertion on the upper part of the manubrium of the malleus, as illustrated in Figure 6-54.

Contraction of the tensor tympani draws the malleus medially and anteriorly. The force is almost at right angles to the direction of rotation of the ossicular chain, and, when acting by itself, the muscle increases the tension of the tympanic membrane, as the name of the muscle suggests.

The Stapedius Muscle The stapedius, considerably smaller than the tensor tympani, is about 6 mm in length, with a cross-sectional area of about 5 mm². It originates within a *bony canal* running almost parallel to the facial nerve canal on the posterior wall of the tympanic cavity. Its direction is almost vertical, but the direction of its tendon is nearly horizontal. The muscle fibers originate from the walls of the canal and converge upon a tendon, which emerges through a tiny aperture at the apex of the

pyramidal eminence. The tendon and its attachment to the stapes are shown in Figure 6-58, and a microscopic view of a stapedius muscle and its attachment to the stapes is shown in Figure 6-59.

Contraction of the stapedius exerts a force on the head of the stapes, drawing it posteriorly, at right angles to the direction of the movement of the ossicular chain. Thus, the stapedius and tensor tympani exert force in directions opposite to each other and perpendicular to the primary rotational axis of the ossicular chain.

Action of the Tympanic Musculature Although a number of persons have some voluntary control of their tympanic musculature, its contraction is usually reflexively[7] mediated by sound energy. Most information regarding the behavior of the tympanic musculature has come from animal experiments. In 1878, for example, Hensen inserted a thin metal sliver into the tensor tympani of dogs and observed the movement of the sliver when the ear was stimulated with sound. Pollak, in 1886, conducted similar experiments in which he demonstrated that the **acoustic reflex** of the tensor tympani is dependent upon the adequacy of the stimulus. He further demonstrated that unilateral stimulation resulted in bilateral contraction of the tensor tympani, a finding subsequently used in clinical applications of the acoustic reflex (Jepsen, 1963). Kato, in 1913, was able to elicit acoustic reflexes of the tensor tympani and the stapedius. He noted a direct relationship between the duration of the stimulus and the duration of muscle contraction.

---

[7]A **reflex** is an involuntary, relatively invariable adaptive response to a stimulus.

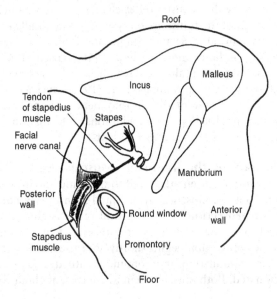

FIGURE 6-58

Schematic of the stapedius muscle and the attachment of its tendon to the neck of the stapes.

FIGURE 6-59

The stapedius muscle and its attachment to the head of the stapes.

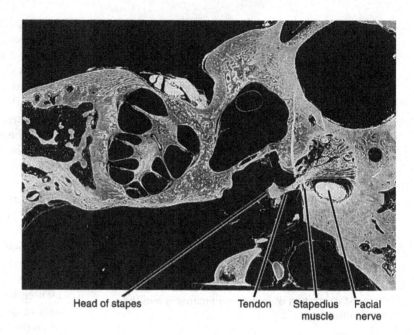

Head of stapes   Tendon   Stapedius   Facial
                                   muscle   nerve

Although the acoustic reflex has been studied less extensively in humans, Lüscher in 1929 was able to observe stapedial reflex movements in a person with a perforated eardrum. He found that a response could be elicited by either ipsilateral or contralateral stimulation and also that contraction could be elicited simply by expectation of a loud sound.

Electromyography has become a useful laboratory technique for investigation of the acoustic reflex. Perlman and Case, in 1939, recorded muscle action potentials from the stapedius muscle in humans. The technique is especially valuable for studying the *latency*[8] of the acoustic reflex.

Because the acoustic reflex changes the mechanical properties of the transmission system of the middle ear, the mechanical resistance (impedance) may be measured by indirect means (Metz, 1946; Jepsen, 1963). This has become a valuable research and clinical tool for studying hearing in humans. Lilly (1973) gives a comprehensive review of the measurement of impedance. Rabinowitz (1981) provides additional information on middle ear impedance measurements.

Functions of the Tympanic Musculature Several functions have been attributed to the tympanic musculature, but the most widely accepted is **intensity control** or **protection.** The acoustical reflex is elicited at sound intensities well above the threshold of hearing. Muscle contraction begins shortly after the onset of the acoustic stimulation and continues until the sound is terminated. Both muscles seem to contract at about the

same time, and although the tensor tympani seems to exert more force, the stapedius seems to be the more effective muscle. In humans the acoustic reflex is elicited at intensities in the vicinity of 80 to 90 dB above the threshold for hearing, with the lowest threshold for the reflex in the frequency range for which the threshold for hearing is lowest (Jepsen, 1963).

The tympanic muscles have been shown to *contribute to the strength of the ossicular chain*. This can be demonstrated by severing the tendons of the muscles. Whereas the ossicular chain is normally quite resistant to mechanical manipulation, it is now loose and flaccid, and inner ear damage can easily result.

> **CLINICAL NOTE:** A similar condition of ossicular chain weakness may be seen in Bell's palsy, where there is temporary paralysis of the stapedius muscle. Low-frequency sounds (even the person's own voice) may seem abnormally loud.

An important limitation to the protection that the tympanic muscles can supply is due to the **latency of the muscle contraction.** There is a certain interval between the time the sound impinges on the eardrum and the onset of contraction of the muscles. Some early experiments by Hensen in 1863, Kato in 1913, and Kobrak in 1932 produced latencies ranging from 0.1 to 0.13 seconds for the stapedius and from 0.01 to 0.29 seconds for the tensor tympani. In summarizing the results of both early and later experimentation, Wever and Lawrence (1954) cite mean values of 0.06 seconds for the stapedius and 0.15 seconds for the tensor tympani.

---

[8]**Latency** is the lag between the stimulus and the response.

Intense sounds, carrying steep wave fronts (transients), such as those resulting from explosions and industrial noise, may impinge upon the ear mechanism and cause damage before the musculature can contract. Too, prolonged exposure to unduly intense sounds (usually man-made), may result in a decrease in protection due to fatigue. Lüscher (1929), Kobrak (1932), and others have noted that upon sustained sound stimulation, a continued contraction was first observed, followed by a gradual decrease until the resting state was reached. A new contraction could only be elicited by changing substantially the frequency of the stimulus. In similar experiments, Kato (1913) and Wërsall (1958) found the tensor tympani to be the more easily fatigable of the tympanic muscles.

Because the ossicles have been constructed in part for the protection of the inner ear, a difficulty arises in the transmission of vibratory energy across the joints, from one ossicle to the other, without having them separate and generate distortion. As Békésy (1960) states,

> If the contact pressure between two vibrating bodies is smaller than the accelerating force acting during the vibration, the two bodies will separate, and the result is like the well-known phenomenon of the bouncing sand grains on a vibrating plate. If the vibrations are small, the elastic ligaments are able to exert a pressure that is sufficiently great that no special measures are necessary. For larger vibrations, however, this is no longer true, and it becomes clear why muscles are present in the middle ear that work opposite to one another and press the stapes against the incus, while at the same time the other ligaments are stretched.

In 1976, Gundersen and Høgmoen used **time average holography**, a special photographic technique that uses a laser beam for a light source to study vibrations of human ossicles. Their observations differ from those of Békésy. *Traction in the tympanic muscles attenuates the vibration amplitudes and reduces the transmission of vibrations from the malleus to the incus.* They attribute the reduction to the movement in the malleoincudal joint and consider the mechanism to be a protective one. The sound pressure levels used to drive the middle ear were on the order of 124 dB. The authors further noted that *contraction of middle ear muscles alters the pattern of movement of the ossicular chain.*

To summarize the functions of the middle ear muscles, normally in a state of minimal tension, they can be reflexively excited by sounds about 80 dB above the threshold for hearing (80 dB sensation level or 80 dB SL). Contraction is not immediate, however, and the latency of the reflex response is at least 10 msec for intense sounds. The forces exerted by the two muscles are almost at right angles to the axes of rotation of the ossicles, and as a result, the efficiency of vibratory energy transmission is reduced on the order of 10 to 30 dB, with the greater effect on low frequencies. The impedance changes due to middle ear muscle contraction have little or no effect on frequencies above 2000 Hz. Because of the latency of reflexive contraction, the middle ear cannot help protect us against transient bursts of high-intensity noise, such as explosions and many types of industrial noises. They do offer a certain protection against stress, fatigue, and inner ear damage due to prolonged exposure to high levels of low-frequency sounds.

Reflexive contraction of the middle ear muscles may also minimize middle ear distortion by facilitating the linkage between the ossicles, particularly at the incudostapedial joint. Holographic photography reveals that the malleoincudal joint breaks up at high-intensity sound levels, action that may well be protective.

Stapes Movement as a Protective Mechanism

In 1936 Békésy noted that at very low frequencies, an increase in sound pressure produces an increase in loudness, up to a certain point, beyond which further increases in sound pressure seem to produce a sudden decrease in loudness. He found, as in Figure 6-60A, that when the ossicles are driven by a moderate sound pressure, the rotation of the stapes is about an axis indicated by the dashed line. Because the footplate is more rigidly fixed posteriorly than it is anteriorly, the stapes rocks about an axis near its posterior edge, much the way a door swings on its hinges.

As sound pressure is increased beyond a certain critical limit, however, the stapes begins to turn about an axis that runs horizontally through the footplate, as in Figure 6-60B. As a result, the cochlear fluids flow only from one edge of the footplate to the other, with much less fluid displacement than when the mode of vibration is through a vertical axis and the footplate is acting like a swinging door. Békésy felt that this *shift of rotational axes*, which seemed to be due to a certain amount of freedom in the suspension of the ossicular chain, was an effective protective mechanism occurring primarily with high-intensity sounds at low frequencies. Békésy's observations were supported by subsequent experiments by Kobrak (1959), Fumagalli (1949), and Kirikae (1960).

Guinan and Peake (1967) also measured ossicular movements, using a microscope and stroboscopic illumination. Their measurements of stapes displacements showed movements that were predominantly *pistonlike*, at sound intensities of 130 and even 140 dB re .0002 dynes/cm^2. In 1970 Dankbaar measured stapes movements in fresh human temporal bones using a device called a *capacitive probe*. He also failed to find Békésy's

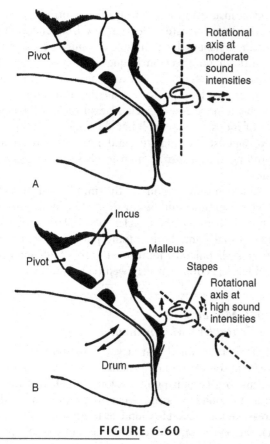

A

B

Pivot

Rotational axis at moderate sound intensities

Incus

Malleus

Pivot

Stapes

Rotational axis at high sound intensities

Drum

FIGURE 6-60

Changes in mode of vibration of stapes due to an increase in sound intensity, according to Békésy. (Courtesy Békésy.)

trapdoor movement, even with sound intensities of 130 dB sound pressure level, but he did find fairly simple pistonlike movements of the stapedial footplate. *The vibration pattern was independent of frequency and intensity.* An additional observation by Dankbaar is that the middle ear works as a *linear vibration transmitter* for sound pressures up to about 100 dB sound pressure level. For higher intensities, the input-output relation tends to become nonlinear.

And finally, in 1977, Høgmoen and Gundersen applied time average holography to measure movements of the human stapes footplate. They confined their investigations to a single frequency (600 Hz) and at high intensity levels detected a departure from the simple pistonlike movement. That is, they found a *tilting action* that amounted to about one-third of the pistonlike movement, a change that would somewhat reduce the efficiency of footplate vibration.

It seems reasonable to conclude that if a change in the mode of stapedial vibration is to offer us protection against high levels of sound, it apparently does so only in a limited manner, and at intensity levels that would already become damaging or painful to our ears.

CLINICAL NOTE: Despite frequent claims that the middle ear reflexes and stapes footplate vibrations may offer us protection from transient noises and high-level industrial noise, the incidence of noise-induced deafness and hearing loss should be ample evidence that our built-in protection is incapable of coping with human ingenuity.

The Transformer Action of the Middle Ear

A well-known principle in acoustics states that *sound waves traveling in a medium of some given elasticity and density will not pass readily into a medium with different elasticity and density but, rather, that most of the sound will be reflected away.* The amount of sound reflected is directly related to the differences in the physical properties between the two media. **Acoustic resistances,** which can be used to calculate sound transmission from one medium to another, can be determined if the **density** and the **bulk modulus of elasticity** of each medium are known. Acoustic resistance, R, is the square root of the product of density, p, and the bulk modulus of elasticity, S, or $R = \sqrt{pS}$. It is expressed in mechanical ohms per cm^2.

Wever and Lawrence (1954) assumed the acoustic resistance of the human ear to be about equivalent to that of sea water. For air, the acoustic resistance is 41.5 ohms, for sea water, 161,000 ohms. The ratio (r) of these resistances is 3880. This means that when a sound wave strikes water at a normal angle, the pressure variation in the wave is large enough to displace the water at the interface by 1/3880 of the displacement of the air. **Energy transmission** can be computed by the formula

$$T = \frac{4r}{(r+1)^2} = 0.001$$

This means that one-tenth of 1 percent of the sound in air will pass into the water, while the remaining 99.9 percent is reflected back. Expressed in decibels, the transmission loss is 30 dB. Wever and Lawrence also point out that if sound waves acted directly on the cochlear fluids, a transmission loss of about 30 dB should occur. This is assuming the fluid columns in the cochlea have the same acoustic resistance as a body of sea water. Actually the fluid columns in the cochlea have acoustic properties that are different from that of sea water. The acoustic resistance (impedance) of sea water assumes an effectively infinite medium, which is far removed from the actual fluid column of the cochlea. Cochlear impedance is determined by the fact that cochlear fluid flows from the oval window to the round window and the impedance depends on the manner of fluid flow and its interaction with the oval and round windows. Direct measurements by Lynch, et al. in the cat suggest a cochlear impedance of about 1.5×10^5 Nsec/M^3 at 1 KHz, a value much lower than Wever and Lawrence's. The interested reader is referred to Pickles (1988), pp. 5 and 17.

Impedance Matching In any system where there is to be efficient or maximum transmission of energy, the resistance (or impedance) of the source ought to match that of the load. In mechanics, **impedance** can be defined in relation to velocity of motion to the force required to produce a certain velocity of motion, or

$$Z = \frac{F}{U}$$

where

   Z = impedance in mechanical ohms (Ω)

   F = force in dynes

   U = velocity in centimeters per second

Frequently encountered impedance-matching devices include the gear train of a bicycle, levers of various types, and the transmission of an automobile. In each of these, high-impedance energy sources—arms, legs, and high-speed engines—are matched to low-impedance loads. Or, to put it another way, the source of energy moves through a great distance with comparatively little force, while the load moves through correspondingly little distance with a great deal of force.

Work, which is *force times displacement*, is the same at the source and at the load, neglecting friction (dissipation), but the force required is much greater at the load than at the source, where displacement is more. In a nutshell, *work at the source is equal to work at the load.*

The middle ear, which is transmitting vibratory energy, functions as an imperfect impedance matching device. In general there are two forms of impedance, **resistance** and **reactance.** One type of resistance is friction.

Reactance can be due to the inertial properties of the middle ear. The mass of the ossicles resists motion in what is known as **mass reactance** (Xm). Stiffness also contributes to the impedance of the middle ear, and it is known as **stiffness reactance** (Xs). Both mass and stiffness reactance are frequency dependent, resistance is not. Reactance and resistance are related to total impedance by the following expression:

$$Z = R^2 + (Xm - Xs)^2$$

For frequencies below 1000 Hz, the stiffness reactance dominates to attenuate transmission, while the mass reactance dominates at frequencies above 2000 Hz to attenuate transmission. At frequencies between 1000 and 2000 Hz, the mass reactance and stiffness reactance cancel, leaving only the resistive component to attenuate transmission.

Another type of impedance, the **characteristic impedance,** is given by the expression $Zc = poc$, where po is the density of the medium and c is the velocity of sound in the medium.

Transmission of Sound to the Inner Ear There are three possible avenues by which airborne sounds can be transmitted to the inner ear. One fairly direct route is by *airborne conduction across the middle ear space.* The sound energy that impinges on the eardrum excites the air contained in the middle ear cavity, an excitation that is transmitted directly to the inner ear. This route is extremely inefficient, simply because the inner ear is fluid filled and the fluid must be driven by vibrating air. As we have seen, a large mismatch exists between the impedance of air and that of the inner ear fluids. At least a 30 dB hearing loss could be expected if this were in fact the transmission route. A second route is *directly through the bones of the skull* to the cochlea and inner ear fluids. We will learn later in the chapter that the skull is constructed so as to minimize bone and tissue conduction of sound energy. The third route requires the *transmission of mechanical vibration through the ossicular chain to the stapes footplate,* and this brings us to the problem the middle ear must encounter. If somehow the impedance of the ear could be made to approach that of air, efficient transmission would result. In order to match the acoustic impedance of air to that of the inner ear fluids (which for the moment we will assume are the same as sea water), we need to find the required **transformation ratio.** It is the square root of the ratio of the two acoustic resistances. Earlier we found the ratio to be 3880:1. Thus, in order to have maximum transmission of sound energy, we must have a mechanism that increases the pressure at the oval window, over what it is at the drum membrane, by a factor of about 63.

Evidence that the middle ear facilitates hearing can be seen from clinical cases where a *disruption of the ossicular chain* results in a hearing loss of 30 dB or greater. Figure 6-61 shows an audiogram of a person with disruption of the ossicular chain and presumably no other ear pathology (bone conduction is essentially normal). In a series of experiments, Wever, Lawrence, and Smith (1948) removed the drum membrane, malleus, and incus from animals, after determining their hearing sensitivity with the structures intact. The hearing loss was greatest for tones in the 500 to 2000 Hz range and in the 5000 to 7000 Hz range. As shown in Figure 6-62, the *average loss was about 28 dB*, which probably represents the **transformer action of the middle ear.**

Audiogram of a person with a disruption of the ossicular chain. The solid lines represent hearing by air conduction for the left and right ears, while the dashed lines represent hearing by bone conduction.

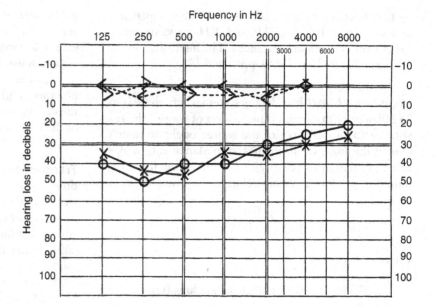

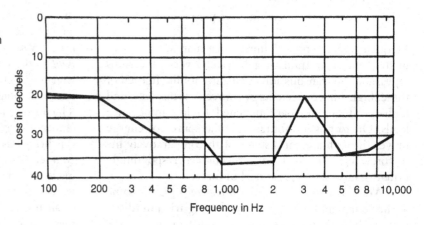

FIGURE 6-62

Loss of hearing sensitivity resulting from removal of the middle ear mechanism in the cat. (After Wever, Lawrence, and Smith, 1948.)

In experiments of this nature, it is important that the stimuli be delivered to the oval window and not to the middle ear in general. Both the oval and round windows open into the inner ear, but on opposite sides of the **basilar membrane** (upon which are located the essential end organs for hearing). Positive pressure on the stapes footplate causes the basilar membrane to move downward, while pressure on the round window will cause the membrane to move in the opposite direction. Sound energy delivered to the middle ear cavity results in the same pressure (except for a slight phase difference) applied to both the round and oval windows, and as a result the basilar membrane is not disturbed.

CLINICAL NOTE: This lack of disturbance of the basilar membrane explains why persons who have no middle ear mechanism may suffer hearing losses (airborne) of 60 dB, rather than the theoretical 28 to 30 dB, unless the round window is occluded or shielded from the middle ear sound vibrations.

We should bear in mind that the normally vibrating drum membrane does indeed set the air in the middle ear cavity into vibration, and even though this vibration is not well absorbed by the inner ear fluids, positive and negative air pressures are exerted against the round window at almost the same instant these pressures are exerted against the oval window. The results are a slight increase in the impedance of the inner ear and a slight reduction in the middle ear transformation function.

In 1863 Helmholtz formulated the transformer action of the middle ear, and his account of it may be found in the fourth edition of his classic *On The Sensations of Tone*, published in 1877. Helmholtz proposed that the transformer action of the middle ear was due to the combined effects of (1) the lever action of the eardrum (which was assigned a dominant role), (2) the lever action of the ossicular chain, and (3) the mechanical advantage due to the ratio of the effective eardrum area to stapedial footplate area. Helmholtz suggested that pressures exerted on the cone-shaped eardrum are transformed into much greater pressures at the apex of the cone by virtue of the **catenary principle,** which is illustrated in Figure 6-63B. As force F impinges on the curved portion of the membrane, it is transformed into a greater force at points V, which, however, are fixed in position. As a result, the point at V_1 moves in the direction of the arrow at H with a force much greater than that impinging on the drum membrane.

Drum Membrane Movement Quantitative descriptions of drum membrane movement are difficult to obtain simply because of the minute displacements that occur in response to sound. At sound intensity levels that are nearly painful, the displacement at low frequencies may amount to about one-tenth of a millimeter, but at comfortable sound intensities (56 dB SPL), displacement is on the order of 5 Å (1 Ångstrom is equal to 10^{-8} cm).

In 1941 Békésy plotted the mode of eardrum vibration; it is shown in Figure 6-64. The closed curves represent equal amplitude (isoamplitude) contours, while the numbers represent the relative magnitude of drum membrane excursion. These results show that *for a frequency of 2000 Hz, the membrane vibrates like a solid disc pivoted on an axis* (shown as a dashed line in Figure 6-64). Békésy found that the greatest amplitude of vibration occurs near the lower edge of the membrane for fre-

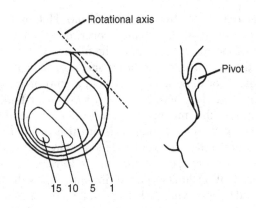

FIGURE 6-64

Mode of vibration of the drum membrane for a 2000-Hz tone. Lines delineate isoamplitude regions while the numbers represent relative amplitude. (Courtesy Békésy.)

quencies up to about 2500 Hz. *At higher frequencies the pattern broke up and the membrane vibrated segmentally.*

In 1968 Tonndorf and Khanna studied the pattern of membrane vibration using time average holography. The pattern shown in Figure 6-65 represents drum membrane vibration for a frequency of 525 Hz, at 120 dB SPL. The isoamplitude contours show that maximum vibration occurs in the upper rear quadrant. If the numbers assigned to each contour are multiplied by a factor of 10^{-5}, the actual displacement (in centimeters) can be determined. Maximum displacement in this illustration amounts to about 1 micron. The segmental type of vibration seen in holographic photography is only somewhat compatible with the vibratory pattern suggested by Helmholtz. Khanna and Tonndorf (1972) found the "buckling" to be a comparatively small factor in the total transformer action of the middle ear.

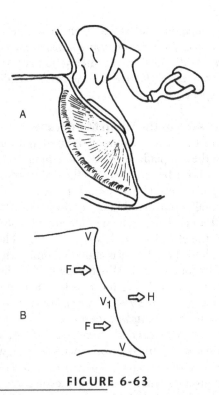

FIGURE 6-63

(A) Illustration of curved drum membrane as required for the catenary principle of Helmholtz. (B) Schematic of catenary principle. Helmholtz supposed this principle was responsible for an increase in force F at point H. This buckling of the membrane is not a significant contributor to the transformer action of the middle ear.

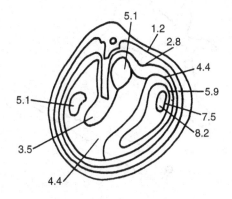

FIGURE 6-65

Holographic representation of drum membrane vibration for a frequency of 525 Hz at 120 dB sound pressure level. Maximum vibration occurs in the upper-rear quadrant. If the numbers assigned to each isoamplitude region are multiplied by 10^{-5} the actual displacement can be determined. (After Tonndorf and Khanna, 1968.)

Lever Action of the Ossicular Chain Helmholtz envisioned the ossicular chain as constituting a lever system. As shown in Figure 6-66, the fulcrum is at point *C*, with the lever arms being the distances *CA* and *CB*. Measurements of these lever arms yield a ratio of 1.5 to 1, which is in close agreement with subsequent findings. This means the amplitude of movement by the lenticular process of the incus, compared with that of the manubrium of the malleus, would be reduced by a ratio of 1.5 to 1, with a corresponding increase in force.

In 1930 Dahmann placed tiny mirrors on the ossicles and by observing deflections of light was able to describe the movements of the ossicular chain. In Figure 6-67A, the rotational axis of Dahmann runs from the anterior process of the malleus through the point of attachment of the short process of the incus to its ligament, while the lever arms run perpendicular to this axis. In B, the line, *AB*, is the malleolar lever arm and *CD* is the incudal arm. Measurements of these lever arms yield a ratio of 1.31 to 1, which means the force at the lenticular process would exceed the force applied to the manubrium by a comparable ratio.

Wever and Lawrence (1954) also investigated the action of the ossicular chain, by measuring the electrical output of the inner ear when the ossicular chain was stimulated at audio frequencies by a mechanical vibrator. Vibrations had maximum effects when they were applied to the manubrium of the malleus and to the long process of the incus, and they had minimal effects when applied to points that agree very closely with the rotational axis described by Dahmann. Wever and Lawrence obtained a lever ratio on the order of 2.5 to 1. If any of these values is representative of the mechanical advan-

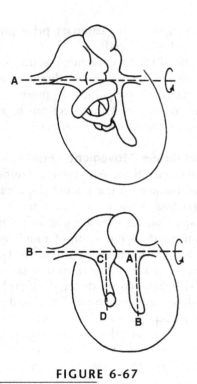

FIGURE 6-67

The ossicular chain lever system as described by Dahmann (1930). The axis of rotation is shown in A. In B, the lever arms are *CD* and *AB*.

tage provided by the ossicular chain, *they do not adequately account for the transformer action of the middle ear structures.* Additional transformer action is provided by the differences in *effective areas of drum membrane and stapes footplate.*

Effective Area of the Drum Membrane Since the periphery of the drum membrane is fixed and rigidly fastened to the tympanic annulus, something less than the total area must be regarded as effective in transmitting vibrations. Békésy (1941) found that about two-thirds of the total drum membrane area was effective. Since the total area of the human drum membrane is about 90 mm^2, the effective area is about 55 mm^2. The area of the footplate of the stapes is about 3.2 mm^2, which gives a ratio of about 17 to 1. When expressed in decibels, it amounts to 24.6 dB. We must realize that *although the force exerted on the drum membrane is the same as the force exerted on the stapes footplate, the pressure at the stapes is increased by a factor equal to the ratio of the effective areas.*

Pressure is defined as force per unit area, when the force acts at right angles (normal) to a surface, while **force** is given by the product of pressure and area, or $F = PA$. In Figure 6-68A, the weight (force of gravity) is distributed over the entire base, and the pressure is not very great. In Figure 6-68B, however, the pressure is much greater, simply because the area of contact is much

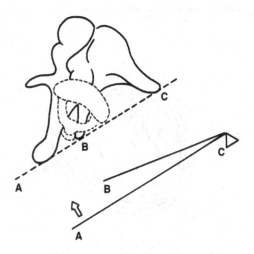

FIGURE 6-66

Schematic of ossicular chain lever system as described by Helmholtz. The fulcrum is at point *C*, with the lever arms being the distances *CA* and *CB*.

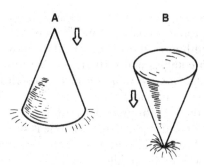

FIGURE 6-68

Illustration of force and pressure. In A, the weight (force of gravity) is distributed over the entire base, and the pressures (force per unit area) is not very great. In B, the pressure is much greater because area is so much less. The downward force is the same in each instance.

less. The *downward force*, however, is the same in each instance. As shown in Figure 6-69, the total force acting on the drum membrane is equal to the pressure multiplied by the area, or $F = PA$. The force is conducted by the ossicular chain to the stapes footplate, where the pressure is given by the force divided by the area, A_2, or

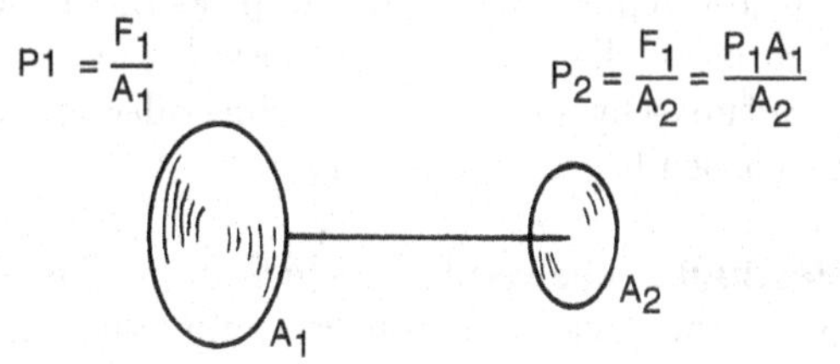

$P1 = \dfrac{F_1}{A_1}$ $P_2 = \dfrac{F_1}{A_2} = \dfrac{P_1 A_1}{A_2}$

FIGURE 6-69

Pressure increase due to differences in area. The total force acting on the drum membrane is equal to the pressure multiplied by the area or $F = FA$. The force conducted to the stapes footplate is the force divided by the area A_2.

$$P_2 = \frac{F}{A_2} = \frac{P_1 A_1}{A_2}$$

Thus, pressure is the product of the ratio of the two areas. Using an ossicular chain lever ratio of 1.31 to 1, as obtained by Dahmann, the *combined ratio provided by the transformer action of the middle ear is the product of the ossicular lever ratio and the effective areal ratio*, or

$$14.0 \times 1.31 = 18.3 \text{ to } 1$$

The total mechanical advantage afforded by the middle ear amounts to 25.25 dB. If we include the *buckling effect* of the drum membrane, which increases pressure by about two times, the overall increase amounts to about 31 dB.

Frequency Dependency of Pressure Transformation
The pressure transformation is frequency dependent, however. Békésy found that the *natural frequency of the middle ear* was between 800 and 1500 Hz. This was determined by the period of the transient response at the manubrium, when the ear is stimulated by a compressional wave from a spark. The overall pressure transformation of the middle ear is shown in Figure 6-70. It indicates that the increase in pressure at the stapes, as compared to the drum membrane, is 20 dB or more, up to about 2500 Hz.

The pressure transformation decreases above this frequency, but we must not overlook the contributions of the resonance of the auricle and external auditory meatus, in the range of from 2000 Hz to about 5000 Hz, a frequency range important for the reception of speech.

Pressure Differences Across the Cochlear Partition
It is generally assumed that vibrations of the ossicles produce pressure in the cochlear fluids, but we must ask the obvious question: Is this vibratory energy in fact

FIGURE 6-70

Average pressure transformation of the middle ear. (Courtesy Békésy.)

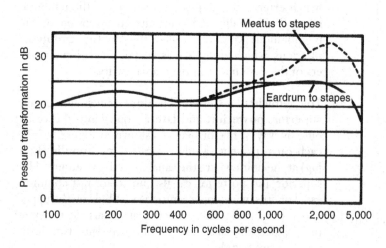

transmitted to the cochlear fluids? In 1974 Nedzelnitsky reported an experiment in which sound pressure measurements were made in the cochlear fluids of anaesthetized cats. Stimulus levels ranging from 40 to 105 dB were delivered to the tympanic membrane and a very small-probe microphone was inserted into either the scala vestibuli or scala tympani (to be described later). Pressure differences across the cochlear partition were also measured, as shown in Figure 6-71. Note that the *pressure across the cochlear partition exceeds pressure at the tympanic membrane in the frequency range of from about 100 to 10,000 Hz.* In addition, when the lower graph in Figure 6-71 is plotted as sound pressure level (SPL) as a function of frequency, the *shape* of the curve closely approximates the *minimum audibility curve* (MAC).

Having got sound vibrations safely delivered to the cochlear fluids, our next task will be to examine the structure of the inner ear. Then we will be faced with two remaining problems: one deals with the manner in which sound vibrations are transmitted within the inner ear and converted to neural impulses, and the other has to do with the manner in which these neural impulses are conducted to the auditory area of the brain.

The Inner Ear

The inner ear may be divided into two cavity systems, one of which houses the organs of equilibrium and the other the essential organ of hearing. Although this division is based on function, the two systems enjoy an intrinsic anatomical relationship. The inner ear contains two labyrinthine systems. One, called the **osseous labyrinth,** is a complex and tortuous series of excavations; the second, *contained within the first,* is a series of communicating membranous sacs and ducts collectively known as the **membranous labyrinth.** The location of the inner ear within the temporal bone is shown in Figure 6-72. We should note that these structures attain their full size by the middle of fetal life.

The Bony Labyrinth

The bony labyrinth consists of a system of canals and cavities within the dense *petrous* (L. hard, stony) *portion* of the temporal bone. At one stage in fetal life, a bony capsule immediately surrounding the membranous labyrinth is distinguishable from the adjacent cartilage (which later becomes ossified). Removal of the cartilage reveals the **otic** (or **periotic**) **capsule** (Figure 6-73A). The capsule consists of three parts: the **vestibule, semicircular canals,** and the **cochlea** (L. snail shell). With further ossification of the fetal cartilage, the otic capsule becomes assimilated into the homogeneous petrous bone and no longer exists except in textbooks. In some rodents such as the guinea pig, the cochlea projects into the middle ear cavity, as shown in Figure 6-74. This provides easy access to the turns of the cochlea for research purposes and partly explains why guinea pigs and chinchillas are so frequently chosen for research animals.

The Vestibule   The vestibule, which forms the central portion of the bony labyrinth, is continuous with the semicircular canals and with the cochlea. Ovoid in shape, it measures about 5 mm in its anteroposterior and vertical dimensions and about 3 mm across. Its lateral or tympanic wall (which forms part of the vestibular wall of the middle ear cavity) is perforated by the **oval window.** Its medial wall presents a number of small perforations, in addition to the orifice of the **vestibular aqueduct,** which extends to the posterior surface of the temporal bone. This small canal transmits an extension of the membranous labyrinth called the **ductus endolymphaticus,** which terminates as a cul de sac within the layers of the dura mater in the cranial cavity.

The Semicircular Canals   The three semicircular canals, **superior, posterior,** and **lateral,** open into the vestibule by way of five orifices. As shown in Figure 6-73B, each canal presents a dilation called an **ampulla** (L. a jug) at the point where the canal joins the vestibule. The superior and posterior canals join to form a common canal or crus, which opens into the vestibule on the upper and medial wall. The semicircular canals lie in three planes, perpendicular to one another—any two form nearly a right angle.

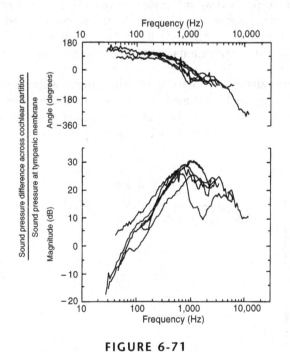

FIGURE 6-71

Magnitude and phase angle of the transfer function: sound pressure across the cochlear partition/sound pressure at the tympanic membrane. Measurements from six cats are shown. (From Nedzelnitsky, 1974.)

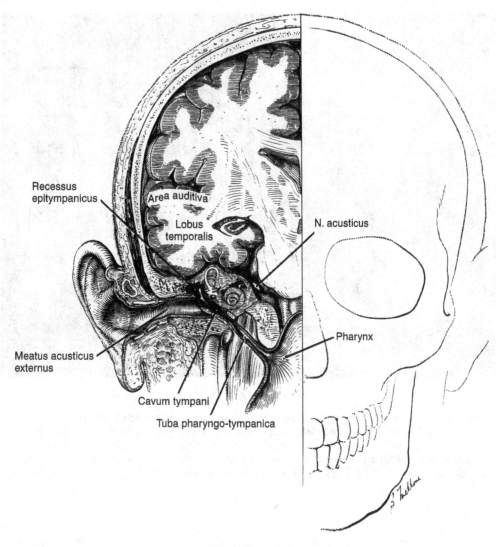

Recessus epitympanicus

Area auditiva

Lobus temporalis

N. acusticus

Meatus acusticus externus

Pharynx

Cavum tympani

Tuba pharyngo-tympanica

FIGURE 6-72

Schematic of the location of the inner ear within the temporal bone. (From *An Atlas of Some Pathological Conditions of the Eye, Ear, and Throat.* Courtesy of Abbott Laboratories, Chicago.)

The Cochlea The medialmost portion of the osseous labyrinth is called the cochlea. It is a bony canal, about 35 mm in length, which is coiled in upon itself around a central core or pillar of bone called the **modiolus** (L. hub). The base of the modiolus is broad, and is located at the bottom of the **internal auditory meatus,** which in life carries the auditory nerve, the facial nerve, nervus intermedius, and the internal branch of the basilar artery. The internal auditory meatus is shown in Figure 6-75, and a section through a cochlea showing the form of the modiolus is seen in Figure 6-76.

The cochlea, which is a continuation of the vestibule consists of a **base** followed by two and five-eighths turns, which terminate at the **apex** or **cupola** (L. little tub). The spiral-shaped canal is partially divided into an *upper duct,* the **scala**[9] **vestibuli,** and a *lower duct,* the **scala tympani,** by a thin bony shelf called the **osseous spiral lamina.** The spiral lamina projects from the modiolar wall (outward with the cochlea as the reference) as shown in Figure 6-76. This division is further completed by the interposition of the *membranous cochlear duct* or **scala media,** which will be discussed in some detail later. Near the apex of the cochlea, the spiral lamina terminates as a hooklike process called the **hamulus,** which assists in forming the boundary of a small opening, the **helicotrema** (Gk. *helix,* coil + *trema,* hole). It establishes communication between the scala vestibuli and scala tympani as shown in Figure 6-76.

[9]**Scala** is a Latin word for staircase.

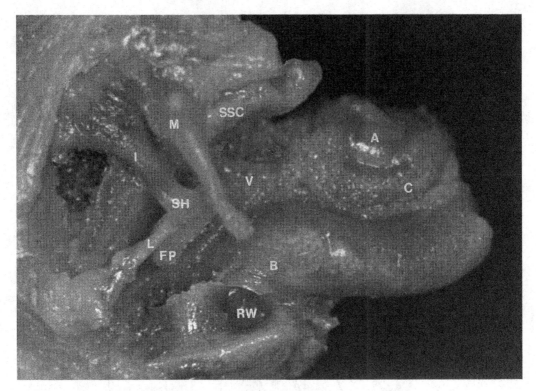

FIGURE 6-73A

The osseous labyrinth and middle ear structures in an early 4-month fetus. The malleus (**M**), incus (**I**), and head of the stapes (**SH**) can be seen along with the ligament of the stapedius muscle (**L**) and the footplate of the stapes (**FP**). The basal end of the cochlea (**B**) with its round window (**RW**) are shown along with the vestibule (**V**) and the second turn (**C**) of the cochlea and the apex (**A**). The lateral semicircular canal (**SSC**) is located to the right of the head of the malleus.

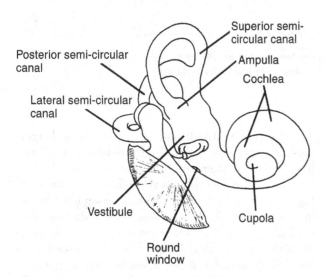

FIGURE 6-73B

The otic capsule, ossicular chain, and drum membrane. Parts of the otic capsule are the cochlea, vestibule, and semicircular canals.

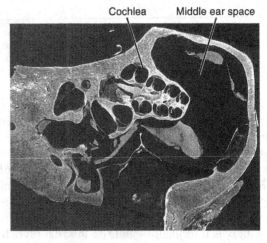

FIGURE 6-74

Section through guinea pig temporal bone illustrating relationship of cochlea to middle ear space. The cochlea protrudes into the space to provide access to its turns. In humans the cochlea is completely imbedded in petrous bone.

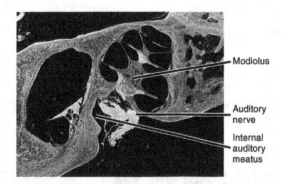

FIGURE 6-75

Section through a cochlea showing auditory nerve and base of modiolus at bottom of the internal auditory meatus.

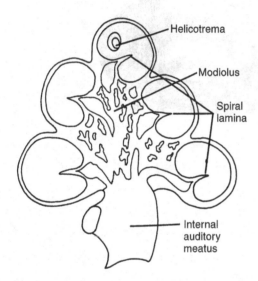

FIGURE 6-76

Schematic section through the bony cochlea, illustrating how the spiral bony lamina partially divides it into upper and lower ducts.

The cochlea has three openings, one of which is the **round window** located at the basal extreme of the scala tympani. The round window opens into the tympanic cavity. In life, however, it is closed off by a thin **secondary tympanic membrane.** In the human middle ear, the round window can be seen as a small opening in the medial wall of the tympanic cavity, tucked in a niche formed by the promontory. *The function of the round window is to permit pressures to equalize between the scala vestibuli and scala tympani.* When the stapes moves in, the round window bulges out. Near the round window, in the scala tympani is a very small aperture, the **cochlear aqueduct,** which is continued to the inferior surface of the temporal bone.

The bony labyrinth is lined with a thin, fibroserous membrane that is closely adherent to the bone. Its free surface is covered with epithelium that probably secretes the ultrafiltrate of blood called **perilymph.** A clear, watery fluid, it is similar to the cerebrospinal fluid that bathes the brain and is similar to extracellular fluid in its ionic composition. Perilymph fills the scala vestibuli, scala tympani, and the perilymphatic spaces within the vestibule and around the semicircular canals.

The Membranous Labyrinth

The membranous labyrinth is shown in Figure 6-77, and its relation to the bony labyrinth is shown in Figure 6-78. The membranous labyrinth is filled with an ultrafiltrate of blood known as **endolymph,** which is similar to perilymph but has an ionic composition similar to intracellular fluid.

Thus we have an endolymph-filled membranous labyrinth, completely contained within the bony labyrinth, which in turn is filled with perilymph. In places the membranous labyrinth is adherent to the walls of its bony confines by delicate tabs of tissue. The membranous labyrinth has three divisions: the **semicircular canals,** the **utricle** and **saccule,** and the **cochlear duct (scala media).** The cochlear duct comprises the system for hearing, and the utricle, saccule, and semicircular canals comprise the system for equilibrium. The latter can be further divided into a **static system,** which functions in the perception of position in space in the vertical plane, and a **kinetic system,** which functions in the perception of rotation and acceleration of the head.

The Membranous Semicircular Canals The membranous semicircular canals are similar in shape to the osseous semicircular canals in which they are housed. The membranous canal system has five openings, all entering the saclike **utricle,** which is located in the vestibule. The **membranous ampullae** correspond in their location to the osseous ampullae and are characterized by marked dilations. The ampullae contain small aggregations of connective tissue, upon which are situated highly developed ciliated sensory cells, the **crista ampularis.** The cilia of these cells are imbedded in a gelatinous mass, which contains minute crystalline grains of carbonate of lime. This mass, called the **cupola,** together with the ciliated or **hair cells,** forms the sense organ located in each ampulla. Very slight movements of the head or the body to which it is attached produce disturbances of the endolymph, which in turn affect the hair cells. The hair cells are supplied by the vestibular branch of the acoustic nerve.

The Utricle and Saccule Sensory organs are also found in the utricle and saccule. Similar to those in the

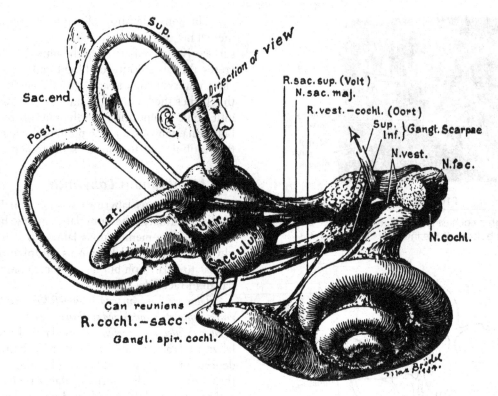

FIGURE 6-77

The membranous labyrinth. (From Wever, 1949.)

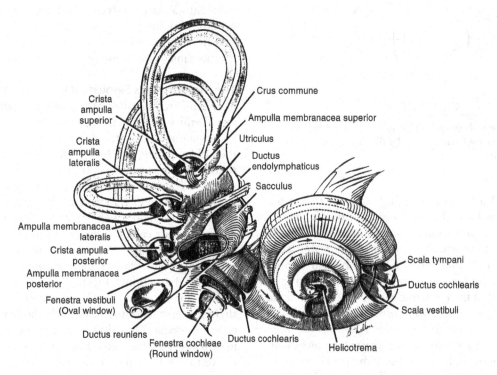

FIGURE 6-78

The membranous labyrinth and its relation to the bony labyrinth. (From *An Atlas of Some Pathological Conditions of the Eye, Ear, and Throat.* Courtesy of Abbott Laboratories, Chicago.)

ampullae, their epithelial cells, hair cells, and gelatinous cupola constitute the **maculae.** They are supplied by the terminal fibers of the saccular and utricular branches of the vestibular part of the acoustic nerve. The maculae respond to linear forward and sideways movements of the head. The labyrinth is fundamentally an organ of reflex action for the maintenance of equilibrium, and is important in the preservation of a constant field of vision. Normally, this function is accomplished in an automatic manner, without preliminary or accompanying sensation, as is the case with vision per se, or audition.

As shown in Figure 6-79, the utricle and saccule communicate indirectly by way of the utricular and saccular ducts which join to form a common **endolymphatic duct.** It, you will recall, courses through the vestibular aqueduct to end in a blind pouch located between the layers of the dura mater.

The saccule and cochlear duct communicate directly by means of the **canal reuniens,** which some authorities believe to be obliterated in the adult human. Because of its small size, high-frequency disturbances of endolymph are prevented from being transmitted from the cochlea to the structures in the vestibule (Vinnikov and Titova, 1964).

The Cochlear Duct (Scala Media) The **cochlea** is a bony, spiral-shaped cavity, about 35 mm in length, and incompletely divided into a **scala vestibuli** and **scala tympani** by the **osseous spiral lamina.** It is a narrow shelf of bone arising from the modiolar side of the cochlea, as shown in Figure 6-76. This division is completed by the membranous **cochlear duct** or **scala media,** a spirally arranged tube about 34 mm in length that complies with the general shape of the osseous cochlea, and lies along its outer wall (see Figure 6-80). As shown in Figure 6-81, its floor is formed by the **basilar membrane,**

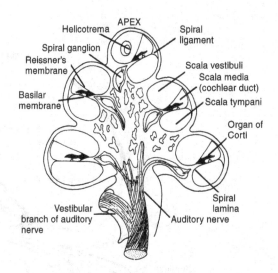

FIGURE 6-80

Schematic section of cochlea, illustrating modiolus in relation to other structures, including cochlear duct or scala media. The cochlear canal is incompletely divided into upper and lower ducts by the bony spiral lamina.

which extends from the spiral lamina to the outer wall of the cochlea. It is attached to a thickened spiral ligament, which as shown in Figure 6-81, lies along the outer wall of the cochlea.

The **cochlear duct** is of ectodermal origin and contains endolymph. The fluid spaces on either side of the cochlear duct (scala vestibuli and scala tympani) are of mesodermal origin and contain perilymph.

The relationship between the vestibule, scala vestibuli, scala tympani, and the cochlear duct is shown in Figure 6-82, with the cochlea uncoiled. Note that the bony spiral lamina and basilar membrane (heavy line) which divide the cochlea into an upper and lower duct are joined with the **vestibule** at the basal end in such a manner that the only direct communication is between the scala vestibuli and the vestibule. The scala tympani (lower duct), on the other hand, is also terminated basally at the bony wall of the vestibule, but it does not communicate with the vestibule proper, except through the helicotrema at the apex. The **vestibular membrane** (of Reissner), which forms the roof of the cochlear duct, terminates blindly at the vestibular wall and also at the apex. As a result, the cochlear duct becomes a *closed tube,* its only outlet being the tiny **ductus reuniens.** The vestibular membrane is composed of one layer of ectodermal epithelium that faces the cochlear duct and the endolymph and one mesothelial layer that faces the scala vestibuli and the perilymph.

The Spiral Lamina (Spiral Plate). The spiral lamina is a very narrow shelf of bone at the apical end, becoming gradually wider toward the basal end. It consists of

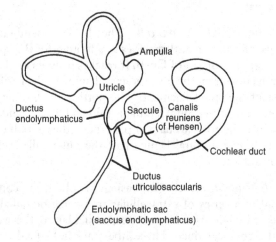

FIGURE 6-79

Schematic of the membranous labyrinth.

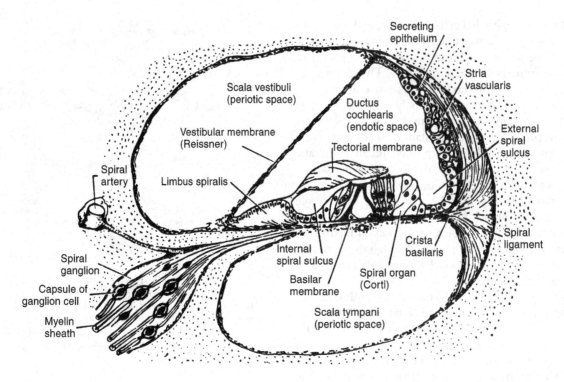

FIGURE 6-81

Illustration of the division of the cochlea into the scala vestibuli, scala media (cochlear duct), and the scala tympani. (From S. S. Stevens, eds., *Handbook of Experimental Psychology,* John Wiley & Sons, Inc., New York, 1951.)

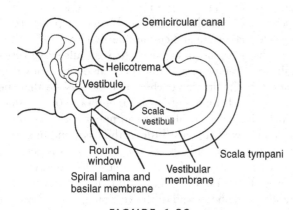

FIGURE 6-82

Schematic of the hearing mechanism, illustrating the relationship between the vestibule, scala vestibuli, scala tympani, and the scala media. The scala media is located between the vestibular membrane (of Reissner) and the spiral lamina and basilar membrane.

two thin plates of bones, between which are canals for the transmission of the peripheral fibers of the auditory nerve. The upper layer of bone is continuous with a thickening of periosteum known as the **spiral limbus.** It is shown in Figure 6-81. The spiral limbus is markedly concave at its outer edge, forming the **internal spiral sulcus** and at the same time giving rise to an upper ex-

tremity, the **vestibular lip,** and a lower extremity, the **tympanic lip,** which is continuous with the lower plate of bone (often called the **perforata habenula**) and with the basilar membrane.

As shown in Figure 6-81, the outer wall of the cochlea is characterized by a marked thickening of the periosteum known as the **spiral ligament** (of Kölliker). It projects inward to form a shelflike prominence, the **basilar crest.**

The Basilar Membrane. The basilar membrane forms a fibrous layer that serves as a footing for the **spiral organ,** or **organ of Corti.** It reaches from its modiolar attachment on the osseous spiral lamina to the basilar crest of the spiral ligament. The portion of the membrane nearest the spiral lamina is thin and fragile, and is known as the **zona arcuata** or **pars tecta** (the roof). It extends from the spiral lamina past the outer pillar cells (rods of Corti).

Fibrous Structure. The basilar membrane is composed of a series of extracellular transverse or radially directed fibers that course perpendicular to the axis of the cochlear duct. These fibers are imbedded in a rather homogeneous interstitial substance. According to Retzius (1905) there are about 24,000 fibers in the basilar membrane. When viewed from above, without its superstructure, the basilar membrane would resemble a corrugated or "washboard" road. The fibrous layer in the zona arcuata divides into two separate layers under the outer pillar cells (Figure 6-83), and this region, with two fibrous layers, is known as the **zona** or **pars pectinata** (L. comblike).

Tympanic Surface. The tympanic surface of the basilar membrane is covered by a layer of mesothelium through which courses vascular tissue. One of the vessels, larger than the others, is known as the **vas spirale**. The scanning electron microscopy of Angleborg and Engström (1973) reveals *spindle-shaped cells* with long processes running at right angles to the fibrous strands in the pars pectinate. The distribution of these cells varies in the basal, middle, and apical turns, and in addition, their shape is species specific. The significance of this tympanic covering layer is largely speculative. The cells are of interest from a phagocytic standpoint and also with regard to ion exchange through the basilar membrane. Also, these cells may well influence the physical properties of the basilar membrane.

Width. The width of the basilar membrane is variable, a fact that has had tremendous impact on the history of theories of hearing. Results obtained by numerous investigators vary considerably, but those of Wrightson and Keith (1918) are most often quoted. They found the width to vary from 0.16 mm at the basal end to 0.52 mm at the apex. *Although the cochlea is broad near its basal turn and narrow at the apex, the basilar membrane tapers in the opposite direction*, the difference being filled in by the spiral lamina. The illustration (Figure 6-84) by Fletcher (1952) is based on the data of Wrightson and Keith.

These data are in essential agreement with later data of Békésy (1960). The basilar membrane is wider, flaccid, and under no tension at the apical end, while the basal end is narrower and stiffer and may be under a small amount of tension. The change in elasticity is more than one hundredfold (Békésy, 1960). These factors contribute to a stiffness gradient along the basilar membrane that permits propagation of a traveling wave along its extent and is largely responsible for the well-established **place coding** of sound frequencies.

The Spiral Organ (of Corti)

The upper or vestibular surface of the basilar membrane bears an important organ that contains the sensory cells essential to hearing. Although the proper name is the **spiral organ**, the use of the term **organ of Corti** is steeped in tradition. The structure is extraordinarily complex, composed of a series of (mostly) epithelial structures that occupy the length and breadth of the basilar membrane. A cross section of a typical mammalian cochlea and the spiral organ contained within the cochlear duct is shown schematically in Figure 6-81, and a greatly enlarged schematic is shown in Figure 6-85. The cells that comprise the spiral organ may be classified as either *receptive* or *supportive*. The spiral organ will be described grossly, and then the supportive and receptor cells will be described in detail.

Near the osseous spiral lamina may be seen two conspicuous structures, the **inner** and **outer pillar cells** (rods of Corti). They are supportive cells that, when seen in a transverse section of the spiral organ, are widely separated at their bases and converge to meet at the top. They enclose a triangular **tunnel of Corti**, the

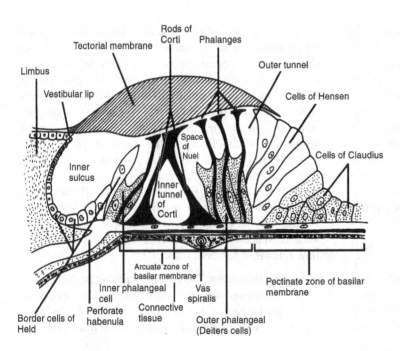

FIGURE 6-83

Schematic representation of the supportive structures of the spiral organ.

FIGURE 6-84

Schematic representation of the dimensions of the basilar membrane and of the scalae of the human cochlea. (From Fletcher, 1953.)

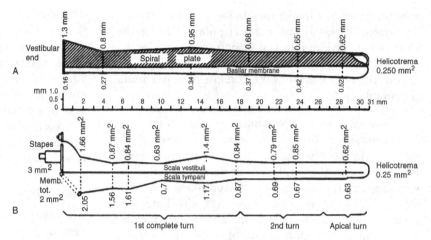

FIGURE 6-85

Illustration of the spiral organ (of Corti). (From Stevens, 1951.)

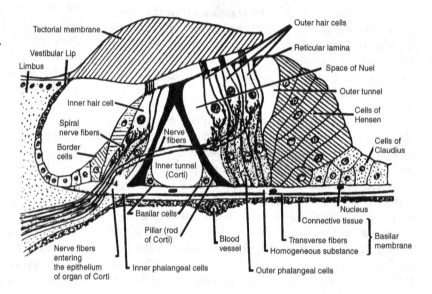

floor of which is formed by the bases of the pillar cells and by the basilar membrane. The tunnel contains a fluid sometimes known as **cortilymph.** On the modiolar side of the inner pillar cells is a single row of **inner hair cells,** which are flanked on the inner side by supportive cells. On the outer side of the pillar cells are three rows of **outer hair cells,** held in position at their bases and tops by a complex network of supportive cells, particularly the **cells of Deiters** and their phalangeal processes. The ciliated tops of the hair cells project beyond a delicate **reticular membrane** and extend toward a fibrogelatinous mass called the **tectorial membrane.**

The Supporting Cells The complex supporting cells of the spiral organ are shown schematically in Figure 6-83. We can begin with structures nearest the modiolus and progress across the basilar membrane to the spiral ligament on the outer side. The surface of the vestibular lip of the spiral lamina is covered with a very distinctive layer of epithelium. Its cells are arranged in parallel rows, and when viewed from the vestibular surface (from above), the lip has a serrated appearance. Early anatomists referred to the cells as "auditory teeth." The cells are epithelial, and Vinnikov and Titova (1964) have shown them to be secretory. They are thought to form the substance of the tectorial membrane, and are continuous with the epithelial lining of the **internal spiral sulcus,** which is composed of large, flat, polygonal cells that are directly continuous with the supporting cells for the inner hair cells. The first few rows of cells bordering the inner hair cells on the modiolar side are known as the **border cells of Held.** They are distinguished by a somewhat flattened head, closely connected with similar flattened heads of adjacent cells.

The Phalangeal Cells. The supporting cells most closely associated with the inner hair cells are structures called phalangeal cells, and they consist of two parts. The main **body** of the cell, with its small basal end, rests directly on the spiral lamina in the region of the **habenula perforate.** The cell body extends to the lower limit of the inner hair cell, and at about that level, a rather rigid process is given off. It extends upward to the level of the apex of the hair cell. This cuticular extension is called a **phalangeal process,** and it expands at its upper limit to form a flattened lamella which contributes to the formation of the **reticular membrane.** In this way, *the inner hair cells are strongly supported at their bases by the bodies of the phalangeal cells, and at their apexes by the phalangeal processes.* The word *phalanx* is from the Greek, "a line or array of soldiers."

The Rods of Corti (Pillar Cells). Probably the most conspicuous of the supporting structures are the inner and outer rods of Corti. As shown in Figure 6-83, the base of the **inner rod** rests at the point of junction of the tympanic lip of the osseous spiral lamina and the basilar membrane, while the base of the **outer rod** rests on the outer limit of the arcuate zone of the basilar membrane. The widely expanded bases of the outer and inner rods, which actually come into direct contact, contain the cell nuclei. The rods converge and meet at the top, forming an acute angle. The inner rods number about 6000 and the outer 4000. The distance between the bases of the inner and outer rods increases from the basal end to the apex of the cochlea, while the angles between the rods and the basilar membrane diminishes.

In a transverse section, as in Figure 6-85, the rods enclose a triangular **inner tunnel of Corti.** Its floor is formed by the expanded bases of the rods and by the subjacent basilar membrane. When viewed from the side, the walls of the tunnel are not solid. Rather, the rods, which are epithelial cells stacked alongside one another, have slitlike spaces between them which permit endolymph to circulate and nerve fibers to pass through as they course toward the modiolus and the nerve cell bodies contained therein. At their heads and bases, however, the rods are continuous. The outer surface of the head of the inner rod presents a deep concavity which accommodates a convexity on the head of the outer rod. In addition, the head of the inner cell presents a laminar headplate, which overlaps a similar headplate on the outer rod. These headplates bridge a gap between the inner hair cells and the first row of outer hair cells. The thin headplates of the outer pillar cells are also known as **phalangeal processes,** and they unite with the phalangeal processes of other supporting cells to form the **reticular membrane,** a delicate netlike structure which lies over the spiral organ.

The Cells of Deiters. In contact with the bases of the outer rods, but separated from the body or shaft of the cells, is a row of phalangeal cells similar to the inner phalangeal cells described earlier. They are called the cells of Deiters. Although the bases of the first row of the cells of Deiters are in direct contact with the bases of the outer pillars, their main bodies become widely separated above to enclose an inverted, triangular endolymphatic space, the **space of Nuel.** The bases of the Deiters cells rest on the pectinate zone of the basilar membrane. The main body of the Deiters cell is cylindrical; however, it becomes quite complex where it comes into contact with the base of the hair cell it supports. As shown schematically in Figure 6-86, *its shape is modified to form a cup that snugly accommodates the basal end of an outer hair cell.*

At about the level of the cup, or lower head, the cell also gives off an ascending phalanx, which reaches the upper level of the spiral organ between adjacent hair cells. There it quickly expands to form a thin lamella that contributes to the reticular membrane and also separates the apexes of neighboring hair cells. The phalangeal processes course upward at an oblique angle, so they reach the level of the reticular membrane two or three hair cells more apicalward than the main cell body from which they arose.

Thus, we see that the **reticular membrane** (or **lamina**) is not an independent structure, but rather is composed of the inner phalanges, the headplates of the inner rods, the phalangeal processes of the outer rods, and of the Deiters cells. Its function is to lend support to the apexes of the hair cells whose tufts of cilia occupy the spaces in the netlike matrix and project beyond it toward the tectorial membrane.

The Supporting Cells of Henson. Immediately adjacent to the outer row of Deiters cells are five or six rows of tall columnar cells, the supporting cells of Hensen. The narrow bases of the innermost row rest on the basilar membrane in direct contact with the bases of the outer row of Deiters cells. Toward their apex, however,

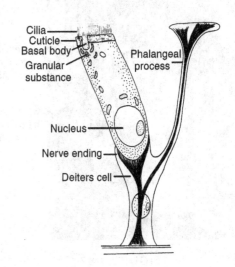

FIGURE 6-86

Schematic of a Deiters cell and outer hair cell.

they are separated slightly from the outer row of hair cells, giving rise to a narrow **outer tunnel.**

The Cells of Claudius and Boettcher. Additional rows of columnar and cuboidal cells, in decreasing height, lie outside Hensen's cells. They are the cells of Claudius and Boettcher which are continuous with a highly vascular layer of epithelium lining the spiral ligament. These latter cells, which are secretory, together with the vascular tissue form the important **stria vascularis.** It probably secretes endolymph, and since the spiral organ does not enjoy a blood supply per se, the nutritive function of endolymph is vital to hearing. The stria vascularis, which extends from the crista basilaris to the vestibular (Reissner's) membrane, has been likened to a *microkidney* and, in addition to producing endolymph, is believed to be the source of a positive 80 mV DC endolymphatic resting potential.

The Receptor (Sensory) Cells The receptor cells of hearing are arranged on either side of the rods or pillar cells: a single row of **inner hair cells** on the modiolar side and three rows of **outer hair cells** arranged in a very regular geometric pattern on the outer side, as shown in Figure 6-87. The inner and outer hair cells differ considerably in their shape, in the arrangements of the **hairs** or **stereocilia,** and in their nerve supplies.

The Inner Hair Cells. The human ear has about 3500 inner hair cells, arranged in a single row between the inner phalangeal cells and the inner rods, with the same angle of inclination as the inner rods. The electron micrograph, shown in Figure 6-88, illustrates the relation between an inner hair cell and its supportive cells. The hair cell is well supported from its base to its free upper extremity, which is oval, capped by a **cuticle,** and provided with a number of sensory hairs or stereocilia. *The basal end of each hair cell is in contact with nerve endings and supportive cells.*

During embryonic development all sensory (and supportive) cells have a single large hair called a **kinocilium** located on their upper free surface. It disappears during the latter part of fetal life, and in adult humans only a structure called the **basal body** remains as a vestige, just beneath a cuticle-free region of the cell surface, on the modiolar side of the cell. The basal body is characteristically surrounded by an aggregate of granular material. Basal bodies, from which a single coarse cilium (kinocilium) arises, are found in adult vestibular cells. The cell body height of the inner hair cell is fairly constant over the extent of the cochlea, but stereocilia vary in length and diameter within an individual hair cell and also among the individual turns of the cochlea. The number of cells also varies along the length of the

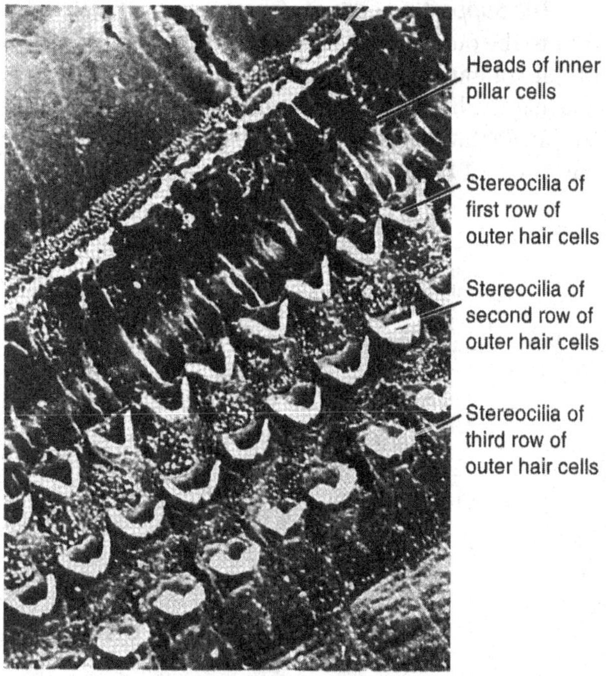

Heads of inner
pillar cells

Stereocilia of
first row of
outer hair cells

Stereocilia of
second row of
outer hair cells

Stereocilia of
third row of
outer hair cells

FIGURE 6-87

Scanning electron photomicrograph of the spiral organ as seen from above illustrating the arrangement of the inner and outer hair cells. (Photograph courtesy Dr. Harlow Ades.)

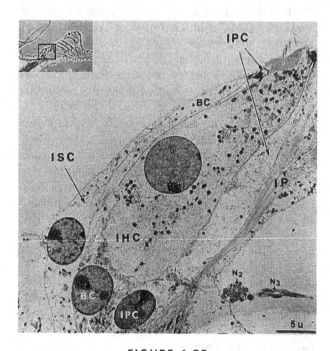

FIGURE 6-88

An electron photomicrograph of an inner hair cell and its supportive cells. **ISC** is an inner supportive cell. **IHC** is an inner hair cell. **IPC** is an inner phalangeal cell and its nucleus. **IP** is an inner pillar, **BC** is an inner border cell, N_2 is spiral tunnel bundle, and N_3 is radial tunnel bundle. (Courtesy David J. Lim, M.D.)

basilar membrane. Bredberg (1968) found about 80 inner hair cells per millimeter at the basal end and 115 cells per millimeter at the apical end.

The cuticle-capped **apex** of an inner hair cell is slightly concave and bears about 48 stereocilia arranged in three or four wavy rows that are oriented *parallel* to the longitudinal axis of the cochlea. Individual cilia are larger in diameter at their upper free ends, and the outer row of stereocilia, on both the outer and inner cells, is the longest. In addition, their length increases from base to apex and the stereocilia of the inner hair cells are coarser than are those of the outer hair cells. Each cilium has a marked constriction at its base and a rootlet that penetrates into the cuticular plate. *The cilia are joined by bridges of very fine fibrils so that all the cilia on one cell tend to move together as a unit, when the longest ones are bent.* The stereocilia are connected sideways by links that run parallel to the cuticular plate. These links run between the stereocilia of the same row as well as between the stereocilia of different rows (Pickles, et al., 1984). This linkage probably serves to couple the stereocilia mechanically. As a result, all stereocilia of a cell tend to move together when deformation occurs (Flock and Strelioff, 1984). A second set of stereocilia links can be found that is a single vertically pointing strand that courses to the adjacent taller stereocilium. When deflected away from the shorter stereocilia, the tips tend to be stretched. Pickles et al. (1984) suggest that stretching of the tip links opens membrane channels in the stereocilia and that relaxation closes the channels. The result may be excitation with stretching and inhibition with relaxation. The cilia also contain **actin** and other proteins, which suggests that they may be able to actively change their mechanical properties or that they may even be motile (Pickles, 1982). The entire hair cell, including the stereocilia, is surrounded by *plasma membrane* (true of both inner and outer hair cells). The cytoplasm of inner hair cells is particularly rich in endoplasmic reticulum and in mitochondria, especially in the apical region.

The Outer Hair Cells. The 13,500 or so outer hair cells share a number of features with the inner hair cells. They are capped with a cuticular membrane from which a number of stereocilia protrude, rising above the reticular membrane; they contain a basal body (remnant of the kinocilium); and the entire cell and its cilia are covered with a well-defined plasma membrane. Outer hair cells, however, are cylindrical in shape, with a rounded, nucleated base (like a mini–test tube) that nestles snugly into the cup-shaped head of the **Deiters cells.** The arrangement of the stereocilia differs from that of the inner hair cells. They are distributed in three or more rows, in the form of the letter V, or W, (Figure 6-89) with the base of the W directed toward the spiral lamina. The angle of the W, which is wide at the basal turn, becomes increasingly

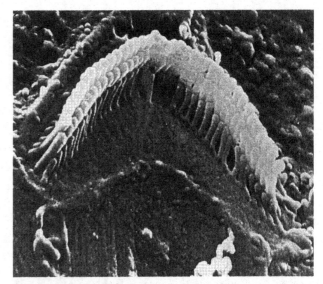

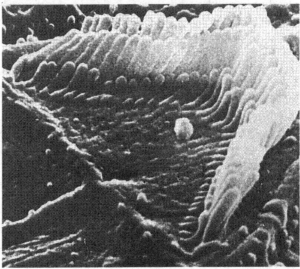

FIGURE 6-89

Electron photomicrograph of stereocilia of outer hair cells, illustrating their graduation in size and their shape. (Photograph courtesy Dr. Harlow Ades.)

acute toward the apex of the cochlea. The outer stereocilium on each cell is considerably longer than the others, and this may have important theoretical implications. For example, the arrangement of the stereocilia on both the inner and outer hair cells suggests that they respond (primarily) to a lateral (radial) shearing movement, a point to be considered later. The length of the outer hair cell bodies increases from about 20 microns basally to about 50 microns apically, but at the same time the number of stereocilia decreases from about 130 per cell basally to about 65 to 70 in the apical turn. The cells are arranged in three parallel rows in the basal turn, four rows in the middle turn, and sometimes at least a suggestion of five rows apically.

The most widely quoted hair cell count was conducted by Retzius in 1905; he estimated about 3500 inner hair cells and from 12,000 to 20,000 outer hair cells. Subsequent counts support the conservative number. The architecture of the hair cells has important implications regarding their highly specialized functions.

The Tectorial Membrane A very delicate looking structure, the tectorial membrane, is connected to the epithelial covering of the vestibular lip of the limbus, as shown in Figure 6-90. It is described as a semitransparent, gelatinous structure, with a density scarcely exceeding that of endolymph. Others see it as a fluid-filled tube; however, it does contain numerous interwoven fibrils (about 90 Å in diameter) that apparently contribute to its physical properties. Like the fibrils of the basilar membrane, the tectorial membrane is completely noncellular, and since it is devoid of a true cell membrane, it probably has no bioelectrical or metabolic functions, but rather *its role is purely mechanical.*

One of the most exquisite descriptions of the tectorial membrane (and cochlea) ever was that of Held in 1926, and only recently have new findings been added to his observations (Iurato, 1962; Lim, 1972). Held recognized five separate substrata in the tectorial membrane, but we can use the description by Lim who divided the membrane into three: (1) the **cover net,** (2) the **fibrous main body,** and (3) the **homogeneous basal layer** or **Hardesty's membrane.** They are shown in Figure 6-91, where the tectorial membrane is also divided into a **limbal, middle,** and **marginal zone.** A ridge called **Hensen's stripe** is located on the undersurface of the tectorial membrane, just above the region of the inner hair cells. In Figure 6-91, Hardesty's membrane is shown detached (for illustrative purposes) from the fibrous layer or main body. A marginal band and marginal net were also recognized by Held. Again, for illustrative purposes, the **mar-**

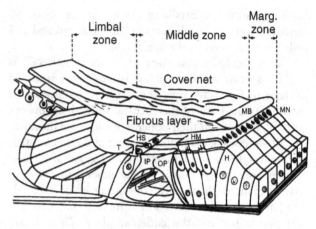

FIGURE 6-91

A schematic of the substrata of the tectorial membrane, illustrating the cover net, fibrous main body, and homogeneous basal layer (Hardesty's membrane, **HM**). The marginal band (**MB**), marginal net (**MN**), Hensen's stripe (**HS**) shown detached from the tectorial membrane (**T**), and inner and outer pillar cells (**IP–OP**). Hensen's supportive cells (**H**) are also illustrated.

ginal net is shown detached from the fibrous main body, even though the marginal zone, Hardesty's membrane, and the marginal net constitute a single marginal complex of the tectorial membrane.

The morphogenesis of this noncellular membrane is not well understood, but it is generally believed that it is the result of secretions of cochlear epithelial cells and that it is maintained by the "auditory teeth" mentioned earlier (Iurato, 1962).

Whether or not the tectorial membrane is somehow attached to the stereocilia has been a subject of debate for over a hundred years, and the arguments continue, partly because the membrane is so subject to distortion and fixation artifacts. It shrivels up, for example, when placed in fixative materials used in microscope slide preparation. However, electron microscopy shows that the membrane is thought to be attached in at least two ways. One is an attachment to the longest stereocilia of the outer hair cells, and the other, illustrated in Figure 6-91, is by means of Hensen's stripe, which attaches to the border cells of Held by fine trabeculae and by means of the marginal network near the last row of Deiters cells, or near Hensen's cells. As shown in Figure 6-92, the longest stereocilia of the outer hair cells have left imprints on the undersurface of the tectorial membrane (Lim, 1972).

From a functional point of view, it appears likely that the stereocilia of the inner hair cells are also in contact with the tectorial membrane, but such a contact has not been verified. It seems reasonable to conclude that at least the longest of the stereocilia on each of the outer hair cells are in contact with the tectorial membrane (Kimura, 1966; Bredberg, 1968).

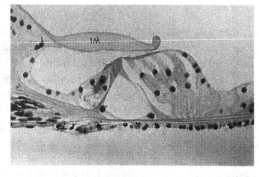

FIGURE 6-90

Bright-field photomicrograph of the spiral organ, illustrating the tectorial membrane (**TM**). It rests on the vestibular lip of the limbus (**L**).

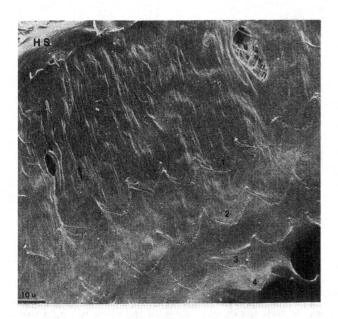

FIGURE 6-92

Electron photomicrograph of the undersurface of the tectorial membrane, illustrating the imprints of the stereocilia of the outer hair cells. The rows are numbered 1–4, and Hensen's stripe (**HS**) is also shown. (From Lim, 1972.)

According to Angleborg and Engström (1973), it seems possible that the contact of the tectorial membrane is fairly extensive before birth, but when hearing begins, the contact is forcefully weakened and only small strands reach from the tectorial membrane to Hensen's cells. This supports earlier findings by Lindemann and Ades (1971).

THE FUNCTION OF THE INNER EAR

Introduction

We are now faced with the problem of propagation of sound within the cochlea and the way in which vibratory energy is transformed into a train of neural impulses. From our description of the inner ear, it is evident that the entire membranous labyrinth forms a closed system. Since the walls of the bony labyrinth cannot yield to pressures and the labyrinthine fluids are practically incompressible, vibrations of the stapes footplate must cause the cochlear fluids somehow to be displaced. The exact mechanism of fluid movements within the cochlea has important theoretical implications and has a direct bearing on the form many of the theories of hearing have taken.

One point of view is that the *movements of the stapes are transmitted directly to the fluid column in the cochlea which responds as a whole—a* **mass-action mechanism.** As illustrated in Figure 6-93, inward movement of the stapes footplate causes the perilymph to flow up the scala vestibuli, through the helicotrema, and then down the scala tympani, where the round window is distended by an amount directly proportional to the inward movement of the stapes. During outward movement, the direction of flow of the fluid column is reversed. Sound energy, transmitted by the vibrating fluid column, is selectively absorbed by the structures on the basilar membrane.

An alternate viewpoint is that the pressure generated in the scala vestibuli is transmitted across the scala media to the scala tympani. As shown in Figure 6-94, such a transmission of pressure results in distortion of the vestibular membrane and, in turn, the basilar membrane. As before, however, there will be displacements of the round window that are out of phase with the direction of movement of the stapes. *The fluid movements may be distinctive for a particular frequency and thus produce*

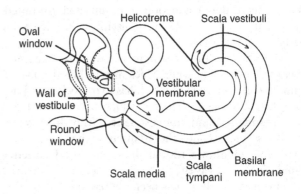

FIGURE 6-93

Schematic of mass-action flow through the cochlea. Inward movement of the stapes footplate causes perilymph to flow up scala vestibuli, through the helicotrema, and down scala tympani, where the round window is distended.

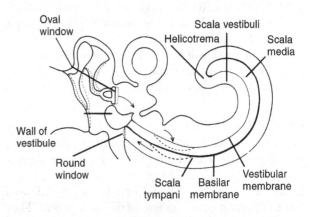

FIGURE 6-94

Schematic of the path of vibrations through the cochlea. Vibrations are transmitted across the scala media, into scala tympani.

distortion of the basilar membrane at a specific frequency-related locus. In either of these mechanisms, disturbances of the hair cells located on the basilar membrane transform the mechanical energy into electrical disturbances that stimulate the fibers of the cochlear nerve.

Theories of Hearing

Introduction

The exact nature of the movements of the cochlear fluids and of the mechanism by which the hair cells are stimulated and the analytic properties of the cochlea—all have been the subject of speculation and intensive research for many years. More than one researcher has devoted an entire lifetime in an attempt to explain the physiology of hearing. To date, even some of the most fundamental questions have not been resolved. No one knows, for example, exactly how the hair cells are stimulated. The hearing mechanism is, to say the least, enigmatic, and it has captured the imagination of, intimidated, frustrated, and challenged virtually every discipline in science for over a hundred years.

During that time research has given rise to a number of theories of hearing, which may be broadly divided into two classes, each of which has two subclasses. They are, first, the **place theories,** which have as subclasses the **resonance** and **nonresonance (traveling wave)** theories; and second, the **frequency theories,** which have the **telephone (nonanalytic)** and the **frequency analytic** theories as subclasses. In most of these theories the primary emphasis has been the passage of vibratory energy through the cochlea and the characteristics of disturbances produced on the basilar membrane. The neurophysiology of the cochlea and the role of the central neural pathway have received less emphasis, and in some instances have been all but excluded in the scheme of the hearing theory. But then, it wasn't until about 1892 that Gustav Retzius suggested that the hair cells are responsible for initiating the neural impulse. He was correct, of course.

Our first task will be to briefly review some theories of hearing, after which some features of the neurophysiology of hearing will be examined.

Resonance Theory

One of the earliest well-formulated theories of hearing was advanced by Helmholtz in 1857. His resonance theory was well received, and no theory of hearing has enjoyed such long-lived popularity. It closely followed three important developments of the same period. They were Ohm's law of auditory analysis, Johannes Müller's doctrine of specific energy of nerves, and the then recent anatomical findings of Corti.

Ohm's law very briefly states that any periodic sound wave consists of the sum of a series of sine (or co-sine) waves whose frequencies are integral multiples of the fundamental frequency. Also, a series of sine waves may be added to form a complex wave, the form of which is specific for any given series when the amplitudes and phase relationships are given. This law formed the very basis for Helmholtz's theory of hearing.

He was also influenced by **Müller's doctrine of specific nerve energy,** which stated that *the effects produced by stimulation of a nerve are specific to the particular sense with which the nerve is associated.* For example, although the eye is normally responsive to light energy, electrical, chemical, or physical stimulation of the visual receptors will produce sensations of light, and not shock or pressure. Müller's doctrine enabled Helmholtz to state that each fiber in the auditory nerve is associated with a specific pitch.

Helmholtz also found support for his theory in the discovery of the **rods of Corti.** He theorized that the outer rods made up a series of individually tuned resonators, with high-frequency resonators located at the basal end of the cochlea and low-frequency resonators in the apical region. He used as his analogy, piano or harp strings, which, as everyone knows, may be set into vibration by singing or playing a loud musical tone into them. According to Helmholtz, a note of a given pitch causes a specific resonator to be set into vibration, and because each resonator is supplied with a separate nerve fiber, pitch analysis is accomplished within the cochlea. In a later presentation of his theory Helmholtz no longer considered the rods of Corti to be the resonators, but, rather, the transverse fibers of the basilar membrane were thought to be the crucial resonating elements.

The analogy of piano or harp strings is still applicable in this, the revised and final form of the Helmholtz resonance theory of hearing. Unfortunately, this analogy, which is erroneous, is still being alluded to in some "authoritative" publications intended for public consumption. As a result, parents and teachers alike go through life supposing they have tiny pianos, harps, or marimbas inside their heads.

Helmholtz's theory was developed at a time when knowledge of the microscopic anatomy and the physical properties of the cochlea were not nearly advanced as they are today. Yet, except for Helmholtz's specification of resonating elements, his theory bears a remarkable resemblance to the current place theories. *The results of intensive research on the physical properties of the basilar membrane make it seem unlikely that actual resonators do exist.* Since Helmholtz located high frequencies at the basal end and low frequencies at the apical end of the cochlear duct, we would expect the transverse fibers to be longer in the apical region than at the basal end. As support for his hypothesis, Helmholtz cited anatomical observations of Hensen, who found that the length of the transverse fibers of the basilar membrane increases from 0.04 mm at the basal end to 0.495 mm at the apical end, a difference of about 12-fold. Subsequent measurements by Keith (1918) and Guild (1927) show that a difference in length does exist, but in the order of 3- or 4-fold. Measurements by Wever (1938) on a large sample (25 ears) indicate a mean width of 0.1 mm at the basal end and 0.5 at the apex, for a variation of about 6-fold. By applying principles derived from the basic laws of physics, we can account for only about 20 percent of the frequency range in human ears.

A second condition necessary to support the theory of Helmholtz is that the *resonators exhibit a high degree of independence from one another*; that is, the radial tension ought to be relatively great with respect to the longitudinal tension. In examining a basilar membrane, Helmholtz failed to find anatomical support for differential tension, and he assumed that the radial tension present in life was lost in death.

In 1941 Békésy examined a basilar membrane from a cadaver to determine the ratio between longitudinal and radial tensions. After gaining access to the tympanic surface of the basilar membrane by drilling away part of the bony wall, he then touched the membrane with a short piece of hair.

To satisfy the conditions for Helmholtz's resonance theory, the depressed area would look something like A in Figure 6-95. If the basilar membrane were constructed of a rank of thin elastic fibers stretching radially from the spiral lamina to the spiral ligament, there would be no coupling between them, and, when depressed by the hair, only a few fibers would be displaced. But, with equal radial and longitudinal tensions, the deformation would be circular, as in Figure 6-95B. Békésy found the ratio of longitudinal to radial (major and minor) to be very small —never exceeding 1:2—and when he cut a slit in the basi-

lar membrane, either radially or longitudinally, the edges of the incision did not pull away into an elliptical opening. Békésy did find, however, that the narrow basal end of the membrane was about 100 times stiffer than the apical end, but that it was not under appreciable tension.

Voldrich, in 1978, replicated the experiment of Békésy. Voldrich's specimens were from guinea pigs, examined within 15 minutes after death. Other specimens were examined 24 hours after death, while still others were fixed in various formaldehyde and lysol (lysoformlosung) solutions and stored under refrigeration, experimental conditions that had been reported by Békésy and others. Voldrich found that the force of a needle, applied to the fresh basilar membrane, produced a narrow, radially oriented depression on all turns of the cochlea. When pressure was applied to basilar membranes dissected up to 24 hours after death, the result was always a circular impression, like a broad shallow crater. *Some profound tissue changes occur within a few hours after death, and they influence the mechanical properties of the basilar membrane.*

Since Békésy obtained his specimens from the prosector of a large hospital, we can assume an interval of at least a few hours between death and time of examination. The speculations of Helmholtz regarding tissue changes at death may have been correct after all.

The findings of Voldrich do not invalidate the criticisms of the Helmholtz theory, simply because the basilar membrane fibers are not resonating elements. On the basis of these more recent findings, we can no longer view the basilar membrane as a gelatinous structure with no mechanical orientation, but rather we see that the radial fibers act as limiting elements which prevent wave propagation in the longitudinal direction. In other words, *the basilar membrane consists of a radially oriented series of relatively independent and uncoupled elements, each with its own mass, compliance, and stiffness, and thus its own response characteristics to oscillating pressure gradients within the cochlear fluids.*

We know, from basic acoustics, that a highly selective (undamped) resonator will be slow to respond to a driving force and equally slow to decay once the force has been removed. If a resonator is to cease vibrating soon after the excitatory force is removed, it must be highly damped, and if that is the case, it loses its sharpness of tuning and responds to a broad range of frequencies rather than just a single or narrow range of frequencies.

Nonanalytic Frequency (or Telephone) Theory

Frequency theories do not endow the cochlea with any analytic function as do place theories. Rather, they suppose the inner ear to be a *transducer*, which transforms vibratory energy into coded patterns of neural impulses, which are then conveyed by the acoustic nerve to the brain where discrimination and analyses occur. Such a

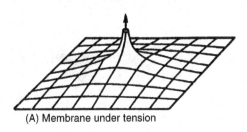
(A) Membrane under tension

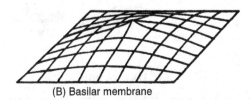
(B) Basilar membrane

FIGURE 6-95

Schematic of impressions produced by a point source on the basilar membrane under radial tension and on a membrane under even tension. (Courtesy Békésy.)

system so closely resembles the basis for the telephone that they are sometimes called **telephone theories.** Although an early frequency theory was outlined by Rinne in 1865, the theory of Rutherford, advanced in 1886, is the most widely known. This theory, as do some earlier frequency theories, supposes that any hair cell may be stimulated anywhere along the basilar membrane by sounds of any frequency or complexity.

Although Rutherford realized his theory was very demanding of the auditory nerve fibers, he apparently did not regard a discharge rate of up to 15,000 impulses per second beyond the limits of any single nerve fiber or hair cell. In fact, Rutherford felt the auditory nerve was specially adapted for very high discharge rates. He also attributed pitch and quality analyses, a capacity that must be acquired through training, to the brain rather than the ear. Rutherford also acknowledged that a gross place mechanism may exist and suggested that his theory and the place theories could be compatible. A number of telephone theories followed Rutherford's, all of them limited by the severe demands they place upon the individual nerve fibers.

Research on the frequency of discharge of single nerve fibers has revealed maximum firing rates that range from 24 to 1000 impulses per second. In 1926 Adrian and Zotterman, among the first to conduct such experiments, obtained maximum discharge rates of 190 impulses per second on frog muscle-nerve preparations. Since that time many similar experiments have been conducted, and the maximum rate has been, with few exceptions, something below 300 impulses per second, when the stimulus was continuous. For brief intervals, a maximum discharge rate may exceed 1000 impulses per second, evidence that fails to support a strict single-fiber theory such as Rutherford's. What we know about the properties of the neural elements, hair cells, and the basilar membrane is simply not compatible with a frequency theory such as Rutherford's.

Standing Wave Theory

Almost everyone is familiar with stationary or standing transverse waves on a rope or string. If a rope is fixed at one end and the other held under a moderate degree of tension, then moved up and down periodically, a *traveling transverse wave* is generated that courses along the rope until it encounters the fixed end, and the wave is reflected back toward the source. For each cycle or "round trip" the displacement must travel over the length of the rope twice, and when the movements are properly timed, the incident and reflected waves combine to form a displacement pattern that appears to be standing still.

Loops and nodes are produced on the rope at very regular intervals, and they appear not to be progressing along the rope. A standing wave pattern is shown in Figure 6-21. Regions of maximum displacement (**loops**) are separated at half-wavelength intervals by regions where no displacement (**nodes**) takes place. Standing waves are generated when the length of the string and the vibratory rate are related in an integral manner. The velocity of a progressive transverse wave is directly related to the square of the tension and inversely related to the square of the mass of the string. The period for a complete cycle is inversely related to the length of the string, and frequency, of course, is the reciprocal of the period.

These same principles have been applied to the basilar membrane. Békésy (1960) has shown that—depending upon the basilar membrane's mass, compliance, and resistance, and their relationship to the frequency of stimulation—either standing or traveling waves can be generated on it.

Pressure Pattern Theory

In 1899 Ewald developed a pressure pattern theory of hearing, in which repeated reflections of an incident wave generated by stapes vibration occurred along the basilar membrane. Ewald assumed that the lowest tone we can hear is 20 Hz and that it produced two loops on the membrane, a half-wavelength apart and separated by a node, as shown in Figure 6-96. Higher-frequency sounds produced an increased number of loops and nodes, all integrally related. Since a 20 Hz tone required two loops and a single node, Ewald's model necessitates that the highest perceptible tone (which he took to be 32,000 Hz) produce 3200 loops on the basilar membrane separated by nodes every 0.01 mm. Even at 20,000 Hz, the spatial distribution of loops and nodes would be quite demanding of the basilar membrane. These patterns of displacement and the spatial separation of the loops are, according to Ewald, interpreted by the brain

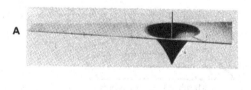

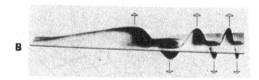

FIGURE 6-96

A point force on a very compliant membrane produces a depression as in A, and the membrane response takes the form of a standing wave, as described by Ewald (B). (After Békésy, 1960.)

as a tone. Since frequency analysis is relegated to the central nervous system, this theory falls into the *nonanalytic* classification.

Traveling Wave Theory

A number of *nonresonance place theories* followed Helmholtz and Ewald, and they all applied hydrodynamic principles to the cochlea. These theories recognize a spatial distribution of basilar membrane displacement, which is frequency dependent, but they are not dependent upon resonating elements in the cochlea. In both the resonance and nonresonance theories, however, frequency analysis occurs within the cochlea.

An early nonresonance place theory advanced by Hurst in 1895 proposed that stapes vibration sets up waves within the cochlear fluids and that these waves move up and down the cochlea. As shown in Figure 6-97, inward movement of the stapes causes basilar membrane displacement, which begins as a bulge at the basal end and moves toward the apex where it is reflected and begins a downward journey. This theory ascribed low-frequency hearing to the basal end and high-frequency hearing to the apical end. Trouble is, it has been shown

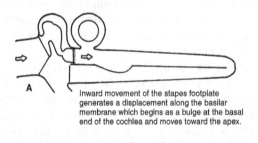

Inward movement of the stapes footplate generates a displacement along the basilar membrane which begins as a bulge at the basal end of the cochlea and moves toward the apex.

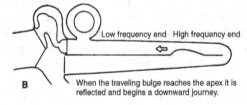

When the traveling bulge reaches the apex it is reflected and begins a downward journey.

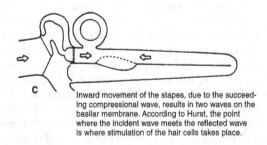

Inward movement of the stapes, due to the succeeding compressional wave, results in two waves on the basilar membrane. According to Hurst, the point where the incident wave meets the reflected wave is where stimulation of the hair cells takes place.

FIGURE 6-97

Schematic of the traveling wave theory of Hurst. (After Békésy, 1960.)

repeatedly that *the location for high tones is the basal end and for low tones the apical end of the cochlea.*

A number of traveling wave theories appeared around the turn of the century; however, a complete review of them is beyond the scope and purpose of this text, and the interested reader is urged to refer to Wever (1949) and Wever and Lawrence (1954).

Frequency Analytic Theory

In 1896 a form of frequency theory called the **frequency analytic** or **hydraulic theory** was advanced by Max F. Meyer (1899). A frequency theory, it nevertheless assigns analysis to the cochlea. This theory is more complex than most, and the reader is referred to Meyer (1899, 1928). A good account of it can be found in Wever (1949).

We should recognize that these early theories are really not theories of hearing in the true sense. Rather, they are all *theories of cochlear dynamics*, and all of them suffered from a lack of empirical data regarding the physical properties of the cochlear partition (the fluids, membranes, and supportive and receptor cells in the scala media).

In 1928, **Dr. Georg von Békésy** embarked on a long series of brilliant and carefully executed experiments in which he attempted to describe the physical properties and behavioral characteristics of the cochlear partition. He worked with ingenious models of the cochlea, and with fresh and preserved human and animal cochleas. In 1961 Békésy was awarded the Nobel Prize in Medicine and Physiology in recognition of his important contributions toward furthering an understanding of the physical mechanisms of excitation in the cochlea.

Békésy's Traveling Wave Theory

In his initial experiments Békésy observed the movements of the basilar membrane in an enlarged mechanical model of the cochlea, a technique used early by Ewald. Békésy discovered that when a rubber "basilar membrane" was suitably constructed, with appropriate thickness, stiffness, and tension, the model would show a very definite pattern of response to vibratory excitation. He also found that, depending upon the properties of the membrane, *displacement patterns could be generated that satisfy the requirements for resonance, traveling wave, or standing wave theories.* By observing basilar membrane displacement patterns in the fresh human cadaver cochlea, Békésy was able to construct an enlarged model that exhibited very similar displacement patterns in response to vibratory excitation.

As shown in Figure 6-98A, the *cochlear model* consisted of a long metal frame, fluid-filled and divided into an upper and lower "scala" by a thin partition with a tapered opening as shown in Figure 6-98B. This opening was covered by a diluted solution of rubber cement to

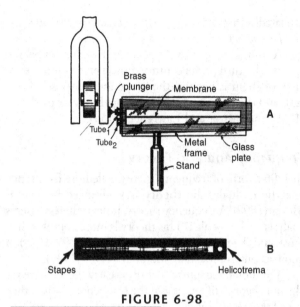

FIGURE 6-98

A model of the cochlea (A) and the partition with the tapered opening that was covered with rubber cement to represent the basilar membrane (B). (Courtesy Békésy.)

represent the basilar membrane, and a small hole representing the helicotrema was drilled in the apical end. Its function was to equalize any static pressure differentials between the two scalae. The basal ends of the two fluid-filled compartments were sealed with rubber membranes, one representing the oval window and the other the round window. A brass plunger was fastened to the oval window to represent the stapes, and it in turn was driven by an electromagnetic tuning fork. The vibrations were sinusoidal. The vestibular membrane (Reissner's) was deliberately omitted because experimentation showed the effect of its presence or absence to be negligible. This model of the cochlea constitutes a closed hydraulic system very much like an animal cochlea. **Pascal's principle** tells us that pressure at any point in a closed-fluid system is transmitted to all other points in the system. Since the cochlear fluids are virtually incompressible, any changes in pressure are transmitted instantaneously throughout the cochlea.

As vibratory energy is transmitted to the cochlear fluids by the stapes, a progressive compressional wave is generated. Perilymph, you will recall, has a viscosity similar to water, while the cochlear partition (the basilar membrane, tectorial membrane, supportive and receptor cells, and endolymph), in its totality, has a viscosity of gelatin.

The difference in physical properties between the perilymph and cochlear partition is so great as to constitute an **interface,** and where an interface exists under conditions just outlined, surface waves occur at the boundary between the two fluids. *Surface waves are generated at the interface.* These waves are not visible in the usual sense since there is no physical discontinuity between the perilymph and cochlear partition. There is only a discontinuity in the physical properties of the perilymphatic fluids and the cochlear partition. As a consequence, when the perilymphatic fluids are driven by a vibrating source (the stapes), a time-space varying pressure gradient is generated along the extent of the interface, and its form is dependent upon the frequency and complexity of the excitation of the perilymphatic fluids and of the velocity of propagation through the fluid.

In other words, as a longitudinal wave travels through the perilymph, it creates a periodic pressure pattern which changes both in time and space, across the cochlear partition. Since the bony walls of the cochlea are unyielding, this time and space varying pressure pattern is transmitted across the cochlear partition to the scala tympani, and finally to the **round window,** which in turn vibrates. Without this pressure release, the incompressible fluids which are confined within the unyielding bony walls of the cochlea would prevent stapes vibration.

Displacement Patterns of the Basilar Membrane

The displacement pattern of the basilar membrane is in response to the pressure pattern that exists at the interface between it and the perilymphatics, and the **traveling wave** represents an energy exchange between the cochlear partition and the surrounding perilymphatics. So now we can direct our attention to the characteristics of basilar membrane displacement in response to vibratory excitation.

Békésy has shown by direct observation, by measurements of the human cochlea, and by his models of it, that the *displacement patterns of the basilar membrane are due to its physical characteristics.* We have seen that the membrane is about 0.1 mm in width basally and about 0.5 mm at the apex. In addition, its *stiffness* increases by about 100 times from the apex to the base. These properties, plus the *coupling* along the membrane from one segment to the next, are the principal determinants of its response patterns. As Békésy has stated,

> In an approximate way we can consider the rubber membrane as divided into several transverse bands, much as conceived of in the resonance theory. Let us suppose that these bands are equal in width (i.e., as measured along the longitudinal dimension of the membrane); but they vary in length at different places along the membrane. Then they can be regarded as separate resonators whose natural frequencies decrease continuously toward the helicotrema. If this system of resonators is exposed to sinusoidal stimulation, the amplitudes of vibration at successive instants will form a group of curves like that of [Figure 6-99].

The traveling wave that Békésy observed is characterized by some unique features, probably the most distinctive one being the *spatial relationship between the*

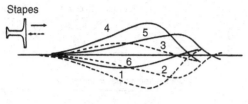

Stapes

FIGURE 6-99

Curves showing successive patterns of amplitude on the basilar membrane of the model during a full sinusoidal vibration. (Courtesy Békésy.)

maximum and the excitatory frequency. That is, the locus of maximum disturbance on the basilar membrane is frequency dependent. In his experiments with models, Békésy noted that at all frequencies an undulating wave began on the basilar membrane nearest the stapes, that it increased in amplitude somewhere along the partition to reach a maximum, and beyond that point the displacement quickly reached zero, as shown in Figure 6-100.

In addition, the amplitude of the waves in the perilymphatic scalae also tend to zero at the same place as it does on the cochlear partition. This is a consequence of the interaction (and energy exchange) between the partition and the perilymph at the interface. We might visualize a spatially distributed energy exchange increasing to a maximum, and here, where the exchange is virtually complete, the displacement falls to zero. The energy has been properly consumed. The **amplitude pat-**

terns on the basilar membrane are spatially distributed, and the point on the membrane where maximum displacement occurs is dependent upon the frequency of excitation. Békésy found that **high-frequency excitation** resulted in bold *maximum displacement at the narrow or basal end*, while **low-frequency stimulation** produced *maximum displacement at the wide or apical end* of the membrane, as illustrated in Figure 6-101.

In order to illustrate *the shape of basilar membrane displacement*, as shown in Figures 6-100 and 6-101, the magnitude of the wave motion is deliberately grossly exaggerated. Estimates of the actual extent of membrane vibration in response to sounds at the threshold of hearing show us that the movement is vanishingly small, about 10^{-3}Å. But, as Dallos (1973) has said, "This extrapolation has been a bone of contention for many years, and a number of authorities profess a disbelief that amplitudes this small could possibly be utilized." A more workable value of displacement is 0.1 Å, which is about the diameter of a hydrogen atom.

Because lower and lower frequencies displace larger and larger segments of the basilar membrane, we begin to see why *low frequencies tend to mask high frequencies*. Since sounds activate not only their frequency-specific points on the basilar membrane, but all the segments extending from the basal end to the maximum, low-frequency sounds activate the high-frequency end of the basilar membrane, in addition to their frequency-specific points. Because of these response patterns to sounds of varying frequencies, the basilar membrane has been

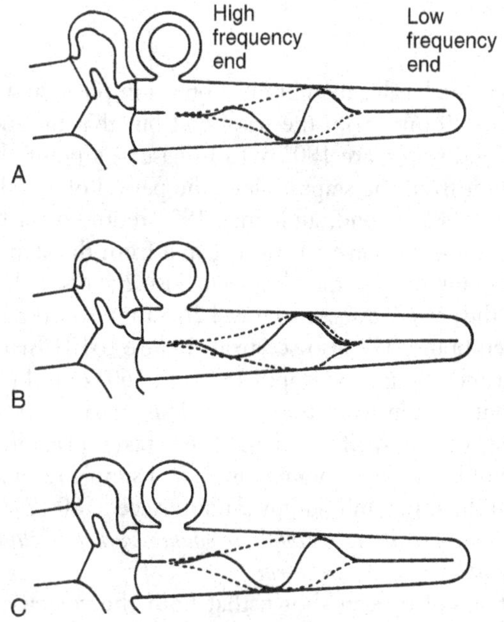

FIGURE 6-100

Schematic of the basilar membrane displacement pattern in the traveling wave theory of Békésy.

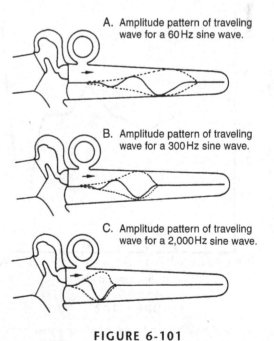

A. Amplitude pattern of traveling wave for a 60 Hz sine wave.

B. Amplitude pattern of traveling wave for a 300 Hz sine wave.

C. Amplitude pattern of traveling wave for a 2,000 Hz sine wave.

FIGURE 6-101

Schematic of amplitude patterns of traveling waves for sinusoidal waves of various frequencies.

likened to an acoustic filter with a shallow (6–24 dB/octave) low-frequency rise and a very steep (in excess of 100 dB/octave) high-frequency cutoff.

Subsequent measures using laser inferometry (Khanna and Leonard, 1982) suggest the band-pass filter characteristics (**tuning curves**) are much steeper than are those suggested by the curves of Békésy. Khanna and Leonard measured the tone intensity required to displace the basilar membrane by a fixed amount (3×10^{-8} cm). In a cat, a tone of 27 kHz (27,000 Hz) requires the least intensity to displace the basilar membrane. The curve, shown in Figure 6-102, represents the responsiveness of the basilar membrane at the 27 kHz point of the cochlear partition. The high-frequency cutoff slope was in excess of 500 dB/octave, which means that basilar membrane displacement is extremely analytic.

The length of time it takes for the displacement wave to propagate along the membrane is of interest; it can be calculated by measuring the phase relationship between stapes vibration and basilar membrane vibration at various locations for various frequencies of excitation. Békésy conducted such an experiment in an attempt to demonstrate that the curves or waves were not the usual resonance curves, but rather some form of traveling wave. In Figure 6-103, the magnitude and place of displacement on the basilar membrane is shown for four different frequencies. Békésy also used the curve for 200 Hz to show basilar membrane vibrations, at two instants of time, separated by a phase angle of 90°, as shown in Figure 6-104. From the lower half of Figure 6-103, we

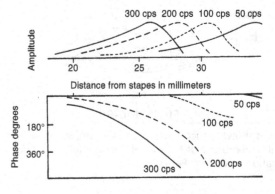

FIGURE 6-103

Amplitude displacement patterns for four low-frequency tones and the phase shift in degrees between stapes and a point on the basilar membrane. (Courtesy Békésy.)

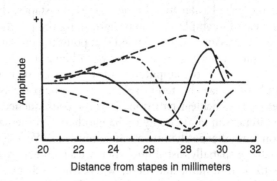

FIGURE 6-104

Cochlear partition displacement for 200 Hz at two instants in time and separated by a phase shift of 90°. (Courtesy Békésy.)

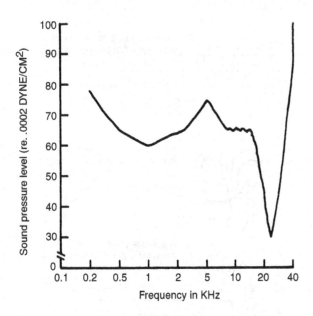

FIGURE 6-102

Tuning curve of basilar membrane of cat, for a frequency of 27,000 Hz. Low-frequency slope (tail) is 86 dB/octave near peak, and high-frequency slope is 538 dB/octave. (After Khanna and Leonard, 1982.)

see that the basilar membrane vibrates in phase at a distance of 20 mm from the basal end but that the membrane and stapes are 180° out of phase at a point about 26.5 mm from the stapes. Since the period of a 200 Hz tone is 0.005 second, and since 180° represents a half-wavelength, the wave has propagated from the stapes to some point on the membrane in just 2.5 msec. It has taken the wave 2.5 msec to travel 26.5 mm over the basilar membrane. We also see from Figure 6-103 that the basilar membrane and stapes are a full 360° out of phase at about 29 mm from the stapes. This means that 180° phase shift (one-half wavelength) has taken place in just 2 mm of basilar membrane. Since, in a simple resonance system the input and output cannot exceed 180°, *Békésy's curves demonstrate that simple resonance cannot account for basilar membrane displacement.*

It has also been shown that both the velocity and wavelength change radically on the cochlear partition from the basal to the apical end. *The velocity and therefore the wavelength decrease with distance from the stapes, and they become infinitesimally small at the point where* the amplitude of displacement falls off to zero. Beyond the point of maximum amplitude displacement, the rate of decrease in all three quantities—amplitude, velocity, and wavelength—is very rapid (Dallos, 1973). This decrease of velocity as a function of distance is a well-known phenomenon in fluids, it occurs in oceans, in swimming pools, in teacups, and in the cochlea.

We might also note that since, in accordance with Pascal's principle, pressure changes in an incompressible fluid are transmitted instantaneously throughout the fluid, it really shouldn't matter where the *source of excitation* is located along the cochlea. It happens to be at the basal end where the stapes is located, but it could just as well be at the apex, or somewhere in between. It wouldn't matter theoretically, and experimentation has shown that it doesn't (Wever and Lawrence, 1954).

The most unique property of the traveling wave is the *location of its maximum*, depending upon the frequency of the excitation source. The higher the frequency of excitation the closer the maximum is to the basal (stapedial) end, and the more constricted is the pattern. As shown in Figure 6-105, at lower and lower frequencies an increasing segment of the displacement pattern appears along the basilar membrane, and at the lowest frequencies, the disturbance is spread over the entire extent of it.

Note in Figure 6-105 that no clear-cut maximum seems to develop at frequencies of 25 Hz, but that at frequencies above about 200 Hz a definite maximum develops at the apical end. At higher and higher frequencies the maximum moves toward the basal end. *This frequency-dependent maximum of membrane displacement is a clear indication that the cochlea performs a mechanical frequency analysis.*

We are dealing with a **place theory,** because each point along the basilar membrane develops a maximum of displacement that is associated with a specific frequency of excitation. Complex stimuli, on the other hand, produce multiple regions of maximum disturbance, in response to a complex time-space pressure gradient in the perilymphatic spaces. Figure 6-106 is a schematic view of membrane displacement at the very instant of maximum. We should note that each point along the basilar membrane that is set into motion vibrates at the same frequency as the excitation force. Thus, we see from the response characteristics of the basilar membrane that for any given frequency, the amplitude of vibration varies from a minimum at the basal end to a maximum at some point along the membrane. Békésy has shown, however, that with the amplitude of stapes vibration held constant, the relative amplitude of displacement at the maximum is fairly constant, irrespective of the frequency of the driving force. Under natural conditions, of course, high-frequency sounds tend to have lower amplitudes of vibration than do the lower-frequency sounds.

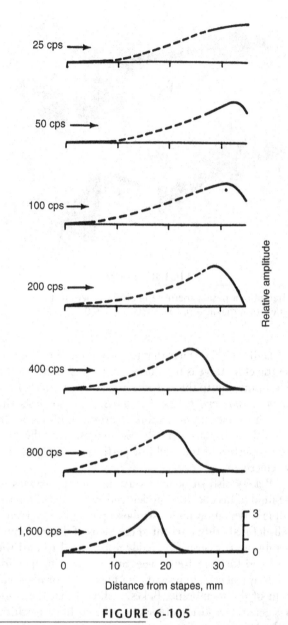

FIGURE 6-105

Patterns of vibration of cochlear partition for seven different frequencies. Dashed lines are extrapolations. (After Békésy, 1960.)

We have seen that the form of the wave of displacement is due to the dimensions and physical properties of the cochlear partition. The single *most important property seems to be the gradual changes in stiffness,* which vary about 100 times from a maximum stiffness at the basal end to a minimum at the apex. In addition, because the entire cochlear partition is attached to the spiral lamina on one side, and to the spiral ligament on the other, plus the fact that it is not under any appreciable tension in its resting state, its rigidity is greater in the radial than in the longitudinal direction. The wave, therefore, assumes a shape much like the one shown in Figure 6-106.

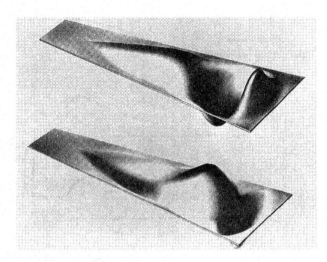

FIGURE 6-106

Schematic of basilar membrane displacement at the very instant of a maximum. (After Békésy, 1960.)

Dallos (1973) states that the pronounced peaking of the traveling wave is not due to simple resonance of the membrane, but to the *exchange of energy between the basilar membrane and the cochlear fluids*. This suggests the traveling wave might exhibit a certain nonlinearity at the peak of displacement. It also suggests that the tuning properties of the cochlear partition are very sharp, or selective.

Békésy also suspended very fine silver particles in the fluid of his cochlear models and, by means of microscopic observation under stroboscopic light, observed a well-defined **eddy current** at the locus of the maximum membrane response. The eddy also moved toward the basal end for high frequencies and toward the apex for low frequencies, along with the maximum of displacement of the membrane. Békésy believed that these eddies generate a steady pressure on the cochlear partition at the locus of maximum membrane response and that this pressure was the actual stimulating agent for the hair cells. Thus, although large portions of the membrane may be displaced, up to a maximum, *the actual location of hair cell stimulation is restricted to the narrow region where the eddy is generated*. Békésy proposed that further frequency analysis takes place in the central pathway.

We should make one additional, very important observation. Békésy found that rather drastic modifications in the resistance of the cochlear fluids, changes in the dimensions of the fluid columns, or changes in the location of the driving force failed to change the vibratory patterns of the membrane and the location of the eddy current. *The crucial factors are the physical properties of the cochlear partition.*

Békésy's findings have provided us with a solid and workable foundation on which to base our constructs of cochlear hydrodynamics and the analytic function of the inner ear. Békésy died in 1972. His contributions are now an important chapter in the long history of auditory physiology.

Analytic Theory

In an early study of auditory nerve responses, Wever and Bray (1930) observed **auditory nerve discharges** that were *synchronous with auditory stimulation* to a frequency as high as 4000 to 5000 Hz. In subsequent studies, Davis, Derbyshire, and Lurie (1934) and Derbyshire and Davis (1935) noted synchronization up to 4000 per second. The results also indicated that the synchronization does not abruptly cease at a specific frequency but, rather, gradually gives way to asynchronous nerve discharges to as high as 15,000 per second. The fact that synchronous nerve discharges failed to reach the upper limits of hearing led Wever and Bray to reject the simple telephone theory. They felt that the *frequency of nerve discharges could not represent pitch throughout the entire hearing range* of from 20 to 20,000 Hz. As a result, the telephone theory was modified to include certain features of both the telephone and place theories.

The Volley Principle One development was the volley principle, which states that when frequency limits are reached for any single nerve fiber, an additional nerve cell and its fibers may come into play. These two nerve cells, discharging alternately, double the response rate of the auditory system. If the frequency increases beyond the limits of the two fibers, three, four, or more nerve cells begin firing, thus raising the frequency limit three- or fourfold. This *alternate firing of individual nerves* has come to be known as **volleying** or the **volley principle,** and a full account of it may be found in Wever (1949). The volley principle is illustrated in Figure 6-107. Wever notes that, when first developed, the **place** and **frequency**

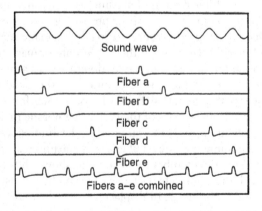

FIGURE 6-107

Illustration of the volley principle. The discharges from fibers a–e combine to provide discharges that are in synchrony with the frequency of the sound wave. (From Wever, 1949.)

theories were exclusive and vigorously opposed conceptions of the action of the inner ear. In the **volley theory** the two traditional conceptions are combined and compromised so that the contributing virtues of each are retained and fused into a single harmonious theory of hearing.

Pitch Analysis. Pitch analysis, for example, is dependent upon the place of disturbance on the basilar membrane and the composite nerve-impulse frequencies. The place and frequency theories are assigned various roles according to tonal region. *Frequency serves for low tones, place for the high ones,* and *both perform in the transition region* between them. Wever notes that the boundaries of the place and frequency regions gradually blend into one another. He suggests that the frequency principle holds for a tonal range of from 15 to 400 Hz, both frequency and place operate in the middle range of from 400 to 5000 Hz, and place alone functions in the high-tone range.

Loudness. Loudness, according to this theory, is dependent upon two factors: the *spatial extent of basilar membrane displacement* and the *number of active fibers.* Intensity representation in the volley principle is illustrated schematically in Figure 6-108. Wever suggests that at low-intensity stimulation, only in a central region of the displaced basilar membrane is sensory action

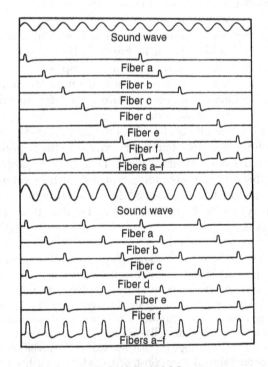

FIGURE 6-108

Schematic of intensity representation in the volley principle. Increased basilar membrane displacement for high-intensity sounds excites increased numbers of nerve fibers. (From Wever, 1949.)

strong enough to excite nerve fibers, but as intensity is raised, adjacent nerve fibers previously inactive are brought into play. Stimulus intensity is represented by the number of active nerve fibers, and by the rates at which they act. Thus, the message that is sent off to the brain consists of a sequence of electrical impulses, which together form some kind of representation of the vibrating motions of the basilar membrane.

According to the volley theory, the representation is best for the low-frequency sounds where a number of neurons convey pitch information and is comparatively poor for the high frequencies where the neurons can supply only a "sketch" of the pitch information. This is probably not a particularly serious shortcoming, however, for neurons leading from the basilar membrane retain their frequency identity in the auditory nerve, the cochlear nuclei, and onto the level of the cerebral cortex.

Although some authors favor evidence for a place or for a frequency theory, others are inclined toward an eclectic view. Regardless, none of the evidence at this time is conclusive. As Dallos (1988) has pointed out, by the 1960s, extensive recordings of the electrical activity in fibers of the auditory nerve (e.g., Kiang, Watanabe, Thomas, and Clark, 1965) showed that the necessary frequency selection was already established at the preneural level of the auditory system. One very important implication of these findings is that no complex neural network for sharpening discrimination was necessary. Once again, Dallos (1988): "The current view is that the phenomenal frequency selective properties of the auditory system are entirely established in the mechanical properties of the cochlea."

We have yet to examine the mechanism by which basilar membrane vibrations are transmitted to the sensory receptors in the spiral organ.

Excitation of the Hair Cells

In some of the earlier theories of hearing, the up-and-down movement of the hair cells and contact of the stereocilia with the tectorial membrane were thought to be the active stimulus for the neural impulses of hearing.

Shearing Action

In 1900, however, ter Kuile developed a theory in which a *lateral shearing action between the reticular and tectorial membranes* was considered the stimulating agent for the hair cells. Békésy has shown that, at least up to moderately high intensities of sound, the entire cochlear partition—including the basilar membrane, its superstructure, and the tectorial membrane—vibrates in phase. Somehow, then, up-and-down movements of the cochlear partition result in a lateral shearing action on the stereocilia. Any membrane or plate which is bent into a curve has produced on it an **inside** and an **outside**

radius, between which a large **shearing force** is generated. Since the inside radius is smaller than the outside radius, the substance between them must slide laterally, as shown in Figure 6-109. This is one mechanism by which shearing forces can be produced. There is another.

The **pivot points** for the tectorial and basilar membranes are shown in Figure 6-110. Because the membranes are hinged at different points, equal vertical displacement of the tectorial and basilar membranes results in a shearing force, the magnitude of which is considerably greater than the vertical force that produces the up-and-down movements. In this way, minute force on the basilar membrane is transformed into a shearing force many times greater. As shown in Figure 6-111, the shearing force causes lateral bending of the stereocilia.

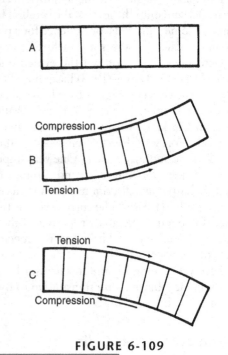

FIGURE 6-109

Bending produces shearing action between inside and outside radii.

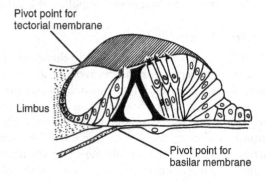

FIGURE 6-110

Schematic of a section of the spiral organ, showing pivot points for the tectorial and basilar membranes.

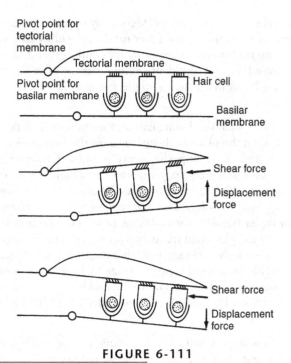

FIGURE 6-111

Schematic illustration of how vertical displacement of the basilar and tectorial membranes produces a shearing force on the cilia of the hair cells.

Thus, the inner ear provides a certain amount of mechanical gain, and that increases the sensitivity of the hearing mechanism.

When we examine the form of basilar membrane vibration, as was shown in Figure 6-106, we see two **curvatures** at the point of maximum displacement, one radial and one longitudinal. Each curvature produces a shearing force. The **radial** curvature produces the principal direction of shear on the rising part of the slope of the displacement envelope, and the other is in the **longitudinal** direction, but it is restricted to the region of the falling slope of the envelope. Dallos (1973) suggests that this very restricted longitudinal shearing wave may account for the sharpness of the tuning (frequency selectivity) on the basilar membrane. He does point out, however,

> The problem with assigning a primary role to the longitudinal shear is that the transducer hair cells are morphologically polarized in a *radial* direction. This polarization is dictated by the essentially radial organization of the stereocilia, which is very pronounced on the outer hair cells and less so on the inner hair cells. It then appears that the hair cells (certainly the outer hair cells) are constructed to be primarily receptive to radial shear. We are clearly confronted with a contradiction that is not now resolvable.

We must keep in mind that the relationship between the two groups of hair cells and the tectorial membrane is somewhat different. If we accept the evidence that suggests that parallel movement of the tectorial and reticular membranes results in a shearing action across the stereocilia, we must examine the microscopic anatomy once again briefly.

Deformation of the Stereocilia

Earlier we saw that only the outermost row of the stereocilia of the outer hair cells seems to make contact with the tectorial membrane. The remaining hairs and the hairs of the inner hair cells do not make such contact, however. At least they do not leave imprints on the tectorial membrane. These free-standing stereocilia are very likely stimulated by the viscous drag of the streaming endolymph during movements of the cochlear partition. The *bending of the outer row of stereocilia is proportional to the displacement of the cochlear partition*, while the *bending of the free-standing outer and inner hair cell stereocilia is proportional to the velocity of basilar membrane movement*. The extent of deflection of the stereocilia is extremely small—in the order of 0.3 nm. A nanometer is one-billionth of a meter. The prefix is from the Greek *nanos*, meaning *dwarf*. Dallos (1988) has shown that, if one scales the dimensions of one cilium up to the height of Chicago's Sears Tower, the movement of the tip of the cilium (0.3 nm) is equivalent to a 2-inch displacement of the top of the Tower. This fundamental difference in mode of stimulation suggests a difference in basic functions.

The exact consequences of the displacement of the hairs are open to some question. It is not known how the hair cell is actually stimulated by the bending action of the stereocilia, and it is not known how neural impulses are initiated. One explanation is that the deformation of the stereocilia results in a change in the electrical resistance of the hair cell. This generates a **receptor current** that flows through the hair cell body, a mechanism thought to be a first step in the initiation of the neural impulse. This means that the hair cell is a resistive element in an electrical circuit, through which current flows.

Earlier we learned that the **endolymph** within the membranous labyrinth is characterized by its high potassium (K^+) ion concentration, as compared to the **perilymph,** which has a high sodium (Na^+) ion concentration. From what we learned in the previous chapter, it should come as no surprise that these fluids differ in their electrical potentials, and that fact is directly related to the change in the electrical resistance of the hair cell body that is thought to take place when the stereocilia are deformed.

Neurophysiology of the Cochlea

We turn now to a brief consideration of the cochlea as a transducer, capable of converting acoustic or mechanical energy into nerve impulses. The discussion here will be rather limited in scope, and the interested reader is referred to Davis (1960, 1962), Dallos (1973), and Pickles (1982).

The Membrane Theory

In order to account for the electrophysiological properties of hair cells, the membrane theory is commonly used. It states that a cell is surrounded by a semipermeable membrane separating a double layer of ions, the positive ions outside and the negative ions inside. At rest the positive and negative charges are stable and a small electrical potential exists between the inside of the cell and its surrounding extracellular fluids. This resting potential usually amounts to about −70 mV. As we learned in the previous chapter, when a cell is excited the membrane breaks down, permitting a rapid exchange of ions, and the surface of the cell becomes depolarized; that is, its electrical charge changes from −70 mV to about +40 mV. *Presumably, this rapid flow of minute quantities of electrical energy serves as the initiator of the nerve impulse.* The excitatory process results in a very sudden diffusion of sodium (Na^+) and potassium (K^+) ions across the cell membrane.

Cell depolarization results in a local potential in the immediate vicinity of the cell, and it also produces a drastic change in the overall electrical resistance of the cell. Immediately after depolarization the ionic cell membrane begins to restore itself, by means of the **sodium-potassium pump** which is powered by adenosine triphosphate (ATP), and in just a few milliseconds is capable of another depolarization or firing. The **neural spike potential** and partial **repolarization** may take as little as 0.5 msec, however, so it is possible that discrete neural events could occur 2000 times per second, for a very short time. A shearing force, acting on the stereocilia of the hair cells, plus the viscous streaming of endolymph, you will recall, are thought to be responsible for an initial disturbance of the cell membrane and the resulting depolarization.

Electrical Potentials

With the development of suitable electrodes, surgical techniques, and electronic instrumentation, many of the electrical properties of the inner ear can be measured. The properties vary, depending on the type of electrode that is used, from where in the cochlea they are measured, and whether or not the cochlea is at rest. Davis (1960) lists four classes of electrical potentials that have been identified and associated with particular sources or bioelectrical potential generators:

1. **DC** (direct current) **resting potentials,** both **intracellular** and **endocochlear.** Resting potentials exist without acoustic stimulation.

2. **CM,** or **cochlear microphonics,** which are alternating current responses to the acoustic stimulation

and are generated at the cilia-bearing end of the hair cells.

3. The **summating potential (SP)** which is direct current, but only appears during acoustic stimulation.

4. The **action potential (AP)** of the fibers of the auditory nerve.

These potentials can probably be recorded best from the guinea pig cochlea. As shown in Figure 6-112, the cochlea protrudes into the bulla, which is a dilated continuation of the middle ear cavity. The bony shell of the cochlea is extremely thin, and the four and a half turns permit access at a number of points.

Resting Potentials In 1950, Békésy reported very small (3 mV) direct current potentials between the perilymphatic scalae and the surrounding cochlear bone. He was curious to find out if normal metabolic processes provided the energy for the stimulus-related electrical events in the cochlea, or if the acoustic stimuli actually provided the energy. Today we know that the *acoustic energy only instigates or triggers the process of local energy conversion to neural impulses.*

By 1952 Békésy had perfected techniques for probing the scalae of the cochlea with microelectrodes. He found a negative 20 mV potential between the two cell layers of the vestibular membrane, while inside the scala media a high positive potential was found. It has since come to be known as the **endocochlear potential** or **EP**; in subsequent experimentation values in the neighborhood of 90 to 115 mV have been found (Peake, et al., 1969). See Figure 6-112.

In 1959 Tasaki and Spiropoulas were able to drain the endolymph from the cochlea and then explore the walls of the scala media with a microelectrode probe.

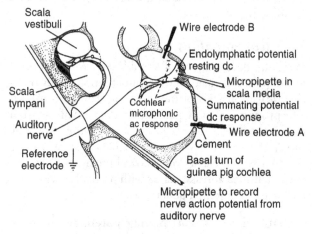

FIGURE 6-112

Schematic of technique of recording cochlear potentials in the guinea pig.

They found the *source of the endocochlear potential to be the stria vascularis.* Other experiments demonstrated the *oxygen dependency of the endocochlear potential*, while *destruction of the hair cells resulted in no detriment to the potential* (Davis, et al., 1958).

Békésy had found in his earlier experiments that, when sound was introduced to the ear, the *endocochlear potential decreased as long as the stimulus persisted.* This change was referred to as **"DC fall,"** and it is most certainly the same as the **summating potential** identified independently by Davis in that same year.

When Békésy invaded the cochlea with his electrodes in 1952, he found that the potential within the spiral organ was *negative* and it amounted to about 40 to 50 mV. He was probably measuring the extremely important negative membrane potential (in this instance due to injury) of the hair cells, although it is possible that the negativity originates from an electrically unique fluid in the spiral organ, which has been labeled **cortilymph.** The ionic concentrations of the extracellular fluid in the spiral organ were found to be similar to that of perilymph, however. Since the endocochlear potential has a value of about 100 mV, the negative 50 mV membrane potential brings a total of about 150 mV across the top of the hair cells, a value probably not exceeded anywhere else in the body. This large voltage could quite easily facilitate triggering the neural impulse by increasing the size of the electrical response of the hair cells.

Stimulus-Related Potentials *Summating Potentials.* With an electrode placed in the scala media, and another in the scala tympani, acoustic stimuli will evoke a direct-current response so that the scala media becomes electrically negative with respect to the scala tympani. These summating potentials, which are best recorded from the region of maximum basilar membrane displacement, were identified some time ago, but they still remain poorly understood.

One reason for this is that *summating potentials are a composite*, made of a number of bioelectric components that are not easily separated. They may also have either positive or negative values. Figure 6-113 shows a composite response from the round window of a guinea pig. It contains a cochlear microphonic, a DC summating potential, and nerve action potential (AP), in response to a high-frequency stimulus of moderate intensity. In addition, this summating potential seems to "mimic" the overall envelope of the stimulus, and that is also illustrated in Figure 6-113. An additional characteristic is that the magnitude of the summating potential doesn't seem to reach any sort of saturation level. That is, its value increases (although not necessarily linearly) with increases of stimulus intensity up to levels that we expect to produce hair cell damage. The summating potentials,

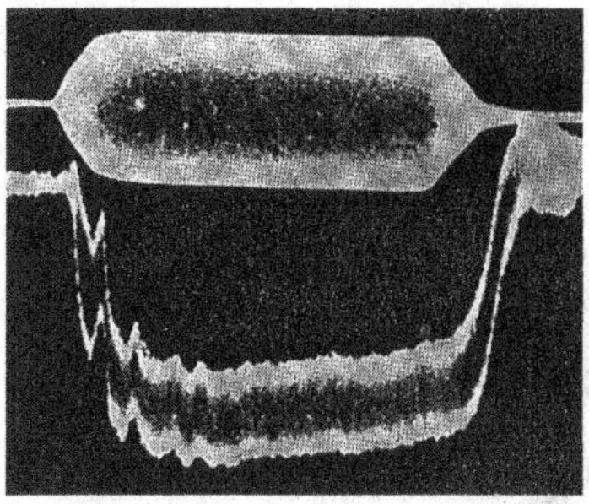
21,500 cps.
60 dB (relative dB)
Cochlear microphonic
plus
Summating potential
plus
Action potential
1 millisecond

FIGURE 6-113

Composite response recorded from round window of a guinea pig, showing high frequency (21.5-kHz cochlear microphonic, top), the DC summating potential (the downward drop of the base line), and the composite recording which includes the nerve action potential. (From Rasmussen and Windle, 1960.)

which *appear to be a product of the outer hair cells*, are closely related to cochlear microphonics.

Cochlear Microphonics. In 1930 Wever and Bray placed an electrode in the auditory nerve of an experimental animal and detected *an electric potential that accurately reproduced the frequency and waveform of the sound stimulus.* When the electrical energy was amplified and channeled into a telephone receiver, Wever and Bray found that speech was reproduced with remarkable fidelity.

Initially they suspected that the electrical activity represented the nerve impulses in the auditory nerve, but subsequent experiments by Wever and Bray (1930), Adrian (1931), and others soon demonstrated that the same electrical activity could be detected by placing an electrode in the vicinity of the cochlea and that a lead from the auditory nerve was unnecessary. Adrian suggested that the cochlea was acting like a *biological microphone*, and the electric energy was not to be confused with the nerve action potentials of the auditory nerve.

The microphonics of the cochlea seem to be generated by the *ciliated bearing end of the hair cells*, or at least seem to be dependent upon the presence of healthy hair cells. Several reasons have been offered in support of this viewpoint. (1) Microphonics continue to be produced after the acoustic nerve has been severed and may persist even though the spiral ganglion cells in the modiolus degenerate. (2) Microphonics disappear, however; when the outer hair cells are destroyed by toxic agents such as streptomycin (Davis, et al., 1958). (3) Certain species of animals with a congenital absence of hair cells lack the microphonics found in animals with healthy inner ears.

Talley (1965) found that an inbred strain of Dalmation that appeared to be deaf (behaviorally) consistently lacked the characteristic cochlear microphonics present in his control animals. Microscopic examination of serial cochlear sections revealed a complete absence of the normal structures in the spiral organ and, in particular, the hair cells and supportive structures. A midmodiolar section through a Dalmation cochlea is shown in Figure 6-114A, and a comparable section through the cochlea of a control animal is shown in 6-114B.

Probably the most compelling evidence that the hair cells are the source of the microphonics is that of Tasaki et al. (1954). They introduced a microelectrode into the scala vestibuli by passing it through the scala tympani, the basilar membrane, and the spiral organ, through the reticular lamina, the tectorial membrane, and finally the vestibular membrane (Reissner's). In the scala tympani, the direct current potential was zero and the amplitude of the cochlear microphonic was quite small. As the basilar membrane and spiral organ were pierced, an irregular direct current shift appeared along with the growth of the microphonic. When the electrode reached the region of the reticular membrane, or passed through it, a large positive endocochlear potential appeared, along with a growth of the cochlear microphonic and a complete 180° shift of phase. When the vestibular membrane was penetrated, the endocochlear potential disappeared and the amplitude of the microphonic was reduced, although the phase remained the same. These results suggested to the authors that *the source of the cochlear microphonics is at the apical, hair-bearing ends of the receptor cells.*

As shown in Figure 6-115, *the amplitude of cochlear microphonics is proportional to that of the stimulus signal throughout a considerable range* (up to about 80 dB SPL). Beyond that, the microphonic amplitude increases less rapidly, and, finally, at about 105 dB SPL, further increases in stimulus amplitude result in an actual decrease in microphonic output. The reason for the decrease in microphonics at high-intensity stimulation is not known. Note in Figure 6-115, that the waveform of the microphonic, throughout the entire range, is distortion free. In addition, there is no real threshold, its determination being limited by the measuring instrumentation and technique.

Also, *the cochlear microphonics demonstrate no adaptation to stimulus, no fatigue, and seemingly no frequency limits*, within reason. Cochlear microphonics, however, are *highly dependent upon the blood supply to the inner ear.* When blood flow is interrupted, they decline rapidly in amplitude to a value approximately 10 percent of that of the original amplitude, where they remain for several hours after blood deprivation or even after death. Sometimes the **high-amplitude (oxygen-dependent) microphonics** are designated **CM-1,** and the **"oxygen-independent" microphonics** are called **CM-2.**

The role of microphonics in hearing has been a subject of speculation and research ever since their discovery.

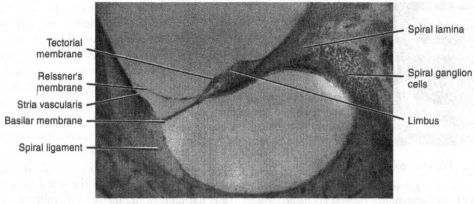

Tectorial
membrane

Reissner's
membrane

Stria vascularis

Basilar membrane

Spiral ligament

Spiral lamina

Spiral ganglion
cells

Limbus

(A) Mid-modiolar section through cochlea of deaf Dalmation

Reissner's membrane

Limbus

Organ of Corti

Stria vascularis

Spiral ligament

(B) Mid-modiolar section through cochlea of normal control animal

FIGURE 6-114

Photomicrographs of normal and abnormal dog cochleas. No cochlear microphonics were recorded from the animal in the top figure. Receptor and supportive cells were also missing. (Courtesy Talley, 1965.)

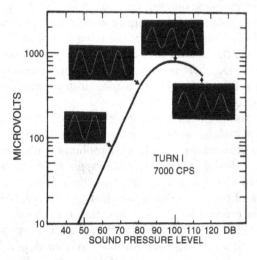

FIGURE 6-115

Input-output curve for the cochlear microphonic response to 7000-Hz tone bursts. Note the absence of distortion. (After Davis, 1960.)

At one time it was thought that they served to stimulate the terminal endings of the auditory nerve, but because microphonics have no latency as opposed to a latency of about 0.5 msec for nerve impulses, this interpretation seems highly unlikely. Besides, Stevens and Davis (1938) point out that it is not essential to assume that microphonics have any real functional significance:

> They are possibly an incidental by-product of the auditory process, an epiphenomenon, like the noise of automobile—but, just as the noise may help us in determining whether or not an engine is running properly, so may the cochlear microphonics serve us in analyzing normal and abnormal functions in the inner ear.

Indeed microphonics are useful in determining the *functional integrity* of the inner ear. They reflect very closely the mechanical events taking place on the basilar membrane. For this reason cochlear microphonics have been used to determine the location of frequency-dependent regions of the basilar membrane.

Cochlear microphonics are easily detected by simply placing a wet-wick or a small metal foil electrode on the round window. This technique has its shortcomings, because only high-frequency microphonics can be recorded very well. This is because the cochlear microphonic is spatially localized in the same way as the traveling wave. An experiment of Tasaki et al. (1952) related the microphonic output to place on the cochlea. Guinea pigs were used because of the accessibility of all four turns of the cochlea.

Microphonics from the first or basal turn were compared with the outputs of the second, third, and fourth turns as frequency was varied. *The time-space pattern of the cochlear microphonics was a bioelectric verification of Békésy's description of basilar membrane displacement at various frequencies.* Note in Figure 6-116 that a 500 Hz tone produces microphonics in both the basal and apical turns, which means that the entire basilar membrane is displaced for low frequencies. A high-frequency tone (8000 Hz) produces microphonics in only the basal turn of the cochlea. This technique, sometimes called **tonotopographical mapping,** has been repeatedly and carefully done over the frequency range of from 60 to 7500 Hz and has led to the formulation of **cochlear frequency maps,** an example of which is shown in Figure 6-117. Note that the high-frequency tones are spread out over the basal region, while the lower frequencies are all crowded into the apical region.

Spatial localization maps can also be generated with a somewhat different technique. If the ear is stimu-

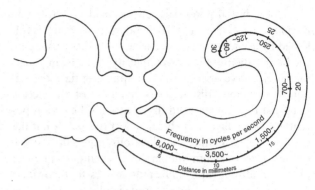

FIGURE 6-117

Frequency location along the basilar membrane.

lated by a tone of extreme intensity until the cochlear microphonics are impaired, presumably the ear has suffered hair cell damage at a frequency-related area on the basilar membrane. It is important to note that the impairment in cochlear microphonics is not confined to the stimulating frequency only, but rather is reflected in a general depression of amplitude throughout the frequency range of the ear. Histological examination of the ears some weeks after the exposure to high-intensity sound reveals some striking findings. *The area of cochlear damage has a direct relationship to the stimulating frequency.* Ears exposed to low-frequency sounds suffer extensive and widespread damage in the apical region, while ears exposed to high-frequency sounds suffer restricted damage in the basal region (Smith and Wever, 1949). These results are just one more verification of a place mechanism.

The Action Potential (AP) or Whole Nerve Potential. The action potential is a stimulus-related electrical activity that takes a form quite different from resting potentials. Even though it is not a true cochlear potential, it can be recorded from either the cochlea or directly from the trunk of the auditory nerve. Electrodes placed in the vicinity of the cochlea, for example, pick up a virtual volley of summated nerve potentials that can be elicited in response to an acoustic event.

If the **auditory stimulus** is a complex one, numerous hair cells are activated along the basilar membrane, and since the displacement travels wavelike toward the apex, nerve impulses are generated at different times at various places on the membrane. As a result, an asynchronous conglomerate of impulses reaches the electrode. Usually, however, a click or a high-frequency tone burst is used as a stimulus. The characteristic pattern begins with a **large negative potential** called N_1. This potential is probably due to very nearly synchronous discharge of a large number of neurons as a result of basilar membrane activity at the high-frequency end. This initial negative potential is often followed by a **second lesser potential** called N_2.

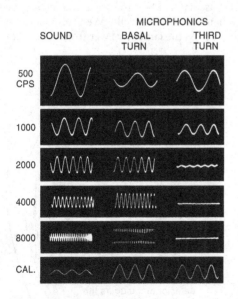

FIGURE 6-116

Cochlear microphonics recorded by electrodes place in the first and third turns of guinea pig cochlea. (After Davis, 1960.)

These initial potentials reflect cochlear activity, in response to a click, at the basal end initially, which is followed by asynchronous discharge as the disturbance on the basilar membrane moves apically. Usually, in studying whole nerve or compound action potentials, the initial synchronous discharge is the part of the action potential that is measured. Even though the action potential heavily favors the basal end of the cochlea, it has certain potential clinical applications, especially since it can be measured from humans, by a technique known as **electrocochleography.** The most successful recordings are obtained when a fine electrode is placed on the promontory of the middle ear. The eardrum is penetrated in order to place the electrode. Action potentials can also be recorded by placing an electrode on the wall of the external auditory meatus, directly on the drum membrane, or in the annular ligament.

The Evoked Cochlear Mechanical Response. In 1978, Kemp placed a tiny loudspeaker and a probe microphone into the sealed ear canal of human subjects. An acoustic click was presented, and 5–15 msec later, a second much smaller click could be recorded, as if the cochlea were returning an echo. This is not a resting or active neural potential, but it suggests that the propagating wave encounters an **interface** somewhere along the basilar membrane and reflects part of the stimulus back toward the source. The **echo** is not found in persons who are sensorineurally deaf, which suggests a cochlear origin for the echo. The echo is not a strong one, and is well below the threshold for hearing. In addition, a click presented to subjects with subjective **tinnitus** (ringing of the ears) triggered a long series of sound pressure fluctuations in the ear canal. The mechanism for the echo is not known, but it is possible that changes in the stereocilia, in response to the pressure wave, constitute an interface, and it is here the reflection occurs, but this is highly speculative.

Transduction in the Cochlea

We have yet to account for the initiation of the actual nerve impulse at the periphery of the auditory pathway. We have seen that the displacement pattern on the basilar membrane is frequency specific and that bending of the stereocilia, either by shearing forces or by viscous streaming, results in a bioelectric change in the hair cell. *Somehow,* the deformation of the hair cells results in a graded electric potential in the nerve fibers that is conducted to the regions of the habenula perforata. Here the myelinated portion of the nerve fiber begins, and here, at the first node of Ranvier, the spike potential is generated and begins its tortuous journey to the cerebral cortex.

Davis (1960) presents a "somehow" that is quite digestible. He asks a very perturbing question first, however: What part do endocochlear potentials, cochlear microphonics, and summating potentials play in exciting the nerve impulses that are represented by the action potentials?

Part of the answer to that question might be found in an experiment by Békésy. He applied forces, by means of a vibrating microelectrode, and found two things. First, he noted that the displacement must be in a radial direction to produce an electrical change. Second, he found that more electrical energy can be released than can be accounted for by the mechanical energy dissipated by the displacement. This is important because it tells us that *the spiral organ is contributing energy and not simply absorbing it.*

Research has shown that both the cochlear microphonic and the summating potential are affected by the magnitude of the polarization of the scala media. If polarization is increased, for example, the cochlear microphonic and the summating potential are increased. What we seem to be confronted with is a polarized and sensitive trigger mechanism that assists in transducing acoustic energy (fluid pressure gradients) into neural impulses.

There is little point in attempting to paraphrase Davis. It is better to take the liberty of quoting him, at the same time giving him full credit for what he suggests. For the hypothesis or model of Davis, refer to Figure 6-118.

> We think of an electric circuit through the hair cells and nerve endings. The current is driven by two batteries and the amount of current is controlled by a variable resistance. One battery is the intracellular polarization of the hair cell and the second battery is the stria vascularis. The variable resistance is provided by the hairs of the hair cells. We assume that the resistance across the cuticular layer from scala media to the

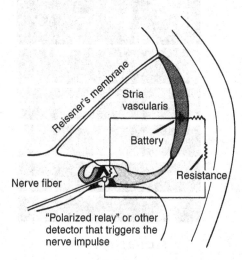

FIGURE 6-118

Davis's model of cochlear excitation. (After Davis, 1960.)

inside of the hair cell varies with the bending (or perhaps the shearing) of the hairs. If the bending of the hairs is an alternate bending to and fro we will have the alternating current output that we call the cochlear microphonic. If it is a steady bending in one direction we have the summating potential. More or less current flows according to how much the hairs are bent.

Our theory assumes that the electric current flows in the proper direction from hair cells through the nerve endings and excites the nerve endings.

The graded potential at the hair cell (voltage across the resistance) is referred to as the **local** or **resting potential,** while the graded neural response of the peripheral unmyelinated part of the nerve fiber is called the **generator potential,** and it initiates the **nerve action potential.**

Responses from the Inner Hair Cells

In 1978 Russell and Sellick were able to place microelectrodes into the spiral organ and record intracellularly from inner hair cells. They were not reliably successful with outer hair cells. The inner hair cells had resting potentials of –25 to –45 mV as compared to resting potentials of –70 mV for neurons. The introduction of sound resulted in both direct current (D.C.) and alternating current (A.C.) changes.

The **DC change** was due to an intracellular depolarization, and the inside of the cell became relatively more positive. Deformation of the stereocilia is thought to result in an inward streaming of potassium ions (K^+), decreasing the negativity of the intracellular fluid. Russell and Sellick (1978) plotted the sound intensity necessary to produce a criterion level of electrical response from the cell to produce a **tuning curve** for that cell, as shown schematically in Figure 6-119. This curve shows that the inner hair cell is very sensitive at one frequency which is known as the **best** or **characteristic frequency,** and the response drops off markedly as the frequency is shifted away from the characteristic frequency. The hair cells may exhibit sharper tuning than the tuning characteristics of the basilar membrane, which would heighten selectivity or increase the frequency discrimination of the cochlea.

It is now thought that frequency selectivity is due to the properties within the cochlea and that the neural events are initiated by the inner hair cells. Earlier research suggests that the traveling wave frequency analysis was not particularly sharp and so the afferent (ascending) neural pathway was given the task of sharpening frequency analysis. Research subsequent to Békésy, however, using refined measurements has shown that the vibration pattern on the basilar membrane is very nonlinear, which means that the amount of membrane displacement does not grow in proportion to an increase in the intensity of sound but at a much shallower rate. In

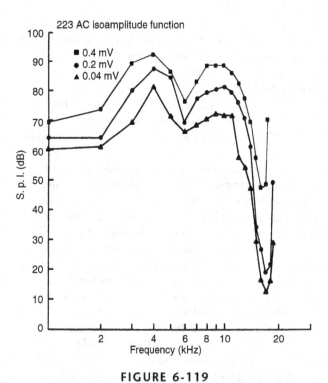

FIGURE 6-119

Tuning curves for an inner hair cell show the sound pressure level to produce a constant amplitude of the electrical response, as a function of frequency. (Based on Russell and Sellick, 1978.)

addition, the nonlinearity is particularly evident in the vicinity of the frequency that produces the optimum response. At lower and higher frequencies, the extent of displacement *is* linear. That is, it is proportional to sound level.

We must remember that, while Békésy was conducting his research, visual observations of basilar membrane displacement were necessary, and, as a result, the observations and measurements were made at extremely high sound levels.

There appeared to be a great disparity between the actual frequency discrimination abilities of a listener and Békésy's traveling wave analysis. Improved measuring techniques have resulted in observations and measurements being made at lower and lower sound intensity levels. One extremely important outcome of these refined observation techniques was that the sharpness of basilar membrane tuning increased at lower and lower sound levels and seems to be optimal at a level comparable with that of quiet conversation. *Sharpness of tuning decreases with an increase in the level of sound intensity*. A second finding relates to the condition of the experimental animal (Khanna and Leonard, 1982). Nonlinearity and responses at low sound intensity levels are possible only in extremely healthy experimental animals. Nonlinearity and fine tuning in the cochlea cannot be observed in the cadaver cochlea, in drained cochleas, in models, or in poorly adapted experimental animals, and this in large part explains the disparity between early and contemporary findings.

The theories of hearing, as we have seen, are essentially based on passive mechanisms. In none of the early theories of hearing is the topic of hair cell and supportive cell maintenance ever considered. The phenomenal fine tuning in the cochlea, and the nonlinearity, strongly imply something in addition to a purely passive and mechanical system. Is there some additional metabolic energy being utilized, and, if so, what is its source? Some investigators strongly support the idea that an active-energy producing mechanism is in part responsible for the mechanical tuning (Kim, 1986). Certain experimental findings almost demand an active metabolic process along the cochlear partition. One such observation is that when brief sound stimuli cease, echoes in the ear canal can be detected. In fact, some subjects (experimental animals, including humans) produce spontaneous emissions of sounds (Zurek, 1981). It is entirely possible that the very processes that produce echoes and emissions from the ear are related to the same mechanisms that result in the sharp tuning of the cochlea. Dallos (1988) states, "Probably the most straightforward means of producing the required sensitivity is to generate a force upon the [cochlear] partition in a direction and with proper timing so as to boost the ongoing movement. Thus the presence of some motor elements within the cochlear partition seems to be required, and the most likely candidate for the role of motor element is the outer hair cell. What structural basis, if any, exists for the notion that the outer hair cell operates as a motor?"

The Role of the Outer Hair Cells   The outer hair cells outnumber the inner hair cells by about 3 to 1, and yet only the inner hair cells seem to generate the responses recorded on the auditory nerve. The outer hair cells are thought to be responsible for the **cochlear microphonic,** but is that their only role?

In addition to the differences in the number of nerve fibers that are supplied by the inner and outer hair cells (95 percent compared with 5 percent), certain structural differences between the two types of cells suggest that the outer hair cells are candidates for a motor element on the cochlear partition. The outer hair cells seem to be capable of storing calcium, which is necessary for either secretory or contractile activity in cells. Also, the apex of the outer hair cells (the cuticular plate) has been found to contain a number of proteins associated with active contractile cells. The proteins include actin and myosin, tropomyosin, and fibrin and alpha-actin. Some of these same proteins are found in the stereocilia of the outer hair cells. Indeed, outer hair cells have been shown to be mechanically active. They are capable of shortening and

lengthening (Brownell, 1983). This electromotility is very rapid, occurring at frequencies as high as the limits of hearing (Dallos, Evans, and Hallworth, 1991; Kalinec, et al, 1992).

Just how outer hair cell motility impacts the motion of the cochlear partition is not known, but recall that the stereocilia of the outer hair cells are imbedded in the tectorial membrane. If a number of outer hair cells move in concert it is entirely possible that the combined movement can influence the motion of the tectorial membrane and thus influence the streaming of the endolymph to the inner hair cells (Iwasa and Chadwick, 1992).

One method for studying the role of outer hair cells is to selectively destroy them. Certain antibiotics, when administered carefully, have been found to destroy outer hair cells before they destroy the inner hair cells.

In 1957 a water-soluble antibiotic **kanamycin** was first isolated and used in the treatment of a certain type of tuberculosis. It is also **ototoxic** and destroys outer hair cells, leaving the inner hair cells normal (presumably). When this happens, the auditory nerve tuning curve shows a marked loss of sensitivity. *The most widely accepted hypothesis is that the outer hair cells somehow increase the sensitivity of the auditory nerve fibers.* Some researchers feel the interaction between the inner and outer hair cells is electrical, others think it is mechanical, while others suspect it to be neural.

In addition, when the outer hair cells are destroyed, the fine-tuning characteristics of the cochlea are reduced or eliminated. Also, many of the nonlinear effects found in the normal ear disappear when the outer hair cells are destroyed (Dallos, Harris, Relkin, and Cheatham, 1980).

Responses from the Auditory Nerve   When a microelectrode is placed into the cochlear nerve, the recordings obtained are from nerve action potentials of a single neural unit. We find, first, that any single neuron has a certain amount of spontaneous activity, and discharges occur presumably in the absence of sound (whatever that means) at rates from a few per minute to almost a hundred discharges per second. About 25 percent of the afferent fibers have spontaneous discharges at a rate less than 20 per second. The remaining fibers discharge between 60 and 80 times per second.

Once the **spontaneous discharge rate** has been determined for a single neural element, we are in a position to find its **threshold,** that is, the minimal stimulus level that produces an increase in the discharge rate, above the spontaneous rate. Suppose, for example, the spontaneous rate of a particular neuron is 10 per second, and our goal is to determine its threshold to 2000 Hz tone. We increase the sound intensity of 2000 Hz tone until an increase in the discharge rate, above the spontaneous rate, is just detected. Further increases in sound intensity result in an increase in discharge rate, as shown by the input-output graph in Figure 6-120. Note that the discharge rate levels off at a certain intensity level and remains fairly constant even though the level of the stimulus is increased. The discharge rate for this neuron increased from its spontaneous rate to almost 100 discharges per second, over a sound level range of from 40 to 80 dB SPL (its **dynamic range**).

We have seen that, except for the highest frequencies, a sound will cause a **displacement pattern** that is distributed over a large portion of the basilar membrane. We should not be surprised to see that any given nerve fiber will respond to a wide range of frequencies. If we attempt to determine the threshold of response of our single neural unit over a range of frequencies, we obtain a **tuning curve** for that neuron, and what we find is that each neuron examined will respond best to a specific frequency. This is reasonable since 90 to 95 percent of the afferent nerve fibers synapse directly with the inner hair cells. As with the inner hair cells, each neuron has its own **characteristic frequency.** As shown in Figure 6-121, a neuron responds to a wide range of frequencies, but best to a specific frequency. Note the low-frequency tail on the lower two curves, indicating that each neuron responds better to frequencies below its characteristic frequency than it does to frequencies above it. A single neural unit with a characteristic frequency below 1000 Hz will usually discharge once per cycle, and in addition, the **neural spikes** appear to have a certain constant phase relationship to the stimulus. This is illustrated in Figure 6-122. In both instances the single unit response is phase related to the stimulus, a response that is called **phase-locked.** Is phase-locking preserved as frequency is increased beyond the response limit for any single neural unit?

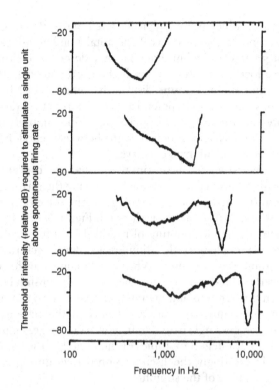

FIGURE 6-121

Tuning curves for single units with different characteristic frequencies.

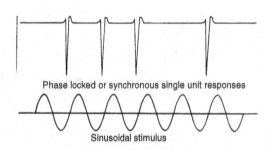

FIGURE 6-122

Illustration of synchronous single neuron responses to a low-frequency stimulus. Top tracing represents the firing pattern of a single neuron while the bottom tracing represents a sinusoidal stimulus. (After W. Yost and D. Nielsen, *Fundamentals of Hearing,* Holt, Rinehart and Winston, New York, 1985.)

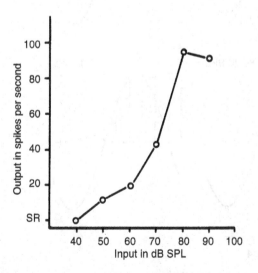

FIGURE 6-120

Input-output function for a single neuron. Output is graphed as discharges per second, as a function of sound pressure level.

Nerve responses can be graphed by means of a **post-stimulus time histogram.** To generate one, a stimulus is presented repeatedly and the occurrence of each action potential is plotted on the histogram by adding the time of arrival of a discharge to a column or bin, relative to time after the onset of the stimulus. Bursts of tone produce an initial burst of discharges followed by a decrease in discharge frequency, which is maintained for the duration of the tone. When the tone burst is turned off, the frequency of discharges drops to zero or near zero after which the spontaneous rate returns. Poststimulus time histograms reveal the total number of discharges at a "point" in time, but they do not reveal the phase-locked synchrony of the discharges (Figure 6-123).

Interval histograms display the time interval between successive spike potentials. The *Y* axis of the graph represents the number of discharges within an interval, while the *X* axis represents the time between neural discharges or the interspike interval.

Phase-locked poststimulus time histograms provide additional information by showing the relationship of the arrival of the discharge to the waveform of the stimulus. An example is shown in Figure 6-124. It is essential that the counting of neural discharges begins at the same phase of the stimulus waveform each time the stimulus is presented. When the stimulus waveform is overlaid on the histogram, the phase relationship between the stimulus and neural discharge pattern can be seen. As frequency is increased beyond the response limits for any single neural unit, neural discharges begin to occur at integral multiples of the period of the stimulus. Interestingly, the discharges only occur during the positive phase of the stimulus.

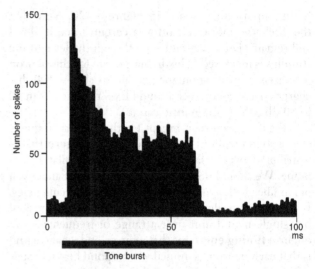

FIGURE 6-123

A poststimulus time histogram. It was made by presenting tone pips many times and incrementing the count at the corresponding point on the histogram whenever an action potential occurred. (From *Discharge Patterns of Single Fibers in the Cat's Auditory Nerve* by N. Y.-S. Kiang, et al., by permission of the M.I.T. Press, Cambridge, Mass., 1965.)

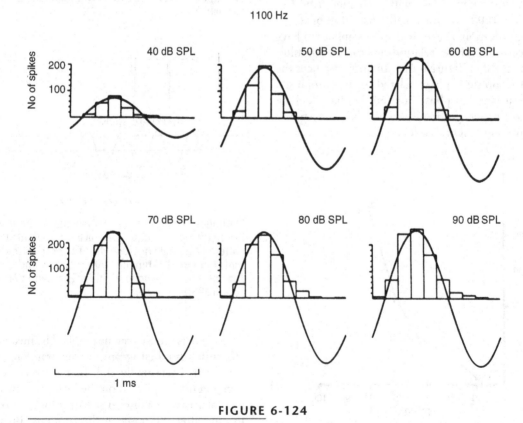

FIGURE 6-124

Period histograms of a fiber activated by a low-frequency tone indicated that the neuron spikes are evoked in only one-half of the cycle. The histograms have been fitted with a sinusoid of the best fitting amplitude, but fixed phase. Note that although the number of spikes increases little above 70 dB sound pressure level, meaning that the firing is saturated, the histogram still follows the sinusoid without a tendency to square or clip. (From Rose et al., 1971.)

The auditory nerve retains the frequency selectivity found along the basilar membrane and in the inner hair cells. The filtering effect of the basilar membrane may be augmented by the hair cells and again by the auditory nerve. This suggests a series of low-pass or band-pass filters that sharpen the tuning of the ear.

The Nerve Supply to the Cochlea

Communication between the peripheral receptor organ of the ear and the central organ, the brain, is established by means of the **auditory** or **eighth (VIII) cranial nerve.** Although the auditory nerve is relatively thick, it contains a surprisingly small number of nerve fibers, about 50,000 in the cat and 30,000 in the human. Upon entering the internal auditory meatus, the auditory nerve abruptly divides into a **vestibular branch** and a **cochlear branch.**

Three innervation components of the cochlea are known. The first and numerically the most important component consists of **afferent bipolar cochlear sensory neurons.** About 95 percent of the spiral ganglion neurons are bipolar and are completely myelinated (including the cell body). They are referred to as **Type I cells.** These cells supply exclusively the inner hair cells. The remaining 5 percent are unmyelinated monopolar neurons and are called **Type II cells.** They supply the outer hair cells.

The second neural component consists of **efferent neurons.** In the cat there are about 1800 fibers, sometimes called **centrifugal,** that arise in the superior olivary complex of the brain stem (to be discussed later).

The third component consists of an **autonomic nerve supply** which probably originates in the superior cervical ganglion and most likely does not enter the spiral organ.

The Afferent Nerve Supply

The cell bodies of the bipolar afferent neurons that supply the hair cells of the cochlea are located within a canal (of Rosenthal) in the modiolus, where they form a long **spiral ganglion.** When the cochlea is seen in a plane parallel to the axis of the modiolus, as in Figure 6-125, the

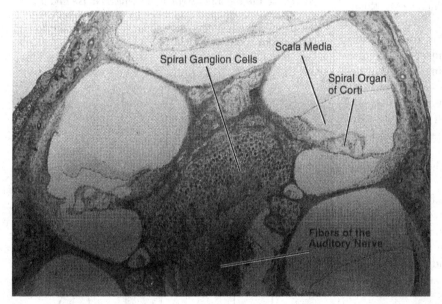

Spiral Ganglion Cells

Scala Media

Spiral Organ of Corti

Fibers of the Auditory Nerve

FIGURE 6-125

Midmodiolar section through cochlea illustrating the spiral ganglion.

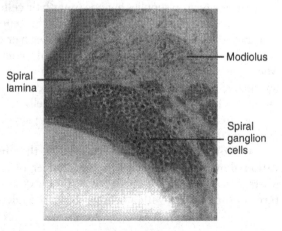

Spiral lamina

Modiolus

Spiral ganglion cells

spiral ganglion is easily identified as an aggregate of nerve cell bodies located near each osseous spiral lamina. The **ganglion cells** are apparently not evenly distributed in the canal. Fewer cells are found in the apical and basal turns than are found in the middle turn.

Each nerve cell body gives rise to two processes, a **central axonal extension** that terminates in the cochlear nucleus of the brain stem and a **peripheral dendritic extension** that terminates at the bases of the hair cells. The endings of the peripheral fibers are small granular enlargements of the dendrite. They reach the basal region of the hair cell body and form typical (about 150 Å wide) **synaptic clefts.** Within the hair cell body, in the region of the synapse, can be seen characteristic presynaptic structures such as **synaptic bars** (Smith and Sjöstrand, 1961) and typical **synaptic vesicles.** The junction between the hair cell bodies and the afferent nerve endings have the form of typical chemically mediated synapses, but the neurotransmitter is not known with certainty. There is, however, some evidence that glutamate, an excitatory neurotransmitter, is the hair cell transmitter. Glutamate receptors have been found in the neurons of the spiral ganglion that contact the inner hair cells (Kuriyama, Albin, and Altschuler, 1993; Ryan, Brumm, and Kraft, 1991).

The processes and cell body of the **spiral ganglion** cells possess a myelin sheath. For the most part the peripheral fibers pass in small bundles, in a direction radial to the axis of the modiolus, through numerous channels between the plates of the spiral lamina, and enter the spiral organ through small perforations on the spiral lamina **(habenula perforata),** where they abruptly shed their myelin. About 30 bare nerve fibers enter the spiral organ through each channel in the habenula perforata. These *naked nerve fibers* can be divided, largely by virtue of their distribution to the hair cells, into two main groups. About 90 percent of these afferent fibers constitute the **radial bundles.** As shown in Figure 6-126, these fibers course from their point of emergence into the cochlear duct in small bundles and, without much deviation, proceed directly to the nearest inner hair cells.

Any one neuron supplies but one **inner hair cell,** but any single hair cell is supplied by about eight neurons. This orderly distribution means that the inner hair cells are represented point for point in the cochlear nuclei, where the central processes or axons of the ganglion cells terminate. This **tonotopographical arrangement** tells us that the basilar membrane, the inner hair cells, and the neurons that supply them constitute a *frequency-dependent sensory system.*

As shown in the graph of Figure 6-127, the **innervation density,** as measured by the number of nerve fibers, is greatest in the upper-basal and lower-middle turns of the cochlea, with a definite decrease in density

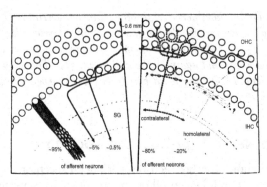

FIGURE 6-126

Schematic of the innervation pattern of the spiral organ (cat). On the left is shown the innervation pattern for the afferent nerve supply. About 95 percent of the afferent fibers are radial fibers and supply only the inner hair cells (**IHC**). The remaining 5 percent of the afferents are the outer spiral fibers which supply outer hair cells (**OHC**) . Each outer spiral afferent fiber supplies about ten outer hair cells in a direction basal to the point of their emergence through the habenula perforata. The efferent innervation pattern is shown on the right. About 80 percent of the efferents are tunnel radial fibers and are crossed. They innervate the outer hair cells. The remaining 20 percent of the efferent fibers are uncrossed and constitute the inner spiral fibers which course under the inner hair cells but are thought not to synapse directly with the bases of the hair cells. Also noted is the spiral ganglion (**SG**). (From Spoendlin, 1974.)

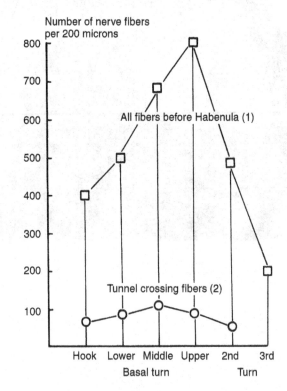

FIGURE 6-127

Nerve fiber density in different turns of the cochlea, at the level of the habenula (1) and at the level of the inner tunnel (2). Afferent plus efferent fibers. (After Spoendlin, 1966.)

of nerve fibers at either end of the cochlea (Guild et al., 1931; Wever, 1949; Spoendlin, 1974).

The course of the remaining 5 to 10 percent of the afferent (Type II) fibers is to the outer hair cells exclusively. They pass between the inner rods or pillar cells, just a few fibers between each cell, cross along the floor of the tunnel of Corti in a radial direction, emerge between the cells of the outer rods, and then turn abruptly and course basally in a longitudinal direction as the **external** or **outer spiral bundle.**

The individual outer spiral fibers give off numerous **secondary** and **tertiary collaterals** that terminate as minute swellings on the sides and bases of about 10 outer hair cells. The arborization and distribution of the collateral afferent fibers is always toward the basal end of the cochlea, along the full extent of the basilar membrane (Figure 6-126). In this way, then, each outer hair cell is innervated by collaterals from many outer spiral bundle fibers, and so theirs is a *diffuse innervation pattern* as compared to the essentially one-to-one pattern of the inner hair cells.

As noted earlier, Type II cells are unmyelinated and they do not seem to possess a central process. A significant difference between the Type I and Type II neurons is their susceptibility to oxygen deficit **(hypoxia).** Type I afferents begin to degenerate after short periods of hypoxia, whereas the Type II cells remain unchanged in numbers and appearance for more than a year (Spoendlin, 1974).

The Efferent Nerve Supply

An **efferent** or **centrifugal pathway** has been known since the end of the nineteenth century (see Held, 1926). Interest in the centrifugal pathway grew with the description by Rasmussen in 1946, of an **olivocochlear bundle,** which courses from the superior olivary complex in the brain stem to the hair cells. There are about 1800 centrifugal fibers in the cat, about 1200 of which are uncrossed. They arise from the superior olive on the same side and form the **uncrossed** olivocochlear bundle. The remaining fibers are from the opposite superior olivary complex and form the **crossed** olivocochlear bundle.

The uncrossed centrifugal fibers that enter the spiral organ form the **inner spiral bundle** which courses immediately beneath the inner hair cells. These fibers synapse with **afferent terminal boutons** on the inner hair cells and rarely do these efferent fibers synapse with the hair cell body.

Crossed centrifugal fibers form the **tunnel radial fibers** which course between the pillar cells and ramify considerably prior to their synapse at the base of outer hair cells. The supply of efferent tunnel radial fibers to the outer hair cells is the most dense in the basal region and least dense apically. This is just opposite to the dis-

tribution of the fibers of the inner spiral bundle, which is most dense at the apical end and has virtually no fibers basally.

The large bulbous nerve endings of the efferent fibers differ from the nerve endings of the afferent fibers, a feature that makes their identification possible. In addition, the **terminal endings** of the efferent fibers which supply the outer hair cells are considerably different from those that supply the inner hair cells. As shown schematically in Figure 6-128, the efferent endings on the outer hair cells are a typical synapse, terminating directly on the base of the hair cell, and separated from it only by the synaptic cleft. Hair cells that receive both afferent and efferent nerve fibers are called **Type A cells,** while those which receive afferent endings only are called **Type B cells.** Type A outer hair cells predominate in the basal end of the cochlea and Type B toward the apex.

The efferent fibers that compromise the **inner spiral bundle** (the uncrossed fibers) synapse, not with the hair cell body directly, but rather, terminate as large bulbous endings on the **afferent nerve endings,** below the inner hair cells. These two different types of endings, which are illustrated in Figure 6-128, have important implications. First, the efferent nerve endings in contact with the bases of the outer hair cells occupy a much larger area than the afferent fibers, and in the basal turn (high-frequency end), they completely dominate the region around the bases of the cells. Second, the distribution of the efferent fibers on the outer hair cells heavily favors the basal or high-frequency end of the basilar membrane. Third, because of the way the uncrossed efferent fibers terminate on the afferent dendrites, and not on the inner hair cell body, the influence of efferent nerve fibers can be expected to affect afferent nerve activity and not the activity of the hair cell itself. As Spoendlin (1974) says, "We would therefore expect the

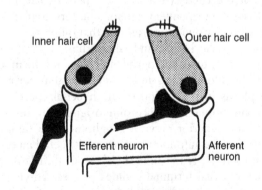

FIGURE 6-128

Schematic of afferent (white) and efferent (black) synapses with inner and outer hair cells. Both afferents and efferents synapse directly with the bases of the outer hair cells, but the efferents synapse below the inner hair cells.

influence of the efferents to be presynaptic directly on the outer hair cells and postsynaptic on the afferent dendrites from the inner hair cells."

Spoendlin's description of the nerve supply, especially of the 90 to 95 percent of the afferent fibers that supply the inner hair cells, was not well received initially, but in recent years has gained widespread acceptance. Many of his experiments have been replicated by other researchers and with supportive results. Often, the nerve count experiments have been conducted by surgically severing the nerve tract (axotomy) which induces degeneration that is observable microscopically. Other experimenters have injected tracers into the nerve tract. Some tracers have been radioactive, and when the tissues are exposed to photographic film, they expose the emulsion to produce **cochlear autoradiographs.** Warr (1975), employing these tracers, has found between 1700 and 1800 cochlear efferent neurons. About 60 percent of the neurons were uncrossed. He also found that the lateral region of the superior olivary complex projects fibers to the inner hair cells of both sides, whereas the medial region of the superior olivary complex projects to the region of the outer hair cells of both sides. This suggests that the *efferent innervation is organized according to the cells of origin in the brain stem rather than as crossed or uncrossed fiber bundles.*

The **neurotransmitter** for the olivocochlear bundle is acetylcholine, and its **inhibitor** is acetylcholinesterase. The effects of stimulation of the olivocochlear bundle can be blocked by the muscarinic and nicotinic cholinergic blockers.

The Autonomic Nerve Supply

Fibers from the sympathetic branch of the autonomic nervous system have been shown to reach the cochlea, but there is no evidence they enter the spiral organ. Histochemical studies reveal that the adrenergic innervation[10] of the cochlea consists of a perivascular and a blood-vessel–independent system. The perivascular network is found around the arterioles that supply the cochlea, such as the basilar and labyrinthine arteries, but does not seem to extend peripherally beyond the modiolus. The blood-vessel–independent system forms a loose plexus in the region of the habenula perforata. These autonomic fibers probably originate in the stellate or the superior cervical ganglion. Some findings suggest that the autonomic nerve activity could increase the ear's sensitivity to sound (Beickert, et al., 1956), but as yet the actual terminal endings of these adrenergic fibers have not been found. It is not known, for exam-

ple, if they form actual synaptic connections with the afferent or efferent nerve fibers of the ear.

Summary

Three types of nerve fibers supply the cochlea: about 30,000 afferent fibers, 1800 efferent fibers of the olivocochlear bundle, and an obscure plexus of sympathetic fibers.

The cell bodies of the **afferent** nerve fibers are located in the spiral canal (of Rosenthal) where they form the **spiral ganglion.** About 90 percent are **radial fibers** which course without arborization to the nearest inner hair cells. Each inner hair cell is supplied by about 8 radial fibers in point-for-point distribution patterns. The remaining 10 percent of the afferent fibers cross the spiral organ to the region of the outer hair cells as the **outer spiral bundle.** The fibers turn toward the basal end and, after extensive arborization, synapse with outer hair cells. Each fiber in the outer spiral bundle innervates about 10 outer hair cells, predominately in the basal or high-frequency end of the cochlea.

About 1800 **efferent (centrifugal)** nerve fibers constitute the **olivocochlear bundle.** Approximately 80 percent of these fibers originate in the contralateral superior olivary complex and are known as **crossed fibers,** while the remaining 20 percent arise from the ipsilateral superior olivary complex and are known as **uncrossed fibers.** The fibers of the crossed bundle ramify considerably, and they course through the tunnel of Corti as **tunnel radial fibers.** By means of a large number of collaterals, they supply a number of outer hair cells, especially in the basal turn.

The uncrossed efferent fibers form the **inner spiral bundle.** After considerable arborization, they supply all 3500 inner hair cells. Their multiple innervation is most extensive apically. The efferent fibers that supply the outer hair cells (tunnel radial fibers) synapse at the base of the hair cell, but in the region of the inner hair cell, the synapses are on the dendrites of the afferent fibers.

Fibers from the **sympathetic** division of the autonomic nervous system also reach the cochlea, but apparently do not enter the spiral organ. Activity of these fibers probably contributes to the homeostasis of the hearing mechanism.

The Role of the Efferent System

Two questions can be raised regarding the function of the **efferent** or **olivocochlear tract.** Does the efferent system affect the sound-transformation function of the cochlea, and is there a reciprocal effect of the two cochleae upon each other? Galambos (1956c) demonstrated that *stimulation of one ear inhibits the nerve impulses generated by the opposite ear,* when the latter is stimulated

---

[10]**Adrenergic innervation** refers to sympathetic nerve fibers which liberate norepinephrine at a synapse when a nerve impulse passes.

simultaneously or with a short delay. In addition, *electrical stimulation of the efferent pathways inhibits electrical activity of the auditory nerve.*

Stimulation of the **crossed olivocochlear bundle** results in a decrease in discharge rates of afferent single neural units, a reduction in the endolymphatic potential in the first turn, and an increase in the cochlear microphonic in the first turn. Stimulation of the **uncrossed bundles** produces inhibition of neural responses but no change in the cochlear microphonic.

The exact nature of the function of the efferent system is not known, but stimulation at various levels of the efferent pathway produces **inhibitory effects,** for the most part. In general, research findings suggest the principal effect produced by activation of the efferent tract is inhibitory. The olivocochlear tract is shown in Figure 6-129.

The Ascending Auditory Pathway

The neurons comprising the auditory pathway do not course uninterruptedly through the brain stem and then on to the auditory cortex of the cerebrum. Rather, there is a succession of at least four neurons between the cochlea and cerebral cortex. Those at the level of the spiral ganglion are called **first-order neurons.** They all terminate in the cochlear nuclei where they synapse with **second-order neurons,** while the nerve fibers that originate with the next synapse are called **third-order neurons,** and so on, to the cortical level.

The **major tracts** of the ascending auditory pathway are shown schematically in Figure 6-130. The word *major* is emphasized because to examine all the collateral pathways, reflex mediating nuclei, reticular formation, and so forth, which are activated by stimulation of the spiral organ, would be a monumental task.

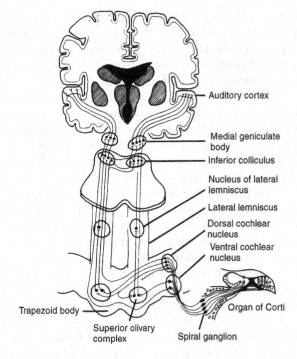

FIGURE 6-130

The major components of the ascending auditory pathway.

The central processes of the spiral ganglion cells pass to the core of the modiolus where they form the **cochlear branch** of the auditory nerve. The most apical fibers follow a straight course and form the core of the nerve, while the basal fibers are added in a twisted fashion to form the periphery of the nerve. The reason for the *twisted feature* seems to be due to the way the ear develops embryologically. The nerve evidently appears rather well developed before the cochlea begins to form. The cochlea begins to develop at the basal end and grows in a spiral fashion toward the apex. As growth progresses, the neural elements are "dragged" along, so that when the structure is completed, the basal fibers have twisted around the apical fibers, and the whole nerve takes on a gross appearance not unlike that of a piece of manila rope. Because of the anatomical architecture of the cochlear nerve, the *high-frequency fibers are the most exposed* and subjected to trauma, while the more essential (for speech reception) *lower-frequency fibers are somewhat protected.*

As the cochlear nerve enters the internal auditory meatus, it is joined by the two divisions of the vestibular nerve to complete the **auditory nerve,** which lies in close proximity to the facial nerve. The auditory nerve is quite short, only about 5 mm in length. It enters the medulla oblongata laterally at the level of the lower pons, where the **cochlear bundle** courses directly to the cochlear nucleus where it divides into two branches. One branch descends to the dorsal part of the nucleus

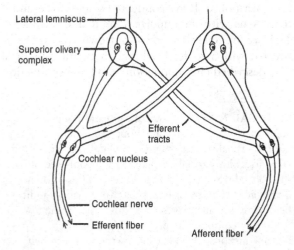

FIGURE 6-129

Highly schematized olivocochlear tract.

(dorsal cochlear nucleus), sometimes referred to as the **acoustic tubercle,** while the other ascends to the **ventral** (or ventral part of the) **cochlear nucleus.** The fibers of both branches terminate in synapses with second-order neurons of the cochlear nuclei.

About half the cell bodies of the second-order neurons send axon fibers across the median plane through the **trapezoid body,** where some terminate by means of synapses with cells in other bulbar nuclei, mainly the **superior olivary complex,** which is located at the same level as, but somewhat lateral to, the trapezoid body.

This *decussation of the nerve fibers* at the level of the cochlear nuclei has important implications. Since about half the fibers from one ear course directly upward from a cochlear nucleus, while the remainder cross over the midline to the cochlear nucleus on the opposite side, nerve impulses from each ear reach both the left and right temporal lobes of the auditory cortex of the brain. For this reason, *destruction of the nerve pathway on one side does not result in complete deafness for the corresponding ear.* The mechanism is reciprocal, as illustrated in Figure 6-130.

The superior olivary complex gives rise to third-order neurons that course upward, forming a tract known as the **lateral lemniscus.** These third-order neurons are accompanied by second-order neurons that pass uninterruptedly through the superior olivary complex. The lateral lemniscus also contains a nucleus, and it forms the point of synapse for some second- and third-order neurons, while other neurons pass uninterrupted from the lenticular nucleus to the inferior colliculus of the midbrain, where synapses may once again take place.

Also, at the level of the inferior colliculus, fibers decussate from one side to the other, through what is called the **commissure of the inferior colliculus.** The inferior colliculus, also known as the inferior quadrigeminal body, contains centers for reflex responses to sound. A few fibers continue through the inferior colliculus to the **medial geniculate body,** which is the thalamic nucleus of the auditory pathway. Most of the fibers of the lateral lemniscus, however, terminate at the medial geniculate body, where they synapse with third- and fourth-order neurons whose axons course through the sublenticular portion of the internal capsule and terminate in the **anterior transverse temporal (Herschel's) gyrus.**

There is good evidence for an orderly correspondence between the cochlea and the **acoustic projection** on the cerebral cortex. The arrangement of the cells within the medial geniculate body and of the fibers that radiate to the cortex is also orderly and predictable, and the tonotopographical arrangement is maintained.

We have seen that the **basilar membrane** is a frequency-selective device with low frequencies causing maximum displacement at the apex and high frequencies causing displacement basally. We have also seen that 90 to 95 percent of the afferent nerve fibers are distributed

in a point-to-point manner to the inner hair cells. Thus, *a frequency-related spatial distribution of receptor and neural elements exists at the very periphery of the auditory nerve pathway.* The question that comes to mind is whether this tonotopographical organization is retained throughout the auditory pathway. The answer is yes.

The picture is not categorical in humans, but tonotopographical organization is quite evident in cats, for example, at the level of the cochlear nuclei, the inferior colliculus, and medial geniculate bodies. The cochlear nuclei have been thoroughly mapped (they are quite accessible), and the individual cochlear nerve fibers are distributed to one of three regions within it. The experimental results are consistent, to the extent that **anteroventral, posteroventral,** and **dorsal cochlear nuclei** and their divisions represent the basilar membrane from base to apex (Figure 6-131). The specificity of this tonotopographical organization is reduced at the cortical level, however. That is, *the tonotopography is more diffuse at the cortical level* than it is in the nuclei and tracts of the ascending pathway. This suggests that the frequency analysis is completed at the lower levels and that the **auditory cortex** is more of an integrative center. A projection of the cochlea onto the temporal lobe is shown in Figure 6-132.

Bone Conduction

So far we have been discussing what is referred to as hearing by air conduction. Another avenue by which we hear sounds is **bone** or **tissue conduction.** Whenever there is direct physical contact between the skull and a vibrating body or when airborne sounds are intense enough, the vibratory energy produces compressions in the skull bones and, as a consequence, disturbances in the ossicular chain and the inner ear.

The importance of hearing by bone conduction is often overlooked. Bone-conducted sound, for example, provides us with an important **feedback** channel by which we are able to monitor our own voices. We are provided with two feedback channels, the system already described (air conduction) and bone conduction.

CLINICAL NOTE: Both the air- and bone-conducted feedback stimulate our ears when we speak, but only the airborne sound stimulates the ears of our auditors. This partially explains why people are often so shocked when they first hear recordings of their own voices. The recording apparatus or other auditor hears only the airborne sounds, and since some low-frequency components produced by the larynx do not become airborne, we hear our own voices as much more powerful and "full" sounding than they appear through a recording system.

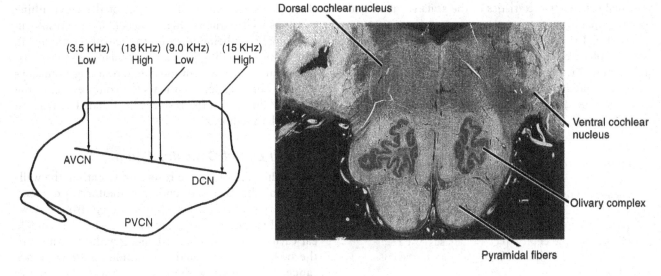

FIGURE 6-131

Tonotopographic organization of the cochlear nucleus of a cat (left). When the nucleus is penetrated with an electrode along the line shown in the illustration, two separate high-low sequences are seen. On the right is a transverse section through the rostral end of a human medulla oblongata. The dorsal and ventral cochlear nuclei and olivary nuclei are identified.

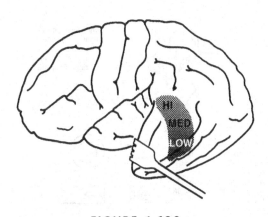

FIGURE 6-132

Schematic projection of cochlea on the temporal lobe, illustrating the preservation of the tonotopographic organization. The temporal lobe has been reflected downward to expose its superior surface.

Other factors, such as phase differences between air- and bone-conducted sounds, and differences in time of arrival to the ear, help augment the differences we detect in hearing our voices "live" and recorded.

When investigation of the bone conduction mechanism was first initiated, it was thought that the pattern of vibration on the basilar membrane was different from that for air conduction. Békésy (1932) found, however, that a tone presented by bone conduction could be so completely canceled by airborne sound, 180° out of phase, that no sound is heard. This means that the vibratory patterns on the basilar membrane for airborne and bone-conducted sounds are the same. The mechanisms by which the disturbances on the basilar membrane are caused are quite different, however. Research suggests three avenues by which bone-conducted sounds result in basilar membrane displacement.

Displacements of the Skull

If a vibrating body is brought into contact with the skull, the bones undergo various types of vibratory patterns (Figure 6-133). These displacements of the skull cause compressions of the fluid within the membranous labyrinth. Basilar membrane displacement is dependent upon

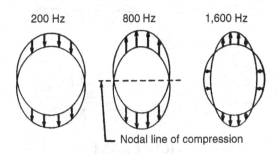

FIGURE 6-133

Illustration of the modes of vibration of the skull bones at various frequencies.

unequal elastic characteristics of the scala vestibuli and scala tympani.

Rejto (1914) and Herzog (1930) pointed out that if the compliance were equal above and below the basilar membrane, the pressures in the scala vestibuli and scala tympani would be the same and the basilar membrane would not be deformed. Occasionally such a condition arises.

CLINICAL NOTE: **Abnormal bone growths** that occlude both the oval and round windows (advanced otosclerosis) or **exudate** with or without accompanying pressure changes may hinder movement of both the round window membrane and the stapes footplate, and although the clinical picture may suggest a sensorineural loss, the problem actually lies in the conduction pathway.

The compliance in the scala tympani is greater than it is in the scala vestibuli, and compression of the cochlear fluids results in a differential pressure between them. Consequently, the basilar membrane is displaced into the scala tympani when positive pressure is being generated, and is displaced into the scala vestibuli when negative pressure is being generated. This is illustrated in Figure 6-134. Since the cochlear ducts are continuous with those of the labyrinth, displacement of the skull bones produces compression of the labyrinthine canals as well as the cochlear ducts (A). This results in additional fluid being forced into the scala vestibuli (B), with a corresponding increase in basilar membrane displacement, (C). The additional fluid resulting from labyrinthine compression augments the compression of the cochlear fluids, and the result is heightened activity on the basilar membrane.

Inertial Lag of Ossicular Chain

When the temporal bone is set into vibration, the walls of the middle ear cavity undergo vibratory movement. The inertia of the ossicles prevents them from following skull vibration; as a consequence, while the middle ear cavity is moving outward, along with the inner ear, the ossicles remain relatively motionless (**mass reactance**). Mechanically, the effect is exactly the same as when the temporal bone remains at rest while the ossicular chain moves in. This inertial effect augments the compression that takes place within the cochlear scalae. Bone conduction due to inertial lag of the ossicular chain is illustrated in Figure 6-135.

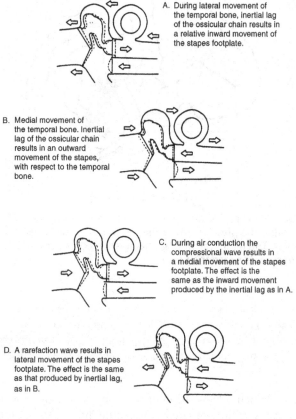

A. During lateral movement of the temporal bone, inertial lag of the ossicular chain results in a relative inward movement of the stapes footplate.

B. Medial movement of the temporal bone. Inertial lag of the ossicular chain results in an outward movement of the stapes, with respect to the temporal bone.

C. During air conduction the compressional wave results in a medial movement of the stapes footplate. The effect is the same as the inward movement produced by the inertial lag as in A.

D. A rarefaction wave results in lateral movement of the stapes footplate. The effect is the same as that produced by inertial lag, as in B.

FIGURE 6-135

Bone conduction produced by inertial lag of the ossicular chain.

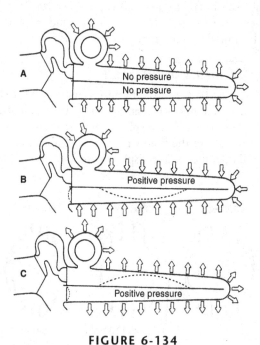

FIGURE 6-134

Schematic of cochlea illustrating displacement of the basilar membrane under conditions of greater compliance in the scala tympani.

Occlusion Effect

A third route by which bone-conducted sounds may be heard results from the nature of the **temporomandibular joint,** shown schematically in Figure 6-136. If a finger is inserted into the **external auditory meatus** while the mandible is being moved, slight displacements in the ear canal wall may be felt. When the bones of the skull are driven by a vibrator, the lower jaw does not follow exactly but lags behind due to its inertia. The mandibular condyle is vibrating at the same frequency as, but out of phase with, the remainder of the skull bones. This results in displacements, at the vibratory rate, of the cartilaginous skeleton of the auditory meatus. Such displacements cause airborne sounds to be generated within the ear canal. These sounds follow the conventional air conduction route. By stopping the ear canal, there arise variations in air pressure that act upon the drum membrane, and the sensation is one of increased loudness. This is easily demonstrated. Simply hum a tone while alternately opening and closing off the external meatus. Note the increase and decrease in the loudness sensation. This is known as the **occlusion effect,** first described by Wheatstone in 1827; it forms part of the basis for the **Weber test** in clinical audiometry. It is important to note, however, that the occlusion effect is confined to frequencies below about 2000 Hz.

This introduction to hearing by no means completes the picture, but it can provide sufficient background information to permit students to pursue some of the important behavioral aspects of hearing that belong to the domain of **psychoacoustics.** They include threshold detection; pitch, loudness, and speech discrimination; masking and distortion effects; and spatial localization.

Hopefully, the contents of this chapter will also have served to sharpen the readers' appetites and to send them in full pursuit of some of their own prodding questions about the exquisite mechanism we call the ear.

BIBLIOGRAPHY AND READING LIST

Adrian, E. D., "The Microphonic Action of the Cochlea: An Interpretation of Wever and Bray's Experiments," *J. Physiol.,* 71, 1931, 28–30.

——, and Y. Zotterman, "The Impulses Produced by Sensory Nerve Endings, Part 2. The Response of a Single End-Organ," *J. Physiol.,* 61, 1926a, 151–171.

——, and Y. Zotterman, "The Impulses Produced by Sensory Nerve Endings, Part 3, Impulses Set Up by Touch and Pressure," *J. Physiol.,* 61, 1926b, 465–483.

Angleborg, C., and H. Engström, "The Normal Organ of Corti," in A. Møller, ed., *Basic Mechanisms in Hearing.* New York: Academic Press, 1973.

Arey, L. B., *Developmental Anatomy,* 7th ed. Philadelphia: W. B. Saunders, 1965.

Beickert, P., L. Gisselsson, and B. Lofström, "Der Einfluss des Sympathischen Nervensystems auf das Innenohr," *Arch. Klin. Exp. Ohr.-Nas.-, Kehlk.-Heilk.* 168, 1956, 495–507.

Békésy, G. von, "Zur Theorie des Hörens. Die Schwingungsform der Basilarmembran," *Physik. Zeitschrift,* 29, 1928, 793–810.

——, "Zur Theorie des Hörens, Über die eben merkbare Amplituden-und-Frequenzänderung eines Tones. Die Theorie der Schwebungen," *Physik. Zeitschrift,* 30, 1929, 721–745.

——, "Zur Theorie des Hörens bei der Schallaufnahme durch Knochenleitung," *Annalen Physik,* 13, 1932, 111–136.

——, "Physikalische Probleme der Hörphysiologie," *Elektr. Nachr. Techn.,* 12, 1935, 71–83.

——, "Zur Physik des Mittelohres und über das Hören bei Fehlerhaftem Trommelfell," *Akustik, Zeitschrift,* 1, 1936, 13–23.

——, "Über die Messung der Schwingungsamplitude der Gehörknöchelchen mittels einer Kapizitiven Sonde," *Akustik. Zeitschrift,* 6, 1941, 1–16.

——, "Über die Frequenzauflösung in der Menschlichen Schnecke," *Acta Oto-Laryngol.,* 32, 1944, 60–84.

——, "Über die Elastizität der Schneckentrennwand des Ohres," *Akustik. Zeitschrift,* 6, 1941, 265–278. Also, "On the Elasticity of the Cochlear Partition," *J. Acoust, Soc. Amer.,* 20, 1948a, 227–241.

——, "Vibration of the Head in a Sound Field, and Its Role in Hearing by Bone Conduction," *J. Acoust. Soc. Amer.,* 20, 1948b, 749–760.

——, "The Vibration of the Cochlear Partition in Anatomical Preparations and in Models of the Inner Ear," *J. Acoust. Soc. Amer.,* 21, 1949, 233–245.

——, "Microphonics Produced by Touching the Cochlear Partition with a Vibrating Electrode," *J. Acoust. Soc. Amer.,* 23, 1951a, 29–35.

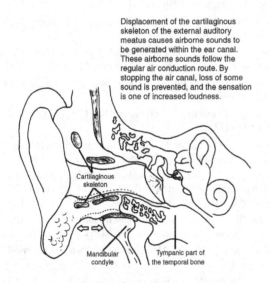

Displacement of the cartilaginous skeleton of the external auditory meatus causes airborne sounds to be generated within the ear canal. These airborne sounds follow the regular air conduction route. By stopping the air canal, loss of some sound is prevented, and the sensation is one of increased loudness.

Cartilaginous skeleton

Mandibular condyle

Tympanic part of the temporal bone

FIGURE 6-136

Schematic of the temporomandibular joint. Displacement of the cartilaginous skeleton of the external auditory meatus causes airborne sounds to be generated within the ear canal. These airborne sounds follow the regular air conduction route. By stopping the air canal, loss of some sound is prevented, and the sensation is one of increased loudness.

——, "DC Potentials and Energy Balance of the Cochlear Partition," *J. Acoust. Soc. Amer.*, 23, 1951b, 578–582.

——, "Cross Localization of the Place of Origin of the Cochlear Microphonics," *J. Acoust. Soc. Amer.*, 24, 1952, 399–409.

——, *Experiments in Hearing*. New York: McGraw-Hill, 1960.

——, and W. A. Rosenblith, "The Mechanical Properties of the Ear," in S. S. Stevens, ed., *Handbook of Experimental Psychology*. New York: John Wiley, 1958.

Bredberg, G., "Cellular Pattern and Nerve Supply of the Human Organ of Corti," *Acta Otolaryngologica* (Stockholm), Suppl. 236, 1968.

Brownell, W. E., "Observations on a Motile Response in Isolated Outer Hair Cells," in W. Webster and X. Altkin, eds., *Neural Mechanisms of Hearing*. Clayton, Australia: Monash University Press, 1983.

Brownell, W. E., "Outer Hair Cell Motility and Otacoustic Emissions," *Ear and Hearing*, 11, 1990, 82–92.

Brownell, W. E., C. R. Bader, D. Bertrand, and Y. Ribakupierre, "Evoked Mechanical Responses of Isolated Cochlear Outer Hair Cells," *Science*, 227, 1985, 194–196.

Dahmann, H., "Zur Physiologie des Hörens: experimentelle Untersuchungen über die Mechanik der Gehörknochelchenkette, sowie über deren Verhalten auf Ton und Lufdruck." *Zeitschrift für Hals-Nasen-Ohrenheilkunde*, 24, 1929, 462–497; and 27, 1930, 329–368.

Dallos, P., *The Auditory Periphery: Biophysics and Physiology*. New York: Academic Press, 1973.

——, "Cochlear Physiology," *Amer. Rev. Psychol.*, 32, 1985a, 153.

——, "Response Characteristics of Mammalian Cochlear Hair Cells," *J. Neuroscience*, 5, 1985b, 1591–1608.

——, "The Role of Outer Hair Cells in Cochlear Function," in M. J. Correla and A. A. Perachio, eds., *Contemporary Sensory Neurobiology*. New York: Alan R. Liss, 1988.

——, "Cochlear Neurobiology: Revolutionary Developments. *ASHA*, 1988, 50–56.

——, B. N. Evans, and R. Hallworth, "Nature of the Motor Element in Electrokinetic Shape Changes of Cochlear Outer Hair Cells," *Nature*, 350, 1991, 155–157.

——, D. M. Harris, E. Relkin, and M. A. Cheatham, "Two-tone Suppression and Intermodulation Distortion in the Cochlea. Effects of Outer Hair Cell Lesions," in G. van den Brink and F. A. Bilsen, eds., *Psychophysical Physiological and Behavioral Studies in Hearing*. Delft, The Netherlands: Delft University Press, 1980.

——, M. C. Billone, J. D. Durrant, C. Y. Wang, and S. Raynor, "Cochlear Inner and Outer Hair Cells: Functional Differences," *Science*, 177, 1972, 356–358.

——, J. Santos-Sacchi, and A. Flock, "Intracellular Recordings from Cochlear Outer Hair Cells," *Science*, 218, 1982, 582–584.

Dankbaar, W., "The Pattern of Stapedial Vibration." *J. Acoust. Soc. Amer.*, Vol. 48, no. 4 (part 2), 1970.

Davis, H., "The Electrical Phenomena of the Cochlea and the Auditory Nerve," *J. Acoust. Soc. Amer.*, 6, 1935, 205–215.

——, "Biophysics and Physiology of the Inner Ear," *Physiol. Rev.*, 37, 1957, 1–49.

——, "Mechanism of Excitation of Auditory Nerve Impulses," in G. L. Rasmussen and W. Windle, eds., *Neural Mechanisms of the Auditory and Vestibular System*. Springfield, Ill.: Charles C Thomas, 1960.

——, "Advances in the Neurophysiology and Neuroanatomy of the Cochlea," *J. Acoust. Soc. Amer.*, 34, 1962, 1377–1385.

——, "An Active Process in Cochlear Mechanics," *Hearing Research*, 9, 1983, 79–90.

——, B. H. Deatherage, B. Rosenblut, C. Fernandez, R. Kimura, and C. A. Smith, "Modification of Cochlear Potentials Produced by Streptomycin Poisoning and by Extensive Venous Obstruction," *Laryngoscope*, 68, 1958, 596–627.

——, A. J. Derbyshire, E. H. Kemp, M. H. Lurie, and M. Upton, "Functional and Histological Changes in the Cochlea of the Guinea Pig Resulting from Prolonged Stimulation," *J. Gen. Psychol.*, 13, 1935, 251–278.

——, A. J. Derbyshire, and M. H. Lurie, "A Modification of Auditory Theory," *Arch. Otol.*, 20, 1934, 390–395.

——, A. J. Derbyshire, and L. J. Saul, "The Electric Response of the Cochlea," *Amer. J. Physiol.* 107, 1934, 311–332.

Derbyshire, A. J., and H. Davis, "The Action Potentials of the Auditory Nerve," *Amer. J. Physiol.*, 113, 1935a, 476–504.

——, and H. Davis, "The Probable Mechanism for Stimulation of the Auditory Nerve by the Organ of Corti," *Amer. J. Physiol.*, 113, 1935b, 35.

DeRossa, L. A., "A Theory as to Function of the Scala Tympani in Hearing," *J. Acoust. Soc. Amer.*, 19, 1947, 623–628.

Doyle, W. J., and S. R. Rood, "Comparison of the Anatomy of the Eustachian Tube in the Rhesus Monkey (*Macaca mulatta*) and Man. Implications for Physiologic Modeling." *Ann. Otol.*, 89, 1980, 49–57.

Engström, H., H. Ades, and J. Hawkins, "Structure and Functions of the Sensory Hairs of the Inner Ear," *J. Acoust. Soc. Amer.*, 34, 1962, 1356–1363.

Ewald, J., "Zur physiologie des Labyrinths, VI, Eine neue Hörtheorie," *Arch. ges. Physiol.*, 76, 1899, 147–188.

Fleming, N., "Resonance in the External Auditory Meatus," *Nature*, 143, 1939, 642–643.

Fletcher, H., "A Space-Time Pattern Theory of Hearing," *J. Acoust. Soc. Amer.*, 1, 1930, 311–43.

——, "On the Dynamics of the Cochlea," *J. Acoust. Soc. Amer.*, 23, 1951, 637–645.

——, "The Dynamics of the Middle Ear and Its Relation to the Acuity of Hearing," *J. Acoust. Soc. Amer.*, 24, 1952, 129–131.

——, *Speech and Hearing in Communication*. New York: D. Van Nostrand, 1953.

Flock, Å., "Contractile Proteins in Hair Cells," *Hearing Res.*, 2, 1980, 411–412.

Flock, Å., and D. Strelioff, "Studies on Hair Cells in Isolated Coics from the Guinea Pig Cochlea. Hearing Res., 15, 1984, 11–18.

Flock, Å., R. Kimura, P. G. Lundquist, and J. Wersäll, "Morpholgical Basis of Directional Sensitivity of the Outer Hair Cells in the Organ of Corti," *J. Acoust. Soc. Amer.*, Suppl. 34, 1962, 1351.

Fumagalli, Z., "Ricerche morfologische sull' apparato di transmissione del suono," *Arch. Ital. Otol. Rinol. Laryngol.*, 60 suppl. 1, 1949.

Galambos, R., "Neural Mechanisms of Audition," *Physiol. Rev.*, 34, 1954, 497–528.

——, "Some Recent Experiments on the Neurophysiology of Hearing," *Ann. Otol., Rhinol., and Laryngol.*, 65, 1956a, 1053–1059.

——, "Suppression of Auditory Nerve Activity by Stimulation of Fibers to the Cochlea," *J. Neurophysiol.*, 19, 1956b, 424–437.

——, "Neural Mechanisms in Audition," *Laryngoscope*, 68, 1956c, 388–401.

——, and H. Davis, "The Response of Single Auditory-Nerve Fibers to Acoustic Stimulation," *J. Neurophysiol.*, 6, 1943, 39–57.

———, and H. Davis, "Action Potentials from Single Auditory-Nerve Fibers?" *Science*, 108, 1948, 513.

Gerhardt, H. J., H. David, and I. Marx, "Electronenmikroskopische Untersuchungen am musculus tensor tympani des meerschweinchens." *Archiv fur Klinische und Experimentelle Ohren-Nasen und Kehlkopfheilkunde*, 186, 1966, 20–30.

Gray's Anatomy. P. L. Williams and R. Warwick, eds. Philadelphia: W. B. Saunders Company, 1980.

Guild, S. R., "The Width of the Basilar Membrane," *Science*, 65, 1927, 67–69.

———, S. J. Crowe, C. C. Bunch, and L. M. Polvogt, "Correlations of Differences in the Density of Innervation of the Organ of Corti with Differences in the Acuity of Hearing," *Acta Oto-Laryngol.*, 15, 1931, 269–308.

Guinan, J., and W. Peake, "Middle-Ear Characteristics of Anesthetized Cats," *J. Acoust. Soc. Amer.*, 41, 1967, 1237,

Gundersen, T., and K. Høgmoen, "Holographic Vibration Analysis of the Ossicular Chain," *Acta Oto-Laryngol.*, 82, 1976, 16.

Held, H., "Die Cochlea der Sauger und der Vogel," in Bethe (ed), *Handbuch der normalen und pathologischen Physiologie, 11, Receptionsorgane 1*, Berlin, Springer-Verlag, 1926, 467.

Helmholtz, H. von, "Die Mechanik der Gehörknöchelchen und des Trommelfells," *Pflügers Archiv für die Geschichte Physiologie*, 1, 1868, 1–60.

———, *Die Lehre von den Tonempfindungen als Physiologische Grundlage für die Theorie der Musik* 4th ed., 1877, trans., *On the Sensations of Tone*, 2nd English ed. A. J. Ellis. New York: David McKay, 1912.

Hensen, V., "Zur Morphologie der Schnecke des Menchen und der Saugetheire," *Zeitschrift für wissenschaftliche Zoologie*, 13, 1863, 481–512.

———, "Beobachtungen über die Thätigkeit des Trommellspanners bei Hund unk Katze," *Archiv. für Physiologie*, 2, 1878, 312–319.

Herzog, H., "Die Mechanik der Knochenleitung im Modellversuch," *Zeitschrift für Hals-Nasen-und-Ohrenheilkunde*, 27, 1930, 402–408.

Høgmoen, K., and T. Gundersen, "Holographic Investigation of Stapes Footplate Movements," *Acoustica*, 37, 1977, 198–202.

Huggins, W. H., "Theory of Cochlear Frequency Discrimination," *Quarterly Progress Report*. Research Laboratory of Electronics, Massachusetts Institute of Technology, Oct. 1950, 54–59.

———, and J. C. R. Licklider, "Place Mechanisms of Auditory Frequency Analysis, *J. Acoust. Soc. Amer.*, 23, 1951, 290–299.

Hurst, C. H., "A New Theory of Hearing," *Transactions of the Liverpool Biological Society*, 9, 1895, 321–353.

Iurato, S., "Functional Implications of the Nature and Submicroscopic Structure of the Tectorial and Basilar Membrane," *J. Acoust. Soc. Amer.*, 34, 1962, 1386–1395.

Iwasa, K., and Chadwick. "Elasticity and Force Generation of Cochlear Outer Hair Cells," *J. Acoust. Soc. Amer.*, 92, 1992, 3169–3173.

Jepsen, O., "Middle-Ear Muscle Reflexes in Man," in J. Jerger, ed., *Modern Developments in Audiology*. New York: Academic Press, 1963.

Kalinec, F., M. Holley, K. Iwasa, D. Lim and B. Kachar, "A Membrane Based Force Generation Mechanism in Auditory Sensory Cells," *Proc. Natl. Acad. Sci.* USA, 89, 1992, 8671–8675.

Kato, T., "Zur Physiologie der Binnenmuskeln des Ohres," *Pflügers Archiv für die Geschichte Physiologie*, 150, 1913, 569–625.

Keith, A., "An Appendix on the Structures Concerned in the Mechanism of Hearing, in Sir T. Wrightson and A. Keith, *An Enquiry into the Analytical Mechanism of the Internal Ear*. London: Macmillan, 1918.

Kemp, D. T., "Stimulated Acoustic Emissions from Within the Human Auditory System," *J. Acoust. Soc. Amer.*, 64, 1978, 1386–1391.

———, "Evidence of Mechanical Nonlinearity and Frequency Selective Wave Amplification in the Cochlea," *Arch. Otorhinolaryngol.*, 224, 1979, 37.

Khanna, S. M., and D. G. B. Leonard,"Interferometric Measurement of Basilar Membrane Vibrations in Cats Using a Round Window Approach. *J. Acoust. Soc. Amer.* 68, 1980, 543.

———, "Basilar Membrane Tuning in the Cat Cochlea," *Science*, 215, 1982, 305–306.

———, and J. Tonndorf, "The Vibratory Pattern of the Round Window in Cats," *J. Acoust. Soc. Amer.*, 50, 1971, 1475–1483.

———, and J. Tonndorf, "Tympanic Membrane Vibration in Cats Studied by Time-Averaged Holography," *J. Acoust. Soc. Amer.*, 51, 1972, 1904–1920.

Kiang, N. Y.-S., T. Watanabe, E. C. Thomas, and L. F. Clark, "Discharge Patterns of Single Fibers in the Cat's Auditory Nerve," *Research Monograph No. 35*, M.I.T. Press, Cambridge, Mass., 1965.

Kim, D. O., "Active and Nonlinear Cochlear Biomechanics and the Role of Outer-Hair-Cell Subsystem in the Mammalian Auditory System," *Hearing Res.*, 22, 1986, 105–114.

Kimura, R., "Hairs of the Cochlear Sensory Cells and Their Attachment to the Tectorial Membrane," *Acta Oto-Laryngol.*, 61, 1966, 55–72.

Kirikae, I., *The Structure and Function of the Middle Ear*. Tokyo: University of Tokyo Press, 1960.

Kobrak, H. B., "Zur Physiologie der Binnenmuskeln des Ohres I. (Untersuchungen zur Mechanik der Schalleitungskette) *Beitr. Anat., etc., Ohr.*, 29, 1932a, 383–416.

———, "Zur Physiologie der Binnenmuskeln des Ohres II." *Beltr. Anat., etc., Ohr.*, 29, 1932b, 383–416.

———, *The Middle Ear*. Chicago: University of Chicago Press, 1959.

Kuile., E. ter, "Die Ubertragung der Energie von der Grundmembran auf die Horzellen," *Archiv für Physiologie*, 79, 1900, 146–157.

———, "Die Richtige Bewegungsform der Membrana Basilaris," *Archiv für Physiologie*, 79, 1900, 484–509.

Kuriyama, R., R. Albin, and R. Altschuler, "Expression of NMDA Receptor in RNA in the Rat Cochlea," *Hear. Res.*, 69, 1993, 215–220.

Lederer, F. L., *Diseases of the Ear, Nose, and Throat*. Philadelphia, F. A. Davis, 1938.

———, and A. R. Hollender, *Textbook of Ear, Nose, and Throat*. Philadelphia: F. A. Davis, 1942.

Lempert, J. E., G. Wever, M. Lawrence, and P. E. Meltzer, "Perilymph: Its Relation to the Improvement of Hearing Which Follows Fenestration of the Vestibular Labyrinth in Clinical Otosclerosis," *Arch. Otol.*, 50, 1949, 377–387.

Lilly, D. J., "Measurement of Acoustic Impedance at the Tympanic Membrane," in J. Jerger, ed., *Modern Developments in Audiology*, 2nd ed. New York and London: Academic Press, 1973.

Lim, D., "Fine Morphology of the Tectorial Membrane," *Arch. Otol.*, 96, 1972, 199–215.

Lindemann, H., and W. Ades, "The Sensory Hairs and the Tectorial Membrane in the Development of the Cat's Organ of Corti," *Acta Oto-Laryngol., Otolaryng.*, 72, 1971, 229–242.

Lorente de Nó, R., "The Sensory Endings in the Cochlea," *Laryngoscope*, 47, 1937, 373–377.

Lüscher, E., "Die Funktion des Musculus Stapedius beim Menschen," *Zeitschrift für Hals-Nasen-und-Ohrenheilkunde*, 23, 1929, 105–132.

Lynch, T., U. Nedzebnitsky, and W. Peake, "Input Impedance of the Cochlea in Cat," *J. Acoust. Soc. Amer*, 72, 1982, 108–130.

Macartney, J. C., S. D. Comis, and J. D. Pickles, "Is Myosin in the Cochlea a Basis for Active Motility?" *Nature*, 288, 1980, 491–492.

Metz, O., "The Acoustic Impedance Measured on Normal and Pathological Ears," *Acta Oto-Laryngol.*, Suppl. 63, 1946.

Meyer, M., "Zur Theorie des Hörens," *Pflügers Archiv für die Geschichte Physiologia*, 78, 1899, 346–362.

———, "The Hydraulic Principles Governing the Function of the Cochlea," *J. Gen. Psychol.*, 1, 1928, 239–265.

Møller, A., *Basic Mechanisms in Hearing*. New York: Academic Press, 1973.

Moore, K., *Clinically Oriented Anatomy*, Baltimore, MD: Williams & Wilkins, 1985.

Müller, Johannes and C. Pouillet. *Lehrbuch der Physik*, 11th ed., vol 1, Brunswick, Germany: Vieweg Verlag, 1934.

Nedzelnitsky, V., "Measurements of Sound Pressure in the Cochleae of Anesthetized Cats," in Zwicker, J. and K. Terhardt, eds., *Facts and Models in Hearing*. New York: Springer, 1974.

Nordlund, B., "Physical Factors in Sound Localization," *Acta Oto-Laryngol.*, 54, 1962, 75–93.

Ohm, G. S., "Über die Definition des Tones, nebst daran geknupfter Theorie der Sirene und ahnlicker tonbildener Vorrichtungen," *Annalen der Physik*, 59, 1843, 497–565.

Peake, W., H. Sohmer, and T. Weiss, "Microelectrode Recordings of Intracochlear Potentials," in *Quarterly Progress Report No. 94*, 293–304, Cambridge, Mass.: M.I.T. Research Laboratory of Electronics, 1969.

Perlman, H. B., and T. J. Case, "Latent Period of the Crossed Stapedius Reflex in Man," *Ann. Otol., Rhinol., and Laryngol.*, 48, 1939, 663–675.

Peterson, L. C., and B. P. Bogert, "A Dynamical Theory of the Cochlea," *J. Acoust. Soc. Amer.*, 22, 1950, 369–381.

Pickles, J., *An Introduction to the Physiology of Hearing*, 2nd ed., London: Academic Press, 1988.

Pickles, J. O., *An Introduction to the Physiology of Hearing*. London and New York: Academic Press, 1982.

———, S. D. Comis, and M. P. Osborne, "Crosslinks Between Stereocilia in the Guinea Pig Organ of Corti, and Their Possible Relation to Sensory Transduction," *Hearing Res.*, 15, 1984, 103–112.

Pollak, J., "Über die Function des Musculus Tensor Tympani," *Medizinisch Jahrbuch*, 82, 1886, 555–582.

Rabinowitz, W., "Measurement of the Acoustic Admittance of the Human Ear," *J. Acoust. Soc. Amer.*, 70, 1981, 1025–1035.

Rasmussen, A. T., "Studies on the VIIIth Cranial Nerve of Man." *Laryngoscope*, 50, 1940, 67–83.

Rasmussen, G. L., "The Olivary Peduncle and Other Fiber Projections of the Superior Olivary Complex," *J. Compar. Neurol.*, 84, 1946, 141–219.

———, and W. F. Windle, *Neural Mechanisms of the Auditory and Vestibular Systems*. Springfield, Ill.: Charles C Thomas, 1960.

Rejto, A., "Beitrage zur Physiologie der Knochenleitung," *Verhandlungen der Deutschen Otologische Gesselschaft*, 23, 1914, 268–285.

Retzius, G., "Die Endigungsweise des Gehörnerven," *Biol. Untersuchung*, 5, 1893a, 35–38.

———, "Weiteres über die Endigungsweise des Gehörnerven," *Biol. Untersuchung*, 5, 1893b, 35–38.

———, *Das Gehörorgan der Wirbeltheire, eine Morphologischhistologische Studien*. Stockholm: Samson & Wallin, 1905.

Rhode, W. S., "Observations of the Vibration of the Basilar Membrane Using the Mossbauer Technique," *J. Acoust. Soc. Amer.*, 49, 1971, 1218–1231.

Rinne, A., "Beitrage zur Physiology des Menschlichen Ohres," *Viertel Jahrschr, J. Prakt. Heilk. Prag.*, 45, 1855, 71–123.

Rood, S. R., and W. J. Doyle, "Morphology of Tensor Veli Palatini, Tensor Tympani, and Dilator Tubae Muscles," *Ann. Otol.*, 87, 1978, 202–210.

Rose, J. E., J. E. Hind, D. J. Anderson, and J. F. Brugge, "Some Effects of Stimulus Intensity on Response of Auditory Nerve Fibers in the Squirrel Monkey," *J. Neurophysiol.*, 34, 1971, 685–699.

Ruggero, M. A., and N. C. Rich, "Application of a Commercially Manufactured Doppler Shift Laser Velocimeter to the Measurement of Basilar Membrane Vibration," *Hear. Res.*, 51, 1991, 215–230.

Russell, E. J., and P. M. Sellick, "Intracellular Studies of Hair Cells in the Mammalian Cochlea," *J. Physiol.* (London), 284, 1978, 261–290.

Rutherford, W. "A New Theory of Hearing," *J. Anat. and Physiol.*, 21, 1886, 166–168.

Ryan, A. F., D. Brumm, and M. Kraft, "Occurance and Distribution of non-NMDA Glutamate Receptor mRNAs in the Cochlea," *Neuro Rep.*, 2, 1991, 543–646.

———, and P. Dallos, "Absence of Cochlear Outer Hair Cells: Effect on Behavioural Auditory Threshold," *Nature*, 253, 1975, 44–46.

Schlosshauer, B. and K.-H. Vosteen, "Ueber die Anordnung und Wirkungsweise der im Conus elasticus ansetzenden Fasern des Stimmulkels," *Zschr. Laryng.*, 642–650, 1957.

———, "Ueber den Verlauf und die Funktion der Stimmulkelfasern," *Zschr. Anat. Entw.*, 120, 456–465, 1958.

Seif, S., and A. L. Dellon, "Anatomic Relationships Between the Human Levator and Tensor Veli Palatini and the Eustachian Tube, *Cleft Palate J.*, 15, 1978, 329–336.

Sellick, P. M., R. Patuzzi, and B. M. Johnstone, "Measurement of Basilar Membrane Motion in the Guinea Pig Using the Mossbauer Technique," *J. Acoust. Soc. Amer.*, 72, 1982, 131–141.

Shaw, E. A. G., "Ear Canal Pressure Generated by a Source Field," *J. Acoust. Soc. Amer.*, 3, 1966, 465–470.

———, "The External Ear," in Keidel and Neff, eds., *Handbook of Sensory Physiology*, Vol. V (1). New York: Springer, 1974.

Sicher, H., and E. DuBrul, *Oral Anatomy*, 6th ed. St. Louis: C. V. Mosby, 1975.

Simpkins, C. S., "Functional Anatomy of the Eustachian Tube," *Arch. Otol.*, 38, 1943, 478–484.

Sivian, L. J., and S. D. White, "On Minimal Audible Sound Fields," *J. Acoust. Soc. Amer.*, 4, 1933, 288–321.

Smith, C. A., "Electron Microscopic Studies of Cochlear and Vestibular Receptors," *Anatomical Record*, 127, 1957, 483.

———, and F. S. Sjöstrand, "Structure of the Nerve Endings on the External Hair Cells of the Guinea Pig Cochlea as Studied by Serial Sections," *J. Ultrastructure Res.*, 5, 1961, 523–526.

Smith, K. R., and E. G. Wever, "The Problem of Stimulation Deafness: The Functional and Histological Effects of a High-Frequency Stimulus," *J. Exper. Psychol.*, 49, 1949, 238–241.

Spoendlin, H., "Ultrastructure and Peripheral Innervation Pattern of the Receptor in Relation to the First Coding of the Acoustic Messages," in A. V. S. De Reuck and J. Knight, eds., *Hearing Mechanisms in Vertebrates*, pp. 89–125. Boston: Little, Brown, 1968.

——, The Innervation of the Cochlear Receptors, in A. Moller, ed., *Basic Mechanisms in Hearing*, 185. New York: Academic Press, 1973.

——, "Innervation Patterns in the Organ of Corti of the Cat," *Acta Otol.*, 67, 1969, 239–254.

——, *The Organization of the Cochlear Receptor*, New York: Springer-Karger, 1966.

——, "Neuroanatomy of the Cochlea," in Zwicker and Terhardt, eds., *Facts and Models in Hearing*. New York: Springer, 1974.

Stevens, S. S., ed., *Handbook of Experimental Psychology*. New York: John Wiley, 1951.

——, and H. Davis, *Hearing, Its Psychology and Physiology*. New York: John Wiley, 1938.

Talley, J., "Hearing Mechanisms in the Behaviorally Deaf Dalmation Dog," Unpublished Master's thesis, University of Illinois, Champaign, Ill., 1965.

Tasaki, I., and C. Spiropoulos, "Stria Vascularis as Source of Endocochlear Potential, *J. Neurophysiol.*, 22, 1959, 149–155.

——, H. Davis, and D. Eldredge, "Exploration of Cochlear Potentials in Guinea Pigs with Microelectrode," *J. Acoust. Soc. Amer.*, 26, 1954, 765–773.

——, H. Davis, and J. Legouix, "The Spacetime Pattern of the Cochlear Microphonics (Guinea Pig), as Recorded by Differential Electrodes," *J. Acoust. Soc. Amer.*, 24, 1952, 502–518.

Tonndorf, J., and S. Khanna, "Some Properties of Sound Transmission in the Middle and Outer Ears of Cats," *J. Acoust. Soc. Amer.*, 41, 1967, 513–521.

——, and S. M. Khanna, "Submicroscopic Displacement Amplitudes of the Tympanic Membrane (Cat) Measured by Laser Interferometer," *J. Acoust. Soc. Amer.*, 44, 1968, 1546–1554.

Vinnikov, Ya. A., and A. K. Titova, *Kortiev organgistofiziologia i gistokhimia*. Moscow: Academy of Sciences, 1961. English ed. New York: Consultants Bureau, 1964.

Voldrich, L., "Mechanical Properties of Basilar Membrane," *Acta Oto-Laryngol.*, 86, 1978, 331–335.

Vosteen, K. H., "New Aspects in the Biology and Pathology of the Inner Ear," *Translations of the Beltone Institute for Hearing Research*, 16, 1963.

Warr, B. W., "Olivocochlear and Vestibular Efferent Neurons of the Feline Brain Stem: Their Location, Morphology and Number Determined by Retrograde Axonal Transport and Acetylcholinesterase Histochemistry." *J. Compar. Neurol.*, 161, 1975, 159–182.

Wërsall, J., "Studies on the Structure and Innervation of the Sensory Epithelium of the Cristae Ampulares in the Guinea Pig," *Acta Oto-Laryngol.*, Suppl. 139, 1958a.

——, "The Tympanic Muscles and Their Reflexes," *Acta Otol.*, 139, 1958b.

Wever, E. G., "The Width of the Basilar Membrane in Man," *Ann. Otol., Rhinolo., and Laryngol.*, 47, 1938, 37–47.

——, "The Stapedius Muscle in Relation to Sound Conduction," *J. Exper. Psychol.*, 31, 1942, 35–43.

——, *Theory of Hearing*. New York: John Wiley, 1949.

——, and C. W. Bray, "Action Currents in the Auditory Nerve in Response to Acoustical Stimulation," *Proceedings of the National Academy of Science*, 16, 1930, 344–350.

——, and M. Lawrence, *Physiological Acoustics*. Princeton, NJ.: Princeton University Press, 1954.

——, M. Lawrence, and K. R. Smith, "The Middle Ear in Sound Conduction," *Arch. Otol.*, 68, 1948, 19–35.

——, and J. A. Vernon, "The Control of Sound Transmission by the Middle Ear Muscles," *Ann. Otol., Rhinol., and Laryngol.*, 65, 1956, 5–10.

Wien, M., "Ein Bedenken gegen die Helmholtzsche Resonanztheorie des Hörens," *Feschrift Adolph Wullner*, Leipzig, 1905, 28–35. (Not seen; reported by Wever and Lawrence, 1954.

Wiener, F. M. "On the Diffraction of a Progressive Sound Wave by the Human Head," *J. Acoust. Soc. Amer.*, 19, 1947, 143–146.

——, and D. A. Ross, "Pressure Distribution in the Auditory Canal in a Progressive Sound Field," *J. Acoust. Soc. Amer.*, 18, 1946, 401–408.

Wrightson, T., and A. Keith, *An Enquiry into the Analytical Mechanism of the Internal Ear*. London: Macmillan, 1918.

Yost, W., and D. Nielson, *Fundamentals of Hearing*, 2nd ed., New York: Holt, Rinehart and Winston, 1985.

Zurek, P. M., "Spontaneous Narrowband Acoustic Signals Emitted by Human Ears," *J. Acoust. Soc. Amer.*, 69, 1981, 514–523.

Zwislocki, Jósef, "Über die Mechanische Klanganalyze des Ohres," *Experientia*, 2, 1946, 415–417.

——, "Theorie der Schneckenmechanik," *Acta Oto-Laryngol.*, Suppl. 122, 1948.

——, "Theory of the Acoustical Action of the Cochlea," *J. Acoust. Soc. Amer.*, 22, 1950, 778–784.

Embryology of the Speech and Hearing Mechanism

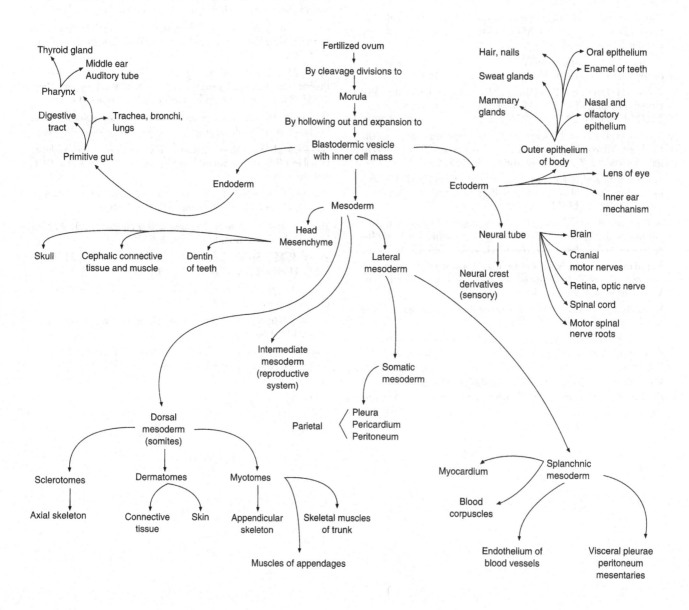

EARLY EMBRYONIC DEVELOPMENT

Mitosis

Because no living organism is immortal, the continuation of any species is dependent upon an unending succession of individuals, each of which possesses the salient characteristics of its species. All animals reproduce, from the simplest protozoan to the most complex mammal. Early forms of life duplicated themselves by a process not unlike fission, much like bacteria and protozoa do today. The process, called **mitosis,**[1] is an example of asexual reproduction in which the parent simply divides into equal parts, usually exact duplicates. Since mitosis is a mechanism that maintains a constant **chromosome,**[2] all offspring have the same number of chromosomes as the parent cell.

Mitotic Cell Division

A mature human is estimated to be composed of approximately 10^{14} cells. These cells not only must be formed and differentiated as the body grows, but also in many instances they must be replaced as they mature and die. In most organisms the process of cell division is essentially the same. Mitosis can be studied in an onion skin, in the root tips of growing plants, or in tissue culture, and the process is essentially the same as that in the living human or growing embryo.

The duplication of genes and chromosomes is the first step in the division of the cell. It is immediately followed by a division of the cytoplasm, with the result that two cells, each identical in genetic characteristics, are formed. Biologists have divided mitotic cell division into five phases, shown in Figure 7-1; in order of sequence they are **interphase** (resting phase), **prophase, metaphase, anaphase,** and **telophase.**

Interphase

The term interphase or resting phase may imply that no activity is taking place in the nucleus of the cell, but this is hardly the case. It is during the interphase that nuclear growth is occurring at an accelerated rate.

Prophase

Toward the end of the interphase the chromosomes, which are not normally visible, begin to take on a granulated appearance. The first sign that cell division is imminent is when the chromosomes become visible as long, thin threads (**chromatids**). This stage of cell division is known as the prophase, throughout which the chromatids become increasingly visible, largely due to the fact that they become shorter and thicker. In addition, the **nucleoli,** which are formed by chromosomes, diminish in size and finally disappear.

Metaphase

The metaphase begins with the disappearance of the **nuclear membrane;** at the same time a new structure appears in the cytoplasm. It is a long, thin chain of protein molecules (the **spindle**) that is oriented between the two "poles" within the cell body. When the spindle is well developed, the chromosomes move randomly through the cytoplasm at first and finally settle in a region midway between the poles of the spindle.

Anaphase

In the anaphase the paired chromosomes are seemingly pulled from the midregion toward opposite poles (presumably by the fine fibrils of the spindle). This migration continues until, at the very end of the anaphase, the chromosomes form a densely packed group at each of the two poles.

Telophase

In the telophase the events that occurred back in the prophase are "replayed," but in reverse order. Thus, a nuclear membrane forms around the chromosomes, which uncoil to form slender threads again, and the nucleoli make their appearance. A cell wall forms in the region of the spindle, which slowly disintegrates leaving two cells, separated from one another and ready to undergo a growth period before the next division is initiated.

Gametogenesis

Sexual reproduction, which is well established in both simple and complex forms of life, involves the union of

---

[1]Gk. **mito-,** thread, or threadlike.

[2]Gk. **chroma,** color. GK. **soma,** body.

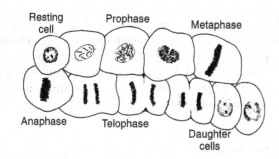

FIGURE 7-1

Schematic representation of the five phases of mitotic cell division.

two sexual germ cells (**gametes**).[3] Two gametes (one male and one female) unite to form a single new cell (a **zygote**)[4] that gives rise to a new individual organism.

In higher-order animals, including humans, the female germ cell is called an **ovum** or **egg**. The human ovum has a diameter of about 200 microns (a micron is 0.0001 mm). The male germ cell (a **sperm**)[5] is about 50 microns in length, including the filament; the head alone is about 5 microns long.

It is important to recognize that when two sexual germ cells unite, their nucleic material and chromosomes are also combined. Every mature human cell contains 46 chromosomes (23 pairs). If mitosis were the only mechanism for the generation of new cells, each human cell would also contain 46 chromosomes, and the zygote, formed by the fertilization or activation of an ovum by a sperm cell, would contain 92 chromosomes, as would the germ cells of the new individual. This means that an individual of the succeeding generation would possess 184 chromosomes, and by the end of the tenth generation each individual would have cells containing 23,332 chromosomes. Without some compensatory mechanism to reduce the number of chromosomes in the gamete, we simply would not remain human beings for very long.

Meiosis

The reduction of the number of chromosomes in the sexual germ cell is accomplished by an extraordinary type of cell division called **meiosis**,[6] which, very grossly, consists of two nuclear divisions during the maturation of the sex cell, with only one division of chromosomes. Before any germ cell is capable of reproduction it must undergo meiosis. That is, the number of chromosomes in the sexual germ cell must be reduced by half.

During the final phases of **gametogenesis—spermatogenesis** for sperms and **oogenesis** for eggs—the number of chromosomes is reduced from the **diploid number** (2N) which is the number found in all body cells, to the **haploid number** (N), just one-half the diploid number, which is the number found in the sex cells. The mature sex cell contains one full set of chromosomes, not two as in the body cells. The mature egg contains 22 ordinary chromosomes plus one sex chromosome (22 + X). Sperm cells, on the other hand, contain either one of two kinds. One group contains 22 + X, while the other contains 22 + Y. Fertilization by one kind of sperm cell (22 + X) results in a female (44 + 2X),

and fertilization by the other kind produces a male (44 + X + Y).

The presence of the **Y chromosome** determines the sex. Gametogenesis is a fascinating process, but beyond the scope of the text. The interested reader is referred to Swanson (1964).

Fertilization

Normally, millions of sperm cells are deposited in the female, and when a mature ovum is present, they stream toward it at a rate of about 75 mm per hour. The first sperm cell that strikes the membrane surrounding the ovum enters, head first, dropping off its tail or filament.

The membrane repairs quickly and sets up a **chemical barrier,** which prevents additional sperm from entering. The fertilized egg is now known as a *zygote*, and when the nuclei of the ovum and sperm unite, the first division of the cell follows shortly thereafter. With the union of the two sex cells, the zygote is in possession of the full complement of 46 chromosomes. The cell division that follows is the **mitotic division** described earlier, and as a result each daughter cell possesses 46 chromosomes.

Much of what is known about early cell division has been learned from animal studies, particularly of the chicken and monkey. It usually procedes as follows:

Initial cell division probably takes place within 24 hours after fertilization. Of the 2 cells, called **blastomeres**,[7] the larger divides so that 3 cells are present after the second division. The other cell then divides, producing 4 cells, and so on, until a rounded mass containing 12 to 16 cells is formed. Such a round mass of cells (a **morula**)[8] has been recovered from the uterine cavity on or about the third day after fertilization. The morula remains in the uterine cavity, bathed in the fluid secreted by the uterine glandular tissue. This fluid eventually passes between the cells of the morula, and as the morula grows, it forms a fluid-filled sphere known as a **blastocyst**.[9] The fluid-filled cavity is called a **blastocoele**.[10] An early form of cell differentiation begins to take place during the blastocyst phase.

A midsection through a blastocyst, shown in Figure 7-2, reveals an outer layer of cuboidal cells (**trophoblasts**)[11] which surrounds an inner cell mass. During this phase of development, the blastocyst becomes attached to the deciduous tissue of the uterine lining in such a way that the inner cell mass (the **animal** or **embryonic pole**) is deepest.

---

[3]Gk. **gam-, gamo-,** marriage, reproductive union.

[4]Gk. **zygo-,** yoked; joined.

[5]Gk. **sperma,** seed.

[6]Gk. **meio-,** decrease in size or number, to make smaller.

[7]Gk. **blastos,** germ. Gk. **meros,** a part.

[8]L. **morus,** mulberry.

[9]Gk. **kystis,** bladder.

[10]Gk. **koilos,** hollow.

[11]Gk. **trophe,** nutrition.

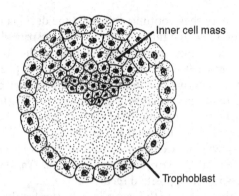

FIGURE 7-2

Schematic section of a blastocyst showing the trophoblast and the inner cell mass.

It is important to note that the trophoblast will not contribute toward the formation of any structures of the developing embryo, but, rather, it forms only the fetal membranes such as the **placenta**,[12] which establishes communication between the mother and embryo by means of the **umbilical cord.** The inner cell mass, on the other hand, forms only embryonic tissue.

Development of the Yolk Sac

The first indication of cell differentiation in the inner cell mass is when certain cells proliferate to form the **endoderm** of the embryo. Proliferation takes place at the periphery of the inner cell mass, between it and the trophoblast. Two distinct layers of endodermal cells become evident. One consists of cuboidal cells and lies against the inner cell mass. These endodermal cells proliferate at the periphery of the inner cell mass and ultimately completely line the inside of the trophoblast to form the **primary yolk sac.** These cells continue to proliferate until the yolk sac completely lines the blastocoele and finally folds or buckles. This folding causes the sac to be constricted so that it consists of two parts, a primary yolk sac that later atrophies and disappears, and a **secondary yolk sac** that persists for some time.

About the time the yolk sac is being formed, cells from the inner surface of the trophoblast proliferate to form a loose network of **extraembryonic mesoderm** which does not contribute to formation of the embryo. This developing mesoderm, the **magma reticulare**,[13] fills the blastocoele and pushes the primary yolk sac away from the trophoblast whereupon the sac shrivels and atrophies. The remaining secondary yolk sac is confined to a small area in the vicinity of the inner cell mass.

[12]Gk. **placenta,** a flat cake.
[13]L. **reticulare,** netlike.

Development of the Amniotic Cavity

During this same period, certain cells in the inner cell mass begin to secrete fluid, so that a layer of cells becomes separated from the inner cell mass. The result is a fluid-filled cavity, the **amnionic cavity,** which is covered by **amnionic membrane,** or simply the **amnion.**[14] The early amnion and its relation to the inner cell mass is shown in Figure 7-3. At the same time as the amnion is being formed, cells in the floor of the amnionic cavity become tall and columnar to form a layer of **ectoderm.** When this has taken place, the inner cell mass is known as the **embryonic disc.** It consists of columnar ectodermal cells in the floor of the amnionic cavity and a subjacent layer of cuboidal endodermal cells which forms the roof of the yolk sac, as shown in Figure 7-4.

[14]Gk. **amnion,** lamb.

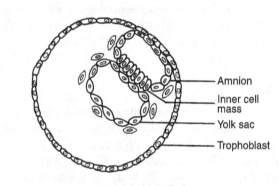

FIGURE 7-3

The early amnion and its relation to the inner cell mass and yolk sac.

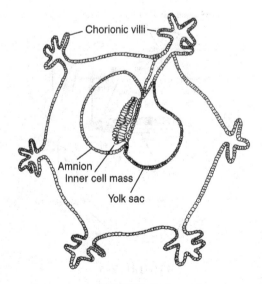

FIGURE 7-4

Schematic of inner cell mass and adjacent structures.

While these changes have been taking place, extra-embryonic mesoderm has continued to proliferate so that it almost completely fills the blastocoele. This extraembryonic mesoderm forms two layers of tissue, one of which (the **somatopleuric extraembryonic mesoderm**) comes in contact with the outside of the yolk sac. The relationship of extraembryonic mesoderm to the embryonic disc is shown in Figure 7-5.

Establishment of Maternal/Fetal Communication

While the blastocyst is implanting and the yolk sac and amnion are being formed, rapid and significant changes are taking place in the trophoblast, which is rapidly growing. **Enzymes,** produced by the cells of the trophoblast, erode the deciduous tissue of the uterine lining and facilitate interstitial implantation of the blastocyst. Proliferation of the trophoblast produces two types of cells. One type, the **syncytiotrophoblast,** proliferates so rapidly that the individual cells do not form cell boundaries. The other type, the **cytotrophoblast,** does produce cell boundaries.

The Villi

As proliferation of the trophoblast continues, fingerlike processes (**trophoblastic villi**) begin to extend out in all directions from the blastocyst, but later, when somatopleuric extraembryonic mesoderm invades them, they are called the **chorionic villi.** As shown schematically in Figure 7-4, villi at first develop all over the surface of the blastocyst. Later, however, they degenerate, except at the region of the inner cell mass (**animal** or **embryonic**

pole), where they continue to invade the decidua of the uterus and become more complex. This restricted area, where villi continue to develop, is known as the **chorion frondosum.**[15] It forms the fetal portion of the placenta, while the maternal portion is formed by the deciduous uterine tissue immediately surrounding the blastocyst. Eventually the chorionic villi invade the maternal blood supply, and when the fetal blood vessels grow into the chorionic villi, an exchange of oxygen and nourishment from the mother to the embryo is possible. Waste materials pass in the opposite direction.

By the middle of the second week after fertilization, the embryo is surrounded by three layers of tissue, which are, from without to within, the deciduous tissue of the uterus, the chorion, and finally the amnion.

The Body Stalk

Extraembryonic mesoderm extends from the chorion frondosum to the embryonic disc by means of a body stalk. As the amnion and yolk develop, the body stalk elongates to form the connective tissue of the umbilical cord, through which the fetal blood courses to the chorionic villi.

The Primitive Streak and Notochord

While the yolk sac and amnion are being formed, the embryonic disc consists only of a layer of ectoderm and of endoderm. The columnar ectodermal cells in the floor of the amnionic cavity (dorsum of the embryonic disc) begin to proliferate rapidly, particularly at the future caudal end of the embryonic disc (the end near the body stalk) to form the primitive streak as shown in Figure 7-5.

The significance of the primitive streak lies in the fact that it is capable of forming not only new ectoderm and endoderm, but **intraembryonic mesoderm** as well. A layer of mesodermal cells begins to grow out laterally from the primitive streak between the ectoderm and endoderm. Thus, the embryonic disc becomes trilaminar. At the head or cephalic end of the primitive streak (away from the body stalk), a small area of proliferating cells produces a node, **Hensen's node,** from which a strip of cells grows cephalically along the midline axis of the embryo between the ectoderm and endoderm. This midline strip of cells, sandwiched between the ectoderm and endoderm, is known as the **notochord.**[16] It is the primitive axial skeleton of the embryo.

The notochord continues its growth cephalically, but is stopped near the extreme limits of the embryonic disc where the ectoderm and endoderm are in such in-

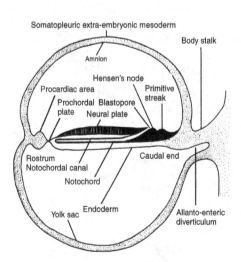

FIGURE 7-5

Diagrammatic representation of a bilaminar embryonic disc as seen in a longitudinal section. Extraembryonic mesoderm is shown in stipple.

[15]Gk. **chori,** fetal membrane, skin. L. **frondosus,** leafy.

[16]Gk. **noto-,** back.

timate contact that the notochord is unable to separate them. This small area of tightly bound ectoderm and endoderm, called the **prochordal plate,** forms the **buccopharyngeal membrane,** to be discussed later. Just ahead of the prochordal plate, an area of intraembryonic mesoderm produced from the primitive streak continues to proliferate until finally it forms an intermediate layer between the ectoderm and endoderm everywhere in the embryonic disc except in the procardiac area, where it is found only in the midline.

Development of the Neural Tube

As the intraembryonic mesoderm continues to grow laterally, it finally meets and becomes continuous with the extraembryonic mesoderm that forms the chorion. During this stage of development a thickening of the ectoderm occurs in an area immediately overlying the notochord. This thickening is called the **medullary** or **neural plate,** the lateral margins of which grow upward to form the paraxial **neural folds,** between which lies the **neural groove.** Eventually the neural folds meet at the midline, fuse, and form the **neural tube,** from which all the future central nervous system is developed. The ectoderm once again becomes a continuous layer over the dorsum of the embryo. These developments, shown schematically in Figure 7-6, usually have occurred by the beginning of the third week.

Formation of Somites

About the beginning of the third week, mesoderm on either side of the neural tube and notochord (paraxial mesoderm) begins a progressive caudal transverse segmentation to form blocks of tissue called somites. They occupy the entire length of the trunk of the embryo on either side of the midline. The somites are subjacent to the ectoderm and are located lateral to the notochord and neural tube. Even in a very early embryo, such as the specimen shown in Figure 7-7, the somites bear a resemblance to the vertebral column. This is reasonable since the vertebrae are adult derivatives of the somites. A schematic transverse section through an embryo showing the relationship of a somite to adjacent structures is shown in Figure 7-8.

In humans, the first pair of somites appears about the sixteenth day after fertilization, and by the end of the fourth week about 30 pairs of somites have made their appearance. There are 3 occipital, 8 cervical, 12 thoracic, 5 lumbar, and from 5 to 8 coccygeal somites. The occipital and coccygeal somites seem to be transitory, because they dedifferentiate and disappear.

The cells in a somite probably have a wider diversity of developmental potentialities than any aggregate of cells in the embryo (Patten, 1946). *The significance of the somites cannot be overemphasized because, except for the*

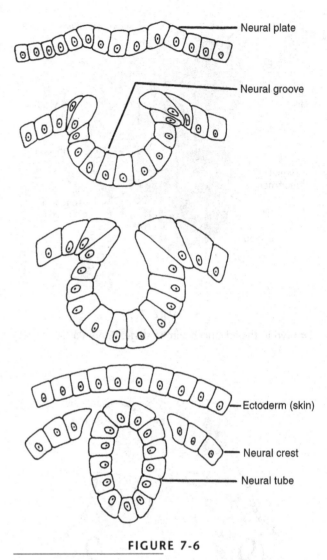

FIGURE 7-6

Schematic of the development of the neural tube and neural crest.

head region, they ultimately give rise to virtually all the connective, muscular, and dermal tissue of the entire body. Initially, the tissue of the somites becomes differentiated into three cell groups.

Sclerotome

The medialmost region of a somite forms a **sclerotome.**[17] The cells of a sclerotome migrate to surround the notochord and the neural tube. *This tissue differentiates into the individual vertebrae, intervertebral discs, and the ribs.* The migration dorsally around the neural tube forms the neural arch of a vertebra, and when the paired migrating sclerotomes meet they join to form the neural spine.

---

[17]Gk. **scleros,** hard. Gk. **tome,** a segment.

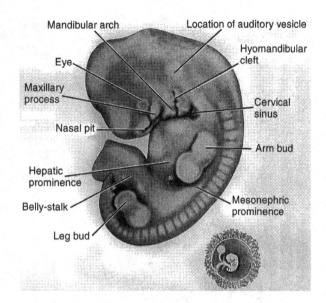

FIGURE 7-7

Embryo in the advanced somite stage. (From Patten, 1946.)

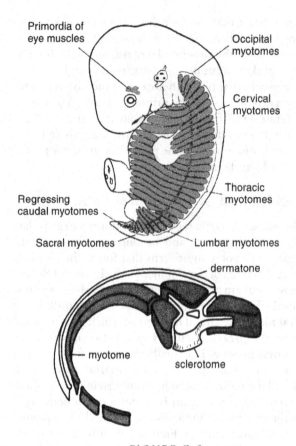

FIGURE 7-9

Diagrams showing the regions into which embryonic myotomes extend. The myotome is shown in gray in the lower illustration.

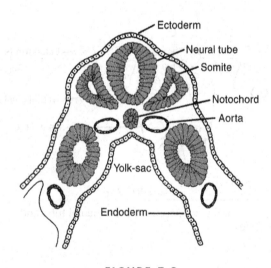

FIGURE 7-8

A schematic transverse section through an embryo, showing the neural tube, somite, and notochord.

Myotome (Myomere)

Cells immediately lateral to the sclerotome become elongated and spindle-shaped, a clue to their final destination. The fairly definite boundaries of these cells contribute to the segmental nature of the human body. Since the tissue *develops into the musculature of the trunk*, these aggregates of cells are known collectively as a myotome or myomere.

Because the fate of the myotomes is of obvious significance to us, we should look into some general features regarding muscle distribution. The gray areas in Figure 7-9 indicate the approximate location and extent of the myotomes when they first differentiate in the somite. The white, ventrally directed extensions from the myotomes suggest the general part of the embryonic body into which the myotome extends. The general orientation of the developing muscle fibers in the myotomes is in a craniocaudal direction.

In certain regions the primordial muscle masses undergo a change in their orientation, and they may even move out of their area of origin. Many muscles of the trunk, however, such as the intercostals and the muscles of the vertebral columns, retain their segmental distribution into the adult form. And, as Patten (1946) points out, even in instances where the changes in muscle distribution are difficult to follow, the cutaneous nerves still exhibit a distribution that illustrates the area in an adult body which are derivatives of the segmental region of the young embryo. This is extremely important in understanding the general organization of the body because *the innervation of the developing muscle is acquired very early, from nerves arising at the same segmental level in the body. So, when changes in the position of a muscle occur, the already attached nerve is simply pulled along with the migrating muscle.* The level of the origin of a muscle is indicated by the segmental level at which the nerve that supplies it arises.

In addition, *the path a nerve follows in reaching a muscle tells us something about the path taken by a migrating muscle* in reaching its adult position. A striking example is the **phrenic nerve** which supplies the diaphragm with motor fibers. This nerve emerges from the fourth and fifth cervical nerves of the embryo. As shown in Figure 7-10, its course to the diaphragm is very direct in the flexed embryo as compared to the long course, along the pericardium, the nerve follows in the adult. As stated earlier, changes may occur in the original craniocaudal orientation of the muscle fibers in the myotome. This is widespread in the body, and an example of a change in original direction is seen in the oblique course of the thoracic and abdominal musculature.

An original *single primordial muscle mass may split longitudinally* into two or more muscle masses. The sternocleidomastoid and trapezius, for example, stem from the same primordial muscle mass, and that explains why these muscles are supplied by the same (spinal accessory) nerve.

There may also be a *tangential splitting of an original primordial muscle mass into two or more muscle layers.* Examples of the results of tangential splitting are seen in the familiar oblique and transverse abdominal musculature and in the intercostal muscles.

Certain portions of successive myotomes may fuse to form a single muscle, a splendid example is seen in the rectus abdominis, which is formed by fusion of the ventral portions of the last six or seven thoracic myotomes.

We have just seen that muscle primordia may migrate to segmental levels different from those of their origins. Patten (1946) cites the **lattissimus dorsi** as an example. It arises from cervical myotomes and ultimately migrates to the lower thoracic and lumbar vertebrae, and to the iliac crest. Facial muscles, which are branchiomeric in origin, exhibit similar migratory trends, as we shall see.

One final and important point is that there may be *degeneration of portions, or an entire muscle segment.* When degeneration occurs, a muscle tends to become converted into connective tissue. A great many of the strong **aponeurotic sheets** in the body can be attributed to muscle degeneration. Examples are the abdominal aponeuroses and the galea aponeurotica which connects the occipitalis and frontalis muscles.

Dermatome

The most lateral portion of a somite forms the dermatome which develops into the **dermis** or **chorium** of the skin. There is strong supportive evidence, however, that many of the cells in the dermatome contribute to developing musculature.

The Flexion of the Embryo

During the latter part of the third week, a very significant development occurs: the flexion of the embryo, in which *a reversal of the direction of growth of the head and tail ends* occurs. Because of the extremely rapid growth of the intraembryonic structures, they cannot maintain themselves in a platelike position, and the entire embryo is thrown into a series of folds. Very rapid growth of the cephalic end of the embryo causes a **cephalic fold** in which the prochordal plate (now known as the buccopharyngeal membrane) is folded under the embryonic head.

This flexion also carries the procardiac area under the developing head, so that both the buccopharyngeal membrane and the developing heart are ventral to the neural plate. What was the original rostral wall of the procardiac area is now the caudal wall. Successive stages of flexion of the embryo are shown schematically in Figure 7-11.

While the embryo is flexing in a sagittal plane, it also flexes along the lateral margins and becomes cylindrical. In order to account for lateral flexion and subsequent developments, it is necessary to elaborate on the developmental progress of the intraembryonic mesoderm thus far. It becomes divided into three parts: the paraxial mesoderm alongside the notochord (which is ectoderm), the intermediate mesoderm, and the lateral plate mesoderm.

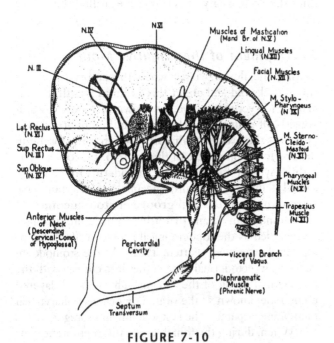

FIGURE 7-10

Illustration of relation of cervical nerves to transverse septum (diaphragm) in an embryo. (From Patten, 1946.)

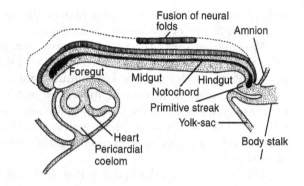

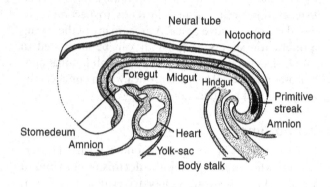

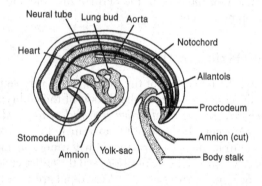

FIGURE 7-11

Schematic sagittal section of human embryos during the longitudinal flexions and the establishment of the digestive tract.

The lateral plate mesoderm divides into two layers, thus producing a cavity, the **intraembryonic coelom.** It subsequently becomes divided into the **pericardial, pleural,** and **peritoneal cavities** in the developing embryo. The upper layer of the lateral plate mesoderm, called the **somatopleuric intraembryonic mesoderm,** is in contact with the ectoderm of the dorsum of the embryo. The lower layer of the lateral plate mesoderm, called **splanchnopleuric intraembryonic mesoderm,** is in contact with the endoderm. Sagittal and lateral flexion of the embryo constricts the yolk sac, which in effect is taken into the body of the embryo, as shown in Figure 7-11, and forms part of the midgut. Formation of the remainder of the gut is also shown schematically in Figure 7-11.

DEVELOPMENT OF THE STRUCTURES FOR SPEECH AND HEARING

Early Development of the Facial Region and Palate

Derivatives of the Three Primary Layers of Tissue

During the flexion phase of development the embryo consists of three layers of tissue: ectoderm, mesoderm, and endoderm. They ultimately give rise to all of the structures of the body (see Figure 1-9).

Ectoderm Ectoderm, as we have seen, is the outermost layer, and it forms the epidermis of the skin, much of the teeth, the entire nervous system, hair, nails, and epithelial tissue.

Mesoderm The intermediate layer is mesoderm, and it ultimately gives rise to most of the connective tissue in the body; that is, it forms the bones, muscles, blood vessels, and cartilages of the body.

Endoderm Endoderm, the deepest of the three layers, gives rise to the epithelial lining of the entire digestive tract (except for the linings of the mouth and pharynx, which are formed by ectoderm) and the epithelial lining of the entire respiratory tract. Because endoderm lines the body cavity, it is sometimes called the "inner skin."

Development of the Primitive Mouth

During the flexion stage, when the embryo is about three weeks old and about three mm in length, the facial area is very primitive. As shown in Figure 7-12, it consists of a smooth, relatively undifferentiated bulge known as the **prosencephalon,**[18] which is the forebrain or anterior brain vesicle of the embryo. It is covered by a thin layer of ectoderm and mesoderm. Immediately caudal (tailward) to the prosencephalon lies a transverse furrow known as the **oral groove** or **stomodeum.**

Stomodeum means **primitive mouth,** and it might be regarded as the topographical center of the developing facial structures (Patten, 1961). As the stomodeum deepens, its ectodermal floor comes into contact with the endodermal lining of the foregut. This two-cell layered membrane, known as the oral plate or buccopharyngeal membrane, separates the stomodeum and foregut.

When, during the fourth week, this membrane ruptures and is absorbed by surrounding tissue, communi-

---

[18]Gk. **proso,** before.

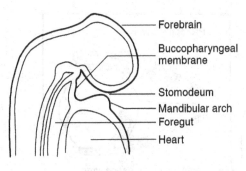

- Forebrain
- Buccopharyngeal membrane
- Stomodeum
- Mandibular arch
- Foregut
- Heart

FIGURE 7-12

Schematic sagittal section through the head of a three-week embryo, showing the forebrain, buccopharyngeal membrane, stomodeum, mandibular arch, foregut, and heart.

cation is for the first time established between the oral groove and the foregut.

The Branchial Arches and Their Derivatives

The lateral walls of the anterior part of the foregut in the **branchial region** become differentiated into a series of transversely placed elevations with depressions between them. The depressions, known as **branchial grooves** or **gill clefts,** are not true clefts, however, because the space is filled in with ectoderm and endoderm. The mesoderm has been pushed aside so that the ectoderm and endoderm are in direct contact. Later, the mesoderm again penetrates between the two layers. The branchial grooves are so closely homologous with similar true gill clefts of fishes and some amphibians that the term gill cleft seems appropriate.

As the paired (right and left) elevations between adjacent branchial grooves grow, they meet at the midline in such a manner that each pair forms a **branchial arch.** According to Gray (1973), six branchial arches make their appearance, but of these, only the first four are visible externally.

The Mandibular Arch The first of the branchial arches is known as the mandibular arch. It ultimately gives rise to the lower lip, the muscles of mastication, the mandible proper, the anterior portion of the tongue, and some of the structures of the middle ear.

The Hyoid Arch The second branchial arch, known as the hyoid arch, gives rise to such structures as the upper body and lesser horns of the hyoid bone, the stapes, and the muscles of facial expression.

Arches 3 to 6 The remaining branchial arches are designated only by number and have no names assigned to them. The **third arch** gives rise to the lower body of the hyoid bone and to the posterior portion of the tongue. The **fourth** and **fifth branchial arches** give rise to the

cricoid and arytenoid cartilages of the larynx and cartilages of the trachea. The caudal portions of the branchial arches (**caudal arches**) give rise to palatine muscles and the pharyngeal constrictors, but the precise contributions are unknown and a source of much disagreement. The derivatives of the branchial arches are shown in Figures 7-13 and 7-14. The **first branchial groove** eventually develops into the concha of the auricle and into the external auditory meatus.

Development of the Facial Region

The Third and Fourth Week

The ventral aspect of the forebrain, shown stippled in Figure 7-15, is crucial to the development of the face.

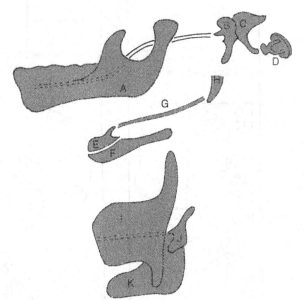

Name of Structure	(mandibular) I	(hyoid) II	III	IV	V	VI
A. mandible	x					
B. malleus	x					
C. incus	x					
D. stapes		x				
E. body of hyoid bone		x				
F. major horn of hyoid			x			
G. stylohyoid ligament		x				
H. styloid process		x				
I. thyroid cartilage				x		
J. arytenoid cartilage					x	
K. cricoid cartilage						*

*The precise derivation of the cricoid cartilage is not known, but it probably is from the mesenchyme of Arch VI.

FIGURE 7-13

Schematic illustrating the skeletal derivatives (osseous and cartilaginous) of the branchial arches. (From: Zemlin, E. and W. Zemlin, *Study Guide Workbook to Accompany Speech and Hearing Science: Anatomy and Physiology,* Champaign, Ill., Stipes Pub., 1988.)

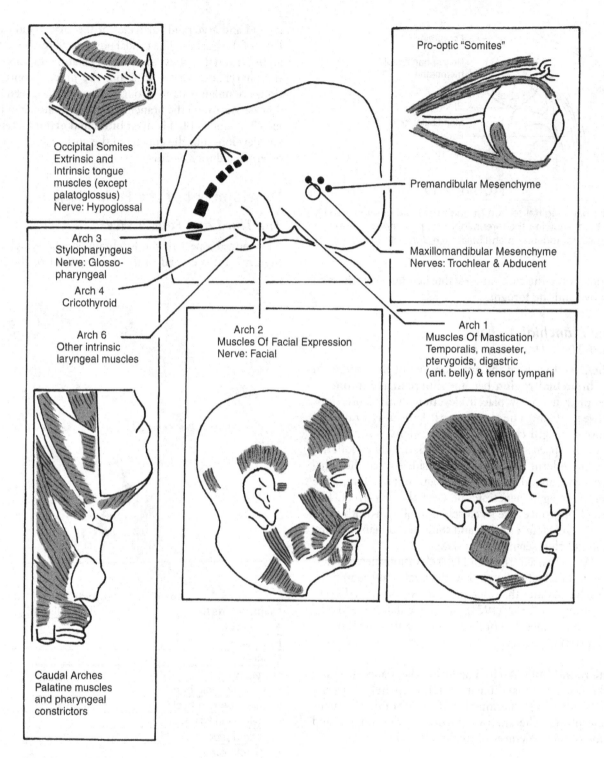

FIGURE 7-14

Schematic illustrating the muscular derivatives of the branchial mesenchyme and the preotic and postotic cranial "somites." (Based on Gray, 36th British edition.)

Although it is relatively undifferentiated during the third week, it eventually develops into the **frontonasal process.** During this same period the first branchial or mandibular arch appears as a single transverse bar located immediately caudal to the oral groove. Some limited proliferation may have taken place, giving rise to as yet undifferentiated **maxillary processes,** one on either side.

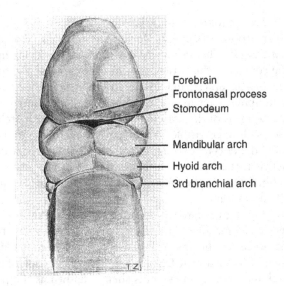

FIGURE 7-15

Ventral view of an embryonic face during latter part of the third or beginning of the fourth week. (Courtesy Therese Zemlin.)

Sometime during the latter part of the third or beginning of the fourth week, two areas, one on either side of the frontal process, begin to proliferate to form thickenings called **nasal** or **olfactory placodes.** Proliferation is of the ectodermal layer. During the fourth week, rapid growth in the areas immediately surrounding the olfactory placodes results in the formation of two **nasal pits.** As shown in Figure 7-16, the nasal pits now divide the previously undifferentiated frontonasal process into a **medial** and two **lateral nasal processes,** one on either side. The olfactory placodes ultimately form the lining of the nasal pits and also the olfactory epithelium which

contains the olfactory sensory cells. Although the maxillary processes continue to develop, they are still relatively undifferentiated from the mandibular arch.

During the fourth week, the hyoid arches appear as two saclike pouches, located in the anterolateral region of what will be the neck. Their continuity is interrupted by the anterior growth of the pericardial swelling. The third branchial arch has grown considerably smaller by the end of the fourth week, when the embryo has attained a length of about 4.5 mm.

The Fifth Week (The Primordial Areas)

The fifth week finds the embryo about 9 mm in length. During this period the branchial arches are at the height of their external development, and the face can now be divided into four primordial areas:

The Frontonasal Process It is still relatively undifferentiated, with the exception of the lateral angles, which are rapidly growing in a caudal direction. During this stage of development the lateral nasal processes do not grow as rapidly as the medial nasal processes. As proliferation of the medial nasal process continues, the two lateral angles become more and more prominent and are known as the **globular processes.** They are shown in Figure 7-17.

The Maxillary Processes Although they are becoming more and more prominent, the maxillary processes cannot as yet be easily differentiated from the mandibular arch from which they arose as cephalically directed

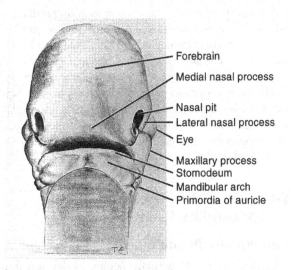

FIGURE 7-16

Ventral view of a five-week embryonic face. (Courtesy Therese Zemlin.)

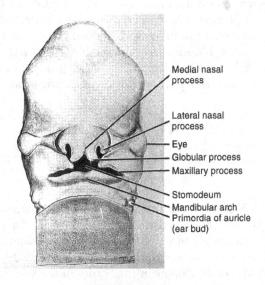

FIGURE 7-17

Ventral view of a six-week embryonic face showing medial and lateral nasal processes and globular process in relation to the maxillary process and stomodeum. (Courtesy Therese Zemlin.)

swellings. The maxillary processes, as shown in Figure 7-17, are located between the lateral nasal processes and the mandibular arch. Sometime during the fifth week, a fusion of the frontonasal and the maxillary processes constricts the opening of the nasal pits.

The Mandibular Arch Due to a pronounced constriction medially, as it crosses the midventral line, the mandibular arch appears as two transverse bars, joined at their medial ends. The mandibular arch, however, is actually a single bar with a free cephalic border. It forms the entire caudal border of the oral pit. This free border is broken only where the mandibular arch is joined with the maxillary processes at the extreme lateral and rostral margins.

The Hyoid Arch During the fifth week of development the hyoid arch is partially interrupted by the ventral bulge of the rapidly growing heart. The hyoid arch, therefore, appears as two saclike processes, one on each anterolateral portion of the neck region.

The Sixth Week

The total length of the embryo remains about the same throughout the sixth week as it was during the fifth, about 9 mm. During this period the medial nasal process forms the entire cephalic boundary of the mouth opening. Also, by the sixth week, the maxillary processes can be identified as wedge-shaped prominences located just caudal to the eye. The eye, which is shown in Figure 7-17, is just beginning to develop laterally.

The medial tips of the maxillary processes are projected toward the caudal ends of the medial and lateral nasal processes. At this stage of development, however, there is no actual fusion with the medial and lateral nasal processes. The maxillary processes are separated from the medial nasal processes by the **oronasal grooves** and from the lateral nasal processes by the **nasooptic grooves.**

CLINICAL NOTE: The oronasal and nasooptic grooves are of special interest because if they fail to be obliterated the face will be malformed.

A fusion of the medial and lateral nasal processes results in a further constriction of the nostrils. The result is a narrowing of the medial nasal process and the beginnings of an anteriorly directed growth. The eyes, which are developing at the border of the lateral nasal process, rostral to the maxillary process, are drawn somewhat anteriorly. At this point, the superior border of the mandibular arch is a continuous ledge forming the caudal border of the mouth.

Except for its extreme lateral portion, the first branchial groove disappears during the latter part of the sixth week. This groove, you will recall, develops into the concha of the auricle and into the external auditory meatus. Several small buds begin to appear at the hyoid-mandibular arch area. These buds are the beginnings of the margins of the auricle. The third and fourth arches are no longer visible. They have been obliterated to form the **cervical sinus,** a temporary structure located between the hyoid arch in front and the thoracic wall behind. Due to the fusion of its walls, the sinus eventually disappears.

During the latter part of the sixth week, fusion between the maxillary and medial nasal processes (globular processes) begins. When this fusion is completed, a shelf of tissue for the first time separates a portion of the oral and nasal cavities. This shelf is known as the **primary palate.**

At the same time as the maxillary and medial nasal processes fuse, the tissue in the area of the globular processes is projected posteriorly into the nasal cavity to form two plates called the **nasal laminae.** During subsequent development, as the nasal pits come closer together, these nasal laminae ultimately fuse to form the **nasal septum,** which divides the nasal cavity into two halves on the median plane. A facial landmark known as the **philtrum** indicates the point of fusion between the maxillary and globular processes (Figure 7-18). The lateral nasal processes do not ultimately form any of the opening of the oral cavity. Rather, they form the alae of the nose.

The Seventh Week

The seventh week sees a pronounced change in the face of the embryo (Figure 7-19). The nasal area is beginning to become prominent, with a corresponding reduction in width. The eyes have moved onto the anterior surface of the face. During this period the mandible has shown little change. *The latter part of the sixth and beginning of the seventh week are important in the development of the palate in the embryo.* Because we are concerned primarily with the formation of the palate, a separate section dealing with the primary and secondary palates follows. Further development of the face of the embryo will be treated only incidentally.

Development of the Primary and Secondary Palates

The Primary Palate

The primary palate actually begins to develop during the fourth week when formation of the olfactory pits is taking place. Beginning at the inferior border of the ol-

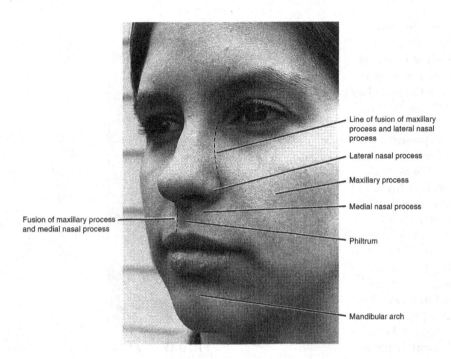

Line of fusion of maxillary process and lateral nasal process

Lateral nasal process

Maxillary process

Medial nasal process

Philtrum

Mandibular arch

Fusion of maxillary process and medial nasal process

FIGURE 7-18

The philtrum indicates the point of fusion between the maxillary and globular processes.

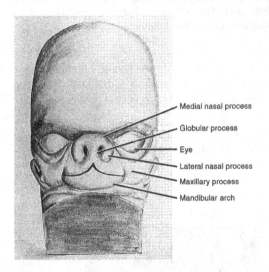

Medial nasal process

Globular process

Eye

Lateral nasal process

Maxillary process

Mandibular arch

FIGURE 7-19

Ventral view of an embryonic face during the latter part of the seventh or the beginning of the eighth week. (Courtesy Therese Zemlin.)

factory pit, the medial nasal process fuses with the maxillary process. During the sixth week fusion between the lateral nasal and medial nasal processes (*globular process*) takes place. Because of the growth of the nasal processes, the olfactory pits are now actual **choanae,** each being closed off by a thin epithelial wall, the **bucconasal membrane.** During the later part of the seventh or early part of the eighth week, this membrane ruptures and is absorbed by surrounding tissues. When this occurs, the pri-

mary choana communicates directly with the oral cavity. *A bar of tissue located between the nasal duct and the oral cavity at the edge between the facial and oral surfaces is the primary palate.* This is the tissue that is formed when, during the sixth week, the maxillary and nasal processes fuse.

Changes in the Mandibular Arch

During the time of the formation of the upper facial regions, an interesting alteration occurs in the mandibular arch. Up until the sixth week it is undifferentiated. Around the beginning of the sixth week, however, *three constrictions appear on the exterior surface of the mandibular arch.* A pronounced constriction known as the **median sulcus** divides the arch into halves. On either side, small furrows called **lateral sulci** develop. These sulci disappear at the same time the nasal and maxillary processes fuse in the upper facial region.

Differential Facial Growth

Differential facial growth accounts for much of the further development of the palate. An example is the rapid growth of the lateral nasal and the maxillary processes relative to the growth of the medial nasal process, which grows more slowly in a lateral direction. While this is taking place, the whole facial area grows in an anterior direction to form the prominence in the nasal region, at the same time causing a movement of the eyes from the anterolateral to the anterior surface of the face. This differential growth is depicted in Figures 7-17 and 7-19. The openings of the nares are closed during this stage of development by proliferating epithelium. The eyes, too, are covered by epithelium until after the development of the lids.

Until about the eighth week, the mouth opening is very wide, becoming smaller with the fusion of the lateral areas of the mandibular arch and the maxillary processes to form the cheeks and at the same time narrowing the width of the mouth opening.

At the time of the development of the primary palate the nasal cavity is a short duct leading from the nostrils to the primitive oral cavity. *The outer and inner openings of the nasal cavity are separated by the primary palate, which will later develop into the upper lip, the anterior portion of the alveolar process, and the premaxillary part of the palate.*

During about the eighth week, *the growth of the head moves into a vertical plane.* This change in direction of growth results in an increase in height of the oral cavity. A direct result of this is that the tissue separating the primitive choana grows posteriorly and in a caudal direction to form part of the future nasal septum.

The oral cavity communicates with the nasal cavities at this time, although an incomplete palate is formed by the primary palate anteriorly and medially directed swellings from the maxillary processes laterally. (We identify this medially directed portion later, in adult anatomy, as the **palatine processes of the maxillae.**) Medially, the oral cavity communicates with the nasal cavity on either side of the nasal septum. A schematic primary palate, as seen from beneath, is shown in Figure 7-20.

The Secondary Palate

In the earlier stages of the formation of the secondary palate, the **tongue** is extended in height so that it almost completely fills the oral cavity and, in fact, touches the tissue that will eventually develop into the nasal septum. This is illustrated in Figure 7-21. Folds of tissue, lateral on either side of the tongue, grow in a downward direction. These folds are the palatine processes of the maxillae. They extend posteriorly to the lateral walls of the pharynx.

The secondary palate is formed primarily by a fusion of the palatine processes of the maxillae. *Fusion can*

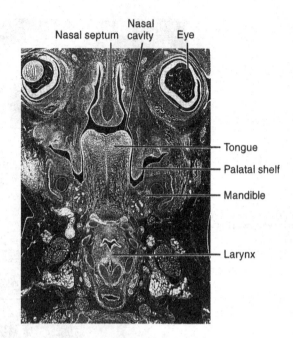

FIGURE 7-21

Frontal section through the face of an embryo during the eighth week. The tongue extends into the nasal cavity thus separating the palatal shelves.

occur, however, only when the tongue has moved down. This downward growth is made possible by a sudden spurt of growth in the mandibular arch. The tongue then drops, leaving a space between the palatine processes. When this occurs, as shown in Figures 7-22 and 7-23, mesodermal cells on the lateral (oral) surfaces of the palatine processes begin proliferating rapidly, causing a change in

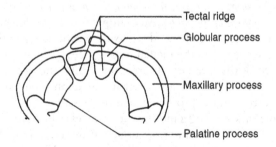

FIGURE 7-20

Schematic of the roof of the mouth of a nine-week embryo illustrating the processes which contribute to the formation of the palate.

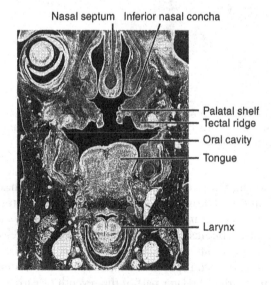

FIGURE 7-22

Frontal section of a nine-week embryo. Rapid growth of the mandible has lowered the tongue to evacuate the space between the palatal shelves.

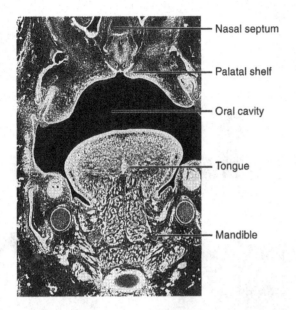

— Nasal septum

— Palatal shelf

— Oral cavity

— Tongue

— Mandible

FIGURE 7-23

Frontal section through the face of an embryo slightly older than that shown in Figure 7-22. The palatal shelves have fused with each other and with the nasal septum.

growth from the vertical to the horizontal plane. The palatine processes fuse with each other and with the nasal septum as well, as shown in Figures 7-23 and 7-24. This fusion takes place in an anterior to posterior direction. The palatine processes form only the soft palate and the medial portion of the hard palate.

As shown in Figure 7-20, the roof of the mouth (**tegmen oris**) is bounded laterally and anteriorly by the **tectal ridge,** which is an inward projection of the globular process. *The tectal ridge is the equivalent of the premaxillary process.* Later in the developmental sequence the alveolar ridge will arise from a layer of mesodermal tissue that is located in a sulcus between the palate and lip.

Summary of Development of the Palate

2nd week:	Appearance of stomodeum or primitive mouth.
3rd week:	Formation of the mandibular arch on either side; maxillary processes bud out from mandibular arch; nasal placodes appear.
4th week:	Rupture and disappearance of buccopharyngeal membrane.
5th week:	Appearance of frontonasal processes; olfactory pits widely separated; appearance of globular processes.
6th week:	Union of lateral nasal with maxillary processes; partial division of stomodeum into an upper and lower cavity.

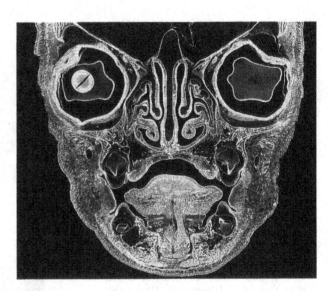

FIGURE 7-24

A frontal section through the face of a five-month fetus.

8th week:	Union of the three portions of the palate commences anteriorly; completion of the upper lip by fusion of globular processes.
10th week:	Completion of union of palatine segments, the uvula being the last to be completed.

CLINICAL NOTE: The embryonic development as just described has been very schematic and highly idealized. Unfortunately, facial development is sometimes interrupted during the period when the fusion between the primitive palate and the palatine processes of the maxillae is normally taking place. As a result, facial deformities of various degrees of severity may occur, the most common of which is **cleft palate.** A cleft may assume any one of a number of forms: **complete, incomplete, unilateral,** or **bilateral.** Some examples are shown in Figure 7-25.

The cause or causes of cleft palate are not known with certainty. Factors such as intrauterine anoxia, toxic poisoning, high concentrations of cortisone, an inherent lack of mesoderm, and heredity seem to be implicated. After an exhaustive study of etiological factors, Fogh-Anderson (1942), in Denmark, concluded that heredity is in all likelihood the most essential etiological factor in cleft palate and cleft lip. Cleft palate occurs in one out of about a thousand births, and it seems that males are far more subject to the deformity than are females. The ratio is about 2 to 1. Males are less subject to the minor palatal defects than are females, but considerably more subject to the severe types of defects, such as complete clefts of the lip and palate.

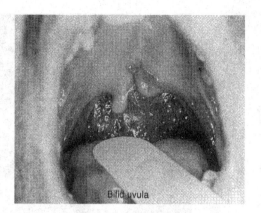

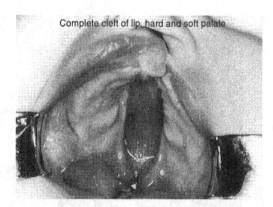

Complete cleft of lip, hard and soft palate

Bifid uvula

FIGURE 7-25

Examples of cleft lip and palate. (Photographs supplied, courtesy Center for Craniofacial Anomalies, Univ. of Ill., Chicago.)

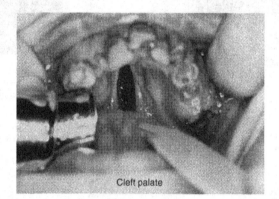

Cleft palate

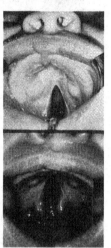

Cleft of soft palate only

Development of the Tongue

The primordial areas that give rise to the mucous membrane of the tongue first appear during the seventh or eighth week. According to Patten (1961), they can best be seen in preparations made by cutting from either side through the branchial arches to the lumen of the pharynx and then removing the brain and oropharyngeal roof so that the floor of the pharynx can be viewed from above as in Figure 7-26.

Embryos in their fifth week often show evidence of paired lateral thickenings (**lateral lingula swellings**) on the internal surface of the mandibular arch. They consist of rapidly proliferating mesoderm (**mesenchyme**) covered by epithelium. A small elevation (the **tuberculum impar**)[19] is located between the lateral lingual swellings. Just behind it, as shown in Figure 7-26, is a second midline swelling known as the **copula**[20] or the **hypobranchial eminence.** It bridges the second and third branchial arches at the midline, and a transverse

groove separates its caudal part that forms the **epiglottis.** Ventrally it approaches the tongue rudiment, spreading ventrally in the form of a "V," and forming the posterior or pharyngeal part of the tongue. In the adult the union of the anterior and posterior parts of the tongue is marked by the **sulcus terminalis,** the apex of which is the site of the **foramen caecum.**

Behind (caudal to) the copula are two swellings, placed on either side of the midline. They are the beginnings of the arytenoid cartilages, and between them may be seen a third midline swelling that will eventually become the epiglottis. These structures are shown schematically in Figure 7-27.

Tissue on either side of the copula proliferates rapidly until, by the end of the seventh week, a distinct tongue-like structure is evident. A small pit, which we later identify as the foramen caecum in the adult, separates the two pairs of bilaterally symmetrical tongue primordia. The cephalic pair (the **anterior lingual primordia**) is located at the level of the first branchial arch, while the caudal pair (the **root primordia**) is located at the level of the second bronchial arch.

At first the tongue is composed only of mucous membrane, but later striated muscle fibers migrate in-

---

[19]L. **tuberculum,** a nodule or small eminence. L. **impar,** unpaired.

[20]L. **copula,** a joining together.

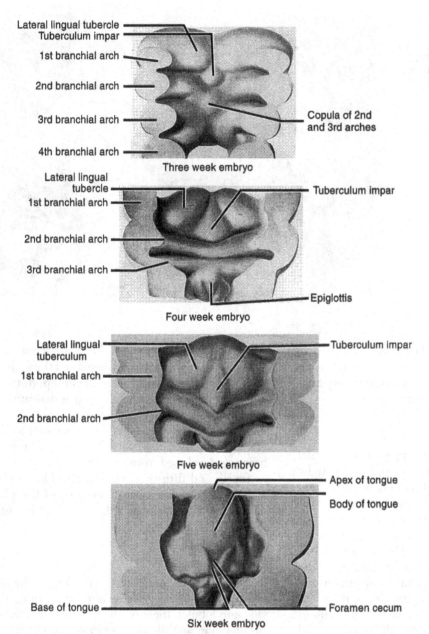

Lateral lingual tubercle
Tuberculum impar
1st branchial arch
2nd branchial arch
3rd branchial arch
4th branchial arch
Copula of 2nd and 3rd arches
Three week embryo

Lateral lingual tubercle
1st branchial arch
2nd branchial arch
3rd branchial arch
Tuberculum impar
Epiglottis
Four week embryo

Lateral lingual tuberculum
1st branchial arch
2nd branchial arch
Tuberculum impar
Five week embryo

Apex of tongue
Body of tongue
Base of tongue
Foramen cecum
Six week embryo

FIGURE 7-26

Floor of the oral cavity and ventral wall of the lower pharynx as seen from above and behind, showing the development of the tongue and adjacent structures. (From Sicher and Tandler, 1928.)

to it, causing a rapid expansion in its dimensions. The musculature does not come from the branchial arches but rather from the three **occipital somites.** When the tongue is well developed, it is composed of two primary muscles, the genioglossus and the hyoglossus. The transverse and vertical intrinsic muscles are derived from the hyoglossus.

Development of the Respiratory System

Caudal to the primitive mouth, the **foregut** becomes widened and flattened dorsoventrally to form the pharynx. Four pocketlike diverticula, the **pharyngeal pouches,** arise from it laterally. Each pouch is located opposite an external branchial groove. Arising medially in the floor of the pharynx at the level of the first and second arches is a band of endoderm called the **thyroid primordium.**

The rudiments of the respiratory system appear in the fourth week as a median **laryngeotracheal groove** on the floor of the pharynx. The groove deepens, and its lips fuse to form the **laryngeotracheal tube.** The fusion begins at the caudal end of the groove and progresses cranially, but the lips at the cranial end of the tube remain separated, providing a slitlike opening into the pharynx. The tube is lined with endoderm, and from this, the epithelial lining of the entire respiratory tract is developed. The cranial end of the laryngotracheal tube develops into the larynx, while the remainder forms the trachea. At the

FIGURE 7-27

Stages in the development of the human larynx. (A) at 5 mm, (B) at 9 mm, (C) at 12 mm, (D) at 16 mm, (E) at 40 mm, (F) sagittal hemisection, at birth. (From Arey, 1965.)

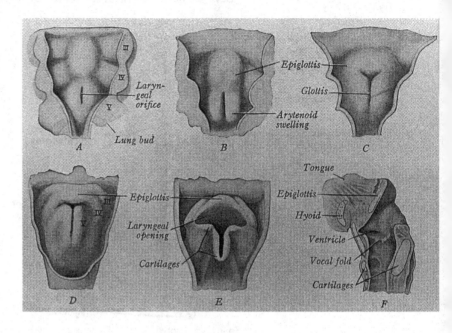

caudal extreme of the tube, two lateral outgrowths arise to form the **main bronchi** and the right and left **lung buds.** The epithelial lining of the entire respiratory tract is derived from the endoderm lining the tube.

The Larynx

The first rudiments of the larynx appear at the cranial end of the laryngotracheal tube, bounded ventrally by the hypobranchial eminence and laterally by the ventral ends of the sixth arches. Two arytenoid swellings appear, one on each side of the groove, and as they enlarge they approximate each other and meet the hypobranchial eminence (which will develop into the epiglottis). Initially the opening into the larynx is a vertical slit, but the enlargement of the arytenoid swellings converts it to a "T"-shaped cleft. At about the seventh week the vertical part of the "T" lies between the arytenoid swellings and the horizontal part lies between the swellings and the epiglottis (Figure 7-27). Soon after the appearance of the cleft the epithelial tissue of its walls adhere to each other, closing off the entrance to the larynx. *The entrance is occluded until the third month, when its lumen is again established by resorption of the tissue.*

CLINICAL NOTE: Failure of this epithelium to resorb explains the presence of congenital **laryngeal webs** and various types of **papillae.**

When the entrance to the larynx has been reestablished, the laryngeal ventricles can be seen. They are bounded cranially and caudally by projecting shelves of tissue that form the ventricular and vocal folds.

The arytenoid swellings differentiate into the **arytenoid** and **corniculate cartilages** and the folds joining them to the epiglottis become the **aryepiglottic folds.** The **cuneiform cartilages** develop as derivatives of the epiglottis.

The **thyroid cartilage,** which appears as two lateral plates joined at the midline by a fibrous membrane, is developed from the ventral ends of the fourth or fourth and fifth branchial arches. The caudal ends give rise to the **constrictor muscles of the pharynx.** The **cricoid cartilage** is a derivative of the fifth arch (Figure 7-13).

The Lungs

The right and left lung buds appear before the laryngotracheal groove has been converted into a tube. They divide into lobules, three on the right and two on the left. Proliferation and division continues and at six months the alveoli begin to form. Three phases of **lung tissue differentiation** are recognized: **glandular, canalicular,** and **alveolar.**

In the glandular phase, the bronchial divisions are differentiated but the epithelial tissue resembles glandular tissue. In the canalicular phase, the respiratory segments and other parts are delineated and establish a relationship with the expanding vascular system. The lungs are not functional at this stage, which may extend into the sixth month. The alveolar phase extends from six months, but new bronchi and alveoli continue to be formed after birth. During their development the lungs migrate in a caudal direction, and at birth the bifurcation of the trachea is located at the level of the fourth thoracic vertebra.

Development of the Outer Ear (and the Hyoid Bone)

The Cartilages of the Branchial Arches

The mandibular (first branchial) arch, presents dorsal and ventral cartilaginous elements. The dorsal cartilage is known as the **palatopterygoquadrate bar.** Any structure with such an impressive name should be expected to persist into the adult form, and although it is a prominent structure in reptiles, it is transient in humans.[21] Its contributions, if any, are a subject of much debate. The ventral cartilaginous element of the mandibular arch (**Meckle's cartilage**) extends from the developing otic capsule into the mandible and meets its fellow from the opposite side. Its dorsal end forms the malleus and incus,[22] and although the cartilage itself disappears, its sheath remains as the anterior malleolar and the sphenomandibular ligaments.

---

[21]Many embryonic structures are transient, and their presence is thought to have an **inductive role.** That is, the presence of structures induces growth and development in its environment that would not take place in the absence of the structure. For example, if the notochord is removed from an embryo, the vertebral column will fail to develop.

[22]There is evidence that the palatopterygoquadrate bar may contribute to the incus and possibly the major wing of the sphenoid bone.

The cartilage of the hyoid (second branchial) arch is known as **Reichert's cartilage.** It also extends from the otic capsule to the midline ventrally. The dorsal end separates and becomes enclosed in the developing tympanic cavity as the **stapes.** It also gives rise to the styloid process of the temporal bone, the stylohyoid ligament, and the lesser horns and upper body of the hyoid bone. The ventral portion of arch 3 gives rise to the greater horns and lower body of the hyoid bone.

The External Ear

The first and second arches and the first branchial groove contribute to the formation of the external ear. The **auricle** develops around the first branchial groove and is derived from tissue of the mandibular and hyoid arches. At about six weeks, six small elevations (**hillocks**) appear—three on the caudal border of the first arch and three on the second arch—along with an elongated elevation called the **auricular fold.** These hillocks are numbered in Figure 7-28, and their contributions to the adult form are also shown. This "classical view" has been challenged to the extent that the entire auricle, except for the tragus, is said to develop from the hyoid arch.

The **external auditory meatus** represents the first branchial groove. The ectodermal floor of the groove is in contact with the endoderm of the first pharyngeal pouch. This contact is lost when growth of the head

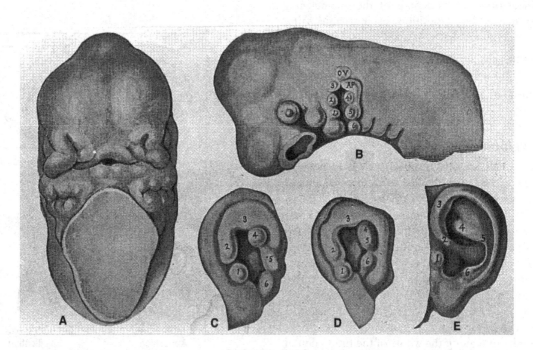

FIGURE 7-28

Embryonic development of the auricle. **AF**, Auricular fold; **OV**, otic vesicle; 1–6 elevations on the mandibular and hyoid arches which become 1, tragus; 2, 3, helix; 4, 5, antihelix; 6, antitragus. (From Arey, 1965.)

tends to separate the meatus from the middle ear cavity. Toward the end of the second month, the groove deepens to produce a funnel-shaped pit. From the bottom of this pit an ectodermal plate grows even deeper until it reaches the wall of the tympanic cavity. During the seventh month the plate splits, and the resultant cleft constitutes the deepest portion of the external auditory meatus. The tympanic membrane develops where the blind end of the external meatus abuts against the wall of the tympanic cavity. The adult tympanic membrane is a fibrous sheet covered by ectodermal epithelium externally and by endodermal epithelial internally.

The skeletal and muscular derivatives of the branchial arches are given in Figures 7-13, and 7-14.

Development of the Teeth

The Development Sequence

The developmental sequence is essentially the same for deciduous and permanent teeth, and the life cycle of a tooth, whether it be deciduous or permanent, may be considered in four periods: **growth, calcification, eruption,** and **attrition.**

Growth—the beginning formation of the tooth bud, specialization and arrangement of cells to outline the future tooth, and deposition of the enamel and dentin matrix.

Calcification—the hardening of the enamel and dentin matrix by deposition of inorganic salts, largely calcium.

Eruption—the migration of the rather fully developed tooth into the oral cavity.

Attrition—the wearing away of the enamel on the contact and occlusal surfaces of the erupted tooth.

Early Development

The teeth, which are modifications of ectoderm and mesoderm, begin to show the first signs of development during the fifth or sixth week of embryonic life (11 mm embryo). The initial stage of tooth growth is the formation of the **tooth bud** from the epithelial tissue contained in what will eventually become the jaws and associated connective tissue. During the fifth or sixth week, the **oral epithelium** is separated from the subjacent connective tissue (mesoderm) by a thin basement membrane. Certain cells in the basal layer of the epithelium begin to proliferate at an accelerated rate, which results in a thickening of epithelium along the whole of the future dental arch. This growing epithelium extends into the mesoderm (from which bone and other connective tissues will develop) to form a thin strand of tissue called the **dental lamina.** *During about the seventh week oval swellings begin to develop in the dental lamina. These swellings are known as tooth buds, and their positions correspond to the future locations of the primary teeth.*

The Cap Stage

Once the development of a tooth bud is initiated, its cells begin to proliferate faster than adjacent cells. The proliferation is differential, however, and the *unequal growth results in an invagination of the deeper surface of the tooth bud.* This is illustrated in Figure 7-29. The developing tooth is now said to have entered the cap stage.

As proliferation continues, the dental cap begins to surround and engulf mesoderm. This mesoderm, which will eventually be located inside the tooth, is known as the **dental papilla.** At this stage the dental cap is surrounded by mesoderm (which ultimately forms the **cementum** of the tooth and the **periodontal tissue**), and

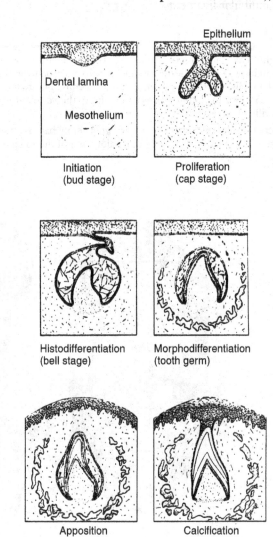

FIGURE 7-29

Schematic representation of the growth of a tooth. (From *Atlas of the Mouth,* Courtesy American Dental Association.)

it also surrounds mesoderm (which gives rise to the **dental pulp** and contributes to the formation of **dentin**).

The Bell Stage

While the papillae are being formed, changes are occurring in the cells of the special dental germ or cap. The cells become differentiated into three distinct layers. Those in contact with the papillae undergo modifications and acquire the ability to form enamel; they are identified as **enamel cells (ameloblasts).** The cells in the outer layer of the cap are called **external enamel epithelium.** These cells, plus the cells in the intermediate layer, become modified to form **enamel pulp.** When these changes have been completed, the special dental germ (dental cap) is spoken of as the **enamel organ.** *At this stage of development the enamel organ has assumed a bell shape.* The tooth has transcended the cap stage and has entered the bell stage. A tooth in the advanced bell stage is shown in Figure 7-29.

The Tooth Germ

Concomitant with the development of the dental organ and papilla, there is a modification of the mesoderm immediately surrounding the developing tooth. The cells become extremely dense and give rise to a fibrous layer of tissue known as the **dental sac.** *The dental organ and its contained dental papilla, plus the dental sac, constitute the formative tissues for the tooth and its periodontal tissue. These structures collectively are called the tooth germ.*

Maturation of Enamel

The cells of the inner dental epithelium become arranged to form a complex matrix for the deposition of enamel. When these cells have become fully developed, they are known as **ameloblasts,** and they form the enamel matrix, which is structurally the same as the mature enamel in the erupted tooth, but has a consistency of cartilage. The process whereby the enamel matrix is transformed into enamel is called maturation of the enamel, during which mineral salts are deposited and crystallized. The formation and maturation of the enamel matrix are inordinately complex, and the interested reader is referred to Orban (1957).

Formation of Dentin

All the while enamel is being formed in the enamel organ, changes are taking place in the mesodermal cells of the papillae. The cells in contact with the inner layer of special dental germ become modified to form **odontoblasts.** These cells are responsible for the formation of the dentin of the crown of the tooth. The odontoblasts form a layer of dentin, move toward the center of the papilla and produce a second layer of dentin, move

again and produce a third layer, and so forth.[23] The very center of the papilla does not undergo differentiation, but remains as the **pulp** of the tooth. The **root** of the tooth, which is an outgrowth of the dental germ, begins to be formed just before clinical eruption occurs. Growth of the root, however, continues for some time after eruption.

Eruption and attrition of the dentition are topics that have been discussed in Chapter 4, articulation. These phases of the life of a tooth transcend the embryonic development.

DEVELOPMENT OF THE NERVOUS SYSTEM

The embryonic development of the nervous system was discussed briefly in Chapter 5. The purpose of this section is to provide a more complete picture and, in addition, supplementary information that might be helpful.

Early Development

The entire nervous system is of ectodermal origin, as shown in Figure 1-9. The primordial nervous system first makes its appearance in the form of the **neural folds** that lie alongside the dorsal midline of the embryonic disc. The neural folds begin just behind the rostral end of the embryonic disc, where they are continuous with one another, and from there extend back, one on either side of the primitive streak (a temporary structure that gives rise to mesoderm). Between the neural folds is a shallow neural groove that gradually deepens as the folds become elevated. Ultimately the folds meet and fuse in the midline to form the **neural tube,** as shown in Figure 7-6.

Fusion of the Neural Folds

Fusion begins rostrally in the region of the future hindbrain and from there extends both forward and backward. With growth of the embryo in the caudal direction, the neural groove, and later the neural tube, grow in that direction. The open caudal end of the neural tube, the **posterior neuropore,** closes off at about the 25-somite stage. At the same time fusion of the neural tube in the rostral end of the groove has brought the neural tube into the region of the future brain, and at about the 20-somite stage, the terminal opening, known as the **anterior**

---

[23]Upon close examination, a tooth may be seen to contain growth rings, similar to growth rings in the trunk of a tree. The growth pattern and general health of an individual may be ascertained by the calcification pattern and incremental growth rings of a tooth.

neuropore, seals off. A neural plate, primitive streak, somites, and developing neural tube including the neuropores can be seen in Figures 7-30 and 7-31.

Prior to the fusion of the neural folds, a ridge of ectodermal cells appears just lateral to each fold. This **neural crest** or **ganglion ridge** is important because it gives rise to spinal and cranial nerve ganglia, and the ganglia of the sympathetic trunk of the autonomic nervous system. Also, on either side of the neural groove, there is an upward growth of mesoderm that soon invades the space between the neural tube and the overlying ectoderm that forms the dorsum of the embryo. In effect, *the ectoderm that gives rise to the nervous system has migrated toward the interior of the embryo.* Upon completion of the fusion of the neural folds, ectoderm once again forms a continuous layer over the dorsum of the embryo, as shown in Figure 7-6, and it is separated from the neural tube by the interposed mesoderm.

Derivatives of the Neural Tube

The rostral part of the neural tube is somewhat broad and flat, and it ultimately forms the brain, while the narrow caudal portion forms the spinal cord. The lumen of the tube forms the ventricles of the brain and the central canal of the spinal cord.

Primitive Medullary Epithelial Cells

At first, the wall of the neural tube is composed of but a single layer of columnar ectodermal cells whose nuclei are located toward the lumen side of the cell. They are known as the primitive medullary epithelial cells, from which most of the cells in the future nervous system are developed. The fate of the primitive medullary epithelium and the forms its cells may take provide an important avenue for an understanding of the development of the nervous system.

Differentiation of Primitive Medullary Cells

Types of Differentiation

One form of cell differentiation may occur when the nucleus migrates toward the middle of the cell, whose body then takes on a spindle shape. Such a cell, called a **spongioblast,** gives rise to an **astrocyte,** which is a particular type of **supportive** or **neuroglial cell.**[24]

These cells send out cytoplasmic extensions that join those of other neuroglial cells to *form a network of supportive fibers.* Because neuroglial tissue stems from primitive medullary epithelium, it is found only in the spinal cord and brain.

Another form of cell modification occurs when the cytoplasm of the cell shrinks away from the outside of the neural tube and moves toward the nucleus at the lumen side of the tube. Such a cell may have one of two fates. It

---

[24]Gk. **glial,** gluelike.

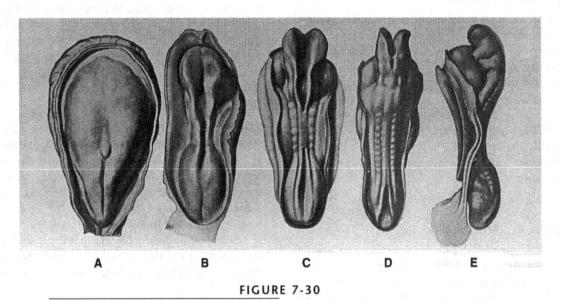

A   B   C   D   E

FIGURE 7-30

Developmental stages of the human neural groove and tube (Streeter). All but (E) are in dorsal view. (A) Presomite embryo, with neural plate and primitive streak (× 40). (B) At 3 somites with deep neural groove. (C) At 7 somites, with closure beginning midway (× 31). (D) At 10 somites, with closure of neural tube beginning midway (× 31). (E) At 19 somites, with closure complete except for neuropores at each end (× 20).

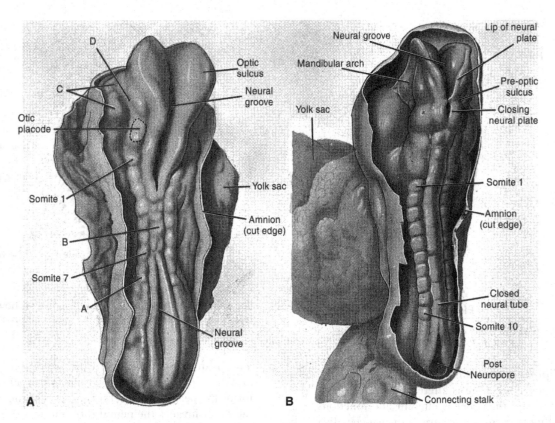

FIGURE 7-31

(A) The dorsal aspect of a reconstruction of a 7-somite human embryo of about the twenty-second day. The early optic sulcus in prosencephalic region. (1) Partially segmented paraxial mesoderm, (2) roof of neural tube, (3) pericardial area, (4) branchial arch region. (B) The dorsal aspect of a reconstruction of a 10-somite human embryo of about the twenty-third day. The bulge visible on either side below the mandibular arches is produced by the pericardium. The elevations on yolk sac wall are due to blood islands. (From Hamilton, Boyd, and Mossman, *Human Embryology,* Williams & Wilkins, 1945.)

may *remain unchanged and form an epithelial cell lining the cavity of the neural tube,* or it may *form a germinal cell that undergoes rapid mitotic cell division.* The daughter cells may form **medulloblasts,** which can differentiate into either astrocytes or **oligodendrocytes,**[25] or they may form **glioblasts** which differentiate into neuroglial cells or into **neuroblasts** (primitive nerve cells).

Neurons

A neuron is composed of a **cell body** (or soma) and its extensions or **nerve processes,** of which there are essentially two types: (1) multiple, short, thick arborizations of the cytoplasm of the cell body called **dendrites** and (2) a single, long thin filament called an **axon.** Dendrites are **afferent** in function, carrying nerve impulses toward the cell, while axons are **efferent** in function,

carrying nerve impulses away from the cell. Although there may be thousands of dendrites on a nerve cell body (which increases its surface area markedly), there is usually but one axon emerging from a nerve cell body. Axons may branch to produce *collaterals,* but typically we think of just one axon per nerve cell, and it may be up to 120 cm in length. Although neurons can be found in a wide variety of shapes and sizes, almost all of them can be classified into one of three types, based primarily on their structure. *Neuroblasts differentiate into **unipolar,** **bipolar,** or **multipolar** neurons.*

Unipolar neurons appear to possess a single axon (Figure 7-32), one limb efferent and the other afferent. A single extension is attached to the cell body, but it quickly divides into two long processes, one of which conducts toward the cell body (the dendrite) and one which conducts away from the cell body (the axon). Structurally, these two processes are identical. These cells are found in the cerebral and cerebellar cortexes, and in the spinal cord (spinal and cranial nerve ganglia).

---

[25]Gk. **oligo-,** little or deficiency.

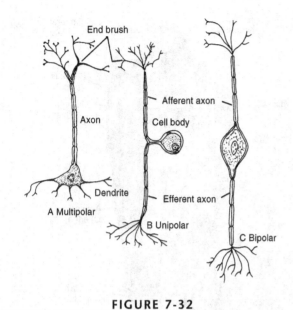

FIGURE 7-32

Illustration of the three common types of neurons.

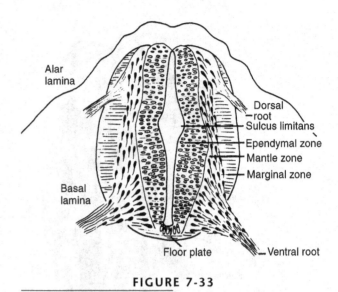

FIGURE 7-33

Section of spinal cord of a four-week embryo showing the sulcus limitans, ependymal, mantle, and marginal zones.

Bipolar neurons have an extension on either pole of the cell body. One is afferent and so functions as a dendrite, and the other is efferent and functions as an axon. Bipolar neurons are primarily associated with the special senses (vision, hearing, balance, taste, and smell).

Multipolar neurons have a large number of dendrites (usually quite short) and a single long axon.

Differentiation of the Neural Tube

Because of the rapid growth of the cells, the central canal of the neural tube takes on a lozenge shape when seen in cross section, the widest portion, or lateral sulcus, being called the **sulcus limitans.** As shown in Figure 7-33, it divides the lateral wall into a **dorsal zone** (the **alar lamina**) and a **ventral zone** (the **basal lamina**). The lateral walls of the neural tube are connected dorsally and ventrally by the thin dorsal roofplate and the ventral floorplate, whose cells retain their epithelial characteristics.

Cells of the basal lamina (neuroblasts) become motor in function while *cells in the alar lamina become sensory.* Neuroblasts in the basal lamina begin to send out processes that course toward the periphery as motor nerve fibers, and they eventually form the ventral (motor) roots of the spinal nerves.

Differentiation of the Neural Crest

Earlier it was pointed out that the neural crest (the ectoderm on either side of the neural tube) gives rise to nerve tissue and, in particular, forms the dorsal root ganglia and dorsal (sensory) roots of the spinal nerves.

The primitive nerve cells in the neural crest develop processes, one of which grows out to the periphery and forms the peripheral (afferent) process of the cell, while the other invades the neural tube and forms the central (efferent) process of the cell.

Myelin-Forming Cells

Oligodendroglial cells are unique because they are responsible for the formation of myelin around the nerve fibers of cells in the brain and spinal cord. **Myelin** is a white, fatty substance that surrounds nerve fibers. It does not appear until the nerve processes are well developed, and it acts as an electrical insulator, ensuring isolated conduction within any given nerve fiber. Thus the *dorsal root ganglion cells and their processes are formed outside the embryonic central nervous system.*

It may be worth noting that while these peripheral fibers may be myelinated, the myelin cannot stem from oligodendroglial cells (which are confined to the neural tube). Presumably, the *myelin sheath on fibers peripheral to the neural tube arises from supportive cells in the neural crest.* These supportive cells give rise to an additional **neurilemmal sheath** which encases peripheral nerves, and since they arise from the neural crest, there are no neurilemmal cells inside the central nervous system.

In addition to dorsal root ganglion cells, the neural crest also gives rise to the ganglia of cranial nerves V through X in the hindbrain region, and the ganglia of the autonomic nervous system. Neural crest cells also produce epidermal pigmentation and cartilage, influence the formation of the axial skeleton, and form the medulla of the adrenal gland.

Zones (Layers) of the Neural Tube

As a result of proliferation and differentiation of the cells in the neural tube, three layers or zones may be defined—an internal (**ependymal**), an intermediate (**mantle**), and an external (**marginal**) zone. The neuroglia and neuroblasts together form the mantle zone, which eventually comprises the gray matter of the spinal cord. Outside the mantle zone is the marginal zone, which is relatively free of developing nerve cells, but into which processes from the mantle zone will extend, eventually forming the white matter of the spinal cord.

Development of the Longitudinal Sulcus and Septum

Continued proliferation of the neuroblasts in the mantle zone of the basal lamina results in obliteration of the ventral part of the central canal, and since growth is also in a ventral direction, swelling occurs on either side of the midline. As a consequence, a longitudinal anteromedian sulcus or fissure is formed. At the same time, proliferation of neuroglia and neuroblasts in the alar lamina compresses and obliterates the dorsal part of the central canal, thus producing a longitudinal posteromedian septum. *Both the longitudinal sulcus and septum persist and are visible in the adult spinal cord.*

Formation of Somatic and Visceral Columns

With continued cell proliferation the central canal is markedly reduced in size, until it occupies only the center of the neural tube. It may even be obliterated. Local proliferation of the neuroblasts in the mantle zone results in aggregates of cell bodies, which form four columns extending the length of the neural tube. Two are found in the alar lamina and two in the basal lamina. As shown in Figure 7-34, one group is located in the dorsal portion of the lateral wall of the alar lamina. It forms the **somatic afferent** (sensory) **column,** which is recognized as the dorsal column or horn in the mature spinal cord. Similarly, a collection of neuroblasts in the basal lamina forms the **somatic efferent** (motor) **column,** which is recognized as the ventral column or horn in the mature spinal cord.

Visceral afferent and **efferent columns** also form in a region just lateral to the sulcus limitans. They are associated with the autonomic nervous system.

Development of the Spinal Nerves

Neuroblasts of the basal lamina send their peripheral processes (**axons**) out through the marginal layer to form the **ventral** (motor) **roots** of the spinal nerves. *These long*

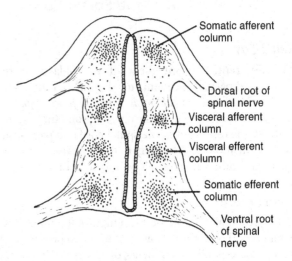

FIGURE 7-34

Formation of columns in the embryonic spinal cord.

axons traverse the peripheral nerves to supply the various skeletal muscles in the body.

Cells in the alar lamina become associated with sensory functions. They receive ingrowing central fibers from the differentiating neural crest cells. These central fibers eventually form the dorsal roots of the spinal nerves. Dorsal horn cells also belong to the sensory side of a reflex arc and are concerned with receiving and relaying impulses from the dorsal root fibers of the spinal nerves. The dorsal root fibers from the spinal ganglion cells (neural crest) enter the spinal cord dorsolaterally, and subdivide the white matter of the marginal zone into **dorsal** and **lateral funiculi.**[26] Similarly, the ventral root fibers separate the lateral funiculus from the **ventral funiculus,** as shown in Figure 7-35. The dorsal funiculus is composed primarily of fibers from the spinal ganglion cells which, after entering the spinal cord, course both rostrally and caudally.

---

[26]L. **funiculus,** a cord.

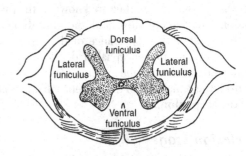

FIGURE 7-35

Division of the spinal cord white matter into dorsal, lateral, and ventral funiculi.

Development of the Spinal Cord

Bell's Law

The differential arrangement of neuroblasts in the spinal cord partially accounts for the rule of thumb that *the dorsal half of the spinal cord is sensory in function and the ventral half is motor.* This basic division, sometimes called Bell's law, is restricted to the spinal cord and part of the brain stem and does not apply to the cephalic portion of the neural tube which develops into the brain.

Neuromeres

A longitudinal section of the embryonic spinal cord would reveal periodic regions of intensified proliferation which correspond to segments of the spinal cord and their sensory and motor roots. Each segment is known as a neuromere, and they are located at intervals that correspond to the somites.

Each neuromere supplies an area of the body that roughly corresponds to a transversely oriented segment of the embryo, and although a nerve fiber may become "lost" in plexuses that develop later, its ultimate termination in a segment of the body is retained. The muscles that the ventral root supplies develop from the somatic myomeres, which lie in close proximity to the developing neuromeres. The first axons that emerge from the neural tube grow into the muscles and establish a path that subsequent fibers will follow. Generally, the tip of the growing nerve fibers follows the course of previously laid down blood vessels, muscle planes, and connective tissue. The growing nerve fibers exhibit **stereotropism.**[27] Once a pathway has been established by the initial nerve fibers, others may follow to form a nerve bundle, and their path will be less haphazard than was that of their predecessors.

The Primary Brain Vesicles

The rostral portion of the neural tube begins to enlarge and differentiate even before the neuropores have closed. Initially three dilations or primary brain vesicles appear. As shown in Figure 7-36, they are known as the **prosencephalon, mesencephalon,** and the **rhombencephalon.** Shortly after the appearance of the three primary brain vesicles, the prosencephalon develops diverticula on either side at its cephalic extreme to form the **telencephalon;** the remainder of the prosencephalon is known as the **diencephalon.**

The Flexion Stage

Because of unequal growth in the embryo and in the differentiating brain, it is thrown into a series of folds or

[27]Gk. **stereo,** solid, three-dimensional. Gk. **tropos,** a turning.

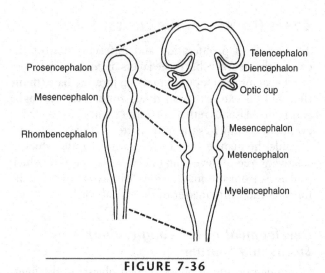

FIGURE 7-36

Differentiation of the neural tube to form the brain vesicles. The cavities represent the developing ventricles. (After Brodmann, 1909.)

flexures. Their location corresponds, in part, to the flexures of the embryo as a whole.

The first to appear is the **cephalic flexure** which occurs in the midbrain region. The prosencephalon makes a sharp "U"-shaped bend ventrally over the rostral end of the notochord and foregut. This causes the midbrain to protrude dorsally as shown in Figure 7-37.

At about the same time, a **cervical flexure** appears at the junction of the brain and spinal cord. For a while the hindbrain and spinal cord form a right angle and the entire head flexes ventrally at the level of the future neck. This flexure gradually disappears as continued body growth occurs.

A third flexure, the **pontine flexure,** also occurs, but it, like the cervical flexure, straightens and virtually disappears. The diencephalon and telencephalon, however, are permanently set at angular relations to each other. These flexures are used as descriptive landmarks in developmental anatomy of the nervous system.

Throughout the flexure stage the mesencephalon remains relatively unchanged, but the rhombencephalon differentiates into the **metencephalon** (cephalic portion) and the **myelencephalon** (caudal portion). The **isthmus,** a constriction that appears in the neural tube between the mesencephalon and the metencephalon, is sometimes used as a reference landmark. The three primary brain vesicles and their subsequent subdivisions are shown in Figures 7-36 and 7-38, and the early brain and its adult derivatives are shown in Table 7-1.

The Rhombencephalon

The subdivisions of the rhombencephalon are the myelencephalon and the metencephalon.

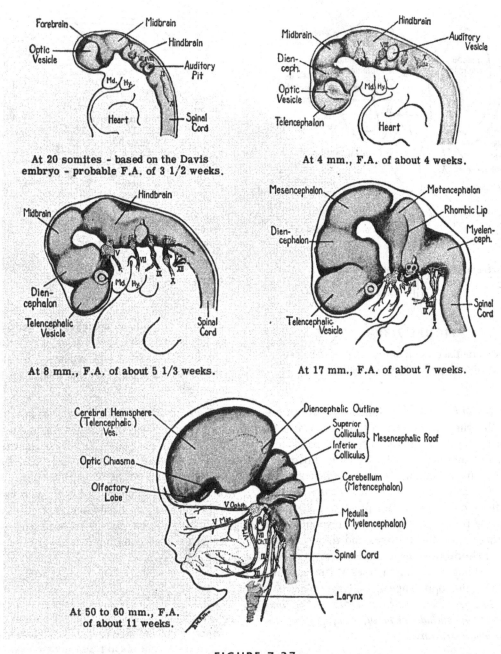

FIGURE 7-37

Five stages in early development of brain and cranial nerves. Cranial nerves are indicated by Roman numerals: V, trigeminal; VII, facial; VIII, acoustic; IX, glossopharyngeal; X, vagus; XI, accessory; XII, hypoglossal. Abbreviations: F.A., fertilization age; Ch.T., chorda tympani of facial nerve; Hy., hyoid arch; Md., mandibular branch of trigeminal nerve; V Max., maxillary branch; V Ophth., ophthalmic branch. (From Patten, 1953.)

The Myelencephalon Initially, the **medulla oblongata,** which is the most caudal part of the brain, is very similar to the spinal cord. It is characterized by roof- and floorplates and by sides containing the basal and alar laminae. In Figure 7-39, the roofplate has become stretched out and very much thinned. The floorplate remains relatively unchanged, however, so the sides are held together ventrally. As a consequence, the sulcus limitans, which

persists, now separates the medially placed basal lamina from the laterally placed alar lamina. A ridge, known as the **rhombic lip,** is formed where the roofplate joins the alar lamina. This ridge is the anlage[28] of the cerebellum.

_____

[28]**Anlage,** meaning predisposition; in embryology, the first structure or cell group indicating development of a structure.

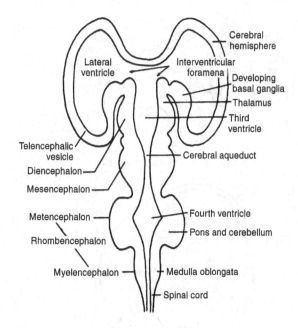

FIGURE 7-38

Schematic of differential growth of the telencephalic vesicles and their relationship to the diencephalon.

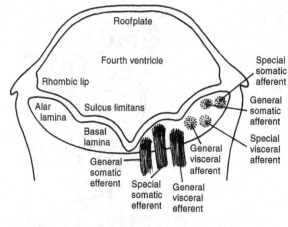

FIGURE 7-39

Schematic transverse section through embryonic hindbrain showing columns of neuroblasts.

The Functional Pattern. The functional pattern remains much the same in the myelencephalon as it is in the spinal cord. The alar lamina is sensory, the basal lamina is motor, and autonomic nuclei are located between them, along the sulcus limitans. *One major difference from the spinal cord is the loss of the segmental nature*, even though the floor of the hindbrain presents a series of seven temporary transverse furrows. Corresponding in position to these **rhombic grooves** and their external bulgings called **rhombomeres** is a lateral row of nerves on either side. They are cranial nerves V (trigeminal), VII (facial), IX (glossopharyngeal), X (vagus), and XI (accessory). *These nerves are all associated with the branchial arch derivatives which include the facial, pharyngeal, masticatory, and laryngeal structures.*

The Reticular Formation. It is also in the region of the myelencephalon that the well-defined demarcation between white and gray matter begins to break down into a mixture called the reticular formation. Although nerve fibers crossing every which way break up the usual pattern, certain specific nuclear masses and tracts can be identified.

Cerebrospinal Fluid. We should note that the roofplate is nonnervous in its structure, and a vascular mesenchyme (the pia mater) known as the **tela choriodea** lies on the ependymal roof. It forms the **choroid plexus** of the fourth ventricle, which is responsible for formation of cerebral spinal fluid. Localized resorptions of the roofplate result in paired lateral apertures (**foramina of Luschka**) and a medial aperture (**foramen of Magendie**) that permit communication with the subarachnoid space.

CLINICAL NOTE: The foramina of Luschka and the foramen of Magendie are an important part of the cerebrospinal circulation system. Failure of these foramina to appear can result in *congenital noncommunicating* (or *obstructive*) *hydrocephaly*.

TABLE 7-1

Adult derivatives of the primary brain vesicles

Primary Vesicle	Subdivision	Derivatives	Cavity
Prosencephalon	Telencephalon	Cerebral cortex, striate bodies, and rhinencephalon	Lateral ventricle and part of third ventricle
	Diencephalon	Thalamus and hypothalamus	Third ventricle
Mesencephalon	Mesencephalon	Collicular structures and cerebral peduncles	Cerebral aqueduct
Rhombencephalon	Metencephalon	Pons and cerebellum	Fourth ventricle
	Myelencephalon	Medulla oblongata	Fourth ventricle and part of central canal
Medulla spinalis		Spinal cord	Central canal

Differentiation of the Alar Laminae. Sensory fibers from the cranial nerves VI (facial), IX (glossopharyngeal), and X (vagus) grow from their respective neural crest ganglia into the alar lamina to form the **solitary tract** in the marginal zone. This is a descending tract containing primary visceral afferent fibers. Alar lamina neuroblasts migrate into the marginal zone, surround the solitary tract, and form the receptive sensory nuclei for cranial nerves IX and X. The **olivary nuclei** are also derivatives of the alar lamina of the medulla. They arise from cells which migrate from the alar lamina into the basal lamina.

Differentiation of the Basal Lamina. The basal lamina of the myelencephalon differentiates a little earlier than does the alar lamina. Basal lamina neuroblasts give rise to the **motor nuclei of origin** for certain cranial nerves. Laterally, near the sulcus limitans, can be found an indistinct nucleus (**nucleus ambiguous**) from which cranial nerves IX (glossopharyngeal), X (vagus), and XI (accessory) acquire their special visceral efferent (motor) fibers that supply musculature of the branchial arch derivatives.

The Metencephalon The metencephalon (Figure 7-40), a part of the hindbrain, is located below the isthmus, a constriction that separates it from the mesencephalon. Caudally the metencephalon is limited at the pontine flexure.

Structure of the Metencephalon. Basically its structure is similar to that of the myelencephalon, with two important exceptions, namely the **pons** and **cerebellum.** The cerebellum is an important integrating and coordinating center for body position and movement. The pons can be thought of as the principal transmis-

sion pathway between the cerebral cortex and cerebellum, and between the cerebellar hemispheres.

The primitive metencephalon is initially composed of roof- and floorplates and a basal and alar lamina on either side. The roof, however, becomes thinned and transformed into a thin layer of white matter on the rostral side of the developing cerebellum, and into nonneural ependyma caudal to the cerebellum. These regions are called the superior and inferior medullary velum. Between them, the roofplate of the metencephalon becomes integrated into the substance of the cerebellum and at the same time forms the roof of the fourth ventricle.

Differentiation of the Alar and Basal Laminae. The alar lamina, an important contributor in the metencephalon, develops sensory relay nuclei for cranial nerve V (trigeminal) as well as for some of nerves VII (facial) and VIII (acoustic). It also contributes significantly to the development of the cerebellum and to the **cerebellar peduncles** as well. The peduncles are three pairs of stalks that connect the cerebellum with the other parts of the brain.

Neuroblasts in the basal lamina, on the other hand, differentiate into motor nuclei of origin for cranial nerves V (trigeminal), VI (abducent), and VII (facial). The roof of the pons becomes the floor of the fourth ventricle while the pontine nuclei, which become enveloped by cells of the basal lamina, are actually derivatives of migrating cells from the alar lamina. Arey (1966) has made an observation well worth noting:

> Since in early embryos the hind-brain lies directly above the pharynx, foregut and heart, it is natural that the centers concerned with the regulation of chewing, tasting, swallowing, digestion, respiration and circula-

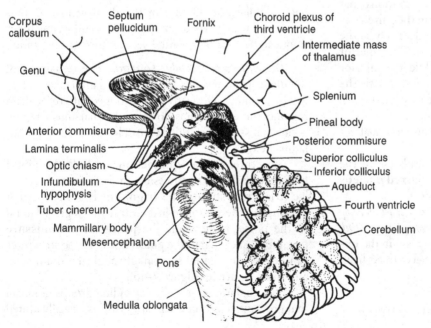

Corpus callosum
Genu
Anterior commisure
Lamina terminalis
Optic chiasm
Infundibulum hypophysis
Tuber cinereum
Mammillary body
Mesencephalon
Pons
Medulla oblongata
Septum pellucidum
Fornix
Choroid plexus of third ventricle
Intermediate mass of thalamus
Splenium
Pineal body
Posterior commisure
Superior colliculus
Inferior colliculus
Aqueduct
Fourth ventricle
Cerebellum

FIGURE 7-40

Details of the brain stem and third ventricle. Beginning caudally, the myelencephalon is shown as the medulla oblongata, the metencephalon is shown as the pons and cerebellum, with the mesencephalon located just rostral. In adult neuroanatomy, the cerebellum is usually not included as part of the brain stem.

tion remain located in the hind-brain, even though the organs innervated become considerably dislocated in position.

The Cerebellum. The cerebellum, which is a derivative of the metencephalon, deserves some special attention. As early as the fifth week, that part of the alar lamina adjacent to the roofplate begins to thicken and it bends over laterally to form the prominent rhombic lip that is the anlage of the cerebellum. The rhombic lip folds down over the alar lamina, covering it, the solitary tract, and the root of the trigeminal nerve (V). The lateral extensions of the alar lamina and rhombic lips are due to the pontine flexure, and by the eighth week the rhombic lips have thickened to the extent that they begin to bulge into the fourth ventricle and partially obliterate it. These proliferations ultimately fuse to form the **vermis of the cerebellum,** while the lateral portions of the rhombic lip form the **cerebellar hemispheres.**

The Mesencephalon

As seen in Figure 7-40, flexion of the neural tube does not result in any great change in the gross structure of the mesencephalon, so initially it retains the characteristics of the spinal cord. This is also true, you will recall, of the myelencephalon and the metencephalon. The region dorsal to the cerebral aqueduct forms the **tectum** and the region ventral to the aqueduct forms the **tegmentum.**[29]

The cavity of the mesencephalon becomes constricted to form the **cerebral aqueduct,** which establishes communication between the third and fourth ventricles. Neuroblasts near the aqueduct (from the basal lamina) develop into the motor nuclei of origin for the oculomotor (III) and trochlear (IV) cranial nerves.

Thickening of the roof (tectum) on either side of the midline produces two longitudinal elevations that undergo a transverse constriction to form the paired **superior** and **inferior colliculi,** known collectively as the **quadrate bodies** (corpora quadrigemina). The superior colliculi are associated with vision, while the inferior colliculi receive fibers from nuclei associated with the cochlear bundle of the acoustic or auditory nerve (VIII). Auditory fibers are found coursing from the inferior to the superior colliculi, providing for auditory-visual reflexive responses.

At the same time aggregates of neuroblasts in the tegmentum form two prominent nuclei, the **red nucleus** and the **black nucleus (substantia nigra).**

As differentiation of the brain occurs, nerve tracts develop and pass either up or down through the mesencephalon to link the hindbrain with the cerebral cortex. Fairly late in the initial development of the brain, very large nerve tracts from the telencephalon pass down the ventral part of the mesencephalon, and they form the cerebral peduncles that are located in the tegmentum of the mesencephalon.

The Prosencephalon

The subdivisions of the prosencephalon are the diencephalon and the telecephalon.

The Diencephalon Progressing in a rostral direction, the next division of the brain is the diencephalon—that part of the forebrain which remains after the development of the telencephalic vesicles. The diencephalon is very prominent during the second month of embryonic life, but the expanding telencephalon soon encapsulates it.

According to Arey (1965), the diencephalon is "almost wholly given over to various kinds of correlations, and through it pass all the nervous impulses that reach the cerebral cortex with the single exception of those from the olfactory organs."

The walls of the diencephalon differentiate into a dorsal roofplate while the sides and floor consist of alar lamina (Arey, 1965). The basal lamina and floorplate encountered at all the previous levels may not extend as far rostral as the diencephalon. This is not certain, however.

The Third Ventricle. In substance the diencephalon is largely gray matter derived from the mantle layer and grouped into nuclei. The cavity of the diencephalon forms the third ventricle. Initially the ventricle is quite large, but the rapidly growing lateral walls compress it almost to oblivion. The roofplate of the diencephalon is ependymal, and with growth and partial obliteration of the third ventricle, it, along with the vascular pia mater, folds into the tela choriodea or choroid plexus of the third ventricle.

At about the seventh week the **pineal body** evaginates caudally, at the end of the third ventricle. This structure, which has a complex neuroendocrine function, can be seen in a sagittal section through the brain.

Derivatives of the Alar Lamina. The remainder of the diencephalon stems from the alar lamina, according to some sources. Derivatives are grouped into three main regions: the epithalamus dorsally, the thalamus laterally —on each side of the third ventricle—and the hypothalamus below.

Structures of the **epithalamus** include the pineal body, the posterior commissure, and trigonum habenulae (triangular strap). The **trigonum** is a nucleus that develops in the roofplate just rostral and slightly lateral to the pineal body, while the **posterior commissure** develops just caudal to the pineal body. These structures can be seen in sagittal sections through the brain stem and third ventricle (Figure 7-40).

The **thalami** are rapidly expanding groups of nuclei that grow into close approximation and are usually united

---

[29]L. **tectum,** any rooflike structure. L. **tegmen,** a cover or roof.

across the third ventricle by a bridge of gray matter called the **massa intermedia** (adhesio interthalamica). *The thalamus is the principal avenue by which all impulses from cutaneous, visual, and auditory senses are relayed to the cerebral cortex:* A phylogenetically old part of the thalamus is instrumental in mediating pleasure and painful sensations.

The **hypothalamus** of the embryo presents the **optic cups** and their **stalks,** as seen in Figure 7-41, and the **infundibulum of the pituitary gland** (hypophyseal body). In addition, the hypothalamic structures include the **tuber cinereum** and **mammillary bodies,** which can be seen in Figure 7-42.

The Telencephalon The telencephalon consists of a medial portion and two expanded lateral portions. The lateral portions are the cerebral hemispheres, each of which contains a lateral ventricle. The medial portion is continuous with the structures of the diencephalon.

The Cerebral Hemispheres. Initially the walls of the hemispheres remain typical of the primitive neural tube with ependymal, mantle, and marginal zones. During the third month, however, neuroblasts migrate to the periphery from the mantle and ependymal zones. They collect in the deeper layer of the marginal zone and so form the outer layer (**gray matter**) of the cerebral cortex.

The nerve processes (which become myelinated) pass, for the most part, toward the depths of the brain to form the **white matter,** but its rate of growth is much less rapid than the gray matter.

Similar cell migration and growth occur in the cerebellum. The cells in the telencephalon are probably a product of the expanded alar lamina. Basal lamina and

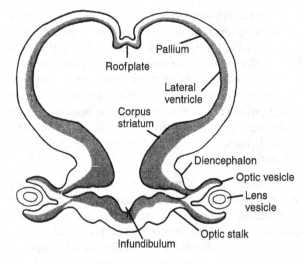

FIGURE 7-41

Human telencephalon at 10 mm, as seen in a transverse section. The hypothalamus develops from the region at the bottom of the illustration and the optic stalk and optic vesicle grow out from it. (After Patten, 1953.)

floorplate are lacking, while the roofplate contributes to the formation of a choroid plexus. The roofplate is confined to the midline of the greatly expanded hemispheres that consist of enlarged alar laminae.

The growth pattern of the hemispheres, which are partially separated by a deeply penetrating cleft, the **longitudinal fissure,** is a significant departure from the formation of the remainder of the brain.

The cerebral hemispheres are quite prominent structures by the sixth week, and they continue to grow rapidly

FIGURE 7-42

Schematic of the fully developed brain as seen from beneath.

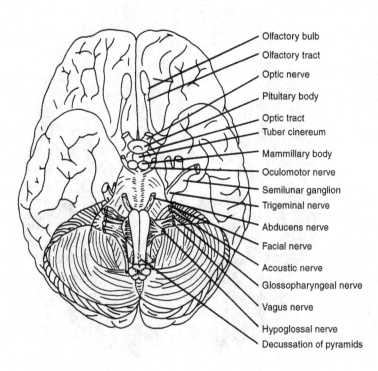

until, by the fifth month of fetal life, they have completely overgrown the diencephalon and mesencephalon and part of the cerebellum. The original rostral limit of the neural tube does not engage in this expansive process, and thus remains relatively stable in its position. This midline region of nonproliferating tissue is known as the **lamina terminalis,** and since the hemispheres are expanding forward on either side of it, the lamina terminalis is soon located at the bottom of the deep longitudinal fissure.

Divisions of a Cerebral Hemisphere. A cerebral hemisphere consists of three functionally distinct parts.

One, the **rhinencephalon,** is phylogenetically quite primitive. The part of the cerebral cortex included in it is called the **archipallium.**[30] The archipallium first appears as a longitudinal ridge on the ventral surface of each hemisphere (beneath what we later identify as the frontal lobes). These swellings, which lie on either side of the lamina terminalis, enlarge into the **olfactory lobes,** which remain small in humans. The archipallium comprises the **hippocampus,** so named because of its resemblance to a sea horse.

The second division of the cerebral hemispheres is the **corpus striatum** (striate bodies). It is anatomically continuous with the thalamus and is functionally related to it, as a high-order relay center. Myelinated nerve fibers passing between the thalamus and cerebral cortex course

through the corpus striatum. These fibers form a somewhat "V"-shaped band which is seen in a section through the brain as the **internal capsule** (Figure 7-43). The upper limb of the internal capsule divides the corpus striatum into the **caudate** and **lenticular (lentiform) nuclei.** The internal capsule emerges from the base of the cerebral hemispheres as one of the cerebral peduncles that is a conspicuous component of the mesencephalon. The corpus striatum elongates, in concert with the growth of the cerebral hemispheres, conforming somewhat to the shape of the lateral ventricle, so that its caudal portion curves around to the tip of the inferior horn of the lateral ventricle. This explains the long slender tail of the caudate nucleus, as well as its name.

Third is the formation of the **white matter.** Earlier it was pointed out that the cerebral cortex was formed by alar lamina cells that migrated from the marginal zone. Much later in the developmental sequence, the white matter is formed by nerve processes that extend into the cerebral hemispheres. Because of the comparatively rapid expansion of the cortical substance, it is thrown into numerous convolutions or gyri that are separated by sulci. The deepest of the sulci are called fissures, and they begin to appear during the fourth month.

The smaller sulci do not appear until the very end of the fetal life. In addition, the cortical region overlying the corpus striatum expands at a slower rate than does the surrounding cortex. As a result this region becomes overgrown by folds of the frontal, parietal, and temporal lobes.

---

[30]Gk. **arche,** beginning. L. **pallium,** cloak.

FIGURE 7-43

Horizontal section through the brain, at a level shown in the insert, to illustrate the relationship of the internal capsule (**IC**) to the lenticular nucleus (Globus pallidus (**GP**) and putamen (**P**)). Also identified are the longitudinal fissure (**LF**), frontal lobe (**FL**), cingulate sulcus (**CS**), corpus callosum (**CC**), caudate nucleus (**CN**), thalamus (**TH**), 3rd ventricle (**3V**), lateral sulcus (**LS**), insula (**IN**), caudate nucleus tail (**CNT**), hippocampus (**HC**), aqueduct cerebral (**AC**), medial (**M**), and lateral (**L**) geniculate bodies, the lateral ventricle-inferior horn (**LV**), inferior colliculus (**IC**), vermis of the cerebellum (**CV**), and cerebellar hemisphere (**CH**).

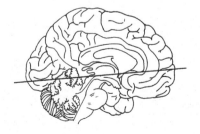

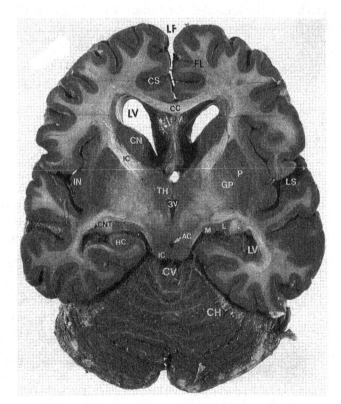

This mechanism explains the prominent **lateral fissure,** and it also accounts for a small region of the cerebral cortex that seems to be buried within the cerebral hemisphere and which can be seen only by separating the folds of the lateral fissure. The region that becomes enclosed is known as the **insula**[31] or **island of Reil,** while the covering folds are called the **opercula.**[32] In the process of this rapid growth, a small strip of gray matter seems to have been separated from the cortex, in the region of the insula. It is called the **claustrum.**[33] In Figure 7-44, the opercula in this four-month fetal brain have not completely covered the insula.

The Commissures. The two hemispheres of the telencephalon are connected by bundles of fibers known as commissures, but not always labeled or identified as such. The optic chiasm is one example of a commissure, the trigonum habenulae is another, and we have encountered the posterior commissure of the diencephalon. There are three commissures in the telencephalon—the corpus callosum, the fornix[34] and the anterior commissure. They arise from the lamina terminalis mentioned earlier.

At about the fourth month a thickening takes place on the lamina terminalis, just in front of the region where the lateral venticles communicate with the third ventricle (interventricular foramen). The lower part of this thickening becomes the **anterior commissure,** while the upper part of the thickening continues to grow caudally, along with the growing hemispheres. It is invaded by two sets of nerve fibers. Transverse fibers connecting the hemispheres pass through its dorsal part, now known as the corpus callosum. A band of longitudinal fibers from the hippocampus begins to invade the ventral part of the lamina terminalis. These fibers arch over the thalamus and course toward the mammillary bodies (located just behind the infundibulum). This commissure is called the **fornix.**

The anterior portion of the lamina terminalis, located between the corpus callosum and the fornix, is not invaded by commissural fibers and becomes known as the **septum pellucidum.**[35]

This description of the embryonic development of the brain is by no means complete, but it does provide a basis for a more comprehensive understanding of the adult nervous system. *A student who has pursued the embryonic development of the human being has an intuitive grasp of body organization and function that can never be attained by just the study of adult anatomy and physiology.*

DEVELOPMENT OF THE INNER EAR

The reception and transmission of sound energy is the function of the external and middle ears. Their development was discussed in part in the section dealing with the development of the outer ear. The end organ for hearing is located in the cochlear duct of the inner ear. The remainder of the inner ear (semicircular canals, utricle, and saccule) is given over to equilibrium.

Early Development of the Inner Ear

The epithelium of the inner ear is a derivative of ectoderm. The inner ear first appears as a thickening of ectoderm, the **auditory placode,**[36] located on either side of the developing myelencephalon. The placodes appear by the middle of the third week (7-somite stage) and by the 9-somite stage the placodes have developed into auditory pits. In 24-somite embryos the pits have closed, leaving hollow **otocysts** (auditory vesicles) embedded in mesoderm. The otocysts soon become detached from the ectoderm from which they arose. The otocyst lies opposite the fifth neuromere, near the facial-acoustic ganglion.

At the point where the otocyst has detached from the ectoderm, the **endolymph sac** extends in a medial direction where it dilates into the **endolymphatic sac.** During the fifth week the otocyst elongates in the dorsoventral direction (Figure 7-45). The slender ventral part is destined to become the **cochlear duct,** while the dorsal

---

[31]L. **insula,** island.

[32]L. **opercula,** a cover or lid.

[33]L. **claustrum** a bar or barrier.

[34]**fornix,** arch.

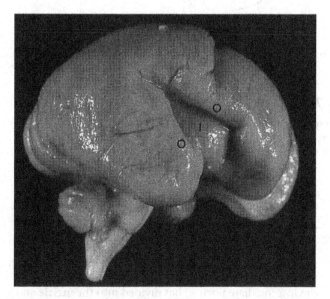

FIGURE 7-44

A four-month fetal brain. The opercula (**O**) have not fully developed, and the insula (**I**) can be seen.

---

[35]L. **pellucid,** to shine through, translucent.

[36]Gk. **placode,** a platelike structure.

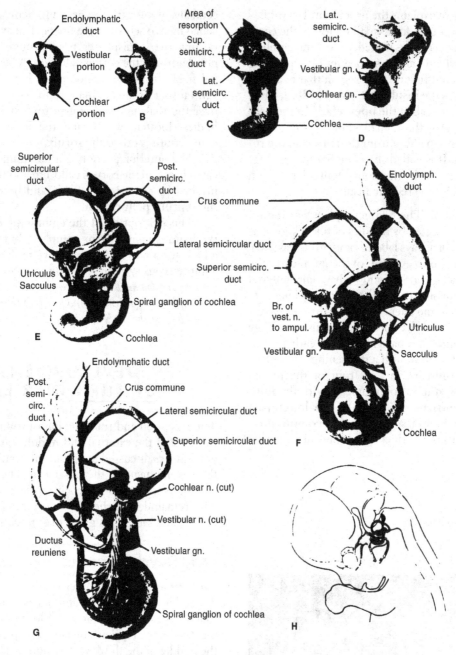

FIGURE 7-45

Development of the membranous labyrinth. (A) 6 mm, lateral view; (B) 9 mm, lateral view; (C) 11 mm, lateral view; (D) 13 mm, lateral view; (E) 20 mm, lateral view; (F) 30 mm, lateral view; (G) 30 mm, medial aspect; (H) outline of head of 30-mm embryo to show position and relations of developing inner ear. (From Streeter, 1922.)

most portion already shows indications of developing into **semicircular canals.** The intermediate region will subdivide into the **utricle** and **saccule.**

By six weeks the semicircular canals are outlined as two flattened pouches. The posterior and superior canals arise from a single pouch at the dorsal limit of the otocyst while the lateral canal emerges as a horizontal outpocketing. The cochlear area has assumed a "J" shape.

By the end of the seventh week the otocyst has been modeled roughly into the membranous labyrinth with its semicircular canals and a cochlea with one turn.

Early in the eighth week the endolymphatic duct and the three semicircular canals are well defined, and the intermediate portion has divided into the utricle and saccule. The cochlear duct has begun to coil giving it a resemblance to a snail shell. As shown in Figure 7-45, the superior and posterior semicircular canals have a common crus or arm, which converges onto the utricle where a dilation, the **ampulla,** is located.

Continued constriction further divides the utricle (which receives the semicircular canals) from the saccule. It remains connected to the cochlear duct by means of a short stalk, the **ductus reuniens.** By the third month the adult form of the inner ear has nearly been completed. Further development results in complete separation of the utricle and saccule, each of which remains attached to the endolymphatic duct by a short slender canal.

The Development of the Membranous Labyrinth

The epithelium of the membranous labyrinth is initially a single layer of columnar cells. Early in the development, fibers of the auditory nerve grow between the cells in regions where subsequent thickening results in the development of the special sense organs. They are the **cristae ampullares** in the ampullae of the semicircular canals, the **maculae** in the utricle and saccule, and the **spiral organ** in the cochlear duct.

In each ampulla (one at the utricular end of each semicircular canal) the epithelium and underlying tissue form a curved ridge, the **crista.** The cells of the epithelium differentiate into supportive and sensory cells.

The supportive cells secrete a jellylike substance (the **cupola**) which covers the sensory cells. The **kinocilia** of the sensory cells project into the cupola. The development of the sense organs in the maculae is essentially the same as that of the crista ampullae. The free surface of these sense organs contains deposits of minerals, the **otoconia.** They provide mass to the top of the cupola, and movements of the head result in an inertial lag that bends the kinocilia of the sensory cells. This results in stimulation of the sensory cells and provides a sense of orientation awareness.

The epithelium of the spiral organ divides into an inner and outer ridge. The cells of the inner ridge become the **spiral limbus** while the outer ridge is the primordium of the spiral organ. Here also, the epithelial cells differentiate into supportive and sensory (hair) cells. Both ridges are covered by an increasingly prominent tectorial membrane that is secreted by the epithelium of the spiral limbus.

The Development of the Osseous Labyrinth

The mesenchyme (mesoderm) surrounding the membranous (epithelial) labyrinth becomes differentiated into a fibrous membrane and later into cartilage. At about the tenth week, the cartilage immediately surrounding the membranous labyrinth undergoes a peculiar *reversal of development.* The cartilage returns to a precartilaginous condition in which the cells lose their boundaries[37] and form a loose network which becomes the **perilymphatic spaces** surrounding the membranous labyrinth. When this has taken place the membranous labyrinth is suspended in the fluid of the perilymphatic spaces.

The cochlear duct is triangular in cross section and its inner angle is attached to the axis (**modiolus**) of the cochlea. Perilymphatic spaces (periotic) develop above and below the cochlear duct. The upper space is the **scala vestibuli** and the lower is the **scala tympani,** each of which is lined by squamous mesodermal cells. The thin partition separating the scala vestibuli from the cochlear duct (scala media) is known as the **vestibular membrane.** It is composed of a single layer of mesoderm on the side of the scala vestibuli, and another single layer, but of epithelium, on the cochlear duct side. The cartilage surrounding the membranous labyrinth is ossified by the fifth month. *By the middle of fetal life the inner ear has attained its full size.*

CLINICAL NOTE: The middle ear of a newborn is usually filled with a gelatinous substance which is absorbed during the first few weeks of extrauterine life. For this reason, hearing acuity of the newborn is not a valid index of the integrity of the hearing mechanism.

BIBLIOGRAPHY AND READING LIST

Arey, L. B., *Developmental Anatomy*, 7th ed. Philadelphia: W. B. Saunders, 1965.

Brodman, K., *Vergleichende Localization der Grosshirnrinde.* Leipzig: Barth, 1909.

Dorland's *Illustrated Medical Dictionary*, 25th ed. Philadelphia: W. B. Saunders, 1974.

Fogh-Anderson, P., *Inheritance of Harelip and Cleft Palate.* Copenhagen: NYT Norkisk Forlag, Arnold Busk, 1942.

Gray, *The Anatomy of the Human Body*, 29th ed., C. M. Goss, ed. Philadelphia: Lea and Febiger, 1973.

Gray's Anatomy, 36th ed., P. L. Williams and R. Warwick, eds. Philadelphia: W. B. Saunders, 1980.

Gray's Anatomy, 38th ed., Churchill Livingstone, 1995.

Hamilton, Boyd, and Mossman, *Human Embryology.* Baltimore: Williams and Wilkins, 1945.

Massler, M., and E. Schour, *Atlas of the mouth.* Chicago: American Dental Assn., 1958.

Myerson, M. C., *The Human Larynx*, Springfield, IL: Charles C Thomas Pub. Co., 1964.

O'Rahilly, R., *Basic Human Anatomy.* Philadelphia: Saunders, 1983.

Orban, B. J., *Oral Histology and Embryology*, 4th ed. St. Louis: C. V. Mosby, 1957.

---

[37]The tissue becomes a **syncytium,** a multinucleated protoplasmic mass.

Patten, B., *Human Embryology*, 3rd ed. New York: McGraw, 1968.

Patten, B., *Human Embryology*, Philadelphia: The Blakiston Co., 1946.

———, "The Normal Development of the Facial Region," in S. Pruzansky, ed., *Congenital Anomalies of the Face and Associated Structures*. Springfield, IL: Charles C Thomas, 1961.

Scammon, R., "The measurement of the Body in Childhood," in J. Harris, ed., *The Measurement of Man*. Minneapolis: Univ. of Minnesota Press., 1930.

Sicher, H., and J. Tandler, "Anatomy for Zahnartz," Vienna and Berlin: Julius Springer, 1928.

Streeter, G., "Development of the Auricle in the Human Embryo," *Contrib. Embryol., Carnegie Inst. Wash.*, 14, 1922.

———, "Developmental Horizons in Human Embryos: Age Group XI, 13–20 Somites, and Age Group XII, 21–29 Somites," *Contrib. Embryol., Carnegie Inst. Wash.*, 30, 1942.

———, "Developmental Horizons in Human Embryos: Age groups XV, XVI, XVII and XVIII, being the third issue of a survey of the Carnegie collection," *Contrib. Embryol., Carnegie Inst. Wash.*, 32, 1948.

Swanson, C. P., *The Cell*, 2nd ed. Englewood Cliffs, N.J.: Prentice-Hall, 1964.

Circulation

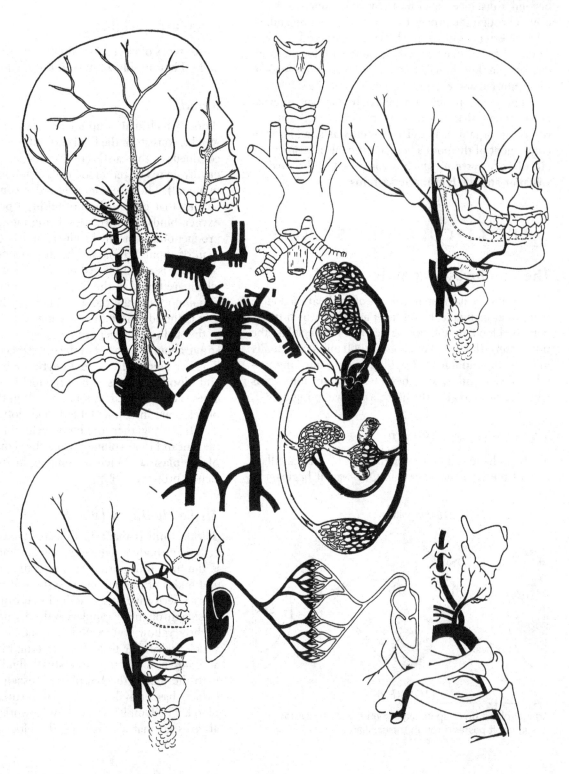

INTRODUCTION

All animal cells are dependent upon a fluid environment to transport the oxygen and nutrients necessary for life and to transport the waste products of cell metabolism. Deprive living animals of their fluid environment and they die.

Diffusion of oxygen and nutrients is not adequate beyond a distance equal to a few cell diameters, however. Through the processes of natural selection and, to a lesser extent, mutation, the circulatory and nervous systems have evolved, and they, along with locomotion, enable complex animals to rapidly adjust to changes in their internal and external environments.

The maintenance of a relatively constant internal environment that is necessary to preserve the integrity of an organism is called **homeostasis,** and a vital component of the body's homeostatic mechanism is the **circulatory system,** which is composed of the **cardiovascular** and the **lymphatic systems.**

THE CIRCULATORY SYSTEM

The Cardiovascular System

The cardiovascular system consists of the **heart,** a double pump that maintains blood flow; **arteries,** which transport the blood away from the heart; and **arterioles,** the tiny vessels which lead to about 60,000 miles of virtually microscopic **capillaries.** Capillaries drain into tiny vessels called **venules,** and they in turn drain into **veins** which return blood to the heart, as shown in Figure 8-1.

The Lymphatic System

The lymphatic system can be thought of as an ancillary part of the circulatory system. One-way, it begins as a

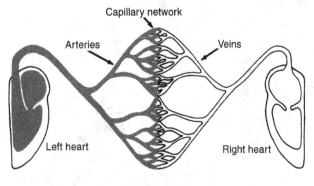

Capillary network

Arteries   **Veins**

Left heart   **Right heart**

FIGURE 8-1

Arterial blood gives up its oxygen and takes on carbon dioxide as it passes through the capillary network.

blind network of **lymph capillaries** that collect **lymph** (tissue fluid) throughout the body. These capillaries feed larger and larger **lymphatic vessels** that finally drain, by way of a one-way valve, into the large veins at the root of the neck. The **spleen, thymus, tonsils,** and **lymph nodes** throughout the body are important parts of the lymphatic system. The lymph transport mechanism is primarily the pumping action of the skeletal muscles.

Circulatory Fluids

Three types of circulatory fluids can be identified in the body. They are **blood, tissue fluid,** and **lymph.**

Blood

Blood, which makes up about 8 percent of total body weight, consists of the fluid and cells transported by, and confined to, the cardiovascular system. Blood contains **erythrocytes** or red blood cells (5 million per milliliter of blood!). They are nonnucleated, biconvex, dislike elements that contain **hemoglobin,** a protein to which oxygen binds. Erythrocytes, being incapable of cell reproduction and normal cellular metabolism, have a life span of about 120 days. The destruction of aging erythrocytes is accomplished by cells called **macrophages,** which are found in the liver, spleen, bone marrow, and lymph nodes, while the site of new erythrocyte production in the adult is in the bone marrow of the chest, base of the skull, and upper arms and legs. Erythrocytes constitute about 99 percent of the cellular elements of blood. The remaining cells are **leukocytes,** or white blood cells, and **blood platelets.** The principal function of leukocytes is defense against foreign cells in the blood, while platelets are instrumental in blood clotting.

Taken together, the blood cells comprise about 55 percent of blood volume, while the remaining (fluid) is **blood plasma,** which is complex in its structure and rich in protein.

Tissue Fluid and Lymph

Tissue fluid is that which is freely circulating among cells in the body and the intercellular fluids, while **lymph** is the fluid transported by and confined to the vessels and nodes of the lymphatic system. It may be thought of as a derivative of tissue fluid that exudes from blood plasma through the capillary walls. Lymph is a clear, but slightly yellow watery fluid, containing **lymphocytes** which are similar to leukocytes found in the blood. In addition to collecting interstitial fluid and returning it to the blood, the **lymphatic vessels** return protein (which has been lost to the interstitial fluid) to the blood. The lymphatic capillary network of the intestine absorbs fat that also reaches the bloodstream. **Lymph**

nodes are important filter sites, and so are instrumental in preventing the spread of infections.

GENERAL FEATURES OF THE CARDIOVASCULAR SYSTEM

Blood flow throughout the body is the result of the pumping action of the heart. As can be seen in Figure 8-2, there are two circuits for blood flow, the **pulmonary** and the **systemic.**

The Pulmonary Circuit

The pulmonary circuit begins with the **right heart.** Two large veins, the **superior** and **inferior venae cavae,** return deoxygenated blood from all parts of the body (except the lungs) to the **atrium** of the right heart, which pumps blood into the **right ventricle.** The superior

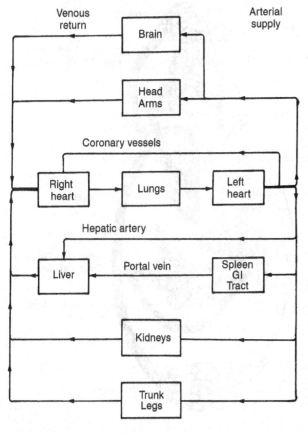

FIGURE 8-2

A block diagram of the adult cardiovascular system, which consists of a pulmonary circuit from the ventricle of the right heart to the lungs and from the lungs to the atrium of the left heart, and a systemic circuit from the left heart to the arteries, capillaries, and veins and, finally, to the atrium of the left heart.

vena cava returns blood to the heart from everything above the diaphragm (except the lungs) and the inferior vena cava from everything below the diaphragm.

By contraction of the right ventricle, the oxygen-poor blood is sent by way of the **pulmonary arteries** to the lungs. Here, about 1000 miles of capillaries and venules closely invest the walls of the pulmonary alveoli, as shown in Figure 8-3, and here the capillary blood is separated from the alveolar air by a barrier only 2 microns thick. Very rapid diffusion of gases takes place, oxygen into the blood and carbon dioxide from the capillaries to the alveoli. We have seen that atmospheric air is replenished in the pulmonary alveoli about 12 times a minute (at rest). Gas diffusion through the alveolar barrier, however, is taking place constantly. At rest the cells of the body consume about 200 ml of oxygen each minute and produce approximately the same quantity of carbon dioxide. We have also seen that at rest pulmonary ventilation amounts to 5 or 6 liters of air per minute. About 20 percent of atmospheric air is oxygen, which means that total oxygen input to the lungs is about 1 liter of oxygen per minute. Of this, about 200 ml diffuses across the alveolar walls into the pulmonary capillaries, while the remaining 800 ml is returned to the atmosphere during exhalation. We should also realize that the so-called oxygen-poor blood, which enters the lungs, actually contains a considerable amount of oxygen. In summary, with each cycle of respiration about 200 ml of oxygen enters 5 liters of pulmonary blood per minute, and it is this blood that is returned to the atrium of the **left heart** by way of the **pulmonary veins.**

The Systemic Circuit

As illustrated in Figures 8-2 and 8-4, the left heart is the pump for the systemic circuit, and it delivers fresh, oxygen-rich blood to cells throughout the body.

Systemic Arteries

Blood leaves the left ventricle by way of the aorta, which quickly divides into a number of arteries. The **aorta** is divided into four parts; the **ascending, arch, descending thoracic,** and **abdominal.**

Ascending Aorta Two very important coronary arteries arise from the ascending aorta, and they return oxygen-rich arterial blood to the muscles of the heart (myocardium).

Arch of the Aorta As the ascending aorta arches over the left bronchus in a dorsal direction, three large blood vessels arise in very quick succession. As shown in Figure 8-5, from front to back, they are the brachiocephalic, left common carotid, and the left subclavian arteries.

FIGURE 8-3

Schematic illustration of the pulmonary artery, capillary network surrounding alveoli in the lung, and pulmonary vein. (From J. E. Crouch, *Functional Human Anatomy,* 3rd edition, 1979. Lea & Febiger, Publisher.)

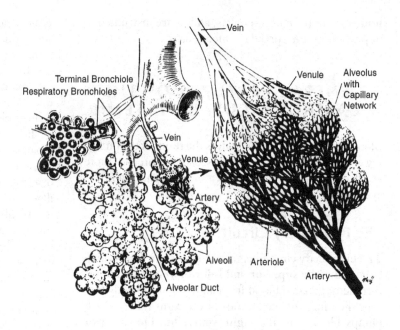

FIGURE 8-4

Schematic representation of the two-heart system of circulation. Oxygenated blood is shown in black; the deoxy-genated blood in white. Arrows indicate the direction of blood flow. (From J. E. Crouch, *Functional Human Anatomy,* 3rd edition, 1979. Lea & Febiger, Publisher.)

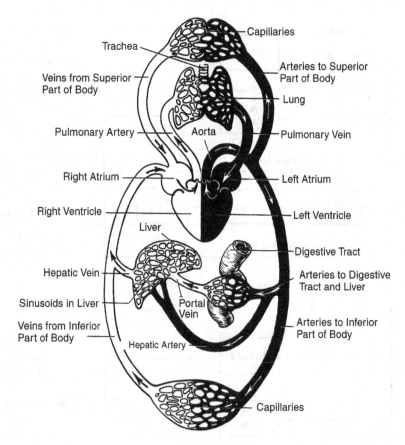

The **brachiocephalic** is a stocky trunk directed upward and to the right. It terminates just behind the sternoclavicular joint where it divides into the right common carotid and the right subclavian arteries.

The **left common carotid** and **subclavian arteries** ascend vertically on the left side of the trachea and esophagus to the level of the left sternoclavicular joint. From this point on, the courses of the left and right common carotids are essentially the same. They ascend the neck vertically just lateral to the trachea and esophagus, and at about the level of the upper border of the thyroid cartilage of the larynx they end, bifurcating into

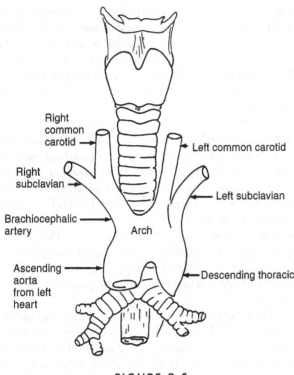

FIGURE 8-5

The aorta is divided into four parts: the ascending, arch, descending thoracic, and abdominal (not shown).

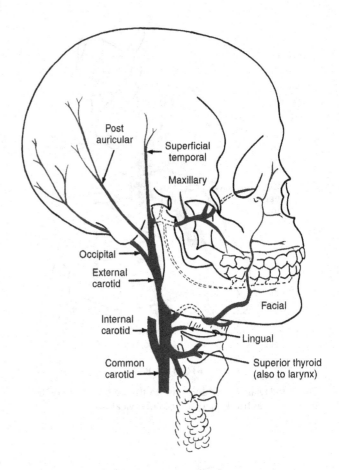

FIGURE 8-6

The common carotid artery divides into the external and internal carotid arteries. Branches of the external carotid are shown, with the exception of the ascending pharyngeal artery. It arises between the posterior auricular and the superficial temporal artery.

the internal and external carotid arteries, as illustrated in Figure 8-6.

The **internal carotid artery** continues its vertical course without giving off collaterals and finally enters the base of the skull through the carotid canal. Here it divides into two large arteries that supply part of the brain and a tiny ophthalmic artery that supplies the eye.

The **external carotid artery** supplies almost all the structures of the head and neck except the contents of the cranial and orbital cavities (brain and eyes), although it does get an "assist" from the subclavian artery, which courses across the root of the neck. The distribution of the external carotid is shown schematically in Figure 8-6, and the blood supply to the various structures it serves will be discussed as we progress through the text.

The **subclavian artery** is the blood vessel of the upper extremity. The vessel arches above the level of the clavicle as it courses toward the axilla, where it is known as the axillary artery, and when it enters the arm, the brachial artery. The subclavian artery gives rise to four collaterals, three near its summit and one, the internal thoracic (mammary), arises from its concave undersurface. As shown in Figure 8-7, the **internal thoracic artery** descends vertically into the thorax, just lateral to the sternum, and as it does so, gives rise to six **anterior intercostal arteries.** They anastomose with the terminal branches of the aortic intercostal arteries, which

arise from the descending thoracic aorta, as illustrated in Figure 8-8.

As it approaches the lower end of the sternum, the internal thoracic artery divides into the **musculophrenic artery,** which supplies the upper surface of the diaphragm and lower intercostal spaces, and the **superior epigastric artery,** which enters the sheath of the rectus abdominis muscle.

The first of the collaterals at the summit of the subclavian artery is the very important **vertebral artery.** It enters the foramen of the sixth cervical vertebra (usually), threads its way up the cervical column, and enters the base of the skull by way of the foramen magnum, where it becomes an important contributor to the blood supply of the brain. The second collateral, the thyrocervical artery, sends a branch called the **inferior thyroid artery** to supply the lower half of the thyroid gland and muscles of the larynx, while other branches supply muscles of the shoulder and back of the neck. The third collateral of the summit of the subclavian artery is the **costocervical**

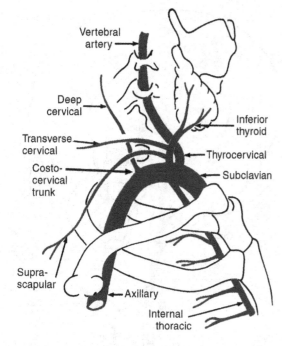

FIGURE 8-7

The subclavian artery gives rise to the vertebral artery, the thyrocervical trunk, and the costocervical trunk.

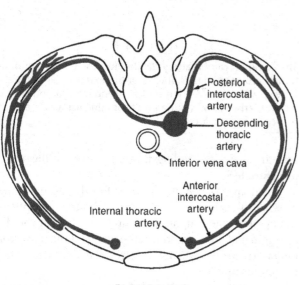

FIGURE 8-8

The anterior and posterior intercostal arteries anastomose not only with each other but with adjacent intercostal arteries.

trunk, which supplies the first and second intercostal spaces with intercostal "arteries" (Figure 8-7).

Descending Thoracic Aorta Eleven pairs of **posterior (aortic) intercostal arteries** arise from the back surface of the descending thoracic aorta. The first nine pairs anastomose with the anterior intercostal arteries (from the internal thoracic artery) as illustrated in Figure 8-8.

The tenth pair of arteries lies below the twelfth rib and is called, appropriately, a **subcostal artery.** The eleventh pair, known as the **superior phrenic artery,** supplies the dorsal upper surface of the diaphragm. The descending thoracic aorta also gives rise to paired **bronchial arteries** that nourish the bronchial tree as well as the esophagus and pericardium.

Abdominal Aorta The continuation of the descending thoracic aorta is known as the abdominal aorta. It bifurcates at the level of the fourth lumbar vertebra into the right and left common **iliac arteries,** which supply the lower limbs. Prior to its bifurcation, however, the back of the abdominal aorta (its dorsal surface) gives rise to five pairs of arteries, the first of which (**inferior phrenic**) supplies the lower surface of the musculature of the diaphragm. The remaining four pairs of **lumbar arteries** supply the posterior abdominal wall.

Three pairs of arteries arise from the sides of the abdominal aorta. They supply the kidneys (and suprarenal glands) and the sex organs. Three unpaired arteries arise from the front (ventral) surface of the abdominal aorta, and they supply the digestive tract, spleen, and associated structures of the abdominal cavity (mesentry, omentum, etc.).

Systemic Veins

The systemic veins drain oxygen-poor and carbon dioxide-laden blood from the tissues of the blood through their capillary beds. Venous vessels that drain into a vein are commonly called **tributaries.** (In some ways the venous system resembles a river and its tributaries.) **Superficial** or **cutaneous veins** are usually not accompanied by a corresponding artery, but the tributaries of the larger blood veins correspond to the branches of its companion artery, and so to discuss them would be largely redundant.

Internal Jugular Vein The pattern of the distribution of the large veins in the cranium, however, is a radical departure from the aortic blood supply, and this topic will receive special attention later. Nevertheless, all veins in the cranium lead to the internal jugular vein, which begins at the jugular foramen at the base of the skull. This large vein, shown in Figure 8-9, descends in the neck, at first in company with the internal carotid and finally the common carotid artery. As it courses downward, the internal jugular receives tributaries that correspond closely with the branches of the external carotid artery.

At the level of the sternoclavicular joint, the right and left internal jugular veins meet the subclavian veins (from the arm) to form the **right** and **left brachiocephalic veins,** both of which course toward the midline.

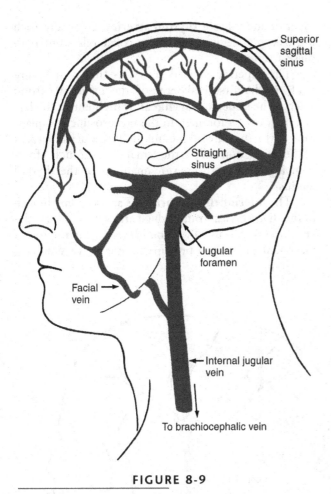

FIGURE 8-9

Schematic of internal jugular vein.

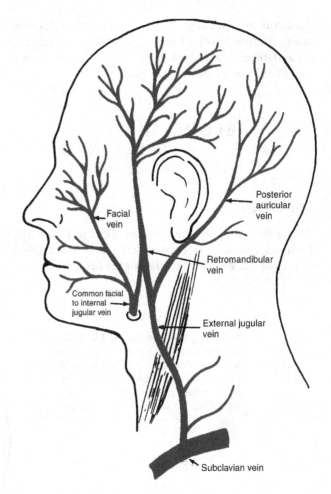

FIGURE 8-10

Tributaries of the veins of the face and neck form the external jugular vein. The confluence of the main and superficial and subcutaneous veins forms the letter "W."

External Jugular Vein The superficial vein of the head and neck is known as the external jugular. Shortly after crossing over the sternocleidomastoid muscle it joins the subclavian, just lateral to the internal jugular, as illustrated in Figure 8-10.

Superior Vena Cava The confluence of the brachiocephalic veins forms the superior vena cava, which drains into the right atrium of the heart. The large superior vena cava also receives the **azygos vein,** which begins in the abdominal region at the level of the second lumbar vertebra. It passes through the diaphragm with the aorta (aortic hiatus). As it courses along the right side of the vertebral column the azygos vein receives tributaries from the intercostal region, from the structures of the mediastinum, and from the pericardium. At the level of the fourth thoracic vertebra, it arches forward to join the superior vena cava. A smaller **hemiazygos vein,** found on the left side of the vertebral column, has a tributary pattern similar to that of the azygos vein (into which the hemiazygos drains).

Inferior Vena Cava The inferior vena cava, the largest blood vessel in the body, is formed by the confluence of

the right and left common iliac veins, at the level of the fifth lumbar vertebra. It receives tributaries corresponding to the arteries that branch from the aorta (except for the digestive tract), and after passing through the diaphragm and pericardium, it enters the posterior-inferior part of the right atrium. And so, the circuit has been completed.

The Heart

The heart begins to contract in the very early days of embryonic life and must continue for the duration of the individual's life. Failure of heart contraction for even a few minutes can lead to irreversible brain damage or even death. At its normal 72 beats per minute, the heart musculature contracts about 100,000 times a day, which adds up to about 2,600,000,000 times in the lifetime of 70 years. In that time the heart pumps 155,000,000 liters (40,951,000 gal) of blood. If you alternately clench and open your fist 72 times a minute, to simulate a pumping action, the muscles involved will begin to feel tired in about 2 minutes. Imagine a muscle complex that must accomplish such a task 24 hours a day, unceasingly, for a lifetime! The remarkable heart commands a measure of respect it often fails to get.

BLOOD SUPPLY FOR THE SPEECH AND HEARING MECHANISM

The Larynx

Two arteries supply the intrinsic laryngeal muscles. Both are branches of arteries that supply the thyroid gland and are known as the **laryngeal branches** of the

superior and inferior **thyroid arteries.** Generally, each intrinsic muscle is supplied by collaterals from both these arteries.

The superior thyroid artery, as shown in Figure 8-11, is the first collateral of the external carotid artery. The **superior laryngeal branch** enters the larynx by way of a foramen in the posterosuperior quadrant of the thyrohyoid membrane in about 60 percent of the population and, in the remainder, through a foramen in the posterosuperior quadrant of the thyroid lamina.

The **inferior thyroid artery** is an ascending branch of the thyrocervical trunk (which arises from the subclavian artery). It is usually accompanied by the **recurrent laryngeal nerve,** the principal motor nerve supplying the larynx.

FIGURE 8-11

Blood supply to the larynx. The superior thyroid artery is the first collateral of the external carotid. The inferior thyroid artery is an ascending branch of the thyrocervical trunk. It arises from the subclavian artery. (See Figure 8-7.)

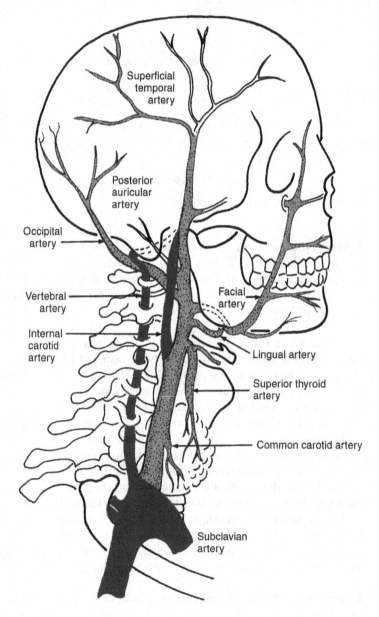

The Face

The muscles of the head, except for the ocular, middle ear, lingual, and pharyngeal, can be arranged into those of the face, and of mastication. For the most part the **facial region** is supplied by two branches of the facial (external maxillary) artery as illustrated in Figure 8-12. The submental branch supplies structures of the **lower lip,** including the musculature that inserts into it. The superior labial artery has an extremely tortuous course along the upper lip. It supplies the membranes, muscles, and glands of the **upper lip** and adjacent structures of the **nose.**

The **facial artery** then ascends along the angle between the nose and eye, ramifying as it does so. The facial artery is characterized by numerous anastomoses, with the artery from the opposite side, and with branches of the **maxillary artery,** which is one of the terminal branches of the **external carotid.** (The other is the superficial temporal artery.)

The **muscles of mastication** are supplied by muscular branches of the maxillary (internal) artery, the eighth

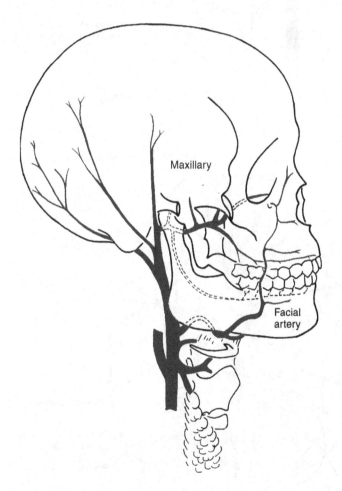

FIGURE 8-12

Blood supply to the face.

of the arterial branches of the carotid. The maxillary artery also gives rise to **inferior** and **superior dental arteries,** and the very important **middle meningeal artery.** (See Figure 8-12.)

The Tongue

Three arteries supply the tongue: the **lingual, ascending pharyngeal,** and the **facial.** The principal artery is the lingual, which is the third branch of the external carotid. The second branch of the external carotid is the ascending pharyngeal artery, and it also supplies branches to tongue muscles. The fourth branch of the carotid is the facial artery (external maxillary), and a collateral of it, called the **submental artery,** supplies musculature in the lower part of the tongue and floor of the mouth. The **lingual** and **ranine** (L. frog) **veins** open into the internal jugular at the level of the hyoid bone.

The Palatine Tonsils

The **tonsillar branch** of the **facial artery** is the principal artery that supplies the palatine tonsil. It may also receive small twigs from the lingual artery and the ascending pharyngeal artery. A large **palatine vein** (external palatine) descends from the soft palate and across the wall of the tonsillar capsule before entering the pharyngeal wall. *This vessel is responsible for the excessive hemorrhage that sometimes occurs during tonsillectomy.* The ascending pharyngeal and facial arteries are in close proximity to the tonsillar capsule, and the internal carotid lies about 25 mm behind and lateral to the capsule.

The Central Nervous System

The Brain

Four arteries, the paired **internal carotids** and **vertebral arteries** (the latter are branches of the subclavian arteries), combine to form the **arterial circle** (of Willis), which is shown in Figure 8-13. The vertebral arteries, which ascend to the base of the brain by way of the transverse foramina of the cervical vertebrae, primarily supply the **cerebellum** and **brain stem** (including the cranial and cervical nerves), while the arterial circle gives rise to three cerebral arteries that supply the **cerebrum.** A useful rule of thumb is that each cerebral artery supplies a surface and a pole of the cerebrum. Thus, the anterior cerebral artery supplies the medial surface and frontal pole, the middle cerebral artery supplies the superior-lateral surface and the temporal pole, and the posterior cerebral artery supplies the inferior surface and occipital pole, as shown in Figures 8-14, 8-15, and 8-16. Each of the three main cerebral arteries in turn gives rise to numerous central arteries. They are perforating arteries that traverse the subarachnoid space and enter the deep

FIGURE 8-13

Schematic of arteries at the base of the brain. The anterior and posterior communicating arteries complete the arterial circle (of Willis). Note that the internal carotid, after branching to give rise to the anterior and posterior communicating arteries, continues as the middle cerebral artery.

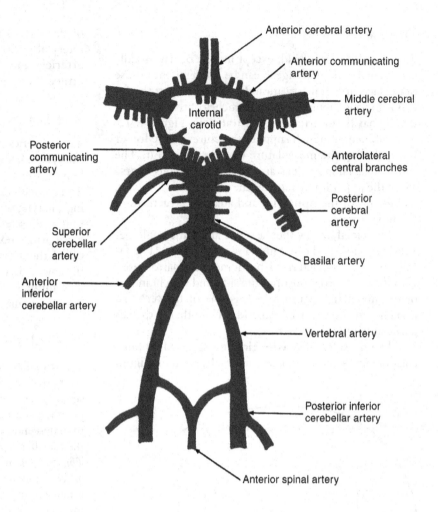

FIGURE 8-14

The arterial circle shown in relation to the base of the brain. Each cerebral artery supplies a surface and a pole of the cerebrum.

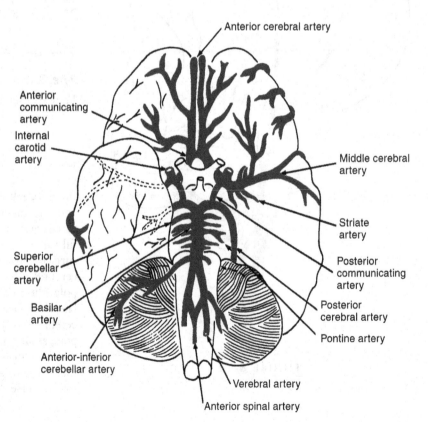

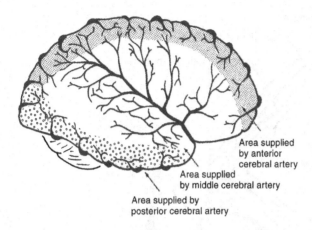

FIGURE 8-15

Lateral schematic of cerebrum and areas supplied by the three principal cerebral arteries.

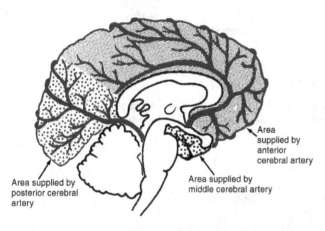

FIGURE 8-16

Sagittal view of the brain, showing areas supplied by the three principal cerebral arteries.

substance of the brain to supply the **basal ganglia, white matter, hypothalamic nuclei,** and so forth. Branches of the basilar and superior cerebellar arteries supply the **brain stem** and the 12 **cranial nerves** that emerge from the base of the brain.

The blood supply to the **dura mater** is the middle meningeal artery, an important branch of the internal maxillary artery, the larger of the two terminal branches of the external carotid (the smaller terminal branch is the superficial temporal artery).

The Spinal Cord

Note in Figure 8-14 that each vertebral artery gives rise to an anterior spinal artery, and they join to form a single **anterior spinal artery.** It descends in the anterior medial fissure of the spinal cord. **Posterior spinal arteries** also arise from the vertebral arteries. They descend along the dorsal aspect of the spinal cord, ramifying as they do so, to form complex (plexiform) networks, especially in the

lower part of the spinal cord. Spinal branches of the vertebral, posterior intercostal, lumbar, and sacral arteries traverse the intervertebral foramina and divide into **medullary** and **radicular branches** which supply the spinal cord, as shown in Figure 8-17. The **veins** that drain the spinal cord are also segmentally arranged and leave by way of the intervertebral foramina.

Cranial Venous Sinuses

Six cranial venous sinuses course between the peritoneal and meningeal layers of the dura mater. These sinuses drain blood from the cranial cavity and are shown in Figure 8-18. They are the superior longitudinal or sagittal sinus, the left and right transverse sinuses, the straight sinus, the cavernous sinus, and the superior and inferior petrosal sinuses.

Superior Sagittal (Longitudinal) Sinus The superior sagittal sinus is a midline structure located at the top of the falx cerebri. It begins over the roof of the nasal cavity and gains in size as it courses backward, receiving numerous superior cerebral veins that drain blood from the surface of the cerebral hemispheres. The sinus terminates at the occipital bone by turning right (usually) and coursing horizontally as the **right transverse sinus,** which follows the margin of the petrous portion of the tentorium cerebelli. As the sinus approaches the base of the petrous portion of the temporal bone, it descends to the jugular foramen as the **sigmoid sinus.**

Straight Sinus Large **internal cerebral veins** receive blood from the interior of the brain. By joining at the midline they form the straight sinus, which courses backward along the right-angled junction of the falx cerebri and tentorium cerebelli. At the occipital region, the sinus turns at a 90° angle to form the **left transverse sinus,** and its course is the same as its fellow on the right.

Cavernous Sinus Large, spongelike cavernous sinuses lie on each side of the body of the sphenoid bone (on each side of the pituitary fossa). Numerous structures such as motor nerves to the eye and the internal carotid artery course through the sinuses, which also receive ophthalmic veins from the orbit of the eye. These sinuses are continued backward as the paired **superior** and **inferior petrosal sinuses.** The inferior sinus makes its exit through the jugular foramen where it immediately joins the **internal jugular vein.** The superior petrosal sinus courses backward to join the beginning of the **sigmoid sinus** on the superior border of the petrous portion of the temporal bone.

Emissary Veins We should note that certain of the cranial venous sinuses receive blood from the outside of the skull by way of emissary veins. They are quite variable, but their channels explain the presence of the posterior

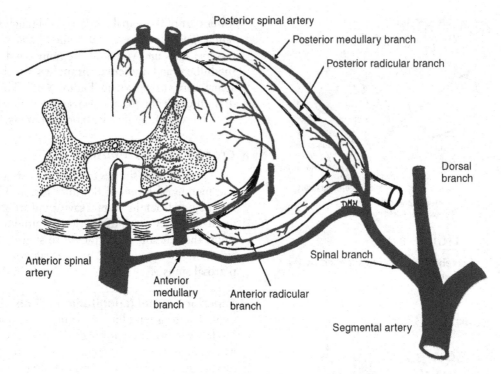

FIGURE 8-17

Spinal branches of the vertebral, posterior intercostal, lumbar, and sacral arteries traverse the intervertebral foramina and divide into medullary and radicular branches, which supply the spinal cord.

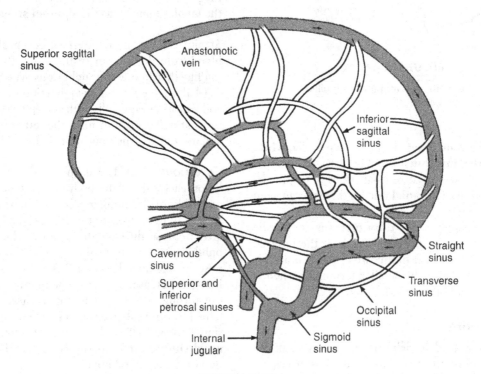

FIGURE 8-18

Schematic of the six cranial venous sinuses. (Adapted from Gray, 36th British ed., 1980, William and Warwick, eds., W. B. Saunders Co.)

condylar foramen on the occipital bone and the mastoid foramen on the temporal bone. Other small and often anonymous foramina that transmit emissary veins can be found on the surface of the calvarium.

The Ear

External Ear

The **arteries** of the external ear are (1) the anterior auricular branch of the superficial temporal supplying the anterior part of the auricle and the external auditory meatus, (2) the auricular branch of the occipital artery, and (3) the posterior auricular branch of the external carotid artery (Figure 8-19). The **veins** of the auricle accompany their corresponding arteries. Both arterial and venous anastomoses are numerous in the skin of the auricle.

Structurally, the **auricle** contains little fat (except in the ear lobe) and but a single layer of blood vessels. As a consequence, the skin is more subject to *frostbite* than any other part of the body. In addition, because of its meager blood supply, the cartilage is *very prone to infection* following trauma.

External Auditory Meatus and Tympanic Cavity and Membrane

The **arteries** that supply these structures are the anterior and posterior auricular branches of the superficial temporal artery, the posterior auricular branch of the carotid, and the deep auricular branch of the maxillary artery.

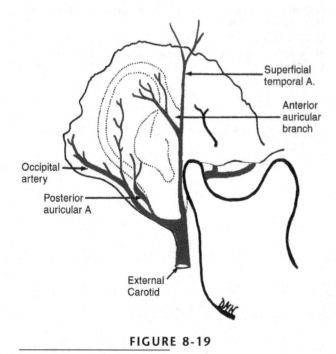

FIGURE 8-19

Blood supply to the external ear.

In addition, the stylomastoid branch of the posterior auricular artery enters the stylomastoid foramen, where it supplies the **facial nerve, tympanic cavity, mastoid antrum** and **air cells,** and part of the **semicircular canals.** In youngsters, a ramus of the stylomastoid branch anastomoses with the anterior tympanic artery to supply the medial surface of the tympanic membrane.

The **ossicular chain** is supplied by small collaterals from the superior branch of the anterior tympanic artery, a branch of the internal maxillary artery. The anterior tympanic artery ascends behind the temporomandibular joint to enter the tympanic cavity through the petrotympanic fissure. It ramifies on the medial surface of the tympanic membrane, forming a vascular circle around it (along with the posterior branch of the stylomastoid artery). The anterior tympanic artery also anastomoses with branches of the caroticotympanic branch of the internal carotid artery. *In early fetal life a stapedial artery passes through the ring formed by the crura of the stapes. It later degenerates leaving the foramen obturator.*

The **veins** of the tympanic cavity terminate in the pterygoid venus plexus and in the superior petrosal sinus. Small veins from the mucous membrane of the mastoid antrum course medially through the arch formed by the superior semicircular canal. They emerge on the posterior surface of the petrous portion of the temporal bone by way of the subarcuate fossa where they open into the superior petrosal sinus. These veins are the remnants of a large **subarcuate vein** in young children and constitute a *pathway for infection from the mastoid antrum to the meninges of the brain.*

Otic Capsule

The **internal auditory** (or labyrinthine) **artery,** together with the **stylomastoid branch** of the posterior auricular (or occipital) artery, supply the entire otic capsule. There are no collaterals of this artery, which is highly variable in origin. In about 38 percent of the human population it arises as a branch of the basilar artery, while in about 46 percent it arises as a branch of the anterior cerebellar artery. The artery passes through the internal auditory meatus and abruptly divides into three branches:

1. The **vestibular artery** supplying the vestibular nerve and parts of the utricle, saccule, and semicircular canals.

2. The **vestibulocochlear artery** supplying the basal turn of the cochlea, parts of the utricle, saccule, in addition to parts of the semicircular ducts.

3. The **cochlear artery,** which enters the modiolus where it subdivides into 12 to 14 twigs that are distributed in the form of a capillary network to the spiral lamina and basilar membrane (Figure 8-20).

FIGURE 8-20

Blood supply to the inner ear.

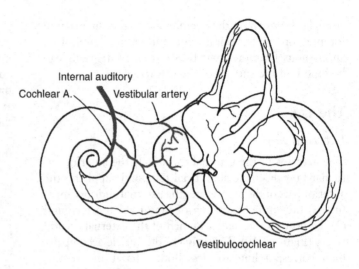

Postscript

With this, the completion of the text material, the reader is probably acutely aware that a complete and comprehensive understanding of the speech and hearing mechanisms is no simple task. It demands, first of all, a thorough knowledge of the basic structures involved, the way they function, and the manner in which they are interrelated. Secondly, it demands a continuous pursuit of new ideas, concepts, and research findings as they appear in the professional literature. Old, well-established, and firmly implanted ideas may have to be cast aside to make way for the new. If I have been at all successful with this textbook, students will come away from it motivated to ask pertinent questions, to seek out new ideas and research findings, and to add them judiciously to their expanding repertories of knowledge. Hopefully the material presented in this textbook will provide the proper basis for each student's construct of the speech and hearing mechanisms. We can never question the validity of that construct, but we can question the validity of the materials upon which that construct is based.

And further, by these, my son, be admonished: of making many books there is no end; and much study is a weariness of the flesh.

Ecclesiastes, 12:12

BIBLIOGRAPHY AND READING LIST

Crouch, J. E., *Functional Human Anatomy, 3rd ed.* Philadelphia: Lea & Febiger, 1979.

Gray, *The Anatomy of the Human Body*, 29th ed., C. M. Goss, ed. Philadelphia: Lea & Febiger, 1973.

Gray's Anatomy, 36th ed., P. L. Williams and R. Warwick, eds., Philadelphia: W. B. Saunders, 1980.

Gray's Anatomy, 38th ed., New York: Churchill-Livingstone, 1995.

Guyton, A. C., *Textbook of Medical Physiology*, 6th ed., Philadelphia: W. B. Saunders, 1981.

Kimber, D. C., C. E. Gray, C. E. Stockpole, L. C. Leavell, and M. A. Miller, *Anatomy and Physiology*, New York: The Macmillan Co., 1966.

a- not, without.

Å symbol for angstrom, a unit of length equal to 10^{-8} cm.

ab- away from.

abdomen that portion of the body lying between the thorax and the pelvis.

abduct to draw away from the midline.

abscess a localized area of pus contained within a cavity.

abscissa the horizontal line in a graph showing the relationship of two values.

ac- *see* ad-.

acetylcholine a chemical substance, released in synaptic regions, that increases the irritability of neurons.

acou-, acu- to hear.

acquired obtained after birth; not congenital.

acr-, acro- extremity, peak.

acromegaly chronic enlargement of the bones and soft tissues of the hands, feet, and face, due to excessive secretion by the pituitary gland.

action potential changes in electrical potential, occurring at the surface of the nerve or muscle tissue at the moment of excitation; consists of a short-duration period of negativity called the spike potential and secondary changes in potential called after-potentials.

acute with sudden onset and of short duration.

ad- (d changes to c, f, g, p, s, or t before roots beginning with those consonants) to, toward.

Adam's apple an anterior projection of the thyroid cartilage, especially in men.

adduct move toward the midline.

aden- gland.

adenoids the enlarged or hypertrophied pharyngeal tonsil.

adenoidectomy excision of adenoids.

adipose fatty, fat.

aditus an entrance.

adrenal near the kidney.

adrenalin a hormone secreted by the medulla of the adrenal gland, also called epinephrine.

aer- air.

aesthe- feeling.

af- *see* ad-.

afferent carrying toward, as toward the central nervous system.

after-potential *see* action potential.

ag- *see* ad-.

agonist a contracting muscle that is opposed by another contracting muscle (its antagonist).

ala- pertaining to wing.

alb- white.

allanto pertains to sausage.

alveolus a small hollow or pit.

ambi- both.

ameboid resembling an amoeba (ameba), which has an indefinite, changeable form and moves by means of pseudopodia.

amnion a membrane surrounding the embryo. (Gk. *lamb*)

amphi- on both sides; on all sides.

amphiarthrodial a yielding joint.

amplitude magnitude; range of movement of a vibrating object.

ampulla a flasklike structure or dilation of a tube.

amygdaloid almond-shaped.

ana-, an- up, back, again.

anastomose to open, one into another.

anatomical position the body standing erect, facing the observer, with arms at the side and palms forward.

andr- man.

androgen male sex hormone.

aneroid *see* barometer.

angi- vessel, blood vessel.

angular velocity in referring to the speed and direction of rotational motion, it is the vector whose magnitude is the time rate of change of the angle θ rotated through. $\omega = d\theta/dt$

anion a negatively charged ion.

ankl- crooked.

anlage predisposition; in embryology, the first structure or cell group indicating development of a structure.

annular ring-shaped.

anode any positively charged electrode.

anomaly a deviation from normal.

anoxia oxygen deprivation.

ansa-, ansi- a handle or loop.

antagonist a muscle that acts in opposition to another.

ante-, anter- front, before.

anterior toward the front; away from the back.

anthropoid resembling man.

anti-, ant- against, counter.

antiresonance a phenomenon in a system in which impedance is tending to infinity.

antrum a cavity or hollow space, especially in bone.

ap- *see* ad-, apo-.

aperiodic not periodic, irregular.

apert- to open.

apex summit or top.

aphasia a collective term meaning the inability to express, recognize, or comprehend language or symbols.

aphonia loss or absence of voice due to failure of vibration of the vocal folds.

apic- extremity, top.

apo- separated or derived from.

aponeurosis a broad sheet of connective tissue that forms the attachment of muscle to bone.

appendicular skeleton the skeleton of the extremities and of the pectoral and pelvic girdles.

apposition the fitting together.

Aq. abbreviation for water.

arachnoid resembling a spider's web.

arch-, archi- beginning, origin.

arcuate arched, bow-shaped.

areola a minute space within tissue.

areolar tissue a meshlike form of connective tissue.

arthr-, arthro- pertaining to joints.

arthroidia a joint permitting only gliding movements.

articulation 1. a joint or juncture of bones. 2. movement and placement of the articulators during speech production.

articulators those structures responsible for modification of the acoustic properties of the vocal tract; i.e. tongue, lips, soft and hard palate, and teeth.

artifact a structure or tissue that has been changed from its natural state by mechanical, electrical, chemical, or other artificial means.

arytenoid resembling the mouth of a pitcher.

as- *see* ad-.

asthenia weakness; loss of strength and energy.

asthm- breathless.

astro-, aster- pertaining to a star.

asper- rough.

aspirate 1. to articulate a speech sound, especially a stop, with audible friction. 2. to remove fluid from a body cavity with an aspirator. 3. to inhale fluid into the bronchi and lungs.

at- *see* ad-.

atavism reversion or the occurrence of a characteristic not usually found in more immediate progenitors.

ataxia lack of muscle control due to incoordination.

atmo- pertaining to steam or vapor.

atmospheric pressure pressure of the atmosphere, which amounts to about fifteen pounds per square inch at sea level.

attenuate to decrease the amplitude or energy of a signal; to decrease.

attrition a wearing down or away by friction.

audi- to hear.

aur- ear.

auto- 1. acting or directed from within. 2. self.

autoimmune directed against the constituents of the body's own tissues.

autonomic self-controlling; functionally independent.

autoradiography making an x-ray of an object or tissue using its own radioactivity.

axial skeleton the skeleton of the head and trunk.

axilla the armpit.

axillary pertaining to the armpit.

axis 1. an imaginary line passing through the center of the body. 2. the line about which a rotating body turns.

axis cylinder the conducting core of a dendrite or axon.

axon the efferent (usually) process of a neuron.

azimuth when pertaining to sound, refers to the angular direction of the sound source in relationship to the listener.

ballistics 1. the study of the motion of projectiles. 2. movements that result from sudden muscle contractions and which are continued by the forces of inertia.

bar- pressure, weight.

barometer an instrument that measures atmospheric pressure.

> *mercury barometer* consists of a glass tube filled with mercury and inverted into a reservoir.
>
> *aneroid barometer* consists of a metal chamber from which the air has been evacuated. Pressure is indicated by the collapsing or bulging of a thin metal wall of the chamber, which in turn moves an indicating pointer.

basal ganglia the striate bodies and the thalamus.

basi- foundation, base.

basilar membrane the membrane in the cochlear duct that supports the organ of Corti.

belly the fleshy portion of a muscle.

Bernoulli's principle in the case of an ideal fluid, as velocity of fluid flow increases, pressure must decrease, so long as total energy remains constant. Pressure is perpendicular to the direction of fluid flow. Thus, if volume fluid flow is constant, velocity will increase at an area of constriction with a corresponding decrease in pressure at the constriction.

bi- two.

bifid divided into two parts.

bifurcate to divide into two branches.

bilateral pertaining to both sides.

biosynthesis building up of a chemical compound in the physiological processes of a living organism.

blade a wide, flat structure.

blast-, blasto- germ; pertaining to bud or budding; often used in embryology.

blastocoele cavity of a blastula.

blastocyst a hollow cell mass; the initial embryonic cell bud.

blastomere one of the cells formed during the primary division of an egg.

blastula a hollow ball of cells, one cell-layer thick.

bolus a rounded mass, usually of food.

bone the dense, hard supportive tissue that comprises most of the skeletal framework.

Boyle's law at any given temperature the volume of gas varies in inverse proportion to the pressure exerted upon it.

brac-, brachi- pertaining to arm.

brachy- short.

branchial pertaining to embryonic gill arches.

breathing the process of inflating and deflating the lungs.

bregma pertaining to the front part of the head; junction of the coronal and sagittal sutures; in infants, the fontanel.

brevis brief, short.

Broca's area an area in the inferior convolution of the frontal lobe of the brain that seems to be related to language or expression of language.

bronch- windpipe.

bronchiole the smallest division of the bronchial tree.

bronchus the primary division of the trachea.

Brownian movement rapid, oscillatory movement, often observed in fluid particles or fine particles suspended in liquids.

bucc- pertaining to cheek.

bulk volume modulus of elasticity when compressional forces acting inward over the surface of a body compress its volume, the coefficient of compression that is determined by the restoring force of the compressed substance is known as the bulk modulus of elasticity; also known as volume modulus of elasticity.

bursa a sac or saclike cavity filled with fluid.

buttock either of the two protuberances that form the rump.

ca. (L. *circa*) approximately.

calcify to harden by the deposits of calcium salts.

calcar- spur-shaped.

callosum hard.

canal a passageway or duct.

canaliculi a number of very small channels.

canine pertaining to dog; tooth next to the incisors.

capill- hairlike.

capit- head.

capitulum a protrusion on the head of a bone.

caps- box or container.

carcin- crab; cancer.

cardiac pertaining to heart.

cardinal vowels eight primary, supposedly invariant sustained vowel sounds that constitute a reference for describing the entire vowel inventory used in a language.

caries molecular destruction of bone or teeth; decay.

carina keel of a boat.

carnivorous flesh eating.

cartilage a nonvascular connective tissue, softer and more flexible than bone.

CAT scan *see* computed tomography.

cata- down; negative.

catheter a tube that is passed into body passages, often for drawing off fluid such as urine.

cathode any negatively charged electrode.

cauda equina shaped like the tail of a horse; collection of vertically directed lumbar and sacral nerve roots.

caudal toward the tail, away from the head.

caudate having a tail.

cav- hollow.

cavity a hollow or space within or between structures.

cecum a blind pouch.

cel-, -cele tumor or hernia.

celiac abdominal; pertaining to belly.

cell body's fundamental unit of structure and function; the smallest unit of life.

cementum a very dense tissue that forms the outer surfaces of the root of a tooth.

cente- puncture.

centi- hundred.

cephalic pertaining to head.

cephalometry science of measuring the dimensions of the human head.

cera- wax.

cerebr- cerebrum, brain.

cerumen waxlike secretion in the external canal of the ear.

cervical pertaining to neck.

cervix the neck of a structure.

cesium, Cs. an alkali similar to potassium and sodium.

chiasma a decussation of fibers, as in the optic chiasma; shaped like the letter X.

choana a funnel-like opening.

chondr-, chondrio- granule, cartilage.

chord-, chordo- cord.

chori- fetal membrane skin.

chorion an embryonic membrane external to and enclosing the amnion; the hard shell of an egg.

choroid a delicate and highly vascular membrane.

chro-, chrom- color.

chron- time.

chronaxie current duration required to excite a neuron or muscle tissue at a current strength twice that of rheobase.

chronic of long duration.

chondr-, chondro- pertaining to cartilage.

chyl-, chym- juice, fluid.

cilia the threadlike cytoplasmic processes of cells, which beat rhythmically.

cinefluorography, cineradiography motion-picture photography of successive x-ray images.

cinematography motion-picture photography.

ciner- ash.

cinerea the gray matter of the nervous system.

cingulum a girdle or zone.

circum- around.

circumduction motion in which the end of a limb describes a circle and the shaft describes a cone.

clas- to break.

claustrum a bar-shaped structure; a thin layer of gray matter lateral to the external capsule.

clav-, clavi- key.

-cle, -cule small.

cleido-, cleid- pertaining to clavicle, key.

clin- to incline.

clinker a mass of uncombustible material, fused together, usually formed during the burning of coal, which has the property of jamming up the works, especially in coal stokers.

clivus a slope.

clon- spasm.

co- together.

coccyx the vestigal, inferior-most portion of the vertebral column, shaped like the beak of a cuckoo.

cochlear microphonics minute quantities of electrical energy generated within the cochlea. The electrical energy has properties analogous to those of the acoustic stimulus.

coel-, -cele hollow.

coelum body cavity.

cognate 1. related by blood. 2. related in origin, as in words having the same root. 3. pair of consonants differing only in the voiced/unvoiced feature.

colliculus a small elevation.

colloid glutinous.

com- with, together.

commissure a joining together; a nerve tract connecting right and left halves of the nervous system.

complemental air air that can be inhaled beyond that inhaled during quiet breathing.

computed tomography (CT scan) combines x-ray imaging and computer analysis of thin cross sections of a structure to develop a three-dimensional view.

con- with, together.

concave resembling the hollow inner surface of a part of a sphere.

concha a shell-like organ or structure.

condenser lens a lens that concentrates light energy; often called a positive lens.

condyle knuckle; a rounded process on a bone.

confluent merging together.

congenital existing at, and usually before, birth; may or may not be hereditary.

conjugate *adj.* joined together; *v.* to inflect a verb in the proper forms.

consonant a speech sound produced by a partial or complete obstruction of a voiced or unvoiced air stream by the articulators.

continuant a speech sound, such as (s) or (m), that remains relatively steady-state over a period of time.

contra-, counter- against, opposed.

contralateral associated with a part on the other side.

convex resembling the rounded external surface of a part of a sphere.

copula pertains to joining together.

coracoid having the shape of a crow's beak.

corium hide.

corniculate like a small horn.

cornu a horn; horn-shaped process.

corona crown.

coronal plane a vertical plane or cut, from side to side, dividing the structure into front and back halves.

corpus, corp- body.

corpus callosum a prominent band of white fibers connecting the right and left cerebral hemispheres.

cortic- bark, rind.

cortex the outer layer of an organ.

cost- rib.

cox- hip.

cps cycles per second. *See* Hz.

crani- skull.

craniometry the science of measuring skulls to establish records for use in comparative studies.

crescendo a gradual increase in intensity or loudness.

crest a ridge, especially a bony prominence.

cretin a person with a congenital lack of thyroid secretion, resulting in hyponormal physical development and mental retardation.

cribriform perforated with small openings like a sieve.

crico-, cric- ring.

crin- distinguish; separate off.

crista crest.

cruciform cross-shaped.

crus leg or leglike part. *pl.* crura.

crypt a narrow pit or recess.

CT scan *see* computed tomography.

culmen a summit; the highest lobule of the cerebellum.

cupula, cupola a vault or dome located on a roof.

cusp a pointed eminence.

cut- skin.

cutaneous pertaining to skin.

cuticle the epidermis.

cymba boat-shaped; the upper part of the concha of the ear.

cyst-, cysto- pertaining to sac or bladder.

cyto-, cyt- pertaining to cell.

cytoarchitecture the cell pattern typical of a region, as in the cerebral cortex.

cyton the cell body of a neuron.

cytoplasm the protoplasm of a cell except for that of the nucleus.

dactyl finger or toe.

dashpot device for cushioning, damping, or reversing motion; consists of a cylinder in which a piston creates pressure or a vacuum.

damping to cause a decrease in amplitude of successive waves or oscillations.

de- down, from, negative.

dead air air in the respiratory tract that does not enter into gas exchange, i.e., air in the mouth, nasal cavities, pharynx, larynx, and trachea.

deci-, dec- ten.

decibel (dB.) a quantitative unit of relative sound intensity or sound pressure, based on the logarithmic relationship of amplitudes or pressures of two sounds, one of which serves as the reference.

deciduous temporary; falling off and shedding at maturity.

declive a lower or descending part.

decussate to cross over, as do nerve or muscle fibers.

deep away from the surface; toward the center.

defecate evacuate the bowel.

degluttition swallowing.

delta triangle.

demi- half.

demulscent an agent that protects a surface from the irritating effects of friction.

dendr- tree, branching.

dendrite the afferent process of a neuron.

dent- tooth.

dentin, dentine the major substance of a tooth, enveloped by enamel on the crown and by cementum on the root.

derm- skin.

dermatome skin area supplied by an individual spinal nerve.

des-, desmo-, -dem band, ligament, bond.

deuter- second.

dextro-, dextr- pertaining to the right side.

di- two, twice.

dia-, di- through, between.

diaphragm a partition separating two cavities.

diarthrosis a moveable articulation between two bones.

diaphysis shaft of a long bone.

diastema a toothless space between two teeth.

diathesis constitutional predisposition.

dichotomize divide into two parts.

dicrotic double beating; pertaining to two clapping, rattling noises.

digastric having two bellies.

digit finger or toe.

digitate having fingerlike branches that may intertwine.

dilate to expand or enlarge.

diphasic occurring in two phases.

diplo- double.

dis-, di-, dif- away, negative, apart.

dissonance a harsh combination of sounds; in music an unresolved combination of sounds.

distal away from the body or from the medial axis.

distend to swell out or stretch out.

diuretic increasing secretion of urine.

diverticulum a blind tube, sac, or process.

dolicho- long.

dorsal toward the backbone.

dorso-, dorsi- back.

drom-, dromo- pertaining to conduction or running.

duc- to lead.

duct a tube, especially for conveying excretions or secretions.

dur-, dura- hard, lasting.

dyna-, dyn- power.

dyne a centimeter-gram-second unit of force.

dys- diseased, faulty, or deficient.

dysostosis defective ossification.

dysphonia any voice impairment, defective phonation.

e- out from.

ec- out of.

echo a returned sound.

ecto- situated on the outside; external.

ectoderm outermost of the three primary layers of the embryo.

-ectomy surgical removal.

eddy current flow that diverges from the main stream of current flow in a fluid.

edema abnormal collection of fluid in tissue; swelling.

edentulous toothless.

edge tone setting an air column into vibration by blowing a stream of air over a sharp edge.

EEG abbreviation of electroencephalography.

ef- out of.

efferent conduction from central region to periphery.

e.g. (L. *exempli gratia*) for example.

-el little.

elasticity the property of returning to initial form following deformation.

elastic tissue connective tissue consisting of yellow elastic fibers.

electrode the surface of contact between a metallic and nonmetallic conductor. A terminal or metal plate through which electrical energy is applied to or taken from the body.

electroencephalography, EEG recording of electric currents generated in the brain.

electromyography, EMG recording the electrical energy generated by active muscles.

embolo-, emboli- wedge; stopper.

embryo early, developing stage of any organism.

emesis vomiting.

EMG abbreviation for electromyography.

eminence projection or prominence, particularly on the surface of a bone.

emphysema an abnormal inflation of an organ or body part with air; usually refers to a morbid lung condition.

en-, em- in.

enarthrosis a joint in which a rounded head of one bone fits into a socket of another, permitting motion in almost any direction; ball and socket.

encephalo- brain.

end organ any terminal structure of a nerve or neuron.

endo-, end- within.

endocrine an internal secretion, originating in one organ and acting on another organ or part.

endothelium a form of epithelial tissue that lines the walls of blood vessels.

ensiform sword-shaped.

entero-, enter- pertaining to intestines.

ento- within or inner.

enzyme a catalytic substance, usually produced by glands, which has a specific effect of promoting chemical change.

ependyma a layer of cells lining the cavities of the brain and spinal cord.

epi-, ep- on or upon.

epidermis the outer nonvascular, nonsensitive layer of the skin.

epiglottis a thin cartilaginous structure that covers the entrance to the larynx.

epinephrine *see* adrenalin.

epiphenomenon 1. a secondary phenomenon. 2. an unusual secondary symptom arising during the course of a disease.

epiphysis an outgrowth, as on a long bone.

epithelium tissue that forms the protecting and/or secreting surfaces of the body.

eponym a person from whom a place or structure takes its name.

erythro- red.

eso- within.

esthet-, esthes- feeling.

estrogens female sex hormones.

et al. (L. *et alii*) and others.

ethmo-, ethm- sievelike; perforated.

etio- cause.

eu- good, well.

evaginate to outpouch or turn inside out.

eversion turning outward or inside out.

ex- out, away from.

excise to remove a part, foreign body, or organ by cutting.

exhale to expel air from the lungs by breathing.

exo- outside, out of.

expectorate to cough up and spit out material from the lungs, bronchi, and trachea.

expire 1. to expel air from the lungs by breathing. 2. to die.

extension an increase in the angle between two bones.

extensor a muscle that straightens or extends a part of the body.

external toward the outside or farther from the midline.

extero- outside.

exteroceptor specialized sense organs that respond to pressure, temperature changes, and pain. The nerve endings are on the surface of the body.

extra- outside of, in addition, beyond.

extrapolate to infer or estimate by extending or projecting known information.

extremity a limb of the body; the distal part.

extrinsic originating outside the part.

extrude to force out or expel; to extend outward.

exudate a discharge of fluid tissue.

facet a small plane area on a structure, usually bone.

facies 1. the appearance of the face. 2. a surface.

falsetto a voice register above the middle or head register.

falx, falc- sickle-shaped.

fascia a sheet of fibrous connective tissue that encases the body beneath the skin and separates muscle bundles from one another.

fascicle, fasciculus a small bundle or cluster, especially of nerve or muscle fibers.

fastigium the highest point or summit, specifically in the roof of the fourth ventricle.

fauces passage from the mouth to the pharynx, surrounded by soft palate, palatine arches, and the base of the tongue.

fenestra a window or small opening.

-ferent, -fer bear, carry.

fiber, fibra-, fibr- elongated; threadlike structure.

fibril a small threadlike component of a compound fiber.

fibrocartilage an elastic cartilage consisting of a predominance of white fibrous tissue.

filum any threadlike anatomical structure.

first-surfaced a mirror with the reflective coating on the side of the glass nearer the light source. Light does not have to pass through the glass, be reflected, and pass out of the glass again.

fission cleaving or splitting into parts.

fissure a cleft or slit.

fistula a tubular passageway formed by disease, surgery, injury, or congenital defect, usually connecting two organs or going from an organ to the surface of the body.

flaccid limp, weak; hypotonus of muscle fibers.

flava yellow.

-flect, -flex to bend.

flexion a decrease in the angle between two bones; bending or being bent.

flexure a series of folds.

flocculent downy, flaky, or wooly.

flocculus a small, but prominent lobe of the cerebellum.

flu-, flux to flow.

focal length the distance from a lens to the point where an infinitely distant source of light will converge to form a common point or focus.

folium a leaflike structure, especially of gray matter in the cerebellum.

follicle a small, secretary cavity or sac.

fontanel, fontanelle a membranous space between the unossified cranial bones; a soft spot.

for- door, opening.

foramen a natural opening, particularly through bone.

force an influence that produces or tends to produce a change in motion.

fore- before, in front.

-form shape.

formant bands regions of prominent energy distribution in a speech sound; broad-band resonant frequencies.

fornix an archlike shape or a vaulted space.

fort- strong.

fossa a pit or hollow.

fossula a small fossa.

fovea a small cup-shaped depression or pit.

fract-, frag- to break.

frenulum, frenum a fold of skin or mucous membrane that limits the range of movement of a structure; bridle-like.

fricative a speech sound generated by friction of air through a restricted opening.

frontal, fronto- anterior position or pertaining to forehead.

funiculus a cordlike structure.

fusiform spindle-shaped.

galea helmet-shaped.

galli cock.

gam-, gamo- marriage, reproductive union.

gamete a sexual germ cell; the female ovum or male sperm cell.

gametogenesis the formation of gametes.

gangli-, ganglio- knotlike.

ganglion a mass of nerve cells located outside the central nervous system.

gastro-, gastr- pertaining to stomach or abdomen.

gemin- twin, double.

gen- to beget.

gene the biological unit of inheritance, which is transmitted by the chromosome.

genetic inherited.

geniculate, genu- bent, like a knee.

genio- pertaining to chin.

ger-, gero- pertaining to old age.

germ a small particle of protoplasm capable of developing into a complete organism.

gest-, -ger to carry, to bear.

gestation pregnancy.

gingiva, gingiv- gums.

ginglymus a hinge joint.

girdle an encircling or confining structure.

glabella the area between the eyebrows; smooth.

gland a cell, tissue, or organ that produces and discharges a substance used elsewhere in the body.

glenoid like a pit or socket.

-glia gluelike tissue or structure.

globose spherical or globe-shaped.

glosso-, gloss- pertaining to tongue.

glottal fry creaky voice produced by phonating at lowest possible pitch.

glottal tone the tone generated by the vibrating vocal folds, to be distinguished from the tone produced by the oscillation or ringing of the vocal tract.

glottis 1. the space between the vocal folds. 2. vocal structure of the larynx.

glow-lamp a light that incorporates the use of inert gases to produce a bright glow. Neon and Xenon are examples of glow-lamps.

gnatho-, gnath- pertaining to jaw.

gomphosis an articulation of a cone-shaped process with an accommodating socket, e.g., the articulation of the teeth with the alveoli.

gonio- pertaining to angle.

gracile, gracilis slender or delicate.

gut intestine or bowel; embryonic digestive tube.

guttural pertaining to throat; produced in the throat.

gyr-, gyro- ring, circle.

gyrus a fold in the cerebral cortex; a convolution.

habenula a frenum or reinlike structure.

halitus the expired breath.

hamulus hook-shaped.

haplo- simple or single.

hapto-, hapt- pertaining to touch.

harmonics the partials of a complex sound which are integral multiples of the fundamental frequency.

head in bone, an enlargement at one end, beyond its neck.

hecto- one hundred.

helico- pertaining to coil.

helio- pertaining to sun.

helix a coiled structure or part.

hemi- half.

hemo-, hema- pertaining to blood.

hepatic pertaining to liver.

herbivorous plant eating.

hermetic air-tight.

hertz (Hz) a symbol to replace the term cycles per second (cps); after Heinrich Hertz, physicist.

hetero-, heter- other or different.

Hg symbol for mercury.

hiatus 1. a perforation in fleshy tissue. 2. any large opening.

hillock a small elevation.

hilum the region where vessels, nerves, etc., enter or leave a part.

histo-, hist- pertaining to tissue.

holo- entire or pertaining to whole.

holography the technique of producing images by wavefront reconstruction, especially by using lasers to record on a photographic plate the diffraction pattern from which a three-dimensional image can be projected.

homeo- pertaining to sameness or constancy.

homo man, human being.

homo- same.

homogeneous consisting of similar parts or elements of uniform quality throughout.

homogenous having a similarity of structure due to descent from a common ancestor.

homunculus a little man.

hormone chemical secretion, usually of an endocrine gland, that is carried by body fluids and specifically regulates a function of another organ.

hyalo-, hyal- pertaining to glass.

hydra a fresh-water polyp.

hydro-, hydr- pertaining to water or hydrogen.

hydraulic moved or operated by a fluid under pressure.

hygro- moist or pertaining to moisture.

hyoid, hyo- U-shaped.

hyper- over, above.

hyperkinesia excessive movement.

hypertrophy an overgrowth or enlargement of an organ or tissue.

hyperventilation excessive respiration resulting in abnormal loss of carbon dioxide from the blood.

hypno- sleep.

hypo- under, beneath, deficient.

hypophysis 1. pituitary gland. 2. an outgrowth.

hypoplasia incomplete or arrested development of a body or part.

hypoxia deficiency of oxygen in inspired air.

hypsi-, hypso- pertaining to height.

Hz *see* hertz.

ibid. (L. *ibidem*) in the place cited.

idio- peculiar, personal, separate, distinct.

idiopathic of unknown causation.

i.e. (L. *id est*) that is.

ilium the broad superior portion of the hipbone. (il*e*um is a part of the small intestine)

immune highly resistant to infectious disease.

impedance the apparent resistance of a mechanical or electrical system to the absorption of energy.

impulse a stimulus carried by the nervous system.

in-, im- 1. in, into. 2. not.

incident *adj.* 1. occurring as a minor concomitant. 2. in physics, falling upon or striking. 3. when pertaining to light and sound, directly from the source.

incident wave a sound wave that falls onto a reflecting or refracting surface.

incisive pertaining to cutting.

incus middle bone in the ossicular chain of the middle ear; anvil.

inert without action.

inertia the tendency of a body to remain in a state of rest or of uniform motion in a straight line, unless acted upon by an external force.

inferior lower or situated beneath; nearer the feet.

inflection modulation of pitch of the voice.

infra- below, beneath.

infundibulum a funnel-shaped structure or passageway.

ingest to take food, etc., into the body.

inguino-, inguin- pertaining to the groin, where the abdominal wall joins the thigh.

inhale to take air into the lungs by breathing.

inherent natural to organism; intrinsic, innate.

inhibit to arrest or restrain a process.

innervation the distribution of nerves to a part.

innominate nameless.

ino- pertaining to fiber.

inscription a mark or line.

insertion the area of attachment of muscle to the bone it moves.

in situ in position.

inspire to take air into the lungs by breathing.

integument a covering, especially the skin.

intensity measure of energy flow per unit of area per unit of time.

inter- between, among, together.

interface a surface that is the common boundary between two parts or spaces.

interdigitation interlocking of fingers or fingerlike parts. The fitting together of cusps of teeth in occlusion.

internal away from the outside, toward the inside.

internuncial serving as a connecting medium, especially in the nervous system.

interstitial pertaining to small spaces in a tissue or structure; situated between.

intra- within.

intrathoracic space the space between the inner thoracic wall and the lung surfaces, the nonexistent intrapleural space.

intrinsic inherent, situated within.

intro- inside, within.

in utero within uterus, not yet born.

inversion the turning inward of a part.

invertebrate without a spinal column.

investment a sheath or covering, usually referring to the connective tissue covering a structure.

ion an electrically charged atom or group of atoms formed by the gain or loss of one or more orbital electrons.

ipsi- self.

ipsilateral situated on or pertaining to the same side.

ischio- pertaining to hip.

iso- equal.

isometric of equal dimensions.

isotonic of equal tension.

-iter a way or tubular passage.

-itis inflammation.

jitter slight cycle-to-cycle variations in vibratory period.

jugular pertaining to neck.

jugum pertaining to yoke or a ridge or depression connecting two structures; union of lesser sphenoidal wings in first year of life.

juxta- near, beside.

karyo- pertaining to nucleus.

kat-, kata- down, against.

kerato- pertaining to horny tissue or to cornea.

kilo- thousand.

kinesthesia the sensation of movement, weight, resistance, and position of muscles.

kinesio-, kine-, kino- pertaining to movement.

koilo- hollow or concave.

kokkyx cuckoo.

kolla- glue.

kymo- pertaining to wave.

kymograph an instrument, consisting of a motor-driven cylinder covered with paper, which records physiological and mechanical variations or undulations.

kyphosis backward curvature of the spinal column, humpback.

kyto- pertaining to cell.

labile gliding; unstable.

labio- pertaining to lips.

labiodental pertaining to lips and teeth.

labyrinth intricate maze of connecting pathways, as in the inner ear.

lacri- pertaining to tears.

lacto- pertaining to milk.

lacuna a small pit or cavity.

lacus a small lake or cavity.

lal-, lalia, lalo- pertaining to speech or babbling.

lambdoid λ-shaped.

lamella a thin plate or scale.

lamina a thin plate or layer.

laminography sectional radiography that shows selected layers of the body.

laparo- pertaining to loin or flank.

laryngo- pertaining to larynx.

latency lag between stimulus and response; seeming inactive.

latent concealed; potential.

latero- pertaining to the side.

lemma husk.

lemniscus a fiber tract within the central nervous system.

lenticular pertaining to or shaped like a lens.

lepto- long, slender, delicate.

leuco-, leuko- white.

levator that which raises or elevates.

ligament a band of fibrous connective tissue which connects bones or holds organs in place.

limbus the border of a structure, particularly of a flat organ or part.

limbic bordering.

limen threshold; boundary line.

limitans limiting.

linea line.

lingua tongue.

lingula a small tongue-shaped structure.

lipid a fat or fatlike substance that is insoluble in water.

litho- stone.

load put under tension in a gross manner.

lobe a rounded portion of an organ, defined by fissures and constrictions.

locus place.

loft *see* falsetto.

logarithm the exponent indicating the power to which a fixed number, the base, must be raised to produce a given number.

logo- pertaining to speech or words.

-logy discourse, study.

longi-, longus long or lengthwise.

loudness the perceptual impression of the intensity of a sound. Sounds may be ordered on a scale extending from soft to loud.

low-pass filter a device, mechanical or electrical, that attenuates high-frequency energy and allows the low-frequency energy to pass through.

lumbar, lumbo- pertaining to loin.

lumen light; the channel within a tube.

luteo- yellow.

lymph a transparent, yellowish fluid derived from blood that carries with it waste from the blood.

lympha clear water.

lyso-, -lysis dissolution; a setting free.

macro- large.

macula a stain or spot.

magma a pulpy mass or a pastelike substance.

magnetic resonance imaging (MRI) a tomographic technique producing cross sectional images of the brain and spine in multiple planes.

mal- defective, bad, wrong.

malar pertaining to cheek or cheekbone.

malleolus a rounded bony process. (L. small hammer)

malleus the largest auditory ossicle, which is shaped like a sculptor's mallet. (L. hammer)

malocclusion any deviation from normal occlusion of the teeth.

mammo- pertaining to the breast or milk-secreting gland.

mandible the lower jaw.

manometer an instrument for measuring the pressure of liquids and gases.

manubrium the upper portion of the sternum. (L. handle)

mass the quantity of matter in a body to which its inertial properties may be ascribed.

masto-, mast- pertaining to breast.

masseter chewer.

mastication chewing.

mater mother.

matrix the place on which anything is formed, or the substance from which it develops. The ground substance of connective tissue.

maxilla the right or left upper jaw.

meatus an opening to a passageway in the body.

medial toward the axis, near the midline.

mediastinum a median partition between two parts of an organ; usually the septum between the two pleural sacs containing all thoracic viscera except the lungs.

medulla the innermost part of an organ or structure, such as bone marrow.

mega-, megalo- great size.

meio- to decrease in number or size.

melano- black.

membrane a thin layer of tissue that binds structures, divides spaces or organs, and lines cavities. (L. thin skin)

meningo- pertaining to membranes, especially those that envelop the brain and spinal cord.

meniscus a crescent-shaped structure.

mental 1. pertaining to the mind. 2. pertaining to the chin.

mero-, mer- part, partial.

mesenchyme connective tissue of the embryo.

mesio- in dentistry refers to the surface of the tooth facing the midline and following the dental arch.

meso-, mes- middle or intermediate.

mesothelium epithelial tissue that lines body cavities.

meta-, met- after, beyond, accompanying.

metabolism sum of physical and chemical processes that produce and maintain a living organized substance; transformation that provides energy to be used by organism.

-meter measure, particularly a measuring instrument.

metopo- pertaining to forehead.

micro-, micr- small size.

microphonic the electric potential produced by a transducer that converts mechanical vibration into electrical energy. *See* cochlear microphonics.

micturate urinate.

mio- less.

milli- thousand, one-thousandth.

mito- threadlike or pertaining to thread.

mitosis asexual cell division.

modality one of the sensory entities, e.g., hearing.

mode, modus manner of action.

modiolus central pillar or columella of the cochlea.

modulate to alter the intensity, frequency, or quality of the voice, as in vibrato or inflection.

modulus a constant or coefficient expressing the degree to which a substance possesses some property.

molar adapted for grinding.

molecule the smallest unit into which a substance can be divided and still retain its characteristics.

monaural pertaining to one ear.

mono- single.

monophasic exhibiting one phase.

-morph, morpho- pertaining to form.

morphogenesis evolutionary or embryological development of the structure of an organism or part.

morphology the study of form and structure of plants and animals; in linguistics, the study of word formations.

morula a solid cellular globular mass. (L. mulberry)

motor unit the muscle fibers supplied by a single axon; may or may not include supplying neuron.

MRI *see* magnetic resonance imaging.

mucin main constituent of mucus.

muco-, muc- pertaining to mucus or mucous membrane.

mucus viscous secretion of mucous glands.

multi- many or much.

mutation 1. any change that represents an evolutionary stage of an organism. 2. the change in the organism that is caused by genetic alterations.

myelin the fatty sheath on the axon of a neuron.

myelo-, myel- pertaining to marrow, myelin, or the spinal cord.

myeloarchitecture the distribution of nerve fibers in an area.

mylo-, myo-, my- pertaining to muscle.

myringo- pertaining to the tympanic membrane.

myxo- pertaining to mucus or slime.

narco pertaining to numbness or stupor.

nares 1. anterior, external. 2. posterior, internal. Orifices of the nose.

naso nose.

neck constricted portion of a structure that serves to join its parts.

necro- pertaining to death or a dead body.

neo-, ne- new or strange.

neonatal pertaining to the first four weeks after birth.

neoplasm abnormal new growth of tissue; tumor.

nephro-, neph- pertaining to kidney.

neural, neuro-, neur- pertaining to a nerve, nervous tissue, or the nervous system.

neurolemma, neurilemma the sheath encasing a nerve fiber.

neutral vowel vowel produced when tongue is positioned toward the center of the mouth—"uh."

nigra black.

noci- to injure.

node a knot, knob, protuberance, or swelling.

nodule, nodulus small node.

noise 1. any unwanted sound. 2. a highly complex sound produced by erratic, intermittent, or statistically random oscillation.

nomen- name.

nomenclature a system of names or terms.

non- absence.

notch an indentation.

noto- pertaining to back.

nuchal nape of the neck.

nucleus 1. the specialized protoplasm of a cell. 2. a group of nerve cells.

nux nut.

nystagmus involuntary spasmodic movement of the eyeball.

ob- against, in front of, toward.

oblique slanting, inclined.

obtuator 1. an organic structure, such as the soft palate, that closes an opening in the body. 2. a prosthetic device serving the same purpose.

occipito- pertaining to the back part of the head.

occlusion the full meeting of the masticating surfaces of the upper and lower teeth.

octa eight.

octave the interval between two sounds with a 2:1 ratio in frequency.

oculo-, ocul- pertaining to eye.

odonto- pertaining to tooth or teeth.

ohm originally, the unit of resistance of a conductor in which one volt produces a current of one ampere (named after G. S. Ohm, German physicist). Also used to denote resistance to the transference of other forms of energy.

olfactory pertaining to the sense of smell.

oligo- little or deficiency.

omo- pertaining to shoulder.

ontogeny the history of the development of an individual organism.

oo- pertaining to egg or ovum.

op. cit. (L. *opere citato*) in the work cited.

operculum a lid or flap.

ophthalmo-, ophthalm- pertaining to eye.

ophthalmoscope a perforated concave mirror used to view the interior of the eye.

opistho- pertaining to behind.

orbicular circular or rounded.

orbit the bony cavity containing the eye.

organ a rather independent part of the body adapted for a specific function.

organic a structural characteristic affecting the function of an organ.

orifice an opening or entrance to a cavity or tube.

origin the place of attachment of a muscle that remains relatively fixed during contraction.

oro- pertaining to mouth.

ortho-, orth- straight, normal, correct.

os 1. pertaining to bone. 2. pertaining to opening or mouth.

oscillo- pertaining to backward and forward movement such as vibration or swinging.

osseous bony, composed of bone.

ossicle a small bone, especially one of the three in the middle ear.

ossify to convert or harden into bone.

osteo- pertaining to bone or bones.

osteoclast large multinuclear cell that resorbs bony tissue.

ostium a mouth or aperture.

otitis an inflammation of the ear.

oto- pertaining to ear.

otoscope a speculum-like device for examining the middle ear.

overtone complex tones, produced by such generators as vibrating strings; contain component frequencies that are integral multiples of the lowest frequency. The first component is the fundamental frequency or first harmonic; the other components are overtones.

ovum egg.

oxidize 1. to combine with oxygen. 2. to increase the valence of an element in the positive direction because of the loss of electrons.

pachy- thick.

palato- pertaining to the roof of the mouth.

paleo- ancient or prehistoric.

pallidus pale.

pallium a mantle or a portion of the cerebral wall.

palpate to examine with the hand, to feel.

pan- all.

papilla a small, nipplelike eminence.

para-, par- beside, beyond, near.

paracentesis the puncture of a cavity to draw off its fluid.

parenchyma the essential tissue of an organ as distinguished from connective tissue.

parietal forming or situated on a wall.

pars a part or portion of an area or structure.

partial in acoustics, a component of a complex tone.

parturition the act of giving birth.

patent open.

patho- pertaining to disease.

pectinate comblike.

pectoral pertaining to the breast or chest.

pedia-, ped- pertaining to child.

pedicle a process or projection that resembles a foot.

pedo- 1. pertaining to child. 2. pertaining to foot.

peduncle a small foot or stalk.

pellucid transparent, translucent.

pelvis a basin-shaped structure.

penniform featherlike in structure.

per- throughout, completely, thoroughly.

peri- around.

pericardium the membranous sac that envelops the heart.

perichondrium a fibrous membrane investing the surface of cartilage.

perikaryon the cell body of a neuron.

period the time required for an oscillating body to make one complete oscillating or vibratory cycle.

periodontal the tissues and structures that surround and support the teeth.

periosteum a fibrous membrane investing the surfaces of bone.

peripheral toward the outward surface or part.

peritoneum serous membrane lining the abdominal cavity.

PET scan *see* positron emission tomography.

petrous resembling stone; hard.

phago-, -phagy pertaining to eating.

phagocyte any cell that ingests microorganisms, foreign particles, or other cells.

phalanx, phalange any bone of a finger or toe.

pharynx the membranous tube connecting the mouth and nares with the esophagus.

phase a particular point of advancement of a cycle, usually expressed in degrees of a circle. One complete cycle = 360°.

philtrum the midline vertical depression of the upper lip, extending from the vermilion border to the nose.

phlebo-, phleb- pertaining to veins.

phonation the production of sound by the vibration of the vocal folds.

phone an individual speech sound.

phoneme the smallest distinctive group or class of phones in a language.

phono-, phon- pertaining to sound, especially the voice.

photo-, phot- pertaining to light.

photocell, photoelectric cell a light-sensitive device that varies resistance in an electrical circuit as illumination varies.

photomicrograph a photograph taken through a microscope.

phren- 1. pertaining to the diaphragm. 2. pertaining to the mind.

phylogenetic pertaining to the complete developmental history of a race or group of animals.

phylum one of the primary divisions of the animal or plant kingdom.

physics science of the laws of nature, especially the forces and properties of matter.

physiology the science of the function of living organisms and their parts.

pia tender, soft.

pineal shaped like a pine cone.

pinna a feather or winglike part; external ear.

pisiform like a pea in size and shape.

pit a depression or indentation.

pitch that attribute of auditory sensation in terms of which sounds may be placed on a scale extending from low to high.

placenta a vascular, spongy tissue, formed by the interlocking of fetal and maternal tissue in the uterus, which allows exchange of nutritive and respiratory products.

placode a platelike structure; in the embryo an anlage of sense organs.

planaria a small, free-living flatworm.

plane a flat, smooth surface either tangent to the body or dividing it.

plano flat.

plantar pertaining to the sole of the foot.

-plasm, plasmo- pertaining to the fluid portion of the blood or to the substance of a cell.

-plasty the shaping or the surgical formation of.

plate a flat structure, particularly a thin layer of bone.

platy- broad or flat.

plethysmograph a device used for measuring changes in the volume of an organ or structure by placing the structure within an airtight container and measuring the displacement of air or water.

pleura *pl.* **pleurae** the serous membrane lining the thoracic cavity and investing the surfaces of the lungs.

pleurisy inflammation of the pleura.

plexus a network of anastomosing vessels or nerves.

plica a fold.

plosive a speech sound produced by building up pressure in the airway and suddenly releasing it.

pneumatised furnished with air cavities.

pneumo- 1. pertaining to lungs. 2. pertaining to air or breath.

pneumograph an instrument for recording the movements of the thorax during respiration.

pneumotachograph device for indicating velocity or quantity of airflow.

pneumothorax the presence of gas or air in the pleural cavity.

pocket a saclike space or cavity.

poly- many or much.

polymorphous having or occurring in several forms.

polyp 1. a projecting growth from mucous membrane. 2. a sedentary type of animal form with a fixed base and a free end with a mouth and tentacles.

pons bridge of tissue connecting two organs.

pontine pertaining to pons.

pore a small opening.

poren-, poro-, porio- pertaining to passage.

positron emission tomography (PET scan) uses principles and radionuclide scanning and computed tomography to study cerebral structure and function.

post- after or behind.

posterior toward the back, or away from the front.

pre- before.

presby- old or pertaining to old age.

pressure the force per unit area exerted at a given point.

pro- before, in front of.

primordial primitive, undeveloped.

procerus long, slender, or high, lofty.

process 1. a prominence or projection, as of a bone. 2. a course of action.

progenitor a parent or ancestor.

progesterone a hormone that prepares the uterus for the fertilized ovum.

prolapse a falling down of an organ or part.

proliferate to grow by multiplication, as in cell division.

promontory a projecting eminence or process.

prone lying face down.

proprio one's own.

proprioception awareness of one's own position, balance, and equilibrium, especially during locomotion.

prosector one who disects anatomical subjects for demonstration.

proso- forward or anterior.

prosody modulation of characteristics of the voice such as pitch, quality, and intensity.

prosthesis 1. an artificial substitute or replacement for a missing part. 2. a device that aids or augments a natural function.

proto-, prot- first.

protean anything that readily changes appearance, character, or principles.

protoplasm basic material of cell composition.

protuberance a projecting part or prominence.

proximal nearest; closer to the body or any point of reference. Opposite of distal.

pseudo- false.

psycho-, psych- pertaining to the psyche or to the mind.

psychogenic of psychological or emotional origin.

ptero- feather, wing.

ptyalo- pertaining to saliva.

puberty the period of sexual maturation and growth.

pulmono- pertaining to lungs.

pulse register *see* glottal fry.

punctiform like a point, or on a point.

pyriform, piriform pear-shaped.

quadri- four.

radio- pertaining to radiation.

radian an angle at the center of a circle subtending its arc, and equal in length to the radius of the circle. Equal to 57.2958°.

radiography a photograph made by projecting roentgen (x-rays) through a part of the body onto a sensitive film.

radionuclide scan uses a Geiger counter and injected radioactive material to evaluate cerebral blood flow and to detect brain pathology.

ramus a branch.

raphe a seam or ridge indicating the line of union of two symmetrical halves.

ratchet a bar or wheel having teeth.

re- back, again, contrary.

recess a small empty cavity or space.

rectus straight.

reflected wave a sound wave that has been cast or thrown back.

reflex an involuntary, relatively invariable adaptive response to a stimulus.

refractory obstinate; resisting ordinary treatment.

refractory period a momentary state of reduced excitability of a nerve or muscle immediately following a response.

register a series of tones that are produced in the same way and having the same quality.

relaxation pressure intrapulmonic pressure due to tissue elasticity, torque, and gravity, which tends to expel air from the lungs.

renal pertaining to kidney.

reniform kidney-shaped.

resonance a structure's absorption and emission of energy at the same frequency band.

resorb to absorb again.

resorption the removal of a substance by absorption.

respiration the interchange of gases of living organisms and the gases of their environment.

respiratory passage the nares, nasal cavities, pharynx, oral cavity, larynx, trachea, and bronchial tubes.

restiform cordlike.

rete- net.

reticular resembling a net.

retract to draw back, shorten.

retro- back, backward, or located behind.

-rhaphy seam, suture.

rheo- pertaining to electric current or to the flow of a fluid.

rheobase a minimal strength of electrical current, which, when left on for an indefinite period of time, produces a nerve stimulation.

rhino-, rhin- nose or noselike.

rhomboid, rhombus an oblique-angled parallelogram.

ribose a pentose sugar occurring in nucleic acids.

ridge an elevation or crest.

rima a chink or cleft.

risorius a cheek muscle that inserts into the angle of the mouth. (L. laughter)

roentgenography *see* radiography.

rostral 1. resembling a beak. 2. toward the head.

rudimentary in an imperfect or early stage of development.

ruga *pl.* **rugae** a wrinkle or fold.

saccule a small bag or sac.

sacro- pertaining to sacrum.

sacrum the fused vertebrae that, with the coccyx, form the interior portion of the vertebral column. (L. sacred bone used in sacrifices)

sagittal 1. arrow-shaped. 2. pertaining to the anteroposterior plane of the body.

saline salty, containing sodium chloride.

saliva fluid secreted by the parotid, sublingual, submaxillary, and other mucous glands in the mouth.

salpingo- pertaining to tube, especially auditory or uterine tubes.

saltatory leaping.

sarco- pertaining to flesh.

sarcolemma elastic sheath investing each striated muscle fiber.

sarcoplasm the longitudinal substance between muscle fibrils.

scala a staircase structure; a subdivision of the cavity of the cochlea, especially of the perilymphatic spaces.

scalene having three unequal sides.

scaphoid boat-shaped.

scapula shoulder blade.

schematic a diagram or model.

schindylesis an articulation where a plate of bone fits into a groove in another bone.

schisto- split or cleft.

sclero- hard.

scolio- twisted or crooked.

-scope an instrument used for examining.

sebaceous containing or secreting fatty matter.

selective permeability characteristic of a membrane that permits only certain substances to pass in or out.

sella a saddle.

semi- half.

semilunar resembling a half-moon or crescent.

semipermeable permitting passage of some molecules and hindering passage of other molecules.

senescent growing old.

sensation a change in the state of awareness due to stimulation of an afferent nerve.

sense organ a specialized sensory nerve terminal activated by a specific stimulus.

septum a partition separating two cavities.

serous characterized by serum.

serrated notched on the edge, like a saw.

serum any watery animal fluid.

sesamoid resembling a sesame seed.

shaft the trunk of any columnar structure, especially the diaphysis of a long bone.

sheath a tubular structure of connective tissue covering vessels, muscles, nerves, etc.

shunt to turn or divert to another course.

sibilant characterized by a hissing sound.

sigmoid shaped like the letter S.

sine a trigonometric function equal to the ratio of the ordinate of the end point of the arc to the radius vector of this end point, the origin located at the center of the circle on which the arc lies, and the critical point of the arc located on the x-axis.

single photon emission computed tomography (SPECT) type of imaging used to improve spatial localization of radionuclide scan.

sinistro- pertaining to the left side.

sink the point where inward current flow occurs during propagation of a nerve impulse.

sinus a cavity or depression within a structure or existing between two adjacent structures. (L. fold, curve)

situs sit or position.

skiff *see* cymba.

socket a hollow into which a movable part fits.

soma-, somato- body.

somatic pertaining to the body and especially the voluntary muscles and skeletal framework.

somatesthesia, somesthesia the consciousness of having a body.

specific gravity the ratio of the mass of a given volume of any substance to that of the same volume of some other substance. Water is usually the standard for liquids and solids, while air or hydrogen is the standard for gases.

SPECT *see* single photon emission computed tomography.

spectrum 1. the band of colors formed when visible light is passed through a prism or other light-dispersing device. 2. in sound, a representation of the amplitude (sometimes also phase) of the components arranged as a function of their frequencies.

speculum an instrument for dilating the orifice of a cavity or tube in order that the interior may be observed.

spheno- pertaining to a wedge or to the wedge-shaped sphenoid bone at the base of the skull.

sphincter a circular band of muscle fibers that close an orifice or constrict a passageway.

splancho- pertaining to viscera.

splenium a bandagelike structure.

spine 1. a thornlike projection. 2. spinal column.

spirometer an instrument for measuring vital capacity, or volumes of inhaled and exhaled air.

spondylo-, spondyl- pertaining to vertebra, or to the vertebral column.

spongio- spongelike.

spuria simulated, false.

sputum matter expelled from the lungs, bronchi, and trachea, through the mouth.

squamous platelike or scaly.

stapes the innermost ossicle of the middle ear. (L. stirrup)

stellate star-shaped or having parts radiating from a center.

steno- narrow or contracted.

stenosis narrowing of a duct or canal.

stereo solid, three-dimensional.

stereognosis the ability to recognize the nature and form of objects by means of touch.

stereotropism tropism in which a solid is the external stimulus.

sterno- pertaining to sternum.

stetho-, steth- pertaining to chest.

stimulus anything that produces functional or trophic reaction in a receptor or in an irritable tissue.

stoma-, stomato- mouth.

stomodeum embryonic mouth.

strain deformation produced by stress.

stratified arranged in layers.

stress the action of forces whereby deformation or strain results.

stria streak or line.

striated striped.

stridor a harsh, high-pitched respiratory sound caused by acute obstruction of the breathing passage.

strobolaryngoscopy examination of the larynx utilizing a stroboscope for illumination. When rate of the flashing light is equal to that of the vibrating vocal folds, they seemingly stand motionless, thus affording a critical inspection.

stroboscope a device that utilizes a short-duration flashing light that seemingly stops or slows down moving objects.

stylo-, styl- pertaining to pillar or to the styloid process of the temporal bone.

sub- under, beneath, deficient.

sulcus a furrow or groove, especially on the surface of the brain.

super- above, excessive.

superficial toward the surface.

superior up, higher, directed upward.

supine 1. lying on the back, face upward. 2. the hand with palm turned forward.

supplemental air (archaic) the air that can be exhaled, beyond that which is exhaled during quiet breathing.

suppurative pus-producing.

supra- above, over, upon.

surface tension a supportive property on the surface of a liquid. An apparent tension in an actually nonexistent surface film due to attractive properties of the liquid molecules.

suture 1. the point or line of junction of two structures or parts in an immovable articulation. 2. the joining of the edges of a wound or incision by stitching.

sym- with, together.

symphysis a site or line of union between two structures. (Gk. a growing together)

syn- with, together.

synapse the region of communication between neurons.

synarthrosis an articulation in which the bones are immovably bound together without any intervening synovial cavity.

synchondrosis an articulation, usually temporary, in which the intervening hyaline cartilage converts to bone before adulthood.

synchrostroboscopy stroboscopic illumination synchronized with the rate of vibration of the vocal folds.

syndesmosis an articulation in which the bones are fixed by means of ligaments.

syndrome a group of symptoms that, when considered together, are characteristic of a condition.

synergy the cooperative action of two or more structures.

synovia, synovial fluid a fluid, resembling the white of an egg, secreted by membranes in an articular capsule.

synthesize combine separate elements to form a whole.

syrinx vocal organ of a bird.

system a combination of parts into functional unity.

systemic pertaining to or affecting the body as a whole.

tag a flaplike appendage.

tectum any rooflike structure.

tegmen a cover or roof.

teinein to stretch.

tela weblike tissue.

tele- pertaining to end or far away.

telencephalon the anterior part of the forebrain.

telereceptors sense organs capable of receiving a stimulus from a distance.

telo- end.

temple lateral portion of the upper part of the head.

temporal 1. pertaining to the lateral portion of the upper part of the head. 2. pertaining to time. 3. temporary, transitory.

tendon a nonelastic band of connective tissue that forms the attachment of muscle to bone.

tensor any muscle that makes a structure or part tense.

tenuous 1. slender. 2. thin in consistency; rarefied. 3. insignificant; unsubstantial.

tertiary third in order.

tetany the blending of discrete muscular contractions to form a sustained contraction.

tetra- four.

tetrahedral having the form of a tetrahedron, which is a solid contained by four plane faces; a triangular pyramid.

thel- nipple.

thermo-, therm- pertaining to heat.

thoraco- pertaining to chest.

thorax the portion of the body, between the neck and the diaphragm, encased by the ribs; the chest.

threshold the point at which a stimulus is of just sufficient intensity to be perceived or to produce an effect.

thyroid resembling a shield.

tissue a colony of cells similar in structure and function.

-tome indicates a cutting instrument.

tomogram an x-ray image of tissue at a specific depth.

tonotopographical topographically arranged according to frequency, as on the basilar membrane.

tonsil an aggregate of lymph nodes and vessels contained in the mucosa of the pharynx.

tonus a normal continuous slight contraction of muscle.

topical pertaining to a particular region; local.

topograph a map, chart, or detailed description of the surface features of an area or figure.

torque a force that produces or tends to produce torsion (twisting) or rotation.

torsio twist.

torso the trunk of the body.

tortuous twisted, turned.

torus a rounded ridge or protuberance.

trabecula a strand of connective tissue resembling a little beam or crossbar.

trachea the tube extending from the larynx to the bronchi.

tracheostomy surgically creating an opening into the trachea through the neck.

tracheotomy cutting into the trachea through the neck.

tract 1. a bundle of nerve fibers having a common origin, function, and termination. 2. a series, group, or system of organs or parts having a common function.

traction drawing or pulling.

tragus a small eminence in front of the external opening of the ear.

trans- through, across, beyond.

transducer a device that absorbs energy and emits energy either in the same form or in another form.

transient constantly changing; a change in steady state.

transillumination to illuminate the interior or lumen of a structure by passing light through the tissue.

transverse crosswise; at right angles to the longitudinal plane.

trapezoid a four-sided figure with two parallel and two diverging sides.

-trema hole.

tremolo exaggerated vibrato.

tri- three.

trifoliate having three leaves or leaflike parts.

trigonum a small, triangular-shaped cavity or structure.

trill 1. in music a rapid alteration of two tones, a whole or half tone apart. 2. in linguistics a rapid vibration of one speech organ against another.

triticeous shaped like a grain of wheat.

trituration to reduce to a powder by grinding.

trochanter a very large, bony process.

trochlea a pulley-shaped part of structure.

trochoid capable of exhibiting rotation around an axis.

tropho- pertaining to nutrition.

trophoblast the outer layer of cells of a blastocyst.

-tropic denoting turning.

tropism orientation of an organism by growth rather than movement in response to an external stimulus.

> *positive tropism* toward the stimulus.
>
> *negative tropism* away from the stimulus.

tuber a rounded swelling or protuberance.

tubercle a small, round projection, especially on bone.

tuberosity a large, rounded projection on a bone.

turbinate scroll-like, spiraled.

turbulence a noise factor; random fluctuation of velocities and pressures.

tympanum 1. middle ear. 2. tympanic membrane (ear drum).

ultra- excess.

umbilicus the navel; central abdominal depression at the region of attachment of the umbilical cord.

umbo the projecting center of a rounded surface.

un- not.

uncinate hooked.

uncus a hood-shaped part or process.

undulation wavelike motion in any medium.

uni- one.

utero pertaining to the uterus; the womb.

utricle 1. a small sac. 2. the larger of the two divisions of the membranous labyrinth of the inner ear.

uvula 1. a pendent, fleshy mass. 2. When used alone, it refers to the uvula palatina, a small, fleshy mass hanging from the soft palate above the back of the tongue.

vacuole a small cavity in the protoplasm of a cell.

vacuus empty.

vagus wandering.

vallecula a shallow groove or depression.

vapor gas, steam, or exhalation.

vas, vaso- vessel or duct, especially those carrying blood or lymph.

vector a quantity having both magnitude and direction; signified by an arrow.

vein a vessel that carries blood from parts of the body to the heart.

velum 1. a thin, veil-like covering or partition. 2. the soft palate.

ventilation the process of supplying oxygen through the lungs.

ventral situated on the lower or abdominal surface.

ventricle a small cavity or pouch.

ventro-, ventri- pertaining to belly or to the anterior aspect of the body.

vermis a wormlike structure, usually refers to the median part of the cerebellum.

version a turning or change of direction.

vertebro- pertaining to a vertebra or to the vertebral column.

vertigo an illusory sensation of movement, dizziness.

vesicle a small sac containing fluid.

vessel a tube or duct conveying body fluid, especially blood or lymph.

vestibule a hollow or cavity forming an entrance to a canal.

vestigial pertaining to a remnant of a structure which, earlier in the species or individual development, was functional.

vibrato small and rapid pitch and intensity changes during singing.

villi fine, vascular processes on the free surface of a membrane. (L. shaggy hair)

virilism masculinity.

viscera soft organs in the body cavities.

viscosity the property of fluid which resists change in the shape or arrangement of its elements during flow.

vital capacity the maximum amount of air that can be exhaled after maximum inhalation.

viz. (L. *videlicit*) namely.

volume modulus of elasticity same as bulk modulus of elasticity.

vomer the inferior-most portion of the bony nasal septum. (L. plowshare)

vowel a vocal sound produced by relatively free passage of the air stream through the larynx and oral cavity.

VU abbreviation for volume units.

wave a progressive disturbance propagated from point to point in a medium without advance of the points themselves.

Wheatstone bridge a sensitive instrument designed to measure the electrical resistance of a component in an electrical circuit.

xiphoid shaped like a sword.

zygo- pertaining to yoked, joined, or junction.

zygote the cell produced by the union of two cells.

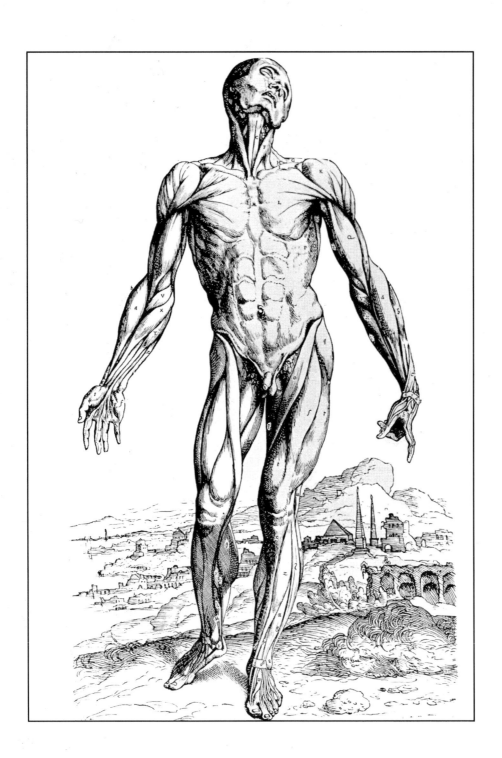